Occupational Health

Management and practice for
health practitioners

Occupational Health

Management and practice for health practitioners

Third Edition

J. Acutt

MA Cur (RAU); BA Cur (UNISA); RGN; RM; CHN; N. Ed; OHN; N. Admin
(Occupational Health Advisor)

S. P. Hattingh

D. Litt et Phil (UNISA); MA (Cur) (UNISA); BA (Cur) Hons (UNISA); B Cur
(I et A) (UP); RGN; RM; Psig N; CH N; N. Admin; N. Ed; OTT; OHN
(Senior lecturer in the Department of Health Studies University of
South Africa

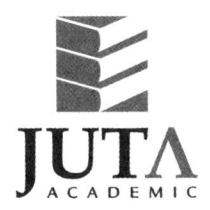

JUTA
ACADEMIC

First Edition 1992
Second Edition 1997
Third Edition 2003

© 2003, Juta & Co, Ltd
PO Box 24309
Lansdowne 7779

This book is copyright under the Berne Convention. In terms of the Copyright Act 98 of 1978, no part of this book may be reproduced or transmitted in any form or by any means, electronic or mechanical, including photocopying, recording or by any information storage or retrieval system, without the permission from the publisher.

Project management: Fiona Wakelin
Subedit: Ethné Clarke
Index: Ethné Clarke
Cover design: The Pumphaus Design Studio
Design and typesetting: McKore Graphics
Printed and bound in South Arica by Creda Communications, Epping

ISBN 0 7021 5699 X

Preface to the Third Edition

The road leading to optimal health extends far beyond the security gate of the industry. To achieve health for the workforce, management and the worker must look at the full circle of life inside and outside the factory walls. Ignorance and often irresponsibility have often contributed unnecessarily to morbidity and mortality not only of the worker, but also in the family and the community. Productive environments are those in which the workers are safe and free from hazards.

In the occupational health sector, a large number of health care professionals as well as other team members contribute to the health and well-being of the worker and, indirectly, the family and the community.

The topics of this book have been carefully selected and are designed to meet the educational needs of a wider spectrum of health care professionals working in industry. The third edition has been updated to enhance knowledge on changes in legislation, prevention in occupational diseases and emergency disaster management. I have no doubt that this book contributes to the body of knowledge in occupational health.

Susan Hattingh (Ed.)
Pretoria 2003

Preface to the Second Edition

During the past decades, the clinical practice of occupational health as a field of study, became increasingly important in South Africa. A great increase in work related health problems, with their resultant impact on family and community life, has created the need for a book which provides for the learning needs of the nurse and other health care workers in the field of occupational health.

The topics for this book have been carefully selected and are designed to meet the educational needs of nursing students in a variety of nursing courses such as the basic, post-basic and graduate training programmes. The second edition has been updated to reflect changes in legislation and the workplace.

A. J. Kotze
Pretoria 1997

Contributors

Our sincere thanks to all the contributors:

Acutt, J.
M.A.Cur, B.A. Cur., R.G.N., R.M., C.H.N., N.Ed., O.H.N., N.Adm., Occupational Health Adviser.

Bergh, Z. C.
M.A. Psych. (Counselling and Industrial Psychology). Senior Lecturer, University of South Africa. Practicing Counselling and Industrial Psychologist.

Hattingh, S. P.
D. Litt et Phil; M Cur (Unisa); B.A. Cur (Hons) (UP), B. Cur (l et A) (UP), R.N., R.M., Psych.; O.T.T., CHN; N.Ed, OHN, N.Admin, Senior Lecturer, University of South Africa.

Kotze, A. J.
D.Litt et Phil (Unisa), M.Cur (Pret), B.Curl (l et A) (Pret), R.G.N., R.M., O.T.T., Int. Care, C.H.N., N.Adm., N.Ed.

Mets, J. T.
M.B. Ch.B. (Leiden), M.R.C.S. (Eng), L.R.C.P. (Lond), D.O.M. (Stell), M.F.O.M. (Eng), M.D. (Pret); F.A.O.M.A. (USA).

Murphy J. P.
MB ChB., DA., DTM&H., DOH., DIP PEC.

2003

Contents

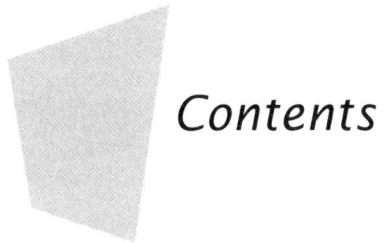

Preface to the third edition v
Contributors vii

1. Concepts of occupational health 1

    1.1 Introduction 1
    1.2 Learning objectives 2
    1.3 Occupational health in history 2
    1.4 Regulation of occupational health in South Africa since 1990 13
    1.5 Occupational health 14
    1.6 The components of an occupational health service 15
    1.7 The role of occupational health 15
    1.8 Organizational models of occupational health services 16
    1.9 The scope of occupational health services .18
    1.10 The objectives of an occupational health service 18
    1.11 The functions and activities of an occupational health service 18
    1.12 Occupational health nursing 19
    1.13 The occupational health team members in South Africa 21
    1.14 Internet Web sites 22
    1.15 Conclusion 23
    1.16 Bibliography 23

2. Legislation in occupational health 25
    2.1 Introduction 25
    2.2 Learning objectives 25
    2.3 Legislation dealing with occupational health in South Africa 26
    2.4 Ethics and the law 26
    2.5 The Constitution of the RSA and the Bill of Rights 26
    2.6 The Health Act, 1977 (No 63 of 1977) 32
    2.7 The Occupational Health and Safety Act, 1993 (No 85 of 1993) 33
    2.8 The Mine Health and Safety Act, 1997 (No 29 of 1996) 41
    2.9 Risk assessment and hazard control 46

2.10 The Compensation for Occupational Injuries and Diseases Act, 1993
 (No 130 of 1993) 49
2.11 The Occupational Diseases in Mines and Works Act, 1973 (No 78 of 1973) .55
2.12 The Basic Conditions of Employment Act, 1997 (No 75 of 1997) 59
2.13 The Employment Equity Act, 1998 (No 55 of 1998) 65
2.14 The Labour Relations Act, 1995 (No 66 of 1995) 67
2.15 The National Economic Development and Labour Council (NEDLAC) Act,
 1994 (No 35 of 12994) 72
2.16 The Unemlpoyment Insurance Act, 1966 (No 30 of 1966) 74
2,17 The Skills Development Act, 1998 (No 97 of 1998) and the Skills
 Development Levies Act, 1999 (No 9 of 1999) 74
2.18 The International Health Regulations Act, 1974, No 28 of 1974)
 (as amended International Health Regulations Act, 2000 (No 51 of 2000)) ..75
2.19 The South African Medicines and Medical Devices Regulatory
 Authority Act, 1998 (No 114 of 1998) 76
2.20 The Drugs and Drug Trafficking Act, 1992 (No 140 of 1992) 76
2.21 The Environmental Conservation Act, 1989 (No 73 of 1989) 76
2.22 The Hazardous Substances Act, 1973 (No 15 of 1973) (as amended Hazardous
 Substances Amendment Act, 1992 (No 53 of 1992)) 77
2.23 The Medicines and Related Substances Control Amendment Act, 1997
 (No 90 of 1997) 77
2.24 The Animal Slaughter, Meat and Animal Products Hygiene Act, 1967
 (No 87 of 1967) 78
2.25 The Domestic Violence Act (No 116 of 1998) 78
2.26 The Foodstuffs, Cosmetics and Disinfectants Act, 1972 (No 54 of 1972) 78
2.27 The Explosive Act, 1956 (No 26 of 1956) 79
2.28 The Nuclear Energy Act, 1982 (No 92 of 1982) 79
2.29 The Merchant Shipping Act, 1951 (No 57 of 1951) 79
2.30 The Human Tissue Act, 1983 (No 65 of 1983) 79
2.31 The Mineral Act, 1956 (No 50 of 1991) 79
2.32 The Water Act, 1956 (No 54 of 1956) 79
2.33 The Atmospheric Pollution Prevention Act, 1965 (No 45 of 1965) 79
2.34 The International Health Regulations Act, 1974 (No 28 of 1974) 80
2.35 Conclusion 80
2.36 List of sources 80

3. Occupational safety 83
3.1 Introduction 83
3.2 Learning objectives 83
3.3 Legislative control of occupational health and safety 84
3.4 Definitions 85
3.5 Basic classification of accidents 88
3.6 Category of injury 90
3.7 Factors that may cause accidents 90

3.8 The domino cause and control sequence 95
3.9 Insured and uninsured costs 99
3.10 Accident prevention 102
3.11 Accident prevention programmes 105
3.12 Leadership by the employer 105
3.13 Safe work habits and practices by employees 106
3.14 Key activities for preventing accidents 107
3.15 Off-the-job safety 109
3.16 The health and safety of the healthcare worker 110
3.17 Ergonomics 110
3.18 The National Occupational Safety Association 117
3.19 The Occupational Health and Safety Act, 1993 (NO 85 of 1993) 119
3.20 Safety committees 121
3.21 The role and functions of the occupational health practitioner in safety
     and accident prevention 123
3.22 Conclusion 125
3.23 Bibliography 126

4. Occupational hygiene 127
4.1 Introduction 127
4.2 Learning objectives 127
4.3 Definition of occupational hygiene 127
4.4 The rationale of oocupational hygiene 128
4.5 Legislative control 128
4.6 The basic principles and procedures of an occupational hygiene programme .129
4.7 The classification and discussion of occupational hazards 131
4.8 The role and functions of the occupational healthcare professional in the
    control of the environment 155
4.9 Conclusion
4.10 Bibliography 157

5. Occupational medicine and occupational diseases 158
5.1 Learning objectives 158
5.2 Occupational medicine 158
5.3 Occupational disease 160
5.4 Main subdivisions of occupational diseases 173
5.5 Shiftwork 211
5.6 Practical exercise 212
5.7 Bibliography 217

6. Occupational health service management ... 220
6.1 Intgroduction ... 220
6.2 Learning objectives ... 220
6.3 The occupational health nurse ... 220
6.4 The appointment of an occupational health nurse in an organization ... 223
6.5 The role of the occupational health nurse ... 225
6.6 Management principles in occupational health ... 226
6.7 The implementation of the occupational health programme ... 232
6.8 Control through adminstration and management ... 233
6.9 Epidemiology as research orientation ... 239
6.10 Benefits of an occupational health service ... 240
6.11 Practical assignment ... 240
6.12 Conclusion ... 240
6.13 Bibliography ... 240

7. Clinical occupational healthcare ... 242
7.1 Introduction ... 242
7.2 Learning objectives ... 242
7.3 The occupational health nursing practitioner ... 243
7.4 Clinical functions of an occupational health nurse ... 244
7.5 Specific occupational health screening tests ... 248
7.6 Primary monitoring to identify unrecognized hazards ... 252
7.7 Providing a treatment service ... 252
7.8 Emergency care and first aid ... 254
7.9 Injuries on duty and occupational diseases ... 255
7.10 Vulnerable employees requiring special care ... 256
7.11 Education ... 257
7.12 Counselling and support groups ... 258
7.13 Rehabilitation ... 258
7.14 Environmental monitoring ... 259
7.15 The nursing process in occupational health nursing ... 259
7.16 Conclusion ... 260
7.17 Bibliography ... 261

8. Health promotion at work ... 262
8.1 Introduction ... 262
8.2 Learning objectives ... 262
8.3 Healthy lifestyles ... 262
8.4 The adult learner ... 263
8.5 Health promotion in the occupational health setting ... 263
8.6 Components of a succesful occupational health programme ... 264
8.7 Health education ... 267
8.8 Selected health promotion programmes ... 270

8.9 Contemporary occupational health programmes in South Africa 274
8.10 Conclusion 276
8.11 Bibliography 277

9. Emergency care and disaster management 278
9.1 Introduction 278
9.2 Learning objectives 279
9.3 What is a disaster 279
9.4 Identifying the risk 280
9.5 Natural disasters 280
9.6 Disasters of human origins 280
9.7 Emergency risks 280
9.8 Legislative control 282
9.9 The disaster management team 290
9.10 Disaster planning 291
9.11 Pre-planning for disaster 293
9.12 Phases of a disaster response 294
9.13 triage 298
9.14 Emergency management of cetain trauma 304
9.15 Communicatiuon during disasters 334
9.16 Management of disaster victims at the hospital 336
9.17 Documentation 337
9.18 Post-disaster management 337
9.19 Death at work 339
9.20 Conclusion 340
9.21 Bibliography 340

10. Epidemiology 341
10.1 Introduction 341
10.2 Learning objectives 343
10.3 What is public health 343
10.4 Conceptualizing epidemiology 344
10.5 The application of epidemiology 353
10.6 Types of epidemiological investigations 358
10.7 Sources of data 364
10.8 The uses of epidemiology in occupational health 364
10.9 Planning an epidemiological study .367
10.10 Ethical considerations in epidemiogical research 368
10.11 Conclusion 368
10.12 Bibliography 369

11. Psychological health and adjustment in the work context 370
11.1 Introduction 370
11.2 Learning objectives 372
11.3 The role of the occupational health worker 372
11.4 Systemic understanding of occupational adjustment 374
11.5 Work and human behaviour 377
11.6 Describing mental health 379
11.7 Aetiology or casual factors in mental health problems 385
11.8 Assessment of occupational mental health 397
11.9 Psychological work dysfunctions 401
11.10 Managing and promoting occupational adjustment 441
11.11 Conclusion 455
11.12 Bibliography 456

12. Environmental health 464
12.1 Introduction 464
12.2 Learning objectives 464
12.3 Conceptualizing health and environment 464
12.4 Interaction between the human race and its environment 468
12.5 Human needs, health and the environment 469
12.6 A sustainable environment and development 471
12.7 Environmental concerns 471
12.8 Demographic transition 472
12.9 Epidemiological transition 473
12.10 Mortality rates 474
12.11 Indicators 475
12.12 The burden of disease 475
12.13 The team approach 477
12.14 Basic requirments for a healthy environment 477
12.15 Ecological issues and their effect on health 483
12.16 The effects of chemical hazards on health 491
12.17 The effects of physical hazards on health 495
12.18 The effects of mechanical hazards on health 499
12.20 Biological hazards and their effects on health 503
12.21 The effects of war 504
12.22 Impact of disasters on health and well-being 505
12.23 Multidimensional diagnostic strategies 510
12.24 Conclusion 513
12.15 Bibliography 513

Addenda and appendices 515
Addenda
Addendum 1: The national drug policy 515

Addendum 2: HIV/Aids and employment: Code of good practice 519
Addendum 3: Notes on the prohibition of pre-employment testing for the
 human immuno-deficiency virus (HIV) Bill 526

Appendices
Appendix 6.1 An example of a Company Policy for a specific health issue 531
Appendix 6.2 An example of a monthly or annual Occupational Health
 Service report 533
Appendix 6.3 An example of an Occupational Health Service audit 536
Appendix 7.1 Man-job specification 545
Appendix 7.2 546

Index 547

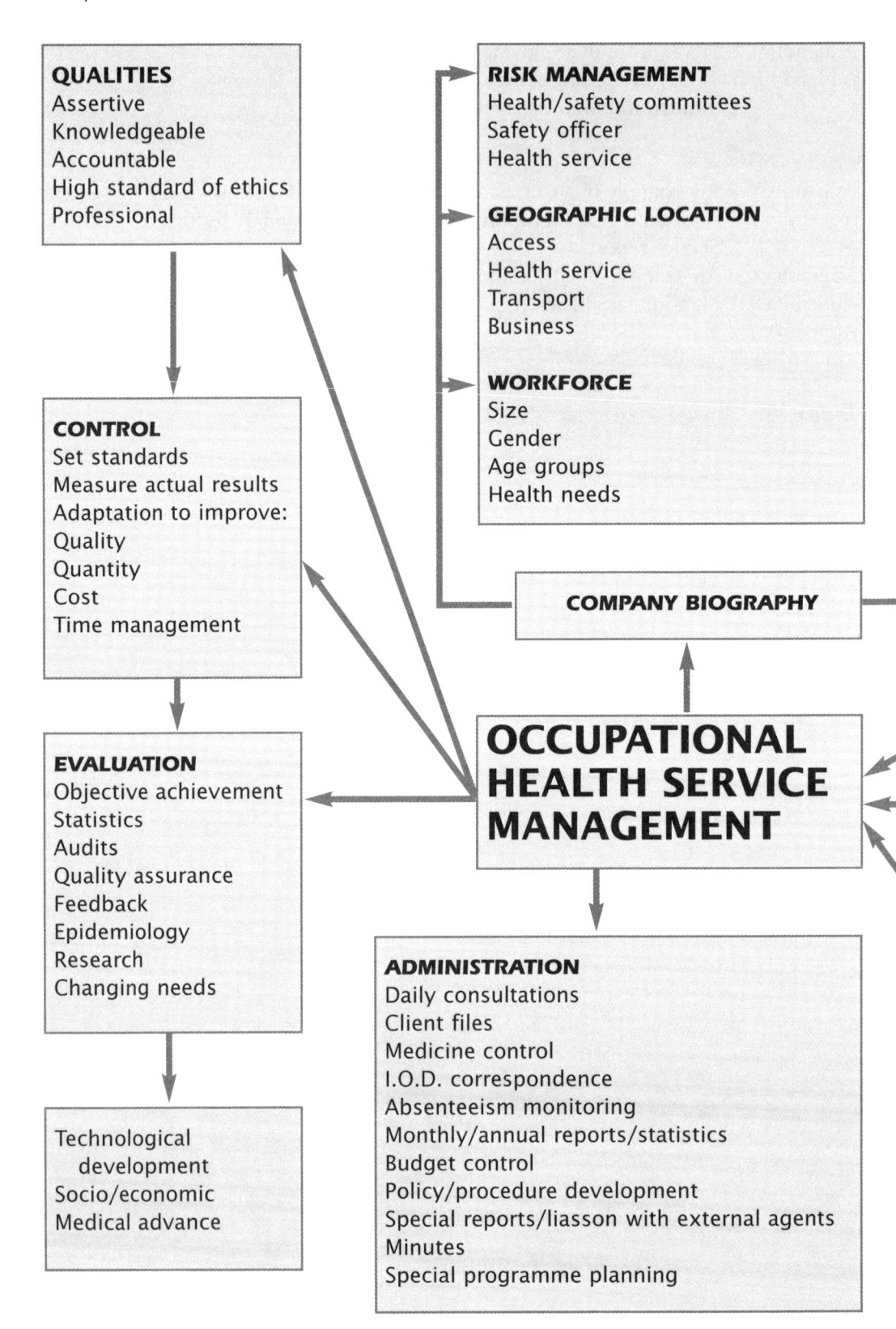

Occupational health

QUALITIES
Assertive
Knowledgeable
Accountable
High standard of ethics
Professional

CONTROL
Set standards
Measure actual results
Adaptation to improve:
Quality
Quantity
Cost
Time management

EVALUATION
Objective achievement
Statistics
Audits
Quality assurance
Feedback
Epidemiology
Research
Changing needs

Technological development
Socio/economic
Medical advance

RISK MANAGEMENT
Health/safety committees
Safety officer
Health service

GEOGRAPHIC LOCATION
Access
Health service
Transport
Business

WORKFORCE
Size
Gender
Age groups
Health needs

COMPANY BIOGRAPHY

OCCUPATIONAL HEALTH SERVICE MANAGEMENT

ADMINISTRATION
Daily consultations
Client files
Medicine control
I.O.D. correspondence
Absenteeism monitoring
Monthly/annual reports/statistics
Budget control
Policy/procedure development
Special reports/liasson with external agents
Minutes
Special programme planning

Occupational health service management

APPLICABLE LEGISLATION
Occupational Health and Safety Act
Compensation
Basic conditions of service
Occupational injuries and diseases
Employment Equity Act
etc.

COMPANY CULTURE
History
Management

NATURE OF BUSINESS
Manufacture
Products
Raw materials

WORKFORCE
Health status
Knowledge of health risks

HEALTH RISKS
Chemical
Physical
Mechanical
Biological
Psychologic

PREVIOUS RECORDS

RESOURCES AVAILABLE
Occupational health team
Facilities
Finance

FINDINGS OF WALK-THROUGH INSPECTION

ASSESSMENT OF HEALTH RISKS

PLANNING: DATA EVALUATION

IMPLEMENTATION
Medical surveillance programme
Emergency programme
Daily primary
  healthcare clinic
  Acute
  Chronic diseases
Health education
Counselling and rehabilitation
Work site inspections
Occupational hygiene
  assessments/monitoring

OCCUPATIONAL HEALTH SERVICE PHILOSOPHY

OCCUPATIONAL HEALTH POLICY

OBJECTIVES
Short term/Long term
Health programme year plan
Clinic activities

Budget
Capital
Operating

POLICY/PROCEDURE MANUAL

EMERGENCY/DISASTER PLAN

PRIORITIES
Highest risks
Clinic equipment
Stocks required

1 Concepts of occupational health

J. Acutt

1.1 Introduction

The relationship between work and health is a two-way process where the working environment may affect the health of the worker and the worker's state of health may have an impact on his/her ability to perform the tasks for which he/she is employed.

Work constitutes an essential element in the lifestyle of most people. In order to address health problems, a complete understanding of the interaction between the various internal and external factors that affect the health of human beings is required. These factors include:
- The workplace, including the design of the workplace
- The community with all its facets
- The group, family and individual interaction.

All these factors are interrelated – harmful effects in the workplace not only affect the worker, but may also influence the family of the worker and the community. Schilling (1973) states that an industry may have adverse effects on the health of neighbouring communities because of the discharge of toxic waste products into the atmosphere, into the water or onto the land, and that the occupational physician's responsibility does not end at the factory gates (Schilling,1973:24). This kind of pollution is still taking place in modern times, as was seen in recent claims for asbestos and mercury poisoning.

At a psychological level, many perceptions have developed around the concept of work-related illness. In earlier years the worker accepted the inevitability of diseases caused by the working environment. It was only after the Industrial Revolution and the success achieved by militant social and political protest and reform that the health and welfare of the worker was regarded as a matter of any importance.

An occupational health service should therefore incorporate into its design a holistic health programme that will anticipate physiological and psychosocial manifestations of disease. An essential part of the programme is that workers accept responsibility for participating in decision-making about their own healthcare needs. Comprehensive measures must be instituted to decrease the threat to health in all spheres of human activity. No one group of health workers can do this alone – a multidisciplinary approach should be followed to achieve the goal of a healthy worker in a healthy community.

1.2 Learning objectives

At the end of this chapter, the reader should be able to:
- Take cognizance of the historical development of occupational health services
- Relate certain important developments in the history of occupational health services to the present-day situation
- Identify important people and groups who have contributed to the development of occupational health services
- Define occupational health and describe its components
- Describe the models for occupational health services
- Describe the scope and objectives of an occupational health service
- Describe the broad functions of an occupational health service.

1.3 Occupational health in history

History reveals that both modern and ancient societies have been slow to recognize and act upon the hazards to which people are exposed in working environments.

Classical Greek literature records the clinical observations of Hippocrates, the celebrated physician of the ancient world. This pioneer of clinical observation in medicine took due note of the appalling working conditions of the time. He urged students of medicine to take into account those factors of the environment that might influence people's health.

Although varying degrees of awareness of occupational health hazards existed throughout history, it is only in modern times that occupational health has become a recognized discipline in the health sciences. Unfortunately, in many communities, this recognition is not yet legally enforceable because of the lack of appropriate legislation and the inadequate infrastructure for health services in the workplace.

The role of the occupational health nurse is inseparable from the history of occupational health. The nurse has a central function in any effective health service in the workplace.

Many examples are known of how people protected themselves from hazardous situations in ancient times. These measures were often ineffective, and neither the employee nor society accepted responsibility for human health in such conditions.

Teleky mentions protective equipment such as arm-protecting plates that were worn by archers to protect their wrists against the recoil of the bow string, and tubes worn on the fingers of the right hand that grasped the bow string. Other such examples are the leather rings that women placed on their heads when they carried water vessels, and the strips of tape worn on the cheeks and lips by the flute players (Teleky, 1948:3). Mining is one of humankind's oldest industries. Many years passed before anything was done to counteract the dangerous conditions that claimed many lives. The hazardous nature of the mining industry was recognized even in antiquity. But the total disregard for the miner's health and safety may be ascribed to the fact that a miner in those times was often a slave, prisoner or criminal, and it therefore never occurred to anyone to improve working conditions. Such miners often made futile attempts to protect themselves by wrapping themselves in bags and sacks, and by using animal bladders to cover their mouths as a protection against the inhalation of the dust that occurs in mines (Schilling, 1973:1).

1.3.1 The Industrial Revolution

Towards the end of the eighteenth century, a great ferment in spiritual, scientific, political and economic ideas took place in Europe (Teleky, 1948:15). Some advances had already taken place in the natural sciences and technology. The latter years of the eighteenth century witnessed political revolution and economic evolution (the French Revolution beginning in 1789).

The cotton and textile industry originally flourished in India. It was introduced by the Moors in Spain and later spread to Europe. Towards the end of the sixteenth century the manufacture of cotton textiles reached England and spinning and weaving thrived as a cottage industry (Schilling,1981). With the advent of water-driven and later steam-driven machines, factories developed all over the countryside. It is said that, by 1810, there were already about 5 000 steam engines in England. Changes in methods of manufacturing – from 'cottage industries' to factories – so unsettled traditional patterns of family and community life that this period eventually became known as the Industrial Revolution (Schilling, 1981:6).

The wealthy and powerful middle classes who owned factories and various enterprises, and who influenced governments, lived lives that were in sharp contrast with those of the working class. As cities developed around the industries workers realized that their labour conferred on them powerful bargaining capabilities. The appalling misery and degradation caused by the living conditions of the working classes were gradually recognized by physicians. These conditions were investigated and opposed by pioneers and reformers, many who came from privileged backgrounds. The reformers sought to bring pressure to bear on governments to eliminate the unacceptable conditions in which most members of the working classes laboured and lived. The influence of these men and women on governments gradually resulted in legislation that brought about improvements in working conditions. Thus the economic, educational, moral and living standards of workers slowly improved. Workers organized themselves into trade unions and learnt to make use of the processes of bargaining to obtain various advantages and facilities. It was, however, a long and slow process that took many decades before real progress was achieved. The initial effects of industrialization on community and individual health may be summarized as follows:

- Disruption of family life because of migrant labour
- A high incidence of social and physical ills, such as prostitution, disease, alcoholism, overpopulation, child abuse, crime and vagrancy
- The appearance of epidemics, aggravated by overcrowded, insanitary dwellings
- Malnutrition caused by failure to adapt from an established rural life to life in towns and cities
- Poverty and unemployment caused by changing conditions of supply and demand, and by an over-supplied labour pool
- Misery and confusion caused by the migration of working people from the established certainties of rural life to the ugliness, degradation and squalor of new industrial towns

- Exposure to specific hazards of occupational diseases and injury
- Exposure to the adverse effects of excessively long working hours
- Exposure to increasingly more dangerous technology in the form of newly developed machines
- Prolonged hours of exposure to the toxic hazards of chemical substances
- Exposure to the pressure of continuous work at a rate totally unsuited to the well-being of workers and often beyond the limits of their physical and psychological capacities.

Schilling (1981:7) writes that forces not dissimilar to those preceding the Industrial Revolution have enabled rapid industrialization to take place in developing countries. These forces include the development of hydro-electric and other forms of power, the end of colonialism, and the financial and technical assistance granted by developed nations (Schilling 1981:6). Problems arising from industrial progress in developing countries today are, in many respects, similar to those that prevailed in the developed world during the period of industrialization. In addition, these countries have to cope with the burdens of pandemic non-industrial diseases. Such situations demand an approach that takes into account the health of the whole community in relation to the changed modes of employment and the changing environment.

1.3.2 The twentieth century

During the Industrial Revolution in Europe, many reports became available of disease and accidents at the workplace. As a result, organized health services were established for workers in large industries such as mining, iron and steel, chemicals, textiles, metal manufacturing, and paper and pulp. The main aims of these health services were the prevention and medical treatment of occupational injuries and diseases.

In the late nineteenth and early twentieth centuries, legislation to protect workers against occupational injury and disease was introduced sporadically. Some of the first regulations addressed problems such as long working hours; accidents and poisoning; dangerous machinery; dust in the mines; air pollution by gases, metal fumes and solvent vapours (Rantanen, 1990:vii).

The First World War aroused a new interest in occupational health as nations strove to cope and survive. Shortages in munitions resulted in a sudden increase in activities in munitions factories and the adoption of very long working hours. A committee was appointed in England to examine the effects that working in these factories had on the health of their workers. The toxic effects of substances that were used in these factories were also studied.

The gradual development of occupational medicine after the economic slump caused by the war was further hampered by deficiencies in the systematic training of doctors in occupational medicine (Schilling, 1973:14).

After the Second World War the focus was on other occupational health factors, such as the influence of heavy physical work, extreme thermal conditions, noise and psychosocial stressors. The 1960s and early 1970s brought the period of semi-automation of manufacturing, which in turn focused concern on physically and psychologically monotonous work.

In the late 1970s the emphasis shifted towards the adverse health effects of exposure to low levels of carcinogenic, mutagenic or teratogenic substances (Rantanen,1990:vii). In the 1980s the main concern centred on the biological and neuropsychological effects of chemicals, as well as the problems caused by the rapid implementation of new technology, such as computers, process automatics and video display units (Rantanen,1990:vii).

Ideally, occupational health services should adjust their goals to the changes in the workplace, particularly those in the highly industrialized countries. This is, however, not always the case in all parts of the world. Accidents such as the Three Mile Island disaster in the, USA in 1979 and the Chernobyl disaster in the former USSR in 1986 where large-scale radiation pollution took place are ample proof of this omission in recent times.

The World Health Organization (WHO) states in a report published in 1990 that, in spite of positive developments in the European Region of the WHO and its Member States, occupational health services are unevenly distributed (Rantanen, 1990:viii). Such developments have been limited to the highly industrialized countries of the European Region and to the most developed areas of industry in these countries. Similar to conditions in South Africa, difficulties are experienced in organizing services for the self-employed, small industries, agriculture and certain mobile sectors such as transportation and construction.

1.3.3 The influence of the Second World War on occupational health

The Second World War and the economic expansion that followed, stimulated the development of occupational health in various parts of the world. This was mainly due to the following factors:

- The increased demand for labour during wartime led to the employment of the disabled as well as the fit.
- Occupational health services placed greater emphasis on assessing degrees of ability to work.
- The development of military equipment, which was adapted to suit soldiers, sailors and air personnel, so that their fighting efficiency was increased, contributed to the development of the science of ergonomics.
- The great need for war labour led to substantial improvements in the rehabilitation of sick and injured soldiers.
- The care of workers became an economic necessity because of the labour shortages.
- Countries that developed quickly because of rapid industrialization gave a high priority to the health of workers, and to safe and hygienic working environments. This contributed to the overall national prosperity of such countries.
- Other factors, such as the realization that a service at the worksite reduces time taken off from work, also influenced the expansion of the occupational health services (Schilling, 1981).

1.3.4 The role of the trade unions

During the twentieth century, a much stronger influence was exerted by trade unions in the interests of obtaining legislation and compensation laws to cover occupational diseases and injuries (Schilling, 1981:22).

In Russia, trade unions have extensive responsibilities for health and safety through their factory inspectors. Trade unions in the United Kingdom contributed towards an Institute of Occupational Health in the University of London.

The General Federation of Labour in Israel established its own health insurance programme – the Kupat Holim – which provides comprehensive medical care for its members who comprise 90% of the working population. It also opened its first Department of Industrial Medicine in Tel Aviv in 1945 (Schilling, 1981:22).

1.3.5 The European Economic Community

The International Labour Organization (ILO) compiled a blueprint for occupational health services to be provided in factories employing more than 200 persons in 1957. All the countries of the now defunct League of Nations were to adhere to the basic recommendations (Ffrench, 1973:7). In 1962 the European Economic Community adopted Recommendation 112, ILO, 1959, namely to provide occupational health services in all industrial, non-industrial and agricultural undertakings and for public services. These services were to be based on statutory requirements, and not voluntary efforts (Schilling, 1981:25).

1.3.6 The development of occupational health services in South Africa

The development of occupational health services is closely linked to the political and socio-economic climate in a country. After the discovery of gold and diamonds in South Africa in the late nineteenth and early twentieth century, many small towns were transformed from predominantly rural agricultural communities into industrial centres.

Large-scale migration from the remaining rural to urban areas within the country and neighbouring regions took place. This social phenomenon caused the upheaval of the traditionally extended family system in the rural areas, bringing along with it all the problems of rapid industrialization. A high crime rate, insufficient infrastructure and the ethnic diversity found in these industrial centres soon developed into a major problem for the service-rendering authorities. Mining activities exposed large numbers of workers to the dangers of high concentrations of silica dust (Baker & Coetzee, 1983:11).

During the period between 1886 and the outbreak of the Anglo-Boer War in 1899, the dangers of silica dust inhalation were ignored and this led to the early death of many mineworkers. Towards the end of 1901, the government mining engineer reported that 18.5% of White miners employed before the war had died.

The first commission of enquiry into phthisis (pulmonary tuberculosis) was appointed by Lord Milner in 1902. The report of this commission showed that the average period for the development of advanced phthisis was less than six years and established occupational health services through prescription of:
- Dust suppression methods which were legally enforced
- Health examinations
- Compensation for silicosis (Baker & Coetzee, 1983:11).

The Mining Regulations Commission was appointed in 1907 to further investigate the problem of dust control in mines. In 1911, a third commission consisting mainly of

Milestones in the development of health through the ages

460–375 BC	Hippocrates, 'the Father of Medicine', taught his students the importance of environmental factors in diagnosing diseases and referred to the poisoning of refiners and extractors of metals.
AD 23–70	Plinius described mercury poisoning.
AD 130–200	Galen documented diseases suffered by miners, fullers and tanners.
1439–154	Aureolus von Hohenheim, alias Paracelsus, described the toxicology of metals.
1494–1555	Georgious Agricola wrote about miners' disease.
1633–1714	Bernadino Ramazinni, known as the Father of occupational medicine, was a physician and professor of medicine in Modena and Padua and: ■ published the first systematic study of trade diseases ■ recommended questioning patients about their occupations ■ and advocated personal prophylaxis, thereby laying the foundations for occupational hygiene.
1750 onwards	The Industrial Revolution brought about: ■ many changes in occupations and social life ■ migration to manufacturing areas with poor living conditions ■ child labour, long work hours and poor working conditions.
1802	The first Factory Bill was introduced in England due to the influence of humanists Robert Owen, Sir Robert Peel, Michael Sadler and physicians Percivall Pott, Thomas Percival and later Charles Turner Thackrah and others.
1819	The first Factory Act limited child employment to nine years of age.
1833	The next Factory Act introduced a Factory Inspectorate in England, with subsequent Factory Acts (1844, 1855, 1864 and 1895) adding stricter control.
1854	The first Mines Act forbade underground work for women and children.
1854	Florence Nightingale and a group of nurses took care of ill and injured British soldiers in the Crimean War.
1878	The first industrial nurse, Phillipa Flowerday, was appointed at J&J Colman.
1884	The Bureau of Labour was established in the United States of America.
1895	Ada Mayo Stewart was appointed as an industrial nurse by Vermont Marble Company.
1897	The first Workmen's Compensation Act was introduced in England.
1898	Thomas Morrison Legge was appointed first Medical Inspector of Factories in England.
1911	The Worker's Compensation Laws were enacted in the United States of America.
1912	The National Council for Industrial Safety was established in the United States.
1914–1918	The First World War required rapid growth in first aid and industrial health services in rapidly growing industries.
1939–1945	The Second World War demanded increased production and workforce.

medical practitioners was appointed to inquire into the incidence of miner's phthisis (tuberculosis) on the mines.

The first legislation was published in 1911. This was the Miners Phthisis Act, which made compensation for phthisis compulsory. The general health of mineworkers received little or no attention at this time. Although large numbers of mineworkers were imported from neighbouring African countries, health conditions on the mines and in the hostels were critical. Facilities were utterly primitive and the diet of workers was inadequate, resulting in conditions such as scurvy, pneumonia and meningitis (Baker & Coetzee, 1983:11).

Finally, due to public pressure, conditions were improved and the Chamber of Mines invited an American expert, Colonel W. C. Gorgas, to visit South Africa. On his recommendation, the Rand Mines Group appointed the pioneer of occupational medicine in South Africa, Dr A. J. Orenstein. He also acted as Surgeon General for the South African Army in the First World War. Baker and Coetzee are of the opinion that Dr Orenstein played a leading role in the development of occupational health services (1983:12).

The Second World War played an important role in the stimulation of the development of industries in South Africa, and, in more recent times, sanctions applied against this country have had a similar effect. Industries developed to provide for the internal needs of the country. During the war, equipment for troops had to be manufactured, and the mines experienced problems in obtaining the necessary machines and equipment. After the war, South Africa, with its reserves of raw materials, offered attractive opportunities to many overseas investors, and this led to an escalation in industrial development.

The first legislation to control conditions in the industry was the Factories, Machinery and Building Works Act, 1941 (No 22 of 1941), today known as the Occupational Health and Safety Act, 1993 (Act 85 of 1993). Also in 1941, the first Workmen's Compensation Act (Act 30 of 1941) was passed and replaced in 1993 by the Compensation for Occupational Injuries and Diseases Act, 1993 (Act 130 of 1993). In 1956 the Pneumoconiosis Research Unit was established. This research unit was later expanded to become the National Research Institute for Occupational Diseases – now known as the National Centre for Occupational Health. The Occupational Diseases in Mines and Works Act, 1973 (No 78 of 1973) was promulgated in 1973.

Research into occupational diseases revealed that conditions in industry left much to be desired. An in-depth investigation was necessary. In 1975, the Erasmus Commission of Enquiry was appointed to report on:

- The nature, incidence and extent of occupational diseases in the Republic of South Africa
- Statutory measures and facilities and their effectiveness
- The manpower situation, with specific referral to occupational health
- Health control in the workplace
- The establishment of health services in the workplace
- The protection of the community against environmental pollution resulting from industries.

This report was very comprehensive and the Commission made many recommendations. The Commission stated that a certain measure of confusion existed in the field of occupational health in South Africa, mainly because legislation relating to occupational diseases had been replicated in many places. This, in turn, had led to the duplication of services in the different government departments responsible for the implementation of such legislation (Erasmus, 1976:8).

In 1977 the government appointed the Wiehahn Commission to examine labour relations and legislation. The findings of the Commission were published in six separate reports. The key role played by employers in labour relations was emphasized, and the Commission gave practical guidelines to employers. It was also recommended that the Department of Manpower be responsible for the overall implementation of the government's manpower policy (Searle, Brink & Grobbelaar, 1988:500).

Many more Acts were subsequently promulgated – these were all finally consolidated into the Occupational Health and Safety Act, 1993 (Act 85 of 1993) and the Mine Health and Safety Act, 1996 (No 29 of 1996).

It is noticeable that the manufacturing industry has developed extensively during the past 40 years. Control over these industries is exercised by the Department of Labour through the following Acts of legislation:
- Occupational Health and Safety Act, 1993 (No 85 of 1993)
- Compensation for Occupational Injuries and Diseases Act, 1993 (No 130 of 1993)
- Labour Relations Act, 1995 (No 66 of 1995) (as amended by Act 12 of 2002)
- Unemployment Insurance Act, 2001 (No 63 of 2001)
- Basic Conditions of Employment Act, 1997 (No 75 of 1997)

(Refer to Chapter 2 for details on legislation.)

The Department of Health regulates and coordinates general health policy. It administers the following legislation which applies to specific sections of occupational health services (refer to Chapter 2):
- The Health Act, 1977 (No 63 of 1977) refers to general preventive and promotive health measures, which also apply to workers, and provides for the notification of conditions, the closing of premises, and the disinfection and evacuation of certain buildings or areas. Local authorities are designated as responsible for environmental health services within their own areas. Their responsibilities include general hygiene, the prevention of nuisances, unhygienic or offensive conditions (these may include factories, industrial or business premises); the prevention of the pollution of water or the atmosphere.
- The Nursing Act, 1995 (No 5 of 1995) (as amended)
- The Medicines and Related Substances Control Act, 1965 (No 101 of 1965) (as amended)
- The Health Professions Act, 1974 (No 56 of 1974)
- The Mental Health Act, 1973 (No 18 of 1973).

The National Health Bill of November 2001 aims to establish a national health system and sets out the rights and duties of healthcare providers.

Various statutory bodies were established under legislation. These bodies are

History of occupational health development in South Africa

Pre-17th century,	African people were mainly hunter-gatherers but gold, copper and iron were also mined, melted and cast, which implies exposure to toxic substances.
1652	Jan van Riebeeck established a halfway station for sailors en route to the East to obtain fresh produce and water in an effort to prevent disease, especially scurvy.
1870	Diamonds were discovered and people worked and lived in poor conditions in the diamond fields at Hope Town and later Kimberley.
1886	Gold was found and mined under poor mining and living conditions on the Witwatersrand and the threat of phthisis from the silica dust was ignored.
1899–1902	The Anglo-Boer War interrupted the mining and highlighted the death toll.
1902	The Milner administration appointed a Commission of Enquiry who found that 19% of rock drillers had died probably from phthisis and recommended dust suppression, health examinations and compensation for phthisis (silicosis).
1907	A Mining Regulations Commission was appointed.
1911	The Miners Phthisis Act was published, enforcing compensation for phthisis.
1913	Public pressure forced the Chamber of Mines to ask for advice from an overseas expert, Colonel W. C. Gorgas, on the health of workers. He recommended the appointment of Dr A. J. Orenstein, Surgeon-General for the South African Army in the First World War.
1914	Dr A. J. Orenstein was appointed by the Rand Mines Group and became known as the Father of occupational health in South Africa owing to his active involvement in regulating the mining conditions and improving health services to the miners, bringing mortality down to 0.26% by 1917.
1939–1945	The Second World War took place.
1941	The Factories, Machinery and Building Works Act (No 22 of 1941) and the Workmen's Compensation Act (No 30 of 1941) were introduced.
1947	The Fertilizers, Farm Feeds, Agricultural Remedies and Stock Remedies Act (No 36 of 1947) was introduced.
1956	The Pneumoconiosis Research Institute was established at the Council for Scientific and Industrial Research under the guidance of Dr A. J. Orenstein. The following Acts were introduced: ■ Explosives Act (No 26 of 1956) ■ Mines and Works Act (No 27 of 1956) ■ Labour Relations Act (No 28 of 1956) ■ The Water Act (No 54 of 1956)

Over the next years the following Acts and legislation were introduced:

1957	Wage Act (No 5 of 1957)
1960	Railways and Harbours Service Act (No 22 of 1960)
1961	Dairy Industry Act (No 30 of 1961)
1964	Shops and Offices Act (No 75 of 1964)
1965	Atmospheric Pollution Prevention Act (No 45 of 1965)
1966	Unemployment Insurance Act (No 30 of 1966)
1967	Animal Slaughter, Meat and Animal Products Hygiene Act (No 87 Of 1967)
1973	Hazardous Substances Act (No 15 of 1973)
1975	Erasmus Commission of Enquiry into health and safety in industry took place.
1977	The Wiehahn Commission investigated labour relations and legislation, and the Health Act (No 63 of 1977) was introduced
1983	Basic Conditions of Service Act (No 3 of 1983)
1983	Machinery and Occupational Safety Act (No 6 of 1983)

(Further development and currently applicable legislation are addressed in Chapter 2.)

responsible for the implementation of the legislation applicable to each area of health under its jurisdiction. Examples of such organizations are:
- The SA Nursing Council
- The SA Health Professions Council
- The Pharmacy Council
- The Medicine Control Council.

The Department of Environmental Affairs controls workplace emissions through the:
- Atmospheric Pollution Prevention Act, 1965 (No 45 of 1965)
- Environmental Conservation Act, 1989 (No 73 of 1989).

The Department of Mineral and Energy Affairs regulates:
- The Mine Health and Safety Act, 1996 (Act 29 of 1996)
- The Occupational Diseases in Mines and Works Act, 1973 (Act 78 of 1973)
- The Nuclear Energy Act, 1982 (No 73 of 1982).

The Department of Agriculture is concerned with farming activities through the:
- Fertilizers, Farm Feeds, Agricultural Remedies and Stock Remedies Act, 1947 (No 36 of 1947)

Two important structures were formed specifically for occupational health matters, namely the Medical Bureau for Occupational Diseases, and the National Centre for Occupational Health, as discussed below.

The Medical Bureau for Occupational Diseases (MBOD)
This Bureau was established in 1973 under the Occupational Diseases in Mines and Works Act (Act 78 of 1973). Its main function is the surveillance of the health of at-risk workers in and at controlled mines and works. To enable the Bureau to fulfil this function, a system of certification was developed.

The Certification Committee considers all applications for certification and deals with cases individually. A complete medical and labour history, as well as the result of special investigations, are presented. Applicants are notified of the committee's finding in writing, and may appeal against the finding to the Reviewing Authority.

The Reviewing Authority reviews the case and may confirm the finding of the committee or may disagree with it. In the latter event, a joint sitting of the two bodies will decide by majority vote on the outcome of the case. These two bodies deal with diseases that are compensatable according to scales laid down by legislation.
Other functions performed by the Bureau are:

Medical services. Over the years the Bureau has built up an experienced team of medical specialists who carry out physical examinations.

Database. This database provided unique opportunities for research into various aspects of occupational diseases. X-rays are taken for screening and diagnostic purposes for all dust-related occupational lung diseases.

Lung function laboratory. This laboratory is the most sophisticated in the country, and workers are put through a battery of tests.

Audiometric screening. This screening is carried out in an attempt to build up a database for the development of standards, as noise-induced hearing loss still remains a widespread problem in the mining industry.

Inspectorate. Inspectors visit mines and works at least once a year and represent the Bureau in a wide range of matters in controlled mines and works.

Epidemiological research unit. This unit conducts research into dust-related diseases.

The National Centre for Occupational Health (NCOH)
This Centre functions under the aegis of the Department of Health. It is well equipped with scientists in a variety of disciplines and provides facilities for the following research, services and teaching functions:

Pathology. Reasearch is a vital function of this section, and relates mostly to the effect of mine dusts and gases on the respiratory system. The Centre carries out postmortem heart and lung examinations on deceased miners on behalf of the Medical Bureau for Occupational Diseases.

Biochemistry. Analytical work is done for any industry on request. A database is being built up and the results should be useful for research into metal toxicity. Blood and urine samples are analysed to detect levels of toxic substances such as lead.

Immunology and microbiology. Advanced and sophisticated tests are currently available that help researchers to better understand immunological mechanisms and their relationship to other factors in microbiology. The field of occupational asthma in factories processing organic and inorganic material is studied extensively.

Occupational medicine and epidemiology. Major themes in the research programme of this unit are occupational health services; occupational mortality; social aspects of occupational diseases, such as compensation and other consequences of accidents; recognition and epidemiological measurement of asbestos-related diseases; and biological measurements.

Occupational hygiene
The work is divided into three main sections, namely:
1 *Services.* This consists mainly of ad hoc investigations into environmental conditions in different types of factories. A report of concomitant advice is usually drawn up after the investigation.
2 *Teaching.* Members of the Institute provide formal and informal training for medical and occupational health students.
3 *Research.* This is pursued as and when other commitments permit it.

1.4 Regulation of occupational health in South Africa since 1990

As can be seen in Chapter 2, many Acts were promulgated after 1990 as a result of ongoing development in occupational health and society. A new direction was followed by the South African government when a general Reconstruction and Development Programme was introduced in South Africa in 1994. In the policy framework, occupational health services are specifically referred to in the document under 'Other healthcare programmes'. The following suggestions were made:

- 'Occupational health services must be greatly expanded and legislation to protect the health of workers must be enforced' (ANC, 1994:48).
- Emphasis must be placed on the protection of the most vulnerable workers, e.g. domestic and farm workers and commercial sex workers.
- Workers must be involved in policy-making processes through their health and safety committees.
- The importance of periodic examinations in the workplace must be emphasized.
- Penalties for violations of occupational health standards must be stricter.
- Laws must conform to International Labour Organization and other international standards.
- Unions and State agencies must be empowered to monitor and enforce safety and health standards at the workplace.
- The compensation system for injured and ill workers must be restructured to ensure a more efficient service.
- A board should be established to deal with preventive and compensatory aspects of worker safety and health.
(ANC, 1994:48–49)

A National Committee on Occupational Health brought out a report in 1996 stating that health services in this country have developed in an ad hoc manner and employers provide services mostly on a discretionary basis (Department of Health, 1996:1). The following services are listed:

- Work-based services provided and funded by the employer in the private sector. Employers provide services for the following reasons: remote settings; inherently dangerous work (mining); the need to reduce absenteeism and increase productivity; certain legal requirements for medical surveillance; the need to screen potential employees; executive medical examinations; and in more recent years, pressure from the trade unions.
- Private-sector primary care providers (non-workplace-based). Where no workplace services exist, employers often make use of private medical practitioners for pre-placement medical examinations, acute medical and injury care, medical surveillance and health advice.
- Workplace-based safety and hygiene activities. There are many people with part-time or full-time responsibility for managing safety, risk or loss control in industrial and mining enterprises in South Africa.
- Workplace-based occupational health services for public-sector employees.
- Public-sector-based occupational medical services are available in Johannesburg,

Cape Town, Durban and Bloemfontein. Workers are referred by occupational health services to these centres for specialized diagnosis and treatment.
- Public-sector-based occupational hygiene and environmental health services. The Department of Health employs industrial hygienists at the National Centre for Occupational Health (NCOH). They provide technical and scientific support to a variety of parties in industry, as well as to other government departments.
- Public-sector laboratory services. The NCOH has an analytic laboratory for analysing environmental and biological specimens. The SA Institute for Medical Research and most academic hospitals offer a range of laboratory services.
- Private and non-governmental organizations offer facilities in each of the categories of services given under the previous paragraphs:
    - injuries or diseases falling under the Compensation for Occupational Injuries and Diseases Act are referred to and treated at private hospitals
    - services for the general rehabilitation of injured or sick workers are available from private practitioners, e.g. physiotherapists and occupational therapists
    - private-sector laboratories are available for biological and environmental samples in all provinces
    - occupational hygiene and safety services – there are a number of associations and affiliations rendering such services, for example the National Occupational Safety Association (NOSA).
- Union-linked non-governmental organizations deal with safety and health issues concerning their members.

1.5 Occupational health

The discipline of occupational health is concerned with the relationship between work and health and was defined in 1950 by a joint committee of International Labour Office and the World Health Organization as being concerned with:
- The promotion and maintenance of the highest degree of physical, mental and social well-being of workers in all occupations
- The prevention among workers of departures from health caused by their working conditions
- The protection of workers in their employment from risks resulting from factors adverse to health
- The placing and maintenance of the worker in an occupational environment adapted to his/her physiological and psychological state.

In 1980 the World Health Assembly emphasized the need for a new perspective integrating occupational health in the primary healthcare of underserved working populations, particularly those in the developing countries (Rantanen, 1990:12).

The WHO Eighth General Programme of Work contains several goals for occupational health programmes to meet the health needs of workers at, or near, their place of work. These are based on appropriate technology and workers' participation. The means of attaining these goals include factors such as:

- The collection of data at a national level on workers' morbidity and working conditions
- The identification of priority risks and hazards at the workplace
- The training and education of occupational health personnel, workers and employers
- The development of occupational health institutions.

The overall strategy of the WHO clearly recognizes the importance of occupational health services in putting 'health for all' strategies into practice. The advantages of this approach – especially in carrying out preventive health activities, reaching high-risk working populations, and introducing primary healthcare through health services provided at the workplace – are appreciated (Rantanen, 1990:12).

1.6 The components of an occupational health service
Occupational health consists of two components, as listed in Table 1.1.

Table 1.1 The components of occupational health

Occupational Hygiene	Occupational Medicine and Occupational Health Nursing
Environmental factors	Human factors
Legislation	Legislation
Hazard	Health screening and placement
■ recognition	Medical surveillance
■ measurement	Health promotion and protection
■ management	Emergency care
■ evaluation	Primary healthcare
■ control	Treatment of diseases
Reports and records	Administration and records
	Rehabilitation
	Epidemiology and research

1.7 The role of occupational health
In an overview of occupational health services in the European Region of the WHO, Rantanen (1990:1) states that the shift from expanding to intensive production services is a consequence of new structures in world economics – a fact that is rapidly changing working life in Europe.

This change involves the following process, which can also be observed in many other industrialized countries:
- An active adaptation to new divisions of work
- Growing economic integration of regions and globalization
- The rapid implementation of technology.

These processes have a direct impact on:
- Working conditions

- The types of industry and occupation
- The content of jobs and the organization of work
- The nature, occurrence and seriousness of health hazards at the workplace.

Economic restraints have slowed the development of health services in general, but more specifically in the occupational health field. The health of the worker is never really the primary objective of any industry. Today the efficient use of available human and financial resources is becoming increasingly important, as occupational health services are faced with an ever-expanding range of problems. Such services must be able to solve the traditional problems of various industries and agriculture, as well as meet the challenges posed by new information technology, highly reactive chemical substances and different types of physical energy.

This range implies an expansion of the traditional scope of occupational health services, a need for greater competence and the adaptation of a multidisciplinary approach to services (Rantanen, 1990:1).

Alongside the changes in the structure of industries and the content of jobs came profound social changes. These are characterized by:
- Changes in attitude toward work
- The evolvement of new value systems
- A growing interest in self-determination by workers
- An increase in the worker's mobility, which enables workers to compare conditions in different jobs and areas.

Workers of today are increasingly eager to participate in decisions about the structure and organization of their work, as well as the quality and the content of the occupational health services provided. All this is reflected in new legislation and in agreements between employers and the trade unions in various fields of labour.

1.8 Organizational models of occupational health services

Organizational models for occupational health services vary within regions, according to national and political traditions, the organization of occupational health and safety, general health services, and the nature of industrial and economic activities in a region. The Europe Regional Office of the WHO describes six basic models found specifically in this region (Rantanen, 1990:25). These models will be discussed briefly.

1.8.1 The Major Industry model

This is a typical model of large units in manufacturing, processing and other large industries. These units have:
- On-site occupational health units
- A multidisciplinary team staffed by full-time experts, which may consist of a physician, nurses, an industrial hygienist, a safety engineer, radiographer, physiotherapist and psychologist.

1.8.2 The Group Service model
Small- and medium-sized undertakings may join to organize occupational health service units of a certain size and quality. Some countries make legal provisions for the establishment of such group service centres by undertakings that are not large enough to warrant their own services. Examples of these services are found in France where a unit may serve different types of undertaking in a given geographical area, or a number of undertakings with the same type of economic activity.

1.8.3 The Private Health Centre model
This model is found in several countries, where physicians in their privately owned health centres provide occupational health services. They function as a group service, and are not managed by the industries concerned. These industries transfer the risk of managing their health programme to the private centres, which are run on the profit principle.

The advantages of this model lie in its flexibility, but the concern for profit may influence the orientation of the activities. A distinct disadvantage is that the undertakings served do not participate in the management of the services provided.

1.8.4 The Community Health Centre model
This model implies the provision of health services by the local public health and/or primary healthcare units. In countries such as Italy, the local health units are legally responsible for providing this service.

Any other community health service may also be used to render the occupational healthcare services in a given area. The specific advantage of this kind of service is the accessibility of the service to the community, and the automatic integration of the service with the primary healthcare services.

On the other hand, local health services may have difficulty handling the occupational health problems of a large number of undertakings engaged in widely varying activities in its area. To meet this problem, the larger municipal health centres employ special occupational health personnel.

1.8.5 The National Health Service model
The occupational health units in this model are located on the business premises, but personnel are employed by the national health service system. These services are mostly found in Eastern Europe. This model effectively combines the elements of occupational health with general services, constituting a comprehensive workers' health service. Concern is, however, expressed that the broader curative activities may receive priority over the preventive aspects of the occupational health service.

1.8.6 The Social Security Institution model
In this model, a social security institution provides the occupational health services. This model operates in a way similar to the group service model. Israel operates a system based on this model with the occupational health service organized and administered by the Health Insurance programme or Kupat Holim of the General Federation of Labour (Schilling, 1981:22).

1.8.7 New models
Many kinds of enterprises, such as the small business, the mobile workplace and the self-employed, constitute a challenge for the occupational health service. Various models are used, such as the community-based primary healthcare unit and mobile units in attempts to serve these workers.

1.9 The scope of occupational health services
Company policy is directly responsible for the scope of services offered in industry. Gardner and Taylor say that the objectives and responsibilities of an occupational health service can only be as good or as bad as the company policy allows (1975:20). Successful health programmes require a commitment from management. A high-quality healthcare progamme should be based on the philosophy of health promotion, the needs of the organization and the health needs of the employees.

1.10 The objectives of an occupational health service
Each company should strive towards the goal of establishing a healthy and safe working environment. At the same time, workers must be motivated to accept responsibility for their own health and that of their families. To attain this goal, an awareness of safe working conditions and a healthy lifestyle are essential requirements. The overall objectives of occupational health services are embodied in five principles, whose terminology is derived from that used to discuss the 'health for all' concept:
1. The protection and prevention principle: protecting workers' health from hazards at work
2. The adaptive principle: adapting work and the work environment to the capabilities of workers
3. The health promotion principle: promoting the physical and psychosocial well-being of workers
4. The curative and rehabilitative principle: minimizing the consequences of occupational hazards, accidents and injuries, and occupational and related diseases
5. The primary healthcare principle: providing general healthcare services for workers and their families at the workplace, or from nearby facilities (Rantanen, 1990:17).

1.11 The functions and activities of an occupational health service
According to the WHO, the most authoritative list of functions of occupational health services comes from the International Labour Organization (ILO) (Rantanen, 1990:19). The following is a summary of these functions:
- Undertaking surveillance of the work environment and working practices that may affect workers' health
- Identifying and assessing the risks of health hazards in the workplace

- Undertaking surveillance of workers' health in relation to their work
- Advising on planning and organization of work, including the design of the workplace and the choice, maintenance and condition of machinery and other equipment used in the work
- Participating in the development of programmes for the improvement of safe work practices, which includes the evaluation of health-related aspects of new equipment and new work processes
- Advising on occupational health, safety and hygiene, on ergonomics, and on safety equipment for individuals and groups
- Promoting the adaptation of the workplace (particularly in vulnerable groups, and those with health problems)
- Contributing to measures of vocational rehabilitation (observing the effect of work on disease or physiological condition, and taking early measures for reassignment or rehabilitation
- Collaborating in the provision of information, training and education in occupational health, hygiene and ergonomics
- Organizing first aid and emergency treatment
- Participating in the analysis of occupational accidents and occupational diseases.

(These functions include the essential elements of a comprehensive occupational health service as set out in the main objectives given in section 1.10.)

1.12 Occupational health nursing

Occupational health nursing is a nursing specialty that provides healthcare to workers, usually at the workplace. The service focuses on health promotion and protection within the context of a safe and healthy work environment. As an independent practitioner, the occupational health nurse makes autonomous nursing judgements to optimize health, prevent illness and injury, and to reduce health hazards in the interests of both the employee and the company (Rogers, 1994:34–35).

In occupational health nursing, the nurse's client is not a patient, in the usual sense, but a worker who is exposed to a work environment that may be hazardous to his/her health.

The nurse is required to care for many groups of workers from different age, gender, socio-economic, educational and cultural backgrounds. He/she is required to solve health problems that extend along the entire continuum of health and illness.

The tasks he/she is called upon to perform require a wide range of skills, including interpersonal, leadership, management and advanced clinical skills.

The nurse lives and works in a matrix of interpersonal relationships between the employer, the worker and the community and practises according to the highest professional standards and ethical principles. See section 6.3.2 in Chapter 6.

Problems are identified and solutions are sought that are compatible with the work environment, management policy and the health system on the one hand, and the individual health, social and environmental needs of the worker on the other hand.

1.12.1 The development of occupational health nursing in South Africa

Historical background

Searle (1982:515) states that occupational health nursing in South Africa dates back to the establishment of the refreshment station and hospital for sailors at the Cape by the Dutch East India Company in 1652.

Although few occupational health services were established at the workplace, it is known that, during the last century, many hospitals were established by industrial concerns, with the specific purpose of caring for the ill worker. The various mining houses were primarily responsible for this development, as they made use of migratory labour and their workforces were very large. This development led to the establishment of services that were mainly of a curative nature. Many of these hospitals are still maintained today.

The primary function of the occupational health nurse in South Africa is aimed at protecting the health of workers in industry, commerce or other types of services that employ large numbers of workers.

Factors that diminish the worker's ability to produce at an optimum level are damaging, not only to the worker and the employer, but to the national welfare of the country. Owing to the expanding South African economy and the relative shortage of skilled labour, the work of the occupational health nurse is of considerable economic significance to the community as a whole (Searle, 1982:515).

Very little is known about the pioneer nurses in the occupational health field of this country. Baker and Coetzee (1983:15) state that the first known industrial nurse in South Africa was a Matron Herron-Brown, who was employed by the United Tobacco Company Ltd, in Cape Town in 1923.

In the report of the Medical Officer of Health for the year ending 1902, mention was made of the lady Sanitary Inspector, a Mrs A. G. Kenyon, who was a trained nurse. Her duty was to visit the workrooms of milliners, dressmakers and places where women were employed, to report on the sanitary conditions in these places. Although the main purpose of these visits was to decrease the high infant mortality rate in the city at the time, it may indirectly be regarded as an occupational health service (Searle, 1965).

1.12.2 The training for occupational health nurses in South Africa

The occupational health nurse in South Africa is a front-line health nurse. He/she anticipates health problems before they are established and their sphere of activity extends beyond the care of the workers. This approach led to the development of certain trends in the training of the nurse for occupational health in South Africa.

Like many aspects of the South African system of health services, the concept of a health visitor was derived from Great Britain. The concept was later expanded to include the Sanitary Inspector. Local authorities or voluntary organizations to promote the general health of people and to improve sanitary conditions in towns and workplaces employed both these categories of ladies. The Witwatersrand Technical Institute first introduced the training course for health visitors in 1926 with the assistance of the SA

Trained Nurses' Association (Searle, 1965). In 1964 the first regulations and syllabus for a National Diploma in Public Health Nursing was drawn up.

Occupational Health Nursing includes aspects of healthcare that are very specific to the occupational field, and for this purpose a more task-oriented course was developed by the leading nurses in this field, with the first course for the Certificate in Occupational Health offered in 1976. At present, we have Diploma and Bachelor of Technology qualifications in Occupational Health Nursing, with the opportunity to obtain a Master of Science and a Doctorate in the specialty at leading South African universities.

The South African Society of Occupational Health Nurse was formed on 30 April 1980. Its main aims are to promote occupational health in industry and to address the needs of the Occupational Health Nurse.

1.13 The occupational health team members in South Africa

Occupational health may be described as a unique discipline because it requires an interdisciplinary team effort to ensure an effective occupational health programme. The team includes representatives from management, workers, hygiene, safety and training and health professionals. It has no leader since each member contributes unique skills to the assessment, planning, implementation and evaluation of the total occupational health programme.

The report of the National Committee on Occupational Health (1996:15) states that an array of other professionals and non-professionals contribute to the day-to-day activities in health and safety, as part of broader job responsibilities. In our present system of occupational health services it is difficult to estimate the number of people involved in occupational health but according to a survey undertaken by the Committee, it appears that occupational health nurses are currently the major cadre of personnel providing services at the workplace. The majority of these nurses have the additional nursing qualification in occupational health.

1.13.1 The top management of the organization

The success of the occupational health and safety programme depends on the moral and financial support of the leaders of the organization. The company health policy is signed by the chief executive officer who provides the finance for staff, equipment, training and health and safety programmes to achieve the objectives of a safe, healthy work environment.

1.13.2 The occupational medical practitioner

The main objective of occupational medicine is to protect the employee from health risks at work and to guide the employer through the maze of legal requirements pertaining to a healthy and safe work environment.

Occupational medicine as a medical specialization is primarily a branch of preventive medicine that requires a thorough understanding of toxicology, emergency medicine, epidemiology and statistics and business skills.

The South African Health Professions Council recognizes the Diploma in Occupational Health as an additional qualification for medical practitioners. The qualification is required to render a legally acceptable service.

1.13.3 The occupational health nursing practitioner
A qualified general nurse with postgraduate training in occupational health nursing provides the basic healthcare aspect of the occupational health programme.

It often makes good business sense to provide primary healthcare facilities for early intervention in illness and the monitoring of chronic diseases, thereby enhancing employee morale and maintaining optimal production. Early symptoms of an occupational disease may be diagnosed during a primary healthcare session, even before the worker links them to his/her work. The nurse co-ordinates the medical surveillance programme according to the exposure levels of individuals and initiates remedial action as required.

1.13.4 The occupational hygienist
Occupational hygiene is the recognition, evaluation and control of environmental factors that arise in the workplace that may cause sickness, impaired health, or discomfort and inefficiency among workers (Schoeman & Schröder, 1994). (See Chapter 4.)

Occupational hygiene practitioners have been trained in occupational hygiene either through short courses at Technicons, or as part of other postgraduate studies at selected universities. In 1993 an Institute of Occupational Hygienists of South Africa was formed with the aim of developing occupational hygiene as a profession.

1.13.5 Workers through their representatives
Employees and their representatives in organized labour and on health and safety committees are included in the occupational health team at a worksite.

1.13.6 Allied professions
Professions allied to medicine include specialities such as psychology, physiotherapy, occupational therapy, audiology and lung function technology. These categories are not essentially employed in the occupational health services but are contracted to assist in the occupational health programme and can contribute to the programme by advising the occupational health team.

The occupational health team meets regularly to evaluate the programme, address shortcomings and plan ahead. It is important to keep up to date with new information, draft bills and legislation as it becomes available and each member is responsible for reporting on developments in their own specialization.

1.14 Internet Web sites
Occupational health is never inert. It is constantly reacting to scientific, medical, technical, economic and legislative development. The occupational health practitioner keeps up to date through reading professional journals and newspapers, attending seminars, short courses, professional meetings and through the Internet.

Applicable Internet Web Sites include:
- Association of Societies for Occupational Safety and Health (ASOSH): http://www.asoh.or
  Through this site there is access to local and world sites covering all aspects of occupational health, hygiene, safety, legislation, statutory bodies, professional associations, etc.
- International Commission on Occupational Health (ICOH): http://www.icoh.org.sg
- International Labour Office (ILO): http://www.ilo.org
- Mining, Medical and Other Health Care Professionals Association (MMOA): http://www.mmoa.org.za
- National Centre for Occupational Health: http://www.ncoh.pwv.gov.co.za
- South African Government departments: http://www.gov.za
- South African Society of Occupational Health Nursing Practitioners (SASOHN): http://www.sasohn.org.za
- South African Society of Occupational Medicine (SASOM): http://www.sasom.org.za
- World Health Organization (WHO): http://www.who.int

1.15 Conclusion

It took many centuries before employers accepted full responsibility for the prevention of health hazards in the workplace. Social and legal constraints and structures to protect the health of the worker are still being developed today. In many countries, well-established services exist, but in some areas in the world, formal structures are still inadequate, resulting in the continued exposure of workers to conditions which are detrimental to their health.

1.16 Bibliography

African National Congress. 1994. A National Health Plan for South Africa. Johannesburg: ¨manyano Publishers.
African National Congress. 1994. Reconstruction and Development Programme. A Policy Framework. Johannesburg: Umanyano Publishers.
Baker, M. & Coetzee, A. C. 1983. *An Introduction to Occupational Health Nursing in South Africa* Johannesburg: Witwatersrand University Press.
Cralley, L. J. & Cralley, L. V. 1985. *Patty's Industrial Hygiene and Toxicology*. Vol III. Second edition 3A. New York: John Wiley & Sons.
Erasmus, R. P. B. 1976.*Commission of Enquiry into Occupational Health*. Pretoria: Government Printer..
Ffrench, G. 1973. *Occupational Health*. London: Medical and Technical Publishing.
Gardner, W. & Taylor, P. 1975. *Health at Work*. London: Associated Busines Programmes.
Girdano, D. A. 1986. *Occupational Health Promotion*. New York: Macmillan Publishing.
Rantanen, J. (ed.) 1990. *Occupational Health Services – An Overview*. Geneva WHO Publications. European Series No 26.

Report of the National Committee on Occupational Health, 1996. Pretoria: Department of Health.
Republic of South Africa Annual Report of Department of Manpower 2001. Pretoria: Government Printer..
Rogers, B. 1994. *Occupational Health Nursing: Concepts and Practice.* Philadelphia: WB Saunders.
Rosenstock, L. & Cullen, M. R. 1994. *Textbook of Clinical Occupational and Environmental Medicine.* Philadelphia: WB Saunders.
Schilling, R. S. F. (ed.) 1973. *Occupational Health Practice.* London: Butterworths.
Schilling, R. S. F. (ed.) 1981. *Occupational Health Practice.* 2nd edition. London: Butterworths.
Schoeman, J. J. & Schröder, H. H. E. 1994. *Occupational Hygiene.* Cape Town: Juta & Company.
Searle, C. 1965. *The History of the Development of Nursing in South Africa 1652–1960.* Pretoria: The South African Nursing Association.
Searle, C, 1982-1992. Unpublished Notes on Scope of Nursing and Midwifery Practice – Discussions SANC Laws Committee.
Searle, C., Brink, H. I. L. & Grobbelaar, W. I. C. 1988. *Aspects of Community Health.* Cape Town: King Edward VII Trust.
Teleky, L. 1948. *History of Factory and Mine Hygiene.* New York: Columbia University Press.
Zenz, C., Dickerson, O. B. & Horvath, E. P. 1994. *Occupational Medicine.* St Louis: Mosby.

2 Legislation in occupational health

S. P. Hattingh

2.1 Introduction

It is important to know that legislation cannot be studied from a textbook alone. Legislation that is relevant today, may change tomorrow. South Africa is in a period of transition and we have seen numerous changes taking place in our community, in our politics and in our legal system. It is the responsibility of every citizen in this country to take note of these changes. The healthcare team is no exception – members have to stay informed about changes in the legal system that control their practice.

This chapter is by no means an exhaustive text, but it gives guidelines to relevant legal aspects.

There are many aspects that cannot be included here. A comprehensive list of sources is given at the end of the chapter for those who study and work in occupational health fields. This list of sources must also be updated from time to time. We recommend that those who require specific details relating to these Acts obtain the details through the relevant departments dealing with the particulars.

It is essential that occupational health professionals keep a policy and procedure manual in their place of work, as well as a manual containing all the relevant industrial and other legislation applicable to the work situation.

Rules form the boundaries for our work and lives. If we as humans do not conform to these set boundaries, we are punished either by society in an informal manner or by the governing body of our country, depending on the nature and severity of our non-conformation. All legislation thus forms part of a total judicial system designed primarily to ensure an ordered society and the protection of the individual within it. Nurses, doctors and other health professionals are subjected to laws of the courts as is the case with all other individuals in a country. They are, however, also professionals who are ruled by ethical principles which may impose more onerous duties. In South Africa, the regulation of professionals is delegated by Parliament to professional bodies.

2.2 Learning objectives

At the end of this chapter, the reader should be able to:
- Name and discuss the legislation dealing with occupational health in South Africa
- Give an overview of the role of the healthcare worker with regard to the most important legislation in industry

- Discuss the rights at work of people suffering from HIV/Aids
- Describe the role of the healthcare worker with regard to the application of legislative conditions in occupational health practice
- Interpret and apply legislation in the workplace.

2.3 Legislation dealing with occupational health in South Africa

Historically, occupational health and safety policy has evolved in the form of major laws governing occupational health and safety. Fragmentation and duplication have occurred, with parallel systems developing in the mining and non-mining industries, and with occupational health a late addition to occupational safety.

2.4 Ethics and the law

Because something is ethical, it does not necessarily follow that it is legal. The ideal situatiuon is for practice to be congruent both with legislation and the ethical values of a practitioner. In reality this is, however, not always possible.

If a worker reports to the medical station in extreme pain and the nurse provides a *prescribed* schedule 5 pain killer, then there is congruence between legislation and ethics. If, however, the nurse is not authorized through the prescription to provide a schedule 5 pain killer, but does so anyway because of the agony of the patient, then there is incongruence between ethics and legislation.

In the occupational health field, pressures both internal (values, lack of assertiveness) and external (management) can result in incongruence and illegal activities. For example an unacceptably high level of noise pollution in a factory is given tacit approval by the on-site healthcare professional who does not report the matter to the authorities because he/she knows the factory management have said they can't afford to make the required preventive alterations. This is illegal.

It must, however, be remembered that even if a healthcare professional is motivated by ethical considerations, the breaking of a law will have repercussions and he/she will have to take full responsibility for his/her actions.

2.5 The Constitution of the RSA and the Bill of Rights

The Constitution of the RSA, 1993, Act 200 of 1993, came into operation on 27 April 1994. This event constituted the most fundamental transformation in South African constitutional history, and also holds profound implications for health.

Chapter 3 of the Constitution contains the Bill of Rights, which is binding on all legislative and executive organs of state at all levels of government. It contains certain rights which are of direct relevance to the formulation of health policy and its implementation through legislation.

Every person is guaranteed the right to an environment that is not detrimental to his/her health or well-being. Children have the right to security, basic nutrition and basic health and social services, while detainees have the right to be detained under conditions consonant with human dignity, which include at least the provision of adequate nutrition, reading material and medical treatment at State expense. No positive duty is placed on the State to provide essential health services to other disadvantaged groups in society, such as women, the disabled and the elderly. However, it is arguable that the protection of human dignity demands that a person be protected from human suffering flowing from a denial of the right to health.

Many of the other rights in Chapter 3 of the Constitution may also have an indirect impact on health and health legislation. The right to life, for example, has clear implications regarding the death penalty, euthanasia and abortion. The tobacco industry has already invoked the right of access to information held by the State in order to gain access to Department of Health documentation on tobacco control, and has objected to regulations requiring health warnings on tobacco packages, on the basis of the right to health.

Also of considerable importance to health legislation and the organization of health services in South Africa is the designation by the Constitution of 'health services' as a legislative and executive competence of provincial government. Section 126 has the effect that while both provincial legislatures and the national Parliament may legislate on health services to the extent that conflict may arise, the provincial laws will prevail. This principle is made subject to certain limited exceptions relating, for example, to ineffectiveness of provincial legislation, the need for national uniformity, and prejudice to economic, health or security interests of other provinces or the country as a whole. Amendments to the legislative and executive competencies of the provinces require special procedures involving special majorities.

2.5.1 Protecting democracy and citizens' rights

> A Constitution ... is drafted with an eye to the future. Its function is to provide a continuing framework for the legitimate exercise of governmental power, and, when joined by a Bill or a Charter of Rights, for the unremitting protection of individual rights and liberties (Strassheim in Coetzee & Pretorius, 1997).

The Constitution, as the supreme law, therefore sets out the structure of government and its powers, as well as the rights of citizens. The Constitutional Assembly's Guide records that 'to protect democracy and prevent the abuse of power', the Constitution:

- Gives [citizens] important fundamental human rights in the chapter on the Bill of Rights, and protects these rights
- Has rules about when elections must take place and ensures that elections take place regularly so that one government cannot decide to stay in power forever
- Sets up national, provincial and local government. These are also called *spheres of government*. These spheres of government work in different places and help to ensure that the country is run properly and that government is close to the people it serves. It also ensures that there is a clear balance of power and that each part of government knows what powers it has
- Sets up a Constitutional Court, which has the final say about what the Constitution means, and which can scrap laws made by the government if they go against the Constitution
- Sets up independent institutions to educate [individuals] about their rights, to

help [them] protect [their] rights and to monitor (check) government to make sure that it is doing its work properly
- Ensures that the police, army and intelligence services protect South Africa and its people (Strassheim, in Coetzee & Pretorius, 1997).

2.5.2 The Bill of Rights

The Bill of Rights is a cornerstone of democracy in South Africa. It enshrines the rights of all people in a country and affirms the democratic values of human dignity, equality and freedom.

The state must respect, protect, promote and fulfil the rights in the Bill of Rights. The rights in the Bill of Rights are subject to the limitations contained or referred to in section 36, or elsewhere in the Bill.

The fundamental constitutional rights of South African citizens are contained in Chapter 2 of the Constitution, from section 7 to section 39. The main rights are briefly considered below, after other associated matters such as the interpretation, application and limitation of the rights themselves.

RIGHTS THAT ARE PROTECTED

Right	Comments
Equality	Every person is equal and has the right to equal protection and benefit of the law. No one, including the SA Government, has the right to treat any individual in a discriminatory manner including race, gender, sex, sexual orientation, pregnancy, marital status, ethnic or/and social origin, colour, age, disability, religion, conscience, beliefs, culture, language or birth. It must, however, be noted that fair discrimination does exist, for example, a company cannot employ a crane operator suffering from epilepsy or a lorry driver who is blind.
Privacy	Every person has the right to privacy. This includes the right not to have: - Their person or home searched - Their property searched - Their possessions seized - The privacy of their communications infringed.
Freedom of religion, belief and opinion	Every person has the right to believe or think whatever he/she wishes. Every person has the right to follow

	any religion he/she wishes. People cannot be forced to participate in religious activities with which they do not agree.
Freedom of expression	A person has the right to express him/herself, and the press has the right to report freely whatever they wish. Parliament may prevent people from spreading propaganda for war or violence. However, care must be taken about the confidential and factual nature of one's expressions, expecially those that hurt people because of race, ethnicity, gender or religion.
Assembly, demonstration, picket and petition	Every person has the right to peacefully gather with others, to peacefully participate in demonstrations, picket and present demonstrations, but people are not allowed to carry weapons while doing so.
Freedom of association	Every person has the right to associate with whomever he/she wishes.
Political right	Every person has the right to join a political party, encourage others to join a political party or to start a political party. Every person over 18 may vote.
Citizenship	Every person has the right to citizenship.
Freedom of movement and residence	Every person is free to live wherever he/she wishes. Every person has the right to a passport and may enter and exit South Africa.
Freedom of trade, occupation and profession	Every person has the right to do whatever work he/she wishes. Note must, however, be taken of the prescriptions and legislation pertaining to trades, occupations and professions.
Labour relations	Everyone has the right to fair labour practices. Every worker has the right: ■ To form and join a trade union ■ To participate in the activities and programmes of a trade union ■ To strike

Occupational health

	Every employer has the right: ■ To form and join an employers' organization ■ To participate in the activities and programmes of an employers' organization Every trade union and every employers' organization has the right: ■ To determine its own administration, programmes and activities ■ To organize meetings and gatherings ■ To form and join a federation Every trade union, employers' organization and employer has the right to engage in collective bargaining. National legislation may be enacted to regulate collective bargaining. To the extent that the legislation may limit a right in this chapter, the limitation must comply with the relevant section. National legislation may recognize union security arrangements contained in collective agreements. To the extent that the legislation may limit a right in this chapter, the limitation must comply with section 36(1).
Environment	Everyone has the right: ■ To an environment that is not harmful to his/her health or well-being ■ To have the environment protected, for the benefit of present and future generations, through reasonable legislative and other measures that: ● prevent pollution and ecological degradation ● promote conservation ● secure ecologically sustainable development and use of natural resources while promoting justifiable economic and social development
Property	Everyone has the right to property.
Housing	Everyone has the right to have access to housing and it is the government's responsibility to try and provide people with proper housing. A person cannot be evicted or a home taken away unless a court has heard the case.
Health, food, water and social security	Everyone has the right to have access to: ■ Healthcare services, including reproductive healthcare ■ Sufficient food and water

	- Social security, including, if they are unable to support themselves and their dependants, appropriate social assistance. The state must take reasonable legislative and other measures, within its available resources, to achieve the progressive realization of each of these rights. No one may be refused emergency medical treatment.
Children	Children under the age of 18 years have special rights. These include the right to: - Family care, or other care - Food, shelter and healthcare - Not to be abused or neglected - Not to be forced to work or given work not suitable for a child
Education	Every person has the right to education. People can set up their own schools, universities and technikons at their own expense. Educational facilities are not allowed to discriminate on the basis of race.
Language and culture	Everyone has the right to use the language and to paticipate in the cultural life of their choice, but no one exercising these rights may do so in a manner inconsistent with any provision of the Bill of Rights.
Culture, religious and linguistic communities	Every person can enjoy freedom of his/her own culture, religion and use his/her own language. They may also set up their own organizations. They must, however, respect the human rights of others in doing so.
Access to information	Everyone has the right of access to: - Any information held by the State - Any information that is held by another person and that is required for exercise or protection of any rights National legislation must be enacted to give effect to this right, and may provide for reasonable measure to alleviate the administrative and financial burden on the state.
Just administrative action	Everyone has the right to just administrative action. This must be reasonable and the procedures must be fair. Every person also has the right to ask for written reasons for any decision that may affect him/her.

Access to courts	Everyone has the right to have any dispute that can be resolved by the application of law decided in a fair public hearing before a court or, where appropriate, another independent and impartial tribunal or forum.
Arrested, accused and detained	In a case where a person is arrested, accused or detained he/she has the right to: ■ Keep silent, not be forced to make a confession ■ Not to be taken to a court within 2 days of being arrested ■ Be released, either on warning or on bail unless there is a good reason to keep a person in jail ■ A lawyer ■ Be kept in proper conditions ■ Be given free food, something to read and medical treatment ■ Speak to and be visited by one's family, religious counsellor or doctor

2.5.3 Application of the Bill of Rights
Constitutional provisions
A provision of great significance is section 8, which sets out the scope of application of the Bill of Rights. It reads as follows:
- The Bill of Rights applies to all law, and binds the legislature, the executive, the judiciary and all organs of state.
- A provision of the Bill of Rights binds a natural or a juristic person if, and to the extent that it is applicable, taking into account the nature of the right and the nature of any duty imposed by the right.
- When applying a provision of the Bill of Rights to a natural or juristic person in terms of subsection (2), a court
  - in order to give effect to a right in the Bill, must apply, or if necessary develop, the common law to the extent that legislation does not give effect to that right; and
  - may develop rules of the common law to limit the right, provided that the limitation is in accordance with section 36(1).
- A juristic person is entitled to the rights in the Bill of Rights to the extent required by the nature of the rights and the nature of that juristic person.

(See also Addenda 2 and 3 for details on HIV/Aids.)

2.6 The Health Act, 1977 (No 63 of 1977)
The Department of Health has not yet issued a new Health Act to replace the Health Act 63 of 1977. It is reluctant to amend legislation on a piecemeal basis and has therefore appointed the National Health Legislation Review Committee to develop a comprehensive, development-oriented Public Health Act.

There are over 100 existing pieces of South African legislation that have an impact on health, as well as a considerable number of international treaties and conventions which may have application to health legislation in South Africa.

New health legislation will therefore be a comprehensive framework which falls within the parameters of the new Constitution, The National Health Plan, the Reconstruction and Development Programme (RDP) and the recommendations of the policy committees of the Department of Health.

With the changing legislation on health, the laws regulating the conduct of health professionals in South Africa will have to be amended.

It is important to also study the National Drug Policy contained in Addemdum I

2.7 The Occupational Health and Safety Act, 1993 (No 85 of 1993)

The Occupational Health and Safety Act, 1993 (No 85 of 1993) (OHSA) came into effect on 1 January 1994 and is the successor to the Machinery and Occupational Safety Act, 1983 (No 66 of 1983) (MOSA). The Occupational Health and Safety Act may be viewed as a preventive Act, as it describes measures that should be taken to prevent accidents and diseases.

The scope of the OHSA is wide and its main objectives are to provide health and safety for persons at work and for those in the community who may be affected by the activities around them. In some cases the members of the public are also covered by this Act.

One of the basic principles in the Act is that it contains guidelines to promote safety and health with regard to the effective management of machinery.

The emphasis on accident prevention can be seen not just in the modernized forms of requirements in relation to particular machinery or processes, but more generally in the importance given to positive steps to assess risks, act upon such assessment and act to eliminate, avoid or lessen perceived risks.

Where no specific regulations are passed in terms of the Occupational Health and Safety Act, 1993 (No 85 of 1993), those pertaining under the Factory, Machinery and Building Works Act, 1993 still apply (Bendix, 1996:149).

An important aspect regarding the OHSA is that it makes provision for employee participation, representation and consultation at its statutory forums and structures. This has to a large extent led to trust rather than distrust between employees and employers.

2.7.1 Key aspects of the Act
The OHSA addresses the following key aspects:
- Scope of OHSA legislation
  - application of OHSA
  - exclusions from OHSA
- Aims of OHSA
- Advisory Council for Occupational Health and Safety
- Non-employees directly affected by employer's operations
- Duties of sellers, suppliers and importers of machinery in workplaces
- Duties of the employer
  - general duty
  - specific duties

- risk assessment
- duty to inform
- Duties of the Chief Executive Officer
- Standards of care that are 'reasonably practicable'
- Employees' duties and responsiblities
- Participative health and safety structures and arrangements
  - Health and Safety Representatives, and their functions
  - Health and Safety Committees, and their functions
- Inspectors, investigations, inquiries and prohibitions
  - inspectors and their functions
  - investigations
  - formal inquiries
  - prohibitions and penalties
- Regulations passed under the Act.

2.7.2 Scope of the Act

The OHSA applies to all workplaces, namely private and public sectors, SA Police Services, SA National Defence Force, universities, parastatals, and agricultural and domestic workers. The OHSA applies where an employment relationship exists between parties and to which the definitions given in the Act apply.

The OHSA specifies the following exclusions, namely:

- Mines, works and mining areas (here the Mine Health and Safety Act, 1997 (No 29 of 1996) applies).
- Labour brokers as defined under the Labour Relations Act, 1995 (No 66 of 1995).
- Shipping vessels as defined under section 2(1) of the Merchant Shipping Act, 1951 (No 57 of 1951).
- Employers exempted by the Minister from the application of Occupational Health and Safety Act, 1993 (No 85 of 1993).

2.7.3 Aims of the Act

Strassheim (in Coetzee & Pretorius, 1997) states that:

> Common law provides that employers have a duty to provide employees with safe working conditions, usually described as a safe working environment, safe machinery and safe methods of work. Employers are required to take reasonable steps to achieve these, and to take reasonable care of employee safety. The standard required of the employer is that of reasonableness, and the test of reasonableness is normally to ask whether a reasonable employer (or person in that position) would have reasonably foreseen that risk existed or harm could occur, and would have acted to avoid the event happening.

The Consitution of South Africa also provides in the Bill of Rights at section 24 that 'everyone has the right to an environment that is not harmful to their health and well-being ...'. The OHSA, although passed before the 1996 Constitution, would be likely to accord with all aspects of it, as well as with the constitutional right to fair labour practices under section 23(1) of the Bill of Rights.

One of the OHSA's major features is the principle that health and safety issues are best addressed and managed in the workplace through joint cooperation between employers and employees. The OHSA recognized the need for employee participation with employers in safety and health issues which directly affect employees. The employee has the right to participate in specific statutory health and safety structures established under the legislation for these structures, namely health and safety representatives and health and safety committees.

2.7.4 Major provisions of the Act

2.7.4.1 The duties of employers

The OHSA imposes a number of duties and prohibitions on both employers and employees. The majority of these duties concern the employer, but the OHSA also spells out those of the employee. The duties of the employer can be described under direct duties and cooperative duties.

In the section dealing with direct duties, the OHSA requires that the employer undertake three activities:

1. Identify the hazards present in the workplace
2. Assess the risks to employees' health and safety posed by these hazards
3. In the light of this assessment, take steps to eliminate or mitigate the hazards.

It is the employer's general duty to provide and to maintain, as far as *reasonably practicable*, a working environment that is safe and without risks to health. The final responsibility for the health and safety of employees and other affected persons rests with the employer.

Cooperative duties that concern the employer are aimed at the promotion of the use of institutions created by the OHSA to directly promote safety and health. In this regard the Act specifically refers to the provision of information, instructions, training and supervision to ensure health and safety at work. The employer also has a duty to ensure that employees do not perform work unless precautions for safety and health have been taken. Regulations in this regard should also be taken into consideration.

The requirement to maintain a safe and healthy workplace requires both an effective system for monitoring the conditions in the workplace and the correction of any shortcomings. It is thus specified that the employer must consult with the health and safety committee.

The nature of maintenance required will depend on the type of manufacturing process, the substances used in manufacturing, and the risks to health and safety associated with the manufacturing process.

The provision of a safe system of work must take into account the fallibility of human nature. The OHSA also specifically refers to an informed employee. An employer must inform an employee of the hazards to his/her health and safety which may result due to his/her work and any article or substance he/she has to produce, process, use, handle, store or transport. An employer must also inform an employee and the safety representatives beforehand of any notification by an inspector of forthcoming inspections, investigations or formal inquiries. The employer must also inform a health and safety representative as soon as reasonably practicable of the occurrence of an incident in the workplace or section of the workplace for which the representative has been designated.

The OHSA also specifically refers to duties that are not subject to reasonable practicability. These include:
- Taking all possible measues to ensure that all the requirements of the OHSA are complied with by every person employed or on the premises under the control of the employer where plant or machinery is in use
- Enforcing measures to act in the interest of health and safety
- General supervision by trained individuals who understand the hazards associated with the work, plant and machinery and who have the authority to ensure that precautions are taken for health and safety
- Informing all employees about their scope of authority.

Although the previous Act (MOSA) was in operation for less than a decade, it was necessary to replace it to modernize health and safety legislation. The most significant changes are the extension of the OHSA to include:
- The regulation of occupational health and hygiene
- A reorientation of the employer's obligations so as to encourage a more active role and approach to the elimination or mitigation of hazards in the workplace
- The obligation of the employer to supply the worker with information on the dangers and hazards present in the work environment
- The provision of training
- An overhaul of the system of safety representatives and committees to include trade union participation in the election of safety representatives
- A requirement for consultation between employers and safety committees on a wide range of safety matters
- The responsibility of employers to prepare written health and safety policies if a Chief Inspectorate directs an industry to do so
- A revision of the general safety duties of employees
- A more preventive approach to health and safety
- A more comprehensive approach to the protection of the public from safety and health hazards emanating from the workplace
- Changes to the system of inquiries into accidents and other incidents that endanger health and safety
- Major increases in the penalties a court can impose upon conviction of a company where a breach of the Act and regulations can be proved.

2.7.4.2 Duties of employees
The OHSA states that every employee is responsible for his/her own health and safety as well as of those who may be affected by the work he/she does. It is expected of an employee to cooperate with the employer in the performance of his/her duties and to carry out any lawful order given to him/her in the interest of health and safety. It is expected of the employee to report any irregularity that may jeopardize the safety and health of him/herself or his/her fellow workers to the employer, his/her mandatary or

a safety representative. The employee must also carry out any lawful order given to him/her and obey the health and safety rules and procedures laid down by the employer or anyone authorized thereto by the employer in the interest of health and safety.

Bendix (1996:151) states that 'the maintenance of safety is the joint responsibility of the employer, the safety representative, the employees and (if one exists) the safety committee'. It must be emphasized, however, that the greater responsibility still rests with the employer.

If the employee is involved in any incident which may affect his/her health, such incident must be reported to the employer or health and safety representative as soon as possible but not later than the end of the particular shift during which the incident occurred.

Other important aspects addressed by the Act are the following:
- Health and safety representatives
- Safety committees
- Reporting of incidents
- General prohibitions
- Victimization
- The duties of doctors to report diseases resulting from employment
- The duties of inspectors
- The rights and duties of chief inspectors
- Offences and penalties
- Acts or omissions of employees or mandataries
- Presumptions and proof of certain facts
- Exemptions
- Agreements entered into
- Regulations.

The Minister may make regulations pertaining to the OHSA which in his/her opinion are necessary or expedient in the interest of health and safety of persons either at work or who may be affected by the activities of persons at work.

The regulations made under the Machinery and Occupational Safety Act shall be considered to have been made in terms of this section of the Act (and thus remain in effect unless amended).

2.7.4.3 General duties of employees
Every employee shall:
- Carry out any lawful order given to him/her and obey the safety rules laid down by the employer or any one in authority, according to the Act and regulations
- Report to a health and safety representative or his/her employer any situation that is unsafe at or near the workplace and that comes to his/her attention.

2.7.4.4 General duties of employers and users of machinery
Every employer or user of machinery shall:
- Have a copy of this Act and the regulations available for employees to peruse (this

does not apply where there are less than 20 employees in employment) and ensure that all employees observe the provisions of the Act and regulations
- Enforce discipline at the workplace in the interests of safety
- Ensure work is performed and machinery is used under proper supervision
- Be aware of all dangers in the workplace and take whatever steps are necessary to remove them or implement precautionary measures
- Ensure all employees are familiar with the dangers in the workplace and what steps are required to deal with and avoid such dangers, and that precautionary measures are taken by employees.

2.7.4.5 Duties of the Chief Executive Officer (CEO)
The general duties of the CEO include the responsibility to ensure that the employer meets its duties under the OHSA to employers, which are incorporated bodies (companies, closed corporations, etc), government departments, organs of state and enterprises conducted by the state. The CEO is responsible for the overall management and control of the business and in relation to departments of state, the head of departments of any department of state is deemed to be the CEO of that department (s 16(4)).

The CEO should also, as far as reasonably practicable, ensure that the duties of the employer are properly discharged. These stipulations apply also to mines, under the Mine Health and Safety Act, 1996 (No 29 of 1996). The CEO may also assign duties to any person under his/her control, however, the assignment of duties to others will not have the effect of absolving the CEO of the legal responsibility for fulfilling those duties or of the liability for not fulfilling them. The employer is also not relieved of the duties and responsibilities delegated to the CEO.

2.7.5 Meaning of 'reasonably practicable'
Strassheim (in Coetzee & Pretorius, 1997:E6.7) states that the phrase 'reasonably practicable' is defined under the Act as:
- The severity and scope of the hazard or risk concerned
- The state of knowledge reasonably available concerning that hazard or risk and of any means of removing or mitigating that hazard or risk
- The availability and suitability of means to remove or mitigate the hazard or risk
- The cost of removing or mitigating that hazard or risk in relation to the benefits derived therefrom.

The author states that two specific elements are involved, namely reasonableness and practicability. Reasonableness is based upon the common law duty measured against the standard of the 'reasonable man'. Practicability will depend on all or some of the four aspects given above and will generally be assessed against facts and circumstances of every instance.

2.7.6 The role of health and safety representatives
According to the OHSA, where 20 or more employees are assigned, the employer must designate a health and safety representative in writing for a specific period. The OHSA

states that the arrangements and procedures or election, period of office and designation of these representatives must be developed by the employer and labour consultant and disputes must be referred for arbitration. The health and safety representative must be a person employed full-time, who is acquainted with the conditions and activities at the workplace.

The functions of the health and safety representative are to:
- Review the effectiveness of health and safety measures
- Identify potential hazards and/or major incidents
- Examine the causes of incidents
- Investigate complaints about health and safety
- Make representations to the employer or Health and Safety Committee on related matters of health and safety
- Inspect the workplace, which could include any article, substance, plant, machinery or health and safety equipment
- Participate in consultations with inspectors at the workplace and accompany inspectors on inspections
- Receive information from inspectors
- Attend meetings held by the Health and Safety Committee
- Visit any site of an incident
- Attend any investigation or journal enquiry
- Inspect any document which the employer is required to keep
- Be accompanied by a technical adviser on an inspection
- Participate in any internal health and safety audit.

The employers are required to provide facilities, assistance and training to be elected.

2.7.7 The role of the health and safety committee

Where two or more health and safety representatives have been designated for a workplace, the employer must establish a health and safety committee. The employer consults with this committee to mitigate, develop, promote, maintain and review measures to ensure health and safety. The committee has meetings at least once every three months.

The functions of a health and safety committee are to:
- Make recommendations to the employer (or inspector) regarding health and safety and keep records
- Discuss any incident at the workplace in which a person was injured, became ill or died
- Report an incident to an inspector
- Perform any other function as prescribed.

2.7.8 Inspectors, investigations, inquiries and prohibitions

Inspectors are overseen by a Chief Inspectorate within the Department of Labour. Their functions include, among others, to enter the premises of an employer without previous notice, to question persons on any matter related to the Act, to view books, records and documents and examine them, and to ask for explanations of what is recorded and documented. The inspector may also inspect any article, substance, plant or machinery and may remove articles, documents, records and books for examination.

Inspectors also have special powers, namely to prohibit an employer from continuing or commencing work using machinery that permit employees from being exposed to any article, substance, organization or condition. The inspector may also block, bar, barricade or fence off any part of a workplace.

Employers are required to report to the Inspectorate any person who dies, becomes unconscious, suffers a loss of a limb or becomes ill to such a degree that he/she is likely either to die or suffer permanent physical defect or is likely to be unable to work for at least 14 days. Reports must also be submitted to the Inspectorate on any major incident that occurred where the health and safety of any person was endangered and where the following occurred:
- The spoiling of a dangerous substance
- The uncontrolled release of a substance under pressure
- The fracturing or failing of machinery, resulting in flying, jacling or uncontrolled moving objects
- The running out of control of machinery.

Inspectors may investigate the circumstances of any incident that resulted or could have resulted in the injury, illness or death of a person. A written report of an accident must be submitted to the **Attorney-General** and the **Chief Inspector**.

The Chief Inspector may direct an inspection to inquire into any incident that has occurred, and may subpoena any person to appear before him/her, to give evidence or produce any book, document or article required to conduct the inquiry.

2.7.9 Regulations under the Act

Various regulations fall under the Act. These regulations include aspects related to buildings, plants, machinery, safety and health equipment, training, safety facilities, health and safety measures, occupational hygiene, biological monitoring, medical surveillance, hazardous articles, substances or organisms, emergency equipment, directives in respect of health and safety in the workplace, etc. Regulations include:
- Facilities Regulations (GN 2362, 5 Oct 1990)
- General Administrative Regulations (GN R1449, 6 Sept 1996)
- Driven Machinery Regulations (GN R295, 28 Feb 1988, GN R2483, 4 Sept 1992)
- Electrical Installation Regulations (GN R2920, 23 Oct 1992)
- Electrical Machinery Regulations (GN R1593, 12 Aug 1988; GN R1185, 1 June 1990)
- Environmental Regulations for Workplaces (GN R2281, 16 Oct 1987; GN R1754, 18 Aug 1989)
- General Machinery Regulations (GN R1521, 5 August 1988)
- General Safety Regulations (GN R1031, 30 May 1986; GN 2245, 7 August 1992)
- Vessels under Pressure Regulations (GN R2919, 234 October 1996)

- Asbestos Regulations (GN R773, 10 April 1987)
- Diving Regulations (GN R12, 4 January 1991)
- Lead Regulations (GN R586, 22 March 1991)
- Regulations Concerning Certificate of Competency (GN R533, 16 March 1990)
- Integration Regulations (GN 639, 28 April 1995)
- Lift, Escalator and Passenger Conveyor Regulations (GN 797, 29 Apr 1994).

2.8 The Mine Health and Safety Act, 1997 (No 29 of 1996)

The occupational health and safety in mines is regulated by the Mine Health and Safety Act, No 29 of 1996, which came into affect on 15 January 1997, and not by the OHSA.

2.8.1 Key aspects of MHSA
The key aspects covered by this Act include:
- Scope of the Mine Health and Safety Act, 1997
- Owner's functions
- Manager's functions
- Duties of occupational health and occupational medical practitioners
- Shift boss's functions
- Delegation of functions and duties
- Risk assessment
- Employee participation
- Health and safety representatives
- Health and safety committees
- Health and safety agreements
- Disclosure of information
- Disputes
- Right to withdraw from dangerous situations
- Inspectorate, investigations and enquiries
- Penalties
- Regulations

Many provisions, principles or concepts of OHSA and the Labour Relations Act, 1995 (No 66 of 1995) are incorporated in the MHSA, such as aspects related to information sharing, employee participation and consultation, statutory powers of inspectors, regulations of disputes and the duties of employers.

2.8.2 Purpose of the Act
The purpose of this Act is to provide for protection of the health and safety of employees and other persons at mines and, for that purpose to promote a culture of health and safety; to provide for the enforcement of health and safety measures; to provide for appropriate systems of employee, employer and State participation in health and safety matters; to establish representative tripartite institutions to review legislation, promote health and enhance properly targeted research; to provide for effective monitoring systems and inspections, investigations and inquiries to improve

health and safety; to promote training and human resources development; to regulate employers' and employees' duties; to identify hazards and eliminate, control and minimize the risk to health and safety; to entrench the right to refuse to work in dangerous conditions; and to give effect to the public international law obligations of the Republic relating to mining health and safety and to provide for matters connected therewith.

2.8.3 Objectives of the Act
The objects of this Act are stated as the following: to protect the health and safety of persons at mines; to require employers and employees to identify hazards and eliminate, control and minimize the risks relating to health and safety at mines; to give effect to the public international law obligations of the Republic that concern health and safety at mines; to provide for employee participation in matters of health and safety through health and safety representatives and the health and safety committees at mines; to provide for effective monitoring of health and safety conditions at mines; to provide for enforcement of health and safety measures at mines; to provide for investigations and inquiries to improve health and safety at mines; and to promote a culture of health and safety in the mining industry; to provide training in health and safety in the mining industry; and to ensure cooperation and consultation on health and safety between the State, employers, employees and their representatives.

2.8.4 The owners' functions
The Act distinguishes between owners and managers in the mining industry. The owner has the following functions:
- Ensuring that the mine is designed, constructed and equipped in order to provide conditions for safe operation, that a healthy working environment is maintained, and that a communication system and electrical, mechanical and other equipment are provided
- Ensuring that the mine is commissioned, operated, maintained and decommissioned in such a way that employees can work without endangering their own or any other person's health and safety
- Compiling an annual report on health and safety that includes statistics on health and safety, as well as annual medical reports
- Appointing managers where the owner is unable to assume the functions
- Paying the costs of all clinical examinations and medical tests required by the Act
- Entering a collective agreement with trade unions with regard to designation of workplaces, health and safety matters and representatives, meetings, training and arbitration.

2.8.5 Functions of the managers
2.8.5.1 General functions
Under the MHSA, managers have a wide range of sometimes onerous and extremely important functions which they are required to fulfil. The most significant general functions in the occupational health nursing context are broadly these:
- *To the extent that it is reasonably practicable*, providing and maintaining a

working environment that is safe and without risk to the health of employees (s 5(1))
- Identifying the relevant hazards and assessing the related risks to which persons who are not employees may be exposed (s 5(2)(b))
- Supplying all necessary health and safety facilities and equipment to each employee (s 6(1)(a)) and, *to the extent that it is reasonably practicable*, maintaining these facilities and equipment in a serviceable and hygienic condition (s 6(1)(b))
- Having sufficient quantities of personal protective equipment available (s (6)(2))
- Taking reasonable measures to ensure that all employees who are required to use personal protective equipment are instructed in the proper use, the limitations and appropriate maintenance of that equipment (s (6)(3))
- Taking steps to staff the mine with due regard to health and safety, in the following ways, *to the extent that is reasonably practicable* (s 7(1)):
  - ensuring that every employee complies with the requirements of MHSA (s 7(1)(a))
  - instituting measures to secure, maintain and enhance health and safety (s 7(1)(b))
  - appointing persons and providing them with the means to comply with MHSA requirements and any instruction given by an inspector (s 7(1)(c))
  - considering an employee's training and capabilities in health and safety before assigning a task to the employee (s 7(a)(d))
  - ensuring that work is performed under the general supervision of a person trained to understand the hazards associated with the work and who has the authority to ensure that precautionary measures laid down by the manager are implemented (s 7(1)(e))
- Appointing any person with qualifications as may be prescribed to perform any aspect of the functions assigned to managers (s 7(2)), although such appointment does not relieve the manager of any duty imposed on managers by MHSA (s 7(3))
- Keeping a record of all occupational hygiene measurements in a manner that can be linked to each employee's record of medical surveillance (s (12(3)).

2.8.5.2 Medical surveillance system
The medical surveillance system has the following functions:
- Establishing and maintaining a system of medical surveillance of employees (s 13(1))
- Ensuring that every system is appropriate considering the actual or potential hazards (s 13(2)(a)); and is designed to provide information the manager can use in determining measures to either eliminate, control and minimize health risks and hazards to which employees are or may be exposed (s 13(2)(b)(i)) or to prevent, detect and treat occupational diseases (s 13(2)(b)(ii))
- Ensuring that medical surveillance consists of an initial medical examination and other medical examinations at appropriate intervals (s 13(2)(c))
- Engaging the part-time or full-time services of (s 13(3)(a)):
  - an occupational medical practitioner (s 13(3)(a)(i)); and if necessary

- other practioners holding a qualification in occupational medicine recognized by the Health Professions Council of South Africa or the South African Nursing Council (s 13(3)(a)(ii))
- Supplying the practitioners with the means to perform their functions (s 13(3)(b))
- Keeping a record of medical surveillance for each employee exposed to a health hazard (s 13(3)(c)).

2.8.5.3 Fitness for work
The worker's fitness for work is decribed in terms of the following:
- Conducting an investigation in terms of section 11(5) if an employee is declared unfit to perform work as a result of an occupational disease (s 13(6))
- Being notified by the occupational medical practitioner if an employee is temporarily unfit to perform work as a result of any occupational disease (s 13(7))
- Note also the MHSA provisions which allow an employee to dispute a finding of unfitness to perform work, by means of an appeal to the Medical Inspector (under section 20 of the Act).

2.8.5.4 Hazardous work
The responsibility of management with regard to the performance of a worker can be summarized as follows:
- Keeping a service record of employees who perform work in respect of which medical surveillance is conducted under section 13 (s 14(1))
- Preparing a health and safety policy document which:
  - describes the organization of work (s 8(1)(a))
  - establishes a policy concerning the protection of employees' health and safety at work (s 8(1)(b))
  - establishes a policy concerning the protection of persons who are not employees but who are directly affected by mining activities (s 8(1)(c))
  - outlines arrangements for carrying out and reviewing policies (s 8(1)(d))
- Consulting with the Health and Safety Committee in developing and revising the Health and Safety Policy and documents (s 8(2))
- Displaying the Health and Safety Policy and documents for employees to read (s 8(3)(a)) and providing these to each Health and Safety Representative (s 8(3)(b))
- Preparing and implementing codes of practice on any matter affecting the health and safety of employees and other persons (s 9(1)), and, if the Chief Inspector requires it (s 9(2)), consulting the Health and Safety Committee when preparing, implementing and revising codes (s 9(4))
- Providing health and safety training, *as far as reasonably practicable*, to ensure that:
  - employees have the information, instruction, training or supervision necessary to enable them to perform their work safely and without risk to health (s 10(1)9a))
  - employees become familiar with work-related hazards and risks and the measures that must be taken to eliminate, control and minimize those hazards and risks (s 10(1)(b))
  - employees are properly trained to deal with risks associated with the work or

risks that have been recorded (s 10(2)(a)), and in measures to eliminate, control or minimize those risks (s 10(2)(b)), as well as in work procedures (s 10(2)(c)) and emergency procedures (s 10(2)(d))
- Ensuring that training takes place before starting work (s 10(3)(a)), or at intervals as determined by the manager in consultation with the Health and Safety Committee (s 10(3)(b)), or before significant changes are made to mine procedures, mining and ventilation, or to the employee's occupation or work (s 10(3)(c) and (d))
- Identifying hazards to health and safety (s 11(1)(a)), assessing them (s 11(1)(b)), recording significant hazards identified and risks assessed (s 11(1)(c)), and making the records available for inspection by employees (s 11(1)(d))
- Determining all measures necessary, after consultation with the Health and Safety Committee, to eliminate any risk (s 11(2)(a)), to control the risk at source (s 11(2)(b)), to minimize the risk (s 11(2)(c)) and in so far as the risk remains, to provide for personal protective equipment and institute programmes to monitor the risk (s 11(2)(d)(i) and (ii))
- Periodically reviewing the hazards identified and risks assessed (s 11(4)), to determine whether further elimination, control and minimization of risk is possible, including the results of:
  - occupational hygiene measurements and
  - medical surveillance
- Investigating every reportable accident, serious illness and health-threatening occurrence (s 11(5)(a)), consulting the Health and Safety Committee on investigations (s 11(5)(b)), conducting investigations in cooperation with the responsible Health and Safety Representative (s 11(5)(c)), and preparing a report in compliance with requirements (which are set out in (s 11(5)(d)(i)–(iii)))
- Consulting with employees and organized labour regarding:
  - Health and Safety Representatives
  - Health and Safety Committees
  - designation of workplaces
  - election of Safety Representatives
- Determining procedures for employees to exercise their rights under section 23(1) to leave dangerous working places, which must incorporate the requirements of section 23(2)(a)–(e).
- Establishing procedures for the appointment under section 7(2) of another person to perform any aspect of the functions assigned to managers. Note, however, that section 7(3) specifically provides that the appointment (by delegation) 'does not relieve the manager of any duty imposed on managers by this Act'. Therefore a manager can delegate the responsibility for performing a statutory function, but cannot by so doing avoid or escape accountability for the duty to perform it and the statutory responsibility for ensuring that it is performed.

2.8.5.5 Occupational health functions of managers

The MHSA sets out specific duties that managers must discharge in relation to a number of key occupational health practices and procedures, including occupational hygiene, medical surveillance, fitness for work, medical record-keeping and annual reporting. These are given below.

2.8.5.6 Occupational hygiene measurements
- Conducting occupational hygiene measurements, by engaging the part-time or full-time services of a person qualified in occupational hygiene techniques to measure levels of exposure to hazards, if required to do so or if necessary following risk assessment (s 12(1)(a) and (b))
- Ensuring that every system of occupational hygiene measurements is appropriate considering the actual or potential hazards (s 12(2)(a)), and is designed to provide information the manager can use in determining measures to eliminate, control or minimize health risks and hazards (s 12(2)(b)).

2.9 Risk assessment and hazard control

The MHSA requires that the employer implement systems to create and maintain a healthy and safe environment to work in. Although the OHSA has a similar approach, Guild, Ehrlich, Johnston and Ross (2001:4) state that the MHSA's obligations in regard to identifying, assessing and controlling risks and hazards are considerably more detailed and rigorous than the equivalent provisions in the OHSA.

The MHSA requires that employers identify health and safety hazards involved in mining activities and covers both hazards to employees and persons who may be directly affected by activities at the mine. A range of mechanisms should be used to identify hazards, including:
- Workplace inspections
- Health and safety audits
- Job safety analysis
- Collection and analyses of accident and occupational disease statistics.

The MHSA also requires that hazards be assessed, and that measures be taken to control these hazards. This assessment, according to Guild et al. (2001:5) must include an evaluation of the severity of the potential harm and the number of persons who are potentially at risk, as well as the methods that are available to control the risk. Risk management must be undertaken by the employee on a systematic and ongoing basis to review and identify risks assessed. The employer must implement engineering or other collective measures to control and minimize risks. Only if this is not reasonably practicable, can the employer rely on issuing personal protective equipment to protect employees.

2.9.1 Investigations
The employer is responsible for conducting all investigations.
Investigations into accidents and health-threatening occurrences play a key role in risk identification and assessment. All reportable accidents, serious illness and health-threatening occurrences must be investigated.

Investigations must be performed in conjunction with the health and safety representative and the health and safety committee. A report must be completed in which unsafe conditions, acts or procedures are identified that could have contributed to the incident and must contain recommendations to prevent reoccurrences.

2.9.2 Training
Training is an integral part of risk assessment and management. It is the duty of the employer to ensure that employees are properly trained and familiar with risks and hazards, and how these should be managed.

2.9.3 Employee participation in risk management
The MHSA stresses the need for intensive employee participation in the risk assessment process. Health and safety representatives have the right to participate in the identification of risks and hazards, as well as in health and safety investigations (Guild et al. 2001:6).

2.9.4 Occupational hygiene
Guild et al. (2001:6) define occupational hygiene as the 'anticipation, recognition, evaluation and control of conditions at a mine that may cause illness or adverse effects to persons'.

The measurement of levels of exposure to the hazards in mines is an essential and integral part of mine management. A mine must engage a qualified occupational hygienist to conduct measurements and record it. These findings assist the employer to take the necessary steps to control and/or minimize the hazards. The recorded information should, where practicable, be linked to each employee's record of medical surveillance.

2.9.5 Medical surveillance
Guild et al. (2001:6) define medical surveillances as 'a planned programme of periodic examination, which may include clinical examinations, biological monitoring, or medical testing of employees by an occupational practitioner or an occupational medical practitioner'.

Biological monitoring is defined as 'a planned programme of periodic collection and analyses of body fluid, tissues, excreta or exhaled air in order to detect and quantify the exposure to or absorption of any substance or organisms'.

Every mine must have a system of medical surveillance for employees exposed to health hazards. This surveillance system must be designed so that it may provide relevant information to the employer for the purpose of controlling the health risk and for preventing, detecting and treating occupational diseases. Every employee must undergo an initial medical examination (bare-line examination) when starting to work at a mine. Thereafter, every employee must be examined at appropriate intervals.

2.9.6 The occupational medical practitioner
Every mine must engage either on a full-time or part-time basis, the services of an occupational medical practitioner to conduct its medical surveillance programme. If required, the mine must also engage additional persons with appropriate qualifications

in occupational medicine to assist the medical practitioner. These practitioners must take every measure reasonably practicable to:
- Promote the health and safety of employees
- Assist employees in matters related to occupational medicine.

The MHSA places significant duties on occupational medical practitioners which are consistent with their professional and ethical obligations as medical practitioners. As an employee, the occupational medical practitioner must also obey lawful and reasonable instructions by the employer. According to Guild et al. (2001:7) this dual obligation placed on the occupational medical practitioner as an employee and as a medical professional creates the potential for difficult situations to emerge. However, employees are obliged to comply only with instructions that are lawful and reasonable. The occupational medical practitioner is not obliged to comply with an instruction that would require him/her to breach the legal or ethical requirements of professional practice. In fact, Guild et al. (2001:8) state that the occupational medical practitioner is obliged to disobey an instruction that would, for example, require him/her to breach a patient's right to confidentiality. The employer is not entitled to take any disciplinary action against the doctor for refusing to comply with the instruction that would require him/her to breach legal or ethical obligations. The MHSA does not contain any procedure for resolving any differences between a mine and an occupational medical practitioner concerning professional duties.

2.9.7 The doctor–patient relationship
Guild et al. (2001:8) pose the following question:

> Does the relationship between the occupational medical practitioner and the employee, who the occupational medical practitioner examines, during a pre-employment or as part of a medical programme differ from a normal doctor–patient relationship?

The following explanation is given:
The MHSA stipulates that employees may appeal against the decisions and findings of the occupational medical practitioner, for example where an employee is found to be examined at the State's expense by an independent medical practitioner.

2.9.8 Confidentiality
The patient's right to confidentiality is not absolute. There are circumstances that require that information be exposed, for example where an employee has an infectious notifiable condition, the relevant authorities must be notified. Another example is where the medical practitioner believes that an employee he/she has examined or treated has contracted a work-related illness, the employee as well as the employer and chief inspector must be notified. It must also be noted that any improper disclosure of confidential information constitutes a criminal offence.

2.9.9 Keeping records and reports
Surveillance records of every employee must be kept and stored safely for a period of at least 40 years after the last surveillance has been conducted. This record must be

delivered to the medical inspector when the employee ceases to be employed by the mine or if required by the Chief Inspector of Mines. Records of employees must be kept confidential and may only be made available in accordance with the ethics of medical practice, if required by law or court order, or if the employee has consented in writing to the release of the information.

Every medical practitioner is required to prepare an annual report analysing the health of employees at the mine, based on the employee's record of medical surveillance. The names of the employees are not exposed.

The employer is liable for the costs of all clinical examinations and medical tests.

2.9.10 Medical examinations
All employees subject to medical surveillance must undergo a medical examination when they leave employment with the mine for whatever reason. An exit certificate must be issued by the occupational medical practitioner.

2.9.11 Other relevant aspects of the Act
The MHSA makes provision for employees' rights and duties in that they must take reasonable care to protect their own health and safety, as well as that of any other person. They must wear their protective clothing and use the health and safety facilities or equipment issued to them. They must also advise their supervisors of any risk to themselves or others.

Employees have the right to leave a working place if they believe there is serious danger to their health or safety.

The employee's participation in health and safety is encouraged through election of health and safety representatives and committees. A safety representative should be elected for every 20 employees, and a health and safety committee should be established at every mine with 100 or more employees.

Tripartite committees consist of consultation between the representatives of mines owners, employees and government. The Mine Health and Safety Council was established to advise the Minister of Mineral and Energy Affairs on all aspects of safety and health in mines.

2.10 The Compensation for Occupational Injuries and Diseases Act, 1993 (No 130 of 1993)
The previous Workmen's Compensation Act, 1941 (No 30 of 1941) has been repealed and replaced by the Compensation for Occupational Injuries and Diseases Act, 1993 (No 130 of 1993) (COIDA). This Act came into effect on 1 March 1994 and falls under the Department of Labour.

The Act allows for compensation to be paid to an employee who, as result of his/her activities at work, is partially or totally disabled or contracts an occupational disease. It also provides for compensation in the event of death of the employee, to be paid out to his/her dependants.

The Act specifically excludes compensation for scheduled diseases contracted by workers doing risk work in controlled mines and works.

Occupational health

The COIDA stipulates the following:
- Who is entitled to compensation
- When a person is entitled to compensation
- How much is compensated
- What procedures must be followed to claim for compensation.

The COIDA covers both accident and compensable diseases sustained at work.

2.10.1 The Compensation Fund
The office of the Compensation Commissioner administers the Act and falls under the Department of Labour.

The Act states that employers must pay a certain amount of money into a central fund each month. The amount depends on how dangerous the industry is, how many workers are employed in the company and the wages paid to the workers.

Employers who do not pay into this fund are:
- The State
- The Provincial Administrations and certain municipalities
- Employers in the construction industry who are generally insured by Federated Mutual Assurance Company, and a large number of mines that are insured by Rand Mutual Assurance Company.

The workers in these workplaces are covered by the COIDA and receive the same benefits. Their employers pay into a different fund and sometimes the forms to be filled in are different. The Compensation Commissioner has to give them permission to pay compensation in each case.

If an employee is injured or dies at work or contracts a disease caused by his/her work (occupational disease), he/she (or his/her dependant) is paid out of this fund.

The fund is subscribed for the following:
- Compensation, cost of medical aid and any other monetary benefits to employees, or on their behalf or in respect of employees in terms of this Act, where no other person is liable for such payment
- To maintain the reserve fund
- To pay for the costs of medical examinations of employees
- To pay for any other general expenses arising out of the application of this Act, for example, travelling expenses and witness fees (Miles, 1996:222).

Events in which the fund will not pay compensation include:
- If the worker is put off work for three days or less. This is generally covered by sick pay which is different from worker's compensation; workers should consult their workplaces about details of sick pay
- If claims are made more than 12 months after the accident or death
- If the occupational disease is reported more than 12 months after the diagnosis

- If the worker's own misconduct caused the accident but if the worker is seriously disabled, or dies in the accident, then the fund will pay compensation.

A reserve fund is established to provide for any unforeseen demands on the compensation fund and to stabilize the tariffs of assessment.

Under some circumstances the Act applies to accidents that take place outside the borders of the country and also injuries/accidents sustained by foreign employees who work in South Africa on a temporary basis.

2.10.2 The Compensation Commissioner

The Minister of Labour appoints a Compensation Commissioner, whose functions are spelt out in the Act. All notices and claims are sent to the Commissioner who then assesses and decides on the right to compensation, the calculations, degree of disablement and who should be liable for the payment of compensation. The Compensation Commissioner has wide discretion. This includes any question relating to a right to compensation, the calculation of earnings, the degree of disablement of an employee, and the amount and manner of payment of compensation.

According to Miles (1996:220) the Commissioner may also enter into any agreement with any person to carry out certain tasks or services relating to this Act. He/she can also establish or subsidize a body or organization whose objectives are to prevent accidents or diseases caused by certain activities, to promote the health and safety of employees, or to rehabilitate employees injured by accidents or suffering from occupational diseases.

The Commissioner may refuse to pay compensation to an injured employee if the employee misrepresented the state of his/her health, in other words if the employee did not fully inform the employer of his/her true state of health and full details were not disclosed. Compensation is also refused when the employee refuses or fails to get medical attention in respect of the injury or disease. Even if a doctor diagnoses and sends proof of the disease that was contracted at work, to the Commissioner, he/she may still refuse to pay out.

2.10.3 The Compensation Board

The Act makes provision for the establishment of a Compensation Board. The Compensation Board comprises 16 members appointed by the Minister. The composition and functions are specified in the Act – the functions of the Board are to advise the Minister about policy matters with regard to the Act, the benefits that must be payable to employees or dependants of employees, and what adjustments should be made to existing pensions.

2.10.4 Compensation to employees

There are two conditions under which an employee or the stipulated legal dependant will be entitled to compensation. These include:
- If the employee has an accident which results in his/her disablement or death
- If the employee contracts either a listed occupational disease or any other disease arising from and in the course of the employment.

For example, if an employee works for a veterinarian and contracts anthrax, it will be presumed that this disease arose out of and in the course of the employee's employment.

It is important to note, however, that employees must report the disease within 12 months of being diagnosed by a doctor, otherwise they cannot claim for compensation. Some diseases take a long time to manifest in diagnosable symptoms. Sometimes the worker has even left the workplace which caused the disease a long time before the disease is discovered. Workers can claim compensation for an occupational disease caused by conditions in a workplace even if they no longer work there.

2.10.5 Compensation for temporary disability
General information: Workers' rights
- If workers are injured in an accident arising out of or in the course of their work, they are entitled to compensation while they are off work.
- A worker cannot decide to stay off work because of a work injury. He/she has to be laid off work by a doctor.
- Temporary disability means that the worker recovers from the accident or sickness.
- The temporary disability can be total or partial: *Total* means that the worker has to stay completely off work for a while. The compensation for this is 1/2 of the monthly wage. *Partial* means that the worker can go to work, but has to do light duty or work fewer hours. If the worker temporarily earns less because of this, he/she will get 1/2 of the difference between the normal wage and the reduced wage.
- If the worker is off work for three days or less, no compensation is paid.
- If the worker is off for more than three days, then compensation is paid for the first three days as well.
- The compensation is paid instead of wages.
- For the purposes of calculating compensation, the monthly wages include regular bonuses and allowances and regular overtime.
- The employer must pay the worker compensation for the first three months off. The employer can claim this money back from the fund at a later stage.

If the worker is off for more than three months, the Commissioner takes over the payments. The worker will receive periodic payments (once a month) from the Commissioner until he/she is fit for duty. The Commissioner will give periodic payments for up to 12 months for temporary disability. If the worker's condition has not improved by then, the Commissioner may agree to continue periodic payments for up to 24 months.

After 24 months the Commissioner may decide that the condition is permanent and give compensation for permanent disability, in which case all doctors' and hospital bills and medication costs are paid by the Commissioner.

Legislation in occupational health

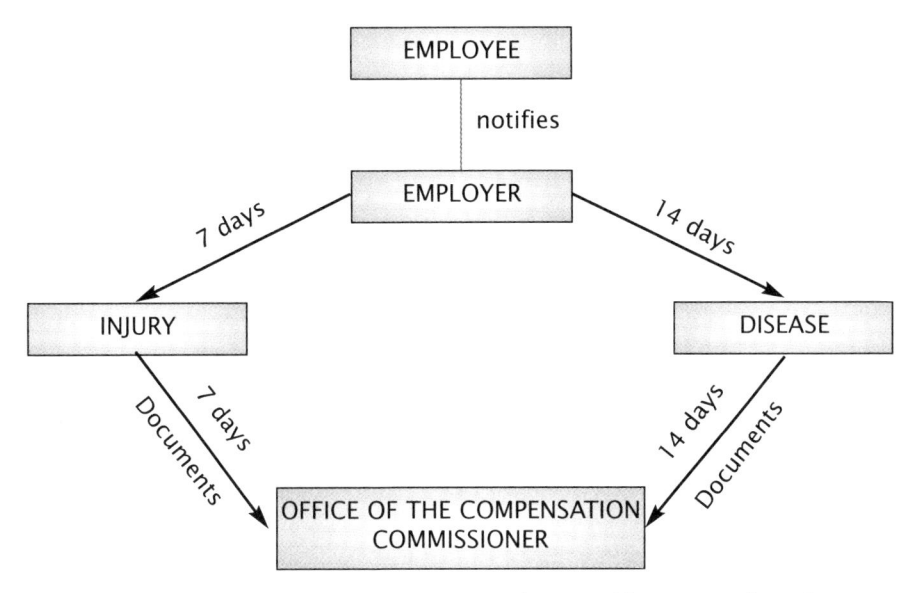

Figure 2.1 Procedure for reporting occupational injury/disease and applying for compensation

Procedures for submitting claims under COIDA

Forms for submitting claims for compensation purposes may be obtained from Rand Mutual or through their website (*www.randmutual.co.za*). An equivalent form for cases not falling under Rand Mutual can be obtained from the Compensation Commissioner in Pretoria (*www.compensation.gov.za*). Forms for occupational diseases are different from those for occupational injury claims.

The procedure for occupational diseases and injuries are reflected in Figure 2.1. The process for submitting occupational disease forms is heavily dependent on appropriate diagnosis by the medical practitioner and the recognition of the occupational-related nature of the disease. The medical practitioner completes the First Medical Report and this is submitted to the employer and to Rand Mutual or to the Office of the Compensation Commissioner within 14 days. The date of commencement of the disease is the date on which the medical practitioner diagnosed the disease for the first time.

If the medical practitioner continues to see the worker for treatment or follow-up, the practitioner completes the Final Medical Report. An estimate of impairment or disability is indicated.

The reports must contain a clear, concise history of the occupational injury or disease, stating signs and symptoms, and should be accompanied by medical tests, such as X-rays. The doctor must give full details of the treatment requested and indicate when the employee is likely to return to work. The Final Medical Report should contain a record of the chance of residual disability of a permanent nature.

Having been informed by the medical practitioner (i.e. received the First Medical Report), the employer must complete the Employer's Report of an occupational disease and submit this to Rand Mutual or the Office of the Compensation Commissioner, within 14 days. A Resumption Report is submitted by the employer if the employee returns to work.

Occupational health

The Act specifies that the employee must inform the employer if he/she believes he/she is suffering from an occupational disease. The employee can complete a Notice of Occupational Disease and Claim for Compensation. This form is essential if the organization in whose employ the worker contracted the occupational disease no longer exists or if the employer refuses to complete an Employer's Report.

2.10.6 Specific aspects included under the Act

2.10.6.1 Noise-induced hearing loss

A new procedure for identifying and evaluating cases of noise-induced hearing loss for compensation was introduced in 2001 in a guideline issued by the Compensation Commissioner, Instruction A1 (RSA 2001).

A baseline audiogram is used as an indication for deterioration in hearing and for calculating hearing loss. Where employees transfer between employers, the recording of a new baseline recording will enable the determination of liability from noise-induced hearing loss.

When submitting a claim for noise-induced hearing loss, the following is necessary:
- The employee's service record (including documented noise-level readings in the areas where the employee worked)
- Diagnostic audiometry (including *all* the specifications)
- A copy of the baseline audiogram.

2.10.6.2 Contact dermatitis

For submission of claims, a dermatologist's opinion is required on Form WCI.53. Patch tests are required in the case of allergic contact dermatitis.

2.10.6.3 HIV and Aids in healthcare workers

The current position is that the Compensation Commissioner will not accept needle-stick injuries as a compensatable injury, nor pay for post-exposure prophylaxis with anti-retroviral drugs, nor for counselling until proven seroconversion has occurred. Needle-stick injuries should thus not be reported to the Commissioner, but must be recorded. The implication for this is that for compensation purposes, every healthcare facility should have in place:
- A written policy on needle-stick or related injuries
- A system of procedures for recording such injuries
- The patient's HIV status should be determined with the necessary consent and counselling
- Follow-up of testing and counselling of the injured worker should take place
- The procedure for submitting a claim should the worker became infected.

2.10.6.4 Post-traumatic Stress Disorder (PTSD)

Under the Act, PTSD is regarded as an injury rather than a disease. Diagnosis of PTSD is considered if the following is present:
- The employee has experienced, witnessed or was confronted by an event that threatened serious injury, physical harm or death
- The person responds with intense fear, helplessness or horror.

2.10.6.5 Motor vehicle accidents
Sometimes motor vehicle accidents cause legal difficulties as they do not occur at the workplace and sometimes occur after official working hours. The issue then is whether the accident arose 'out of' or 'in the course of' employment (Strassheim in Coetzee & Pretorius, 1997:E8.11). The Act deems workers to be covered when travelling to and from work if the vehicle is:
- Provided specifically for this purpose
- Provided at no cost to the worker
- A private vehicle under control of the employer
- Driven by the employer or one of his employees.

An injury on duty involving vehicles requires the submission of the following details:
- Vehicle details and ID
- What the vehicle was being used for
- Driver's licence details
- Any other details related to the accident and injuries
- Details of vehicle insurance.

2.10.7 Schedule 3 of the Act
Schedule 3 of the Act deals with compensation for occupational injuries and diseases. These are summarized in the box on pages 56-58.

2.11 The Occupational Diseases in Mines and Works Act, 1973 (No 78 of 1973)
This Act was written with the objective of consolidating and amending the law relating to the payment of compensation in respect of certain diseases contracted by persons employed in mines and works and matters incidental thereto.

2.11.1 Description of mine and works
According to this Act, a mine is:

> [8] Any excavation in the earth, whether being worked or not, made for the purpose of searching for or winning a mineral; or
> - Any other place where a mineral deposit is being worked and any quarry, including the mining area or other places at or near a mine on which buildings, constructions, mine dumps, dams, machinery or objects are situated and which are used or intended to be used for the following operations or any operation necessary or incidental thereto, namely:
>   - the searching for or winning of a mineral
>   - the crushing, reducing, dressing, concentration or smelting of a mineral
>   - the production of a product of commercial value, excluding a clay or earthenware product or cement, from a mineral, or
>   - the extracting, concentration or refining of any constituent of a mineral.
>
> Provided that if two or more such excavations or places are being worked in conjunction

Occupational health

with one another, they shall be deemed to comprise one mine unless the Chief Inspector as contemplated in the Mine Health and Safety Act, 1996, notifies the owner thereof in writing that such excavations or places comprise two or more mines.

Schedule 3 of the Compensation for Occupational Injuries and Diseases Act, 1993 (No 130 of 1993)

Diseases	Work:
	a Any work involving the handling of or exposure to any of the following substances emanating from the workplace concerned:
Pneumoconiosis-fibrosis of the parencyma of the lung	Organic or inorganic fibrogenic dust
Pleural thickening causing significant impairment of function	Asbestos or asbestos dust
Bronchopulmonary disease Byssinosis	Metal carbides (hard metals) Flax cotton or sisal
Occupational asthma	The sensitizing agents: 1 isocyanates 2 platinum, nickel, cobalt, vanadium or chromium salts 3 hardening agents, including epoxy resins 4 acrylic acids or derived acrylates 5 soldering or welding fumes 6 substances from animals or insects 7 fungi or spores 8 proteolytic enzymes 9 organic dust 10 vapours or fumes of formaldehyde, anhydrides, amines or diamines
Extrinsic allergy alveolotis	Moulds, fungal spores or any other allergenic proteinaceous material, 2.4 tuluene-di-isocyanates
Any disease or pathological manifestations	Beryllium, cadmium, phosphorus, chromium, manganese, arsenic, mercury, lead, fluorine, carbondisulphide, cyanide, halogen derivatives of aliphatic or aromatic hydrocarbons, benzene or itshomologues, nitro- and amino-derivatives of benzene or its homologues, nitroglycerine or other nitric

	its homologues, nitroglycerine or other nitric acid esters, hydrocarbons, trinitrotoluol, alcohol, glycols or ketones, acrylamide or any compounds of the afore-mentioned substances.
Erosion of the tissues of the oral cavity or nasal cavity	Irritants, alkalis, acids or fumes thereof
Dysbarism, including decompression sickness, barotrauma or osteonecrosis	Abnormal atmospheric or water pressure
Any disease	Ionizing radiation from any source
Allergic or irritant contact dermatitis	Dust, liquids or other external agents or factors
Mesothelioma of the pleura or peritoneum or other malignancy of the lung	Asbestos or asbestos dust
Malignancy of the lung, skin, larynx, mouth cavity or bladder	Coaltar, pitch, asphalt or bitumen or volatiles thereof
Malignancy of the lung, mucous membrane of the nose or associated air sinuses	Nickel or its compounds
Malignancy of the lung	Hexavalant chromium compounds, or bischloromethyl ether
Angiosarcoma of the liver	Vinyl chloride monomer
Malignancy of the bladder	4-amino-diphenyl, benzidine, beta naphtylamine. 4-nitro-dipenyl
Leukaemia	Benzene
Melanoma of the skin	Polychlorinated biphenyls
Tuberculosis of the lung	1 Crystalline silica (alpha quartz) 2 Mycobacterium tuberculosis or MOTTS (mycobacterium other than tuberculosis) transmitted to an employee during the performance of healthcare work from a patient suffering from active open tuberculosis
Brucellosis	Brucella abortus, suis or mellitensis transmitted through contact with infected animals or their products
Anthrax	Bacillus anthracis transmitted through contact with infected animals or their products

Q-fever	Coxiella burnetii emanating from infected animals or their products
Bovine tuberculosis	Mycobacterium bovis transmitted through contact with infected animals or their products
Rift Valley Fever	Virus transmitted by infected animals or their products
	b Any work involving the handling of or exposure to any of the following:
Hearing impairment	Excessive noise
Hand-arm vibration syndrome (Raynaud's phenomenon)	Vibrating equipment
Any disease due to overstraining of muscular tendonous insertions	Repetitive movements

According to this Act, 'works' means any place, not being a mine or part of a mine, where any of the following operations and any operation necessary therefor or incidental thereto are carried out and constitute the main operation at such place, namely:
- The moving, transfer or handling of stone, rock, ore, coal or other minerals, including any loading operation at subsidiary sidings
- The crushing, screening, washing, classifying or concentration of any mineral
- The treating of any mineral, in the form obtained from a mine, for the production of coke or for the production of a base metal in any shape or form, including ingots, billets and rolled sections
- The working or treating of mine tailings, deposits or mine dumps for the recovery of any valuble content thereof
- The extracting of any precious metal from any mineral or concentrate
- The refining of any precious metal
- The dyeing of any source material as defined in the Nuclear Energy Act, 1993, (Act No 131 of 1993)
- The making, repairing, re-opening or closing of any subterranean tunnel.

2.11.2 Compensatable disease
This Act describes a compensatable disease as the following:
- Pneumoconiosis
- The joint condition of pneumoconiosis and tuberculosis
- Tuberculosis contracted while the person concerned was performing risk work, or with which the person was already affected at any time within the 12 months immediately following the date on which the person performed such work for the last time

- Permanent obstruction of the airways attributed to the performance of risk work
- Any other permanent disease of cardio-respiratory organs which is attributed to the performance of risk work
- Progressive systemic schlerosis attributed to the performance of risk work
- Any other disease which the Minister, acting on the advice of the committee consisting of the director and not fewer than three other medical practitioners designated by the Minister has, by notice in the Gazette declared to be a compensatable disease and which is attributed to the performance of risk works at mines or works.

The above are all subjected to the opinion of the certification committee for occupational diseases established under this Act. Of notable interest is the definition of tuberculosis included in the Act. Tuberculosis means tuberculosis of the cardio-respiratory organs of a person who has worked at least 200 shifts in circumstances amounting to a risk and where silica dust or any other injurious dust was present, or any sequelae, complication or manifestation thereof, but does not include inactive or calcified foci.

2.11.3 Certificates of fitness, medical and other examinations

According to this Act, certificates of fitness (not exceeding a period of three years) may be required of a person who is employed by a mine or works, or who performs risk work.

Medical examinations must be performed on every person who works at a mine or works and who is not in possession of a current certificate of fitness.

Periodical medical examinations for renewal of certificates of fitness must be awarded to persons who perform risk work. The Minister of Health prescribes the nature and period of examinations as well as the different groups subjected to these examinations.

Medical practitioners have certain roles stipulated in this Act regarding reporting those suffering from compensatable diseases. Also, with regard to postmortem examinations, medical practitioners must remove the cardio-respiratory organs and parts of the body and send these parts to prescribed places for further investigation, if they have obtained the permission of the family.

2.11.4 Certification of compensatable diseases

The Act makes provision for and stipulates the role and functions of an established committee (Medical Certification Committee) who shall perform the review of the medical and/or postmortem certificates for compensation purposes.

2.12 The Basic Conditions of Employment Act, 1997 (No 75 of 1997)

The promulgation of this Act implies that there is a perceived need for protection of employees from malpractice by the employer.

This Act stipulates minimum conditions of employment, which can be further adapted by negotiation between the employer and employee organizations. Among others, it covers items such as sick leave, certificates for sick leave, maximum daily working conditions, hours allowed for overtime, meal intervals, etc. It also prohibits work under certain conditions, such as at a specified age and during pregnancy.

The Act specifically excludes some employees working in certain specified areas or categories, as well as specific people who are earning specified minimum salaries. In 1993, employees working in the agricultural sector and thereafter domestic employees were included under the Act. It further makes provision for a 'regular day worker' who is defined as a domestic worker, employed by the same employer for not more than three days a week and for not less than four consecutive weeks.

The Act is prescriptive in that the transgression of any of its provisions is a criminal offence. Any employer who does not keep to the stipulation may be prosecuted.

The Act is primarily aimed at improving the working conditions of unorganized and vulnerable workers. The Act specifically addresses the problems of:
- Inadequate protection of vulnerable workers, such as part-time, farm and domestic workers
- The lack of mechanisms to set minimum wages for farm and domestic workers
- Child labour
- Excessive long working hours, especially in areas such as in the transport and securitysectors
- Gender discrimination, especially in relation to maternity leave.

The purpose of the Basic Conditions of Employment Act, 1997 (No 75 of 1997) is to advance economic development and social justice by fulfilling its primary objectives, namely:
- To give effect to and regulate the right of fair labour practices conferred in seciton 23(1) of the Constitution by:
  - establishing and enforcing basic conditions of employment
  - regulating the variation of basic conditions of employment
- To give effect to obligations incurred by the Republic as a member State of the International Labour Organization.

The Basic Conditions of Employment Bill are summarized as follows:
(Reference: Strassheim (in Coetzee & Pretorius, 1997))

Who is this Act for?
The Act applies to all workers and employers except members of the National Defence Force, National Intelligence Agency, South African Secret Service and unpaid volunteers working for charities.

This Act must be obeyed even if other agreements differ.

Working time
This section does not apply to senior managers (those who can hire, discipline and fire), sales staff who travel and workers who work less than 24 hours a month.

Ordinary hours of work
A worker may *not* work more than:
- Forty-five hours in any week
- Nine hours a day if a worker works five days or less a week, or
- Eight hours a day if a worker works more than five days a week.

Overtime
If overtime is needed, workers must agree to do it and they may not work more than three hours overtime a day or 10 hours overtime a week.

Overtime must be paid at 1.5 times the worker's normal pay or by agreement get paid time off.

More flexibility of working time may be negotiated if there is a collective agreement with a registered trade union. For example, this would allow more flexible hours for working mothers and migrant workers.
- *Compressed work week*: You may agree to work up to 12 hours in a day and work fewer days in a week. This could help working mothers and migrant workers by having a longer weekend.
- *Averaging*: A collective agreement may permit the hours of work to be averaged over a period of up to four months. A worker who is bound by such an agreement may not work more than an average of 45 ordinary hours a week and an average of five hours of overtime a week over the agreed period. A collective agreement for a averaging has to be re-negotiated each year.

Meal breaks and rest periods
A worker must have a meal break of 60 minutes after five hours work. But a written agreement may lower this to 30 minutes and do away with the meal break if the worker works less than six hours a day.

A worker must have a daily rest period of 12 continuous hours and a weekly rest period of 36 continuous hours, which, unless otherwise agreed, must include Sunday.

Sunday work
A worker who sometimes works on a Sunday must receive double pay. A worker who normally works on a Sunday must be paid at 1.5 times the normal wage. There may be an agreement for paid time off instead of overtime pay.

Night work
Night work is unhealthy and may lead to accidents. Workers who work between 6:00 at night and 6:00 in the morning must receive extra pay or be able to work fewer hours for the same amount of money.

Transport must be available but not necessarily provided by the employer. Workers who usually work between 11:00 at night and 6:00 in the morning must be told of the health and safety risks. They are entitled to regular medical check-ups, paid for by the employer. They must be moved to a day shift if night work causes a health problem. All medical examinations must be kept confidential.

Public holidays
Workers must be paid for any public holiday that falls on a working day. Work on a public holiday is by agreement and paid at double the rate. A public holiday is exchangeable by agreement.

Leave
Annual leave
A worker may take up to 21 continuous days' annual leave or by agreement, one day for every 17 days worked or one hour for every 17 hours worked.
   Leave must be taken not later than six months after the end of the leave cycle.
   An employer may decide to pay a worker instead of giving leave if that worker resigns or goes on pension.

Sick leave
A worker may take up to six weeks' paid sick leave during a 36 months cycle. During the first six months a worker may take one day's paid sick leave for every 26 days worked.
   An employer may want a medical certificate before paying a worker who is sick for more than two days at a time or more than twice in eight weeks.

Maternity leave
A pregnant worker may take up to four continuous months of maternity leave. She may start leave any time from four weeks before the expected date of birth OR on a date a doctor or midwife says is necessary for her health or that of her unborn child. She also may not work for six weeks after the birth of her child unless declared fit to do so by a doctor or midwife.
   A pregnant or breastfeeding worker is not allowed to perform work that is dangerous to her or her child.

Family responsibility leave
Full-time workers employed longer than four months may take three days paid family responsibility leave per year on request when the worker's child is born or sick or for the death of the worker's spouse or life partner, parent, adoptive parent, grandparent, child, adopted child, grandchild or sibling.
   An employer may want proof that this leave was needed.

Job information and payment
Job information
Employers must give new workers information about their job and working conditions in writing. This includes a description of any other related documents.

Keeping record
Employers must keep a record of at least:
- The worker's name and job
- Time worked

- Money paid
- Date of birth for workers under 18 years old.

Payment
An employer must pay a worker:
- In South African money
- Daily, weekly, fortnightly or monthly
- In cash, cheque or direct deposit.

Payslip information
Each payslip must include:
- Employer's name and address
- Worker's name and job
- Period of payment
- Worker's pay
- Amount and purpose of any deduction made from the pay
- Actual amount paid to the worker.

If it is needed to add up the worker's pay, the payslip must also include:
- Ordinary pay rate and overtime pay rate
- Number of ordinary and overtime hours worked during that period of payment
- Number of hours worked on a Sunday or public holiday during that period
- Total number of ordinary and overtime hours worked in the period of averaging, if there is an averaging agreement.

Approved deductions
An employer may not deduct any money from a worker's pay unless:
- That worker agrees in writing
- The deduction is required by law or permitted in terms of a law, collective agreement, court order or arbitration award.

Adding up wages
- Wages are based on the number of hours normally worked
- Monthly pay is 4 and 1/3 times the weekly wage.

Termination of employment
Notice
A worker or employer must give notice to end an employment contract of not less than:
- One week, if employed for four weeks or less
- Two weeks, if employed for more than four weeks but not more than one year
- Four weeks, if employed for one year or more.

Notice must be in writing, except from a worker who cannot write.

Workers who stay in employer's accommodation must be given one month's notice of termination of the contract or be given alternative accommodation until the contract is lawfully terminated.

When a worker is given notice by an employer, it does not stop the worker from challenging the dismissal in terms of the Labour Relations Act or any other law.

Severance pay
An employer must pay a worker who is dismissed due to the employer's operational requirement pay equal to at least one week's severance pay for every year of continuous work with that employer.

Certificate of service
When a job ends, a worker must be given a certificate of service.

Child labour and forced labour
- It is against the law to employ a child under 15 years old.
- Children under 18 may not do dangerous work or work meant for an adult.
- It is against the law to force someone to work.

Variation of basic conditions of employment
Bargaining council
A collective agreement concluded by a bargaining council can be different from this law as long it does not:
- Lower protection of workers in terms of health and safety and family responsibilities
- Lower annual leave to less than two weeks
- Lower maternity leave in any way
- Lower sick leave in any way
- Lower protection of night workers
- Allow for any child labour or forced labour.

Other agreements
Collective agreements and individual agreements must follow the Act.

The Minister
The Minister of Labour may make a determination to vary or exclude a basic condition of employment. This can also be done on application by an employer or employer organization.

Sectoral determinations
Sectoral determinations may be made to establish basic conditions for workers in a sector and area.

Employment Conditions Commission
This Act makes provision for the Employment Conditions Commission to advise the Minister of Labour.

Monitoring, enforcement and legal proceedings
Labour inspectors must advise workers and employers on their labour rights and obligations. They inspect, investigate complaints, question people and inspect, copy and remove records.

An inspector may serve a compliance order by writing to the Director-General of the Department of Labour, who will then look at the facts and agree, change or cancel the order.

This decision may be challenged in the Labour Court.

Workers may not be treated unfairly for demanding their rights in terms of this Act.

General
It is a crime to:
- Hinder, block or try to wrongly influence a labour inspector or any other person obeying this Act
- Get or try to get a document by stealing, lying or showing a false or forged document
- Pretend to be a labour inspector or any other person obeying this Act
- Refuse or fail to answer fully any lawful question asked by a labour inspector or any other person obeying this Act
- Refuse or fail to obey a labour inspector or any other person obeying this Act.

2.13 The Employment Equity Act, 1998 (No 55 of 1998)
The Employment Equity Act seeks to eliminate unfair discrimination in employment and provides for affirmative action to correct the imbalances of the past with respect to access to employment training, promotion and equitable remuneration, especially of Blacks, women and the disabled (Ministry of Labour 1999–2004).

The provisions of the Act apply to all employers, except the military and intelligence services. Employers who employ 50 or more workers will be obliged to develop specific affirmative action plans, formulated in consultation with workers or their representatives, with voluntary targets that will be monitored by government through the submission of employment equity plans (Ministry of Labour, 1999–2004). The Act also establishes an advisory and part-time Commission for Employment Equity, particularly to advise on the formulation of codes of good practice.

The purpose of the Employment Equity Act is to achieve equity in the workplace by:
- Promoting equal opportunity and fair treatment in employment through the elimination of unfair discrimination
- Implementing affirmative action measures to redress the disadvantages in employment experienced by designated groups, in order to ensure their equitable representation in all occupational categories and levels of the workforce.

Occupational health

Chapter II of this Act deals with prohibition of unfair discrimination. Prohibition will be enforced as follows:
- No person may unfairly discriminate, directly or indirectly, against an employee, in any employment policy or practice, on one or more grounds, including race, gender, pregnancy, marital status, family responsibility, ethnic or social origin, colour, sexual orientation, age, disability, religion, HIV status, conscience, belief, political opinion, culture, language and birth.
- It is not unfair discrimination to
  - take affirmative action measures consistent with the purpose of this Act, or
  - distinguish, exclude or prefer any person on the basis of an inherent requirement of a job.
- Harassment of an employee is a form of unfair discrimination and is prohibited on any one ground, or a combination of grounds, of unfair discrimination listed in subsection 1.

2.13.1 Sexual harassment

The South African Constitution protects all citizens against discrimination. The Employment Equity Act, 1998 states clearly that harassment of an employee is unlawful because it is a form of discrimination. It includes harassment based on sex, race, religion and sexual orientation.

Every workplace should have a policy with regard to sexual harassment. Aspects which could be covered in this policy include the following:
- A definition of sexual harassment
- Descriptions of procedures, firstly as prescribed by the Labour Relations Act, and secondly as it applies to the specific workplace
- A brief outline of preventive measures against sexual harassment.

Defining sexual harassment
What is sexual harassment? Does it have to do with sexual attraction between two people who work in the same organization? The answer to this question is a clear NO. Sexual attraction is a matter of choice between people – both of them are willingly engaged in whatever form of interaction they chose to act out the attraction. Sexual harassment, on the other hand, is a situation where one person makes unwanted advances to another person, who feels humiliated, demeaned and stressed as a result of these advances. The person who feels harassed has no choice. In the majority of sexual harassment cases women are the targets, because men usually have more power than women in our society, and therefore in most places of work. Women, on the other hand, have different ways of seducing males and could be as guilty as men on sexual harassment charges.

The following list includes some examples of sexual harassment.
Verbal advance: Your co-worker continues to nag you to go out with him when you've made it clear that you are not interested.
Non-verbal advance: Pictures of naked women and other sexually explicit materials are hung on the walls at work, or a male colleague exposes himself.
Physical advance: Your boss touches you whenever you pass by.

Quid pro quo: Your boss or senior colleague offers you a promotion if you sleep with him.
Sexual favouritism: Only women who respond to a supervisor's advances are given promotion.
Gestures: Winking, blowing kisses, hand sign pretending to outline breasts or indicating sexual intercourse.
Suggestions or innuendos (indirect hints): Colleagues make comments with sexual overtones, or use words with double meanings to ask you to sleep with them.
Jokes or degrading remarks: Sex-related jokes or insults, remarks that offend you as a woman.
Fondling (touching) without your consent.

2.14 The Labour Relations Act, 1995 (No 66 of 1995)

The primary aim of the Labour Relations Act, 1956 (No 28 of 1956) is to provide a statutory framework in which the relationships between the trade unions on the one hand and the employers of employer organizations on the other hand may be regulated.

The greatest significance of this Act is that it was the product of tripartite negotiations between all stakeholders, namely the government, employers and organized labour (NEDLAC – National Economic Development and Labour Council).

2.14.1 Purpose and objectives of the Act

The LRA aims to advance economic development, social justice, labour peace and democracy in the workplace by means of the following objectives:

- To realize and regulate the fundamental rights of workers and employers in the Constitution (section 23), which include the following:
  - every person shall have the right to fair labour practices
  - workers shall have the right to form and join trade unions, and employers shall have the right to form and join employer organizations
  - workers and employers shall have the right to organize and bargain collectively
  - workers shall have the right to strike for the purpose of collective bargaining
  - employers' recognition of lockout for the purpose of collective bargaining shall not be impaired (section 64(1) of LRA).
- To execute the duties of the Republic as a member state of the International Labour Organization
- To provide a framework for trade unions and employees and employers and their organizations to:
  - bargain collectively on terms and conditions of employment, wages and other matters of mutual interest
  - formulate industrial policy
- To promote:
  - orderly collective bargaining
  - collective bargaining at sectorial level
  - employee participation in decision-making in the workplace
  - the effective resolution of labour disputes

Occupational health

2.14.2 Application and scope of the Act
The LRA applies to all employees of the state, universities, technicons, local authorities, SA Police Services, parliamentary workers, agricultural workers, informal sector workers, as well as domestic workers. Only the SA Intelligence Services, SA National Defence Force and the South African Secret Services are excluded from the application of the LRA.

The Act defines an employee as:
- Any person, excluding an independent contractor, who works for another person or for the state and who receives or is entitled to receive any remuneration
- Any person who in any manner assists in carrying on or conducting the business of an employer.

2.14.3 Employer's rights and duties
Strassheim (in Coetzee & Pretorius, 1997:E4.3) states that employers benefit from the new LRA in the following manner:
- Employers have the right to join employers' organizations and participate in the activities of these organizations
- Employers have the right to lock-out workers
- Less production time is lost because there is mutual participation in resolving issues and therefore a decrease in industrial action and labour unrest
- Improved productivity and profitability are possible due to successful restructuring at the workplace through information sharing and consultation
- Joint solution of problems, training and development is possible
- Quick, inexpensive and non-legalistic procedures for the adjudication of dismissal cases are possible
- There is accommodation of the needs of small business.

Trade unions
The LRA contains a range of organizational rights of trade unions which are represented in the workplace. In terms of the Act, the most important aspects include access to the workplace to recruit members, hold meetings, and vote and elect members.

2.14.4 Employee partcipation in the workplace
The LRA specifically aims at promoting labour stability and bringing about positive change in the workplace. To encourage this, the emphasis is placed on the participation of the employee.

Strassheim (in Coetzee & Pretorius, 1997:E4.5) states four considerations to participate, namely:

> ... reasons which caused the LRA to accept the desirability of employee participation to influence or determine issues which affect them in the workplace, may have been NEDLAC participants' positions on four factors:
> 1 Moral considerations (the right of employees to participate)

2 Power considerations (recognition of the collective power of organized labour in the workplace)
3 Union considerations (activities and pressures exerted on management by the trade union in support of demands for greater participation)
4 Political considerations (pressure from political systems for greater participative and inclusive management).

Collective bargaining of employees is an important aspect in the LRA. It is defined as 'a method of determining terms and conditions of employment which utilizes the processes of negotiation and agreement between representatives of management and employees'.

One of the most important features of the LRA is the establishment of *workplace forums*. A workplace forum, according to the LRA, 'must seek to promote the interests of all employees in the workplace, whether or not they are trade union members; and must seek to enhance efficiency in the workplace'. A workplace forum is established in a workplace of 100 or more employees, and holds meetings with the employer, and employees.

Bargaining councils are established in respect of a sector or area by one or more registered trade union/s and employers' organization/s. The powers of bargaining councils are to perform dispute resolution functions; to prevent and resolve labour disputes; to promote and establish training and education schemes; to establish and administer pension, provident, medical aid, sick pay, vacation, unemployment and training schemes or funds; and to develop proposals for submission to NEDLAC.

Statutory councils are formed by one or more registered trade union/s or employers' organizations. The powers are more limited than those of the bargaining councils.

For the employee to be involved in collective bargaing and to participate in joint decision-making, the LRA provides statutory rights to the bodies mentioned above and their members. These rights include:
- To make representations. These are essentially any form of request, suggestion or demand that can be made by the workplace forum on work-related aspects.
- To be consulted by the employer. The employer must consult with the workplace forum on matters such as:
  - restructuring the workplace
  - introducing new technology
  - introducing new work methods
  - making changes in the organization of work
  - undertaking plant closures
  - undertaking mergers and transfers of ownership
  - dismissing employees for operational requirements
  - undertaking job grading, merit, payment of bonuses
  - providing education and training, etc.
- To joint decision-making with the employer. The employer and workplace forum must reach agreement on:
  - disciplinary codes and procedures

- rules relating to the proper regulation of the workplace
- measures to protect and advance persons disadvantaged by unfair discriminations
- changes in trusts or boards and rules regulating social benefit schemes.

The employee, through the workplace forum, also has the right to have information disclosed by the employer. However, there is a limitation to this right and information that is legally privileged and confidential is not disclosed, for example, information which is related to the personal information of an individual which may harm the person in any way, or information which may jeopardize the safety of a company or a country.

Through the workplace forum, employees also have the right to have information disclosed by their employer. However, there are limitations to this right, for example when information that is legally privileged and confidential may cause substantial harm to the employer and employee if it is disclosed, as well as information that is private, personal, or relating to an employee, unless the employee consents to the disclosure.

2.14.5 Dispute resolution

The LRA provides three principal means for the resolution of disputes:

1 Conciliation

Within 30 days of receiving a dispute, the commissioner of the Commission for Conciliation, Mediation and Arbitration (CCMA) must attempt to resolve the dispute by mediation, or by conducting a fact-finding exercise, or by making a recommendation to the disputing parties.

2 Arbitration

In some instances, disputes must be arbitrated by the CCMA or a Bargaining Council, for example:
- Organizational rights
- Disputes about disclosure of information
- Interpretation and application of collective agreemnts
- Interest issues in essential services
- Dismissals, misconducts, incapacity
- Severance pay, promotion, demotion, benefits, training
- Suspension or disciplinary action and failure to re-instate or re-employ.

3 Adjudication

In some instances disputes must be adjudicated by the Labour Court:
- The application or exercise of the right to freedom of association
- Refusal to admit a party to a Bargaining Council
- Strikes and lock-outs, breaches of picketing rules, protest actions
- Automatically unfair dismissals
- Dismissals for operational reasons
- Discrimination.

2.14.6 Essential services

Employees working in essentials services are prohibited to strike. Employees who provide essential services may not lock-out. Essential services are minimum services and maintenance services. In terms of the LRA, a committee has been established to decide and/or make recommendations on whether a service should be designated an essential service for the purpose of labour relations. The LRA stipulates that this committee can ratify any collective agreement which allows the continuance of minimum services in a service that has been designated an essential service.

An essential service is regarded as a service or job which, if interrupted or stopped, would or could endanger the life, personal safety of the whole or part of the population (for example, workers in the health industry, electricity or sewerage systems). It also includes personnel engaged in the parliamentary services or South African Police Service.

Maintenance services are regarded as services which, if interrupted, would result in or cause the material physical destruction of any working area, plant or machinery.

2.14.7 Unfair dismissals

Section 185 of the LRA deals with unfair dismissals. The LRA states that 'every employee has the right not to be unfairly dismissed'. However, the emphasis is on unfairness. An employee may be dismissed if there is a valid or fair reason to do so.

The legal reasons for dismissal include:
- Misconduct, which entails wrongdoing such as bad/poor behaviour
- Incapacity, where a person is unable to do his/her work, poor work performance or through ill health or injury
- Operational requirements due to financial difficulties or reconstructuring of the workplace which may lead to retrenchment or redundancy.

Section 186 of the LRA defines dismissal as meaning that:
- An employer has terminated a contract of employment with or without notice
- An employee reasonably expected the employer to renew a fixed-term contract of employment on the same or similar terms but the employer offered to renew it on less favourable terms, or did not renew it
- An employer refused to allow an employee to resume work after she
  - took maternity leave in terms of any law, collective agreement or her contract of employment, or
  - was absent from work for up to four weeks before the expected date, and up to eight weeks after the actual date of birth of her child
- An employer who dismissed a number of employees for the same or similar reasons has offered to re-employ one or more of them but has refused to re-employ another, or
- An employee terminated a contract of employment with or without notice because the employer made continued employment intolerable for the employee.

A dismissal will only be regarded as fair if:
- The reason for dismissal was a fair reason related to the employee's conduct or capacity or was based on the employer's operational requirements
- The dismissal was effected in accordance with a fair procedure.

Automatic unfair dismissals are as follows:
- An intention, support or participation in a legal strike
- Pregnancy or intended pregnancy
- Discrimination on the grounds of race, gender, sex, ethnic or social origin, sexual orientation, religion, conscience, belief, political opinion, culture, language, marital status or family responsibility.

2.14.8 Schedules included in the Act
The LRA contains the following schedules:
- Schedule 1 deals with the establishment of bargaining councils for the public service sector.
- Schedule 2 gives guidelines for the constitution of a workplace forum.
- Schedule 3 deals with the CCMA.
- Schedule 4 provides flow diagrams of the prescribed route for setting disputes.
- Schedule 5 refers to the amendment of some related laws.
- Schedule 6 refers to Acts that no longer apply in terms of section 212 of this Act.
- Schedule 7 stipulates arrangements for the transition from the old Labour Relations Act to the new one.
- Schedule 8 provides the code of good practice concerning dismissal.

Note should be taken of HIV/Aids and Employment (see Addendum 2).

2.15 The National Economic Development and Labour Council (NEDLAC) Act, 1994 (No 35 of 1994)

Building on the experiences of the previous National Manpower Commission and the National Economic Forum, the National Economic Development and Labour Council (NEDLAC) was created.

NEDLAC has ensured that the significant civil society partners have been included in the policy-making process. Thus, organized business, communities, labour and national government have succeeded, despite divergent views on labour market policies, through an ongoing process of consultation and negotiation, in reaching substantial national consensus on legislation and other measures.

NEDLAC has also made a contribution to the effective resolution of a number of socio-economic protest actions in the education, justice and local government sectors. This is as a result of the application of section 77 of the LRA, which obliges parties to notify NEDLAC and participate in attempts to resolve problems before embarking upon socio-economic protest action (Ministry of Labour, 1999–2004).

2.15.1 Objectives, powers and functions

NEDLAC was launched on 18 February 1996. NEDLAC is a statutory body, constituted by Act 35 of 1994, which stipulates that it must:

- Strive to promote the goals of economic growth, participation and economic decision-making and social equity
- Seek to reach consensus and conclude agreements on matters pertaining to social and economic policy
- Consider all proposed labour legislation relating to labour market policy before it is introduced in parliament
- Consider all significant changes to social and economic policy before they are implemented or introduced to parliament
- Encourage and promote the formulation of coordinated policy on social and economic matters.

In order to fulfil this brief, the Act stipulates that NEDLAC should:

- Make such investigations as it may consider necessary
- Continually survey and analyse social and economic affairs
- Keep abreast of international developments in social and economic policy
- Continually evaluate the effectiveness of legislation and policy affecting social and economic policy
- Conduct research in social and economic policy
- Work in close cooperation with departments of state, statutory bodies, programmes, other forums and non-governmental agencies engaged in the formulation and implementation of social and economic policy.

2.15.2 Representation in NEDLAC

Four major stakeholders in South African society participate in NEDLAC:

1. Organized labour, represented by the Congress of South African Trade Unions (COSATU), the National Council of Trade Unions (NACTU), and the Federation of South African Labour Unions (FEDSAL). Certain specific criteria exist for inclusion of trade union federations. Federation members are appointed to NEDLAC by the Minister of Labour on nominations made by organized labour.
2. Organized business, represented by Business South Africa, the umbrella employers' organization representing 18 constituents. Members representing organized labour are appointed by the Minister of Labour on nominations made by organized business.
3. Government, represented by various departments such as Labour, Finance, Trade and Industry, as well as the Ministry in the Office of the President (the Reconstruction and Development Programme Office). Members of government are appointed to NEDLAC by the President.
4. Community, consisting of five sectors, namely civics, women, rural people, the youth and disabled people. The Minister without Portfolio in the Office of the President, in consultation with NEDLAC's Executive Council, identified these sectors and the organizations that represent them in NEDLAC. Members are appointed by the Minister without Portfolio (South African Trade Union's Library, 2003).

2.16 The Unemployment Insurance Act, 1966 (No 30 of 1966)

2.16.1 Purpose of the Act

The purpose of this Act may be summarized as follows:
- It provides for contributions by employers to an Unemployment Insurance Fund.
- It ensures payment of unemployment benefits to certain persons described in the Act, such as those that become unemployed, who are ill for a long period without an income, or to a woman who has given birth to a child or who legitimately adopts a child.
- It ensures grants/payments of certain amounts of money to dependants of deceased employees.
- It provides for schemes for the combating of unemployment and matters related to unemployment (Miles, 1996:100).

2.17 The Skills Development Act, 1998 (No 97 of 1998) and the Skills Development Levies Act, 1999 (No 9 of 1999)

One of the main causes of our country's economic deficiencies is the low level of skills in an environment that is increasingly experiencing major changes in the workplace, and which relies on methods that require more skills. The skills shortage in our country is reflected by the fact that only 20 per cent (3 million) of our economically active population are skilled or highly skilled, while about 80 per cent (12 million) are semi-skilled, unskilled or unemployed (Ministry of Labour, 1999–2004).

To address these problems, the Skills Development Act (No 97 of 1998) and the Skills Development Levies Act (No 9 of 1999) were passed by parliament at the end of 1998 and beginning of 1999.

Specifically, the Skills Development Act provides for:
- A research and strategic planning unit to gather and disseminate information on labour market skill trends and to promote the planning and prioritization of skills development
- Employment services which will promote people's active participation in the labour market
- Learnerships and other training programmes, which will result in registered qualfications signifying work readiness and which respond to the needs of the labour market
- Coordination of the skills development strategy through Sector and Education Training Authorities (SETA) working with the National Skills Authority and the Minister of Labour, and for these to coordinate with the financing of skills development through a levy grant of 1 per cent.

The Skills Development Levies Act (No 9 of 1999) was passed to put in place an incentive system to promote increased investments by firms in skills development and to ensure funds are available for national skills priorities.

The purpose of the Skills Development Act, 97 of 1998 is listed below.
- Develop the skills of the SA workforce in order to:
  - improve the quality of life of workers, their prospects of work and labour mobility
  - improve productivity in the workplace and the competitiveness of employers
  - improve self-employment
  - improve delivery of social services.
- Increase the levels of investment in education and training in the labour market and to improve the return on that investment.
- Encourage employers to:
  - use the workplace as an active learning environment
  - provide employees with the opportunities to acquire new skills
  - provide opportunities for new entrants to the labour market to gain work experience
  - employ persons who find it difficult to be employed.
- Encourage workers to participate in learnership and other training programmes.
- Improve the employment prospects of persons previously disadvantaged by unfair discrimination and redress those disadvantages through training and education.
- Ensure the quality of education and training in and for the workplace.
- Assist:
  - work-seekers to find work
  - retrenched workers to re-enter the labour market
  - employers to find qualified employees.
- Provide and regulate employment services by:
  - establishing an institutional and financial framework comprising the National Skills Authority, the National Skills Fund, a skills development levy-grant scheme as contemplated in the Skills Development Levies Act, SETAs, labour centres, Skills Development Planning Unit
  - encouraging partnerships between the public and private sectors of the economy to provide education and training in and for the workplace
  - cooperating with the South African Qualifications Authority.

2.18 The International Health Regulations Act, 1974 (No 28 of 1974) (as amended International Health Regulations Act, 2000 (No 51 of 2000)

Companies whose main business is importing and exporting need to take note of this Act. The Act makes provision for the control of Aedes aegypti index; pest control on aircraft, trains and ships; the travellers and crew on any of these means; and freight containers.

Part II of the Act makes provision for the notification and epidemiological information on the first case of disease on any of the above.

Part III deals with sanitary requirements for ports and airports, as well as the following in every airport:
- an organized medical service with adequate staff and equipment

- facilities for transport, isolation and care of infected people
- facilities for efficient disinfection, control of vectors and rodents
- a bacteriological laboratory or facilities for dispatching suspected material
- facilities within the airport for vaccination against smallpox, cholera and yellow fever

Health workers should, however, study the Act carefully as it contains many other provisions that are not included here.

2.19 The South African Medicines and Medical Devices Regulatory Authority Act, 1998 (No 114 of 1998)

This Act was established to provide for the regulation and registration of medicines intended for human and animal use; the regulation and registration of medical devices; the establishment of the South African Medicines and Medical Devices Regulatory Authority; the control of orthodox medicines, complementary medicines, veterinary medicines, scheduled substances and medical devices; the control of persons who may dispense orthodox medicines, complementary medicines and veterinary medicines; for repeal of the Medicines and Related Substances Control Act (1965), the amendmend of the Fertilizers, Farm Feeds, Agricultural Remedies and Stock Remedies Act (1947) and for matters incidental thereto.

2.20 The Drugs and Drug Trafficking Act, 1992 (No 140 of 1992)

This Act is important for healthcare workers who handle any dependence-producing substance, dangerous dependence-producing substance or any undesirable dependence-producing substance.

The Act specifies the occupations in the health sector that may, under conditions of this Act, keep and administer such drugs.

Section 1 of the Act includes all the scheduled substances useful for the manufacture of drugs. Part 2 contains the name of dependence-producing substances, dangerous dependence-producing substances and undesirable dependence-producing substances. (Also study Government Notice No R344 of 1 March 1998 on scheduled substances.) The Prevention and Treatment of Drug-Dependency Amendment Act (No 496 of 1999) is also important.

2.21 The Environmental Conservation Act, 1989 (No 73 of 1989)

The responsibility of every employer and employee rests with the protection and conservation of the environment. It has become evident that there are many aspects with regard to health, safety and conservation that go hand in hand. The above Act falls under the jurisdiction of the Department of Environmental Affairs and provides for the efficient protection and controlled utilization of the environment and several related subjects such as pollution, waste materials, vibration, noise and shock.

2.22 The Hazardous Substances Act, 1973 (No 15 of 1973) (as amended Hazardous Substances Amendment Act, 1992 (No 53 of 1992)

Occupational health professionals, especially hygienists, have an essential task in keeping abreast of hazardous substances and the control of hazardous substances. This Act provides guidelines for the licensing and control of certain hazardous substances and conditions, and falls under the jurisdiction of the Department of Health. The substances and conditions described in this Act are divided into four groups:

Group 1: The hazardous and poisonous substances, e.g. strychnine, are included and may not be sold without a licence.

Group 2: These are mostly household substances that require proper packaging and labelling.

In terms of this Act, Group 1 and 2 substances are substances or mixtures of substances which, in the course of customary or reasonable handling or use, including ingestion, might, by reason of their toxic, corrosive, irritant, strongly sensitizing or flammable nature or because they generate pressure through decomposition, heat or other means, cause injury, ill health or death to human beings.

Group 3: This group covers electronic products capable of dangerous emissions or radiation. Registration is required and premises are inspected.

Group 4: In this section provision is made for dumping and transporting of hazardous substances such as radioactive wastes.

The aims of the Act are to provide:
- Control of substances that may cause injury or ill-health to or the death of human beings by reason of their toxic, corrosive, irritant, strongly sensitizing or flammable nature, or the generation of pressure thereby in certain circumstances
- Control of certain electronic products:
  - for the division of such substances or products into groups in relation to the degree of danger
  - for the prohibition and control of the importation, manufacture, sale, use, application, operation, modification, disposal or dumping of such substances and products
  - for matters connected therewith.

2.23 The Medicines and Related Substances Control Amendment Act, 1997 (No 90 of 1997)

This Act makes provision for manufacturing, keeping, sale of medicines and their compounds, prescribing and registration of medicines. It also prescribes the forms to be used for any application for the registration of any medicine and the particulars of the medicine, which includes the packaging of scheduled substances, labels, sealing, advertising and selling of drugs.

2.24 The Animal Slaughter, Meat and Animal Products Hygiene Act, 1967 (No 87 of 1967)

This Act falls under the Department of Agriculture and deals mainly with hygiene in abattoirs and in the handling of meat. Hygienists and other relevant healthcare professionals who inspect or are employed in industries and places where these activities as indicated in the Act, apply, must take note of the special provisions that the Act makes.

2.25 The Domestic Violence Act, 1998 (No 116 of 1998)

Domestic violence in terms of the Act means physical abuse, sexual abuse, emotional, verbal and psychological abuse, economic abuse, intimidation, harassment, stalking, damage to property, entry into the complainant's residence without consent where parties do not share the same residence, and any other controlling or abusive behaviour towards a complainant where the safety and well-being of the complainant may be in danger.

The State recognizes that domestic violence is a serious social evil; that there is a high incidence of domestic violence within South African society; that victims of domestic violence are among the most vulnerable members of society; that domestic violence takes on many forms; that acts of domestic violence may be committed in a wide range of domestic relationships; and that the remedies currently available to the victims of domestic violence have proved to be ineffective.

The purpose of this Act is to afford the victims of domestic violence maximum protection from domestic abuse that the law can provide; and to introduce measures that seek to ensure that the relevant organs of State give full effect to the provisions of this Act, and thereby to convey that the State is committed to the elimination of domestic violence.

This Act addresses, among others, the following:
- Arrest by a peace officer without a warrant
- Protection orders
- Seizure of dangerous weapons
- Prohibition of publication of certain information, as well as attendance of proceedings at court.

2.26 The Foodstuffs, Cosmetics and Disinfectants Act, 1972 (No 54 of 1972)

This Act protects the health of consumers of foodstuffs, cosmetics and disinfectants, but also concerns the employees in manufacturing industries. The Act falls under the jurisdiction of the Department of Health.

2.27 The Explosives Act, 1956 (No 26 of 1956)
The South African Police Service controls this Act. The Act regulates the manufacture, storage, sale, transport, import, export and use of explosive material (Coetzee, 1995:17).

2.28 The Nuclear Energy Act, 1982 (No 92 of 1982)
This Act falls under the jurisdiction of the Department of Mineral and Energy Affairs and it enables the Atomic Energy Commission to license and control all nuclear activities through its Nuclear Safety Board. It also makes special provision for the regulation of matters related to nuclear damage.

2.29 The Merchant Shipping Act, 1951 (No 57 of 1951)
The Department of Transport enforces this Act and it makes provision for merchant shipping and related matters. It will in all probability be amended in the near future to provide for the health of seamen (Coetzee, 1995:17).

2.30 The Human Tissue Act, 1983 (No 65 of 1983)
This Act is controlled by the Department of Health and deals with those circumstances under which tissue may be removed from a dead body. This Act concerns every occupational health professional. It may be of importance for the diagnosis of occupational diseases which could have contributed to the death of a worker.

2.31 The Mineral Act, 1991 (No 50 of 1991)
This Act falls under the jurisdiction of the Department of Mineral and Energy Affairs. The Act applies to mines and works employees, and their health and safety in these industries.

2.32 The Water Act, 1956 (No 54 of 1956)
This Act addresses the prevention of pollution, in particular by mines and factories. It falls under the jurisdiction of the Department of Water Affairs and its aim is to protect South Africa's water resources.

2.33 The Atmospheric Pollution Prevention Act, 1965 (No 45 of 1965)
The occupational health nurse may have to be responsible for activities regarding atmospheric and water pollution. It is therefore important to have some knowledge about these Acts. The above-mentioned Act falls under the Department of Health and provides guidelines on the prevention of air pollution. As far as industries are concerned, it mainly applies to pollution of the broad environment beyond the immediate working environment (Coetzee, 1995:15).

Any factory may be closed if it does not adhere to the principles laid down by the Act or if the Chief Officer is of the opinion that pollution continues without control or without being checked.

2.34 The International Health Regulations Act, 1974 (No 28 of 1974)

The aim of this Act is to apply the International Health Regulations adopted by the World Health Assembly in the RSA and to provide for incidental matters.

The Act makes provision for the control of the following:
- Notifications and epidemiological information on certain specified diseases and rapid exchange of information
- Control of ports and airports and inspections of ports, ships, airports and aircraft
- Control of vectors (Aedes aegypti)
- Disinfection, disinsecting, deratting and other sanitary operations of cargo, goods, baggage, containers or any other means of preventing vectors and disease-causing organisms to enter the country
- Health measures regarding infected or suspected infected persons
- Vaccination
- Medical examinations of persons on a ship or aircraft, train, road vehicle or any other means of transport, container or any person arriving on an international voyage
- Cargo and goods can be inspected when they are from infected areas and if they are believed to be contaminated by an agent or a disease
- Inspection of animals and disinfection of merchandise
- Postal parcels containing food, linen, bedding, wearing apparel, infectious materials, living insects and animals capable of being a vector of human diseases
- Plague, yellow fever, cholera, small pox, malaria vectors
- Health documents and vaccination documents.

2.35 Conclusion

In this chapter an attempt has been made to show the importance of the legislative control in occupational health. It is by no means a complete text, but should be seen as an introduction to a vast field of knowledge on these aspects.

To conclude, it should again be emphasized that the total practice of the occupational health professional rests on legislation. Without an in-depth knowledge of legislative control in her/his field of work, all efforts to maintain or promote health are fruitless.

2.36 List of sources

ANC. 1994. *The Reconstruction and Development Programme: A Policy Framework*. Pretoria: Government Printers.

Baker, M. & Coetzee, A. C. 1990. *Occupational Health Nursing in South Africa*. Johannesburg: Witwatersrand University Press.

Baldwin, R. & Daintith, T. 1992. *Harmonization and Hazards Regulating Workplace Health and Safety in the European Community.* London: Graham & Trotman.
Bendix, S. 1996. *Industrial Relations in the New South Africa.* Cape Town: Juta.
Bezuidenhout, M. C., Garbers, C. J. & Potgieter, S. 1998. *Managing for Healthy Labour Relations.* Pretoria: JL van Schaik.
Bokat, S. A. & Thompson, H. A. (eds.) 1994. *Occupational Safety and Health Law.* Washington: American Bar Association.
Cheadle, H., Le Roux, P. A. K., Thompson, C. & Van Niekerk, A. 1994. *Current Labour Law.* Cape Town: Juta.
Coetzee, A. M. 1995. *Managing the Health of the People at Work.* Doornfontein: Lex Patria.
Coetzee, S. & Pretorius, A. 1997. *Occupational Health Nursing in South Africa.* Florida: Occupational Health Focus.
Cole, T. A. 1980. *Law and the Individual.* London: Cassell.
De Jager, A., Wild, C. 1993. *Farm Labour. A Guide to Basic Labour Law in the Agricultural Sector.* Cape Town: Juta.
Department of Health (1). January 1996. *National Drug Policy for South Africa.* Pretoria: Department of Health.
Department of Health (2). 1996. *Report of the Committee on Occupational Health.* Pretoria: Department of Health.
De Villiers, D. 1989. *The Small Businessman's Guide to Labour Legislation.* Academia: Pretoria.
Dewar, K. 1991. *A Guide to Employment Law.* Durban: Butterworths.
Dewis, M. & Stranks, J. 1988. *Tolley's Health and Safety at Work Handbook.* Surrey: Tolley.
Du Plessis, L. en Du Plessis, A. G. 1990. *Inleiding tot die Reg.* Kaapstad: Juta.
Fraser, T. M. 1989. *The Worker at Work.* London: Taylor & Francis.
Freedman, W. 1990. *The Law and Occupational Injury, Disease, and Death.* New York: Quorum Books.
Guild, R., Ehrlich, R. I., Johnston, J. R. & Ross, M. H. 2001. *Occupational Health Practice in South African Mining Industry.* Johannesburg: The Safety Research Advisory Committee (SIMRAC).
Gunningham, N. 1984. *Safeguarding the Worker.* London: The Law Company.
Harris, C. 1984. *Occupational Health Nursing Practice.* Briston: Wright.
Habiyambere, V. 'Drugs and Prescribing.' *Africa Health*, May 1996:17–24.
Hermanus, M. 1994. *Occupational Health and Safety Legislation in Southern Africa. A Comparative Analysis.* Cape Town: University of Cape Town Labour Law Unit.
Hunt, J. W. & Strongin, P. K. 1994. *The Law of the Workplace. Rights of Employers and Employees.* Washington: The Bureau of National Affairs.
Industrial Health Research Group. March 1995. *Occupational Diseases and Compensation.* Cape Town: I H R G.
International Labour Office. 1996. *Occupational Safety and Health.* Geneva: ILO.
Jordaan, B. en Rycroft, A. 1994. *Handleiding tot die Suid-Afrikaanse Arbeidsreg.* Kaapstad: Juta.

Kemp, N. 1992. *Labour Relations Strategies: An Interactional Approach.* Cape Town: Juta.
Kloss, D. 1994. *Occupational Health Law.* 2nd edition. London: Blackwell.
Landman, A. A. en Swanepoel, J. P. A. *Arbeidswetgewing.* Pretoria: Digma.
Levy, A. 1992. *Rights at Work. A Guide for Employees.* Cape Town: Juta.
Lyster, R., Clarke, S. & Swiss, S. (eds.) 1992. *Handbook of Public Interest Law.* 2nd edition. Durban: Legal Resources Centre.
Miles, M. 1996. *A Guide to the Industrial Laws of South Africa.* Volume I and II. Johannesburg: Miles.
Mischke, C. & Garbers, C. 1994. *Safety at Work: A Guide to Occupational Health, Safety and Accident Compensation Legislation.* Cape Town: Juta.
Pera, S. A. & Van Tonder, S. (eds.) 1996. *Ethics in Nursing Practice.* Juta: Cape Town.
Rothstein, M. A. 1978. *West's Handbook Series: Occupational Safety and Health Law.* London: West.
Rothstein, M. A. 1984. *Medical Screening of Workers.* Washington: Bureau of National Affairs.
Rutherford, L. A., Todd, I. A. & Woodley, M. G. 1982. *Introduction to Law.* London: Sweet & Maxwell.
Silverston, R. & Williams, A. 1982. *The Role and Educational Needs of Occupational Health Nurses.* Kent: Duncan.
Slaney, B. (ed.) 1980. *Occupational Health Nursing.* London: Croom Helm.
South African trade Unions Library. 2003. *Industrial Relations Directory and Diary.* 28th edition. Johannesburg: Southern Publishers.
Starke, J. G. 1989. *Introduction to International Law.* London: Butterworths.
Strauss, S. A. 1992. *Legal Handbook for Nurses and Health Personnel.* 2nd edition. Cape Town: King Edward VII Trust.
Swanepoel, M. P. A. 1992. *Introduction to Labour Law.* 3rd edition. Johannesburg: Lexicon.
Thompson, C. P. 1991. *Labour Law – The Key Statutes and Regulations.* Cape Town: Juta.
University of the Witwatersrand Centre for Applied Legal Studies: Aids Law Project. 1996. Johannesburg: University of the Witwatersrand.

3 Occupational safety

S. P. Hattingh

With acknowledgement to the National Occupational Safety Association for personal assistance and literature.

3.1 Introduction

Technical advances in machinery and the associated sophisticated procedures, as well as the complicated methods and unique material that are used, demand a greater understanding of safety and awareness of the potential risk.

Comments such as those below often reflect management's attitudes: such negative attitudes in the workplace can affect the entire organization adversely.

> 'I don't have money for this safety business.'
> 'Accidents are caused by plain carelessness.'
> 'Safety is not our business.'
> 'We can't waste money on extra frills such as safety.'
> 'Safety? I'm a man, not a sissy.'
> 'Injuries are part of doing business.'
> 'Taking risks is part of the job.'
> 'Well, you must die of something, eventually!'

The safety of workers is best catered for when the greatest measure of safety precautions, of the best quality, can be provided at the lowest cost.

3.2 Learning objectives

At the end of this chapter, the reader should be able to:
- Discuss what is meant by safety
- Define the following:
  - Accident
  - Employee
  - Workplace
  - Serious physical harm
  - Injury
- Classify the various types of accidents
- Describe the factors that may cause accidents
- Discuss how epidemiology can be applied to safety
- Discuss the domino theory applied to accident causation
- Describe what is meant by the iceberg effect of an accident

Occupational health

- List the reasons why costs escalate when an accident occurs
- Discuss how the occupational health practitioner can contribute to a safety inspection
- Write short notes on the responsibility of management for safety
- Discuss the key activities for preventing accidents
- Discuss the role and functions of safety committees
- Write short notes on: Off-the-job safety
- Define the following concepts: anthropometrics, biomechanics
- Discuss how ergonomics can contribute towards safety
- Discuss the link between ergonomics and health and safety
- Describe how ergonomics may affect work activities
- Indicate how ergonomics principles may be applied at the workplace
- Outline the occupational health worker's role in ergonomics with regard to safety, health and efficiency
- Write an essay on the role and function of the National Occupational Safety Association (NOSA)
- Discuss how safety is promoted by NOSA
- Discuss how the occupational health practitioner can be actively involved in accident prevention and control
- Outline the basic provisions of the Occupational Health and Safety Act, 1993 (No 85 of 1993).

3.3 Legislative control of occupational health and safety

Health and safety legislation at work has come a long way. It could justifiably be described as the Cinderella of the legal, medical and business world. Lawyers were in many ways apathetic about it; doctors regarded occupational health as the poor relation of disease proper; and businesses only got involved on the rare (and ominous) occasion when an inspector visited. Nevertheless, occupational health and safety legislation has undergone rapid revision internationally, as well as within the context of the South African legal system.

The Machinery and Occupational Safety Act, 1983 (No 6 of 1983) has been superseded by the Occupational Health and Safety Act, 1993 (No 85 of 1993) (known as the OHSA), which came into effect in January 1994.

The major revisions contained in the Occupational Health and Safety Act relate to the right of representation of workers through their trade unions on the Advisory Council for Occupational Health and Safety. Employers are now, according to this Act, compelled to consult in good faith with employees over procedures for the nomination or election of safety representatives – the duties and powers of safety representatives are spelt out; and employers have a duty to inform employees about hazards and train them in safe working practices. It is stated in the Act that employers are required to eliminate or minimize hazards and to implement an occupational hygiene programme. The employees too have an active role to play in maintaining occupational health and safety.

In addition, the Act includes numerous provisions previously contained in the General Administrative Regulations. For example, employers are now responsible for the health and safety not only of their own employees, but also of the general public or anyone who might be affected by the activities of employees.

The OHSA thus makes provision for employee participation, representation and consultation, which limits mistrust and enhances optimal cooperation between employers and employees on health and safety issues. The OHSA facilitates joint responsibility and effective employee input and influence at all levels of the workforce. Additional changes include an increase in fines and prison sentences where negligence has been proven and, more specifically, provision for the appointment of health and safety representatives.

It must be emphasized that the law on occupational health and safety at work cannot be examined in isolation. A number of related matters must also be considered as well, such as management, insurance and loss control and social security.

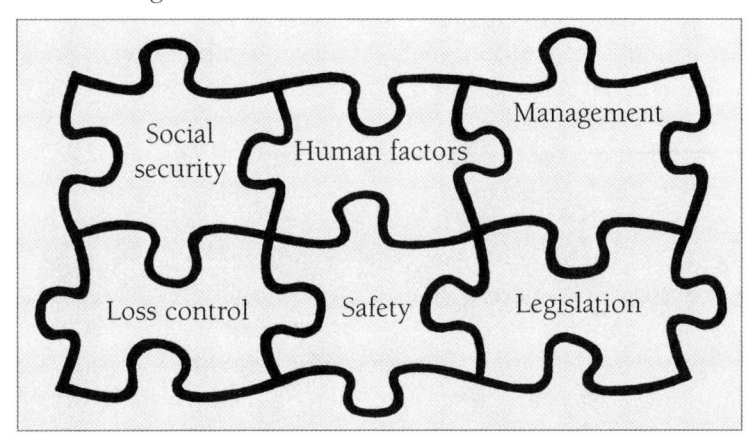

Figure 3.1 The independent nature of occupational health, safety and legislation

In addition, human factors are always present. Human relations and effective human relations management are an integral part of safety management. The level of human relations will determine the extent to which the functioning of the organization will be safe, productive, quality-conscious and cost-effective.

A more detailed discussion on the major provisions of legislation on Occupational Health and Safety is given in Chapter 2.

3.4 Definitions
3.4.1 Safety
Few people seem to agree on the actual meaning of safety and numerous authors, researchers and organizations have attempted to define or describe it. Although definitions vary in length and complexity, there is a common bond that ties them together and involves accident prevention and/or mitigation.

Safety is a condition or state of the human mind which results in the modification of human actions and perceptions, and the designing of the physical environment to reduce the possibility of hazards, thereby reducing accidents.

In the South African context of organized accident prevention, a simplified description of safety would be:

- A work environment that contains no threat to safety and health for the employee and the public at large (employer's and employee's joint responsibility in terms of the Occupational Health and Safety Act)
- A workforce with the necessary knowledge of work safety
- A workforce with a positive attitude to work safety
- A workforce that is physically and mentally healthy
- Correctly placed machinery, equipment and an environment with the maximum ergonomic benefits.

The implication of the above definition is that safety is to be understood as the prevention of accidents and the mitigation of personal injury or property damage that may result from accidents. In addition, the individual must be aware of the broad range of hazardous materials that may cause occupational diseases over a long period, and physical or psychological harm or injury to the worker. Safety also involves precautions against hazards that are not seen or recognized as such.

Safety also involves personal security. It is legitimate to be concerned for one's safety in the face of criminal activity.

Violent crimes occur in the workplace, such as murder, violence, rape, assault and robbery. There may also be property crimes such as burglary, vandalism and theft.

If all these above-mentioned factors are taken into consideration, safety appears to signify more than just accident prevention and/or mitigation. The individual is faced with an assortment of hazards and risks, and there may be a variety of consequences either to the worker or to the management if safety is neglected.

Safety can therefore be defined as it is by Bever (1984:2) as 'a dynamic or ever-changing condition in which one attempts to minimize the risk of injury, illness, death or property damage from the hazards to which one may be exposed in order to maximize success'.

Nevertheless, the importance of occupational health and safety and the responsibility for its maintenance (of both the employer and employee in equal terms) can never be overstated, as recent catastrophic tragedies worldwide, such as the Chernobyl disaster in Russia, have demonstrated. This incident illustrates that occupational health and safety go beyond the workplace and that safety precautions to conserve the environment must be considered at all times.

Figure 3.2 illustrates that safety is the foundation of optimal health. A safety-conscious individual or group is concerned about their health (physical and mental), as well as the environmental conditions that may affect health and safety. The environment is respected and protected in order to restore and maintain optimal health.

3.4.2 Employee

According to the Labour Relations Act, 1995 (No 66 of 1995), an employee is regarded as any person, except an independent contractor, who works for the State or another person and who is entitled to receive renumeration. The definition also includes any other person who in any manner assists in carrying on or conducting the business of an employer.

Occupational safety

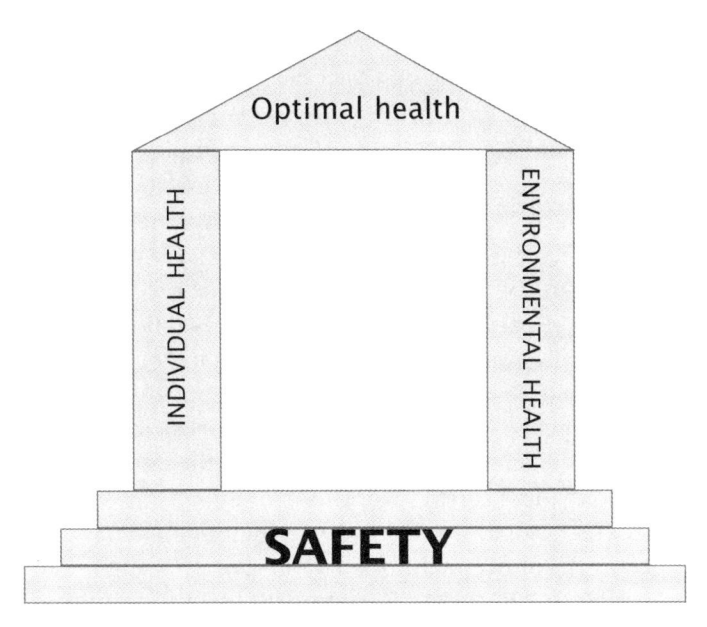

Figure 3.2 Safety as the foundation of optimal health

3.4.3 Workplace
The Labour Relations Act, 1995 (No 66 of 1995), distinguishes between the workplace in the public sector and the private sector (elsewhere).

A workplace in the public sector is a place of work as determined by the responsible Minister where a specific bargaining sector exists. The Minister of Public Service and Administration determines the definition after consultation with the Public Service Coordinating Bargaining Council.

In other areas – the private sector – a workplace is a place where employees work. If an employer conducts two or more operations which are independent of each other because of their size, function or organization, the place or places where their employees work in each independent operation, will constitute a workplace for that operation (Miles, 1996: 271).

3.4.4 Accident/incident
Different authors have numerous and varied definitions of what constitutes an accident. An accident may be defined as a sudden uncontrollable, unplanned, undesirable happening that disrupts the normal functions of persons and causes or has the potential to produce or to cause unintended injury, death or property damage and/or business interruption.

Taking all the definitions into account, an accident can be described simply as an undesired event that has caused or has the potential to cause injury/damage or to disrupt operations.

During an accident where injuries are sustained, there is physical contact or exposure of the body to some object (even another person), substance or any foreign object which is injurious.

87

Whereas an accident is unplanned and unintended, personal injury, property damage or criminal activity, such as violence, assault and robbery, are planned and deliberate.

Accidents/incidents could be said to occur because of poor or inadequate control.

The Compensation for Occupational Injuries and Diseases Act, 1993 (No 130 of 1993) defines an accident as follows: 'An accident arising out of and in the course of an employee's employment and which results in personal injury.' This definition has been analysed repeatedly in court cases and it has become accepted that the expression 'accident' is used in the popular and ordinary sense of the word as denoting an unlooked for mishap or an untoward event which is not expected or designed. 'Arising out of' means there must be a link between the accident and the work, i.e. the employee's employment must be the basis from which the accident arose. 'In the course of' means sustaining an accident whilst doing the work the employee was employed to do, at the place of employment during working hours.

Where the health professional is uncertain whether an incident would qualify as an accident as indicated in the above-mentioned definition, the employer's report must be sent to the commissioner to adjudicate the admissibility and viability of the claim.

3.4.5 Serious physical harm

Serious physical harm is harm of such a nature that it may cause permanent or prolonged impairment of the body in such a way that part of the body is functionally useless or part of the internal bodily system is inhibited in its normal performance. Serious physical harm may also cause psychological and mental damage, which may be irreversible.

3.4.6 Injury

An injury is a harmful condition sustained by the body as the result of an accident and can take any form from a less serious abrasion or bruise to a laceration or a more serious injury such as a fracture, penetration of a foreign body, burns or electric shock, all of which may or may not cause permanent deformation, malfunction and even fatal consequences.

3.5 Basic classification of accidents

In order to be able to effectively control accidents, one should be able to identify what classes of accidents form the major problem.

Eleven basic types of accidents may occur. These accidents may or may not occur independently.

3.5.1 Being struck by falling objects

These accidents occur when a person suffers a blow or impact from a moving object. For example, a person may be struck by a crane's chain, a falling rock, material or equipment falling from above; also shooting accidents, in which one is struck by a bullet.

3.5.2 Stepping on, striking against or being struck by objects
A person may sustain an injury when he/she walks into a solid object which is stationary or moving. For example, a person may collide with a moving vehicle such as a truck or forklift, machinery or equipment.

3.5.3 Caught in, on or between objects
Here different accidents are involved, but the basic principles are the same. For example, 'caught in' accidents may occur when a person's arm, finger or foot is caught between moving machinery or a floor grate or wire mesh screen.

'Caught between' accidents occur when, for example, a tie, coat or ring is caught on a moving machine part, between a fan belt and the pulley.

3.5.4 Falls from above
Falls can take a variety of forms. Falls from above are also called 'falls from a different level'. For example, a person may fall from a ladder, catwalk, stairs or scaffold.

3.5.5 Falls at ground level
Falls at ground level are also called 'falls on same level'. For example, a person may slip on a wet or oily surface, trip while walking, or fall over undesired objects lying around.

3.5.6 Strain, over-exertion or strenuous movements
These accidents occur when bad lifting habits are applied. For example, picking up objects that are too heavy, pulling or pushing something alone when it would have been better to have another person helping or to use some form of mechanical aid such as a hoist, chain hoist, lift or forklift.

3.5.7 Electric contact or exposure
Contact with electricity may result in an accident. For example, contact may be made with a live current or to improperly earthed or live equipment.

3.5.8 Exposure to or contact with harmful substances or radiation
Accidents caused by exposure may be the consequence of contact with too high or too low a temperature, as when working with dry ice, cold storage, melting iron ore, or working in an environment where one is exposed to ice or sun which may result in blindness or burns, sunstroke, etc. Exposure to radiation, toxic agents, waste products, acid burns, and so on, may also cause accidents that fall into this category.

3.5.9 Inhalation
These accidents occur when employees work with noxious substances such as gases, fumes or materials that may cause serious harm when inhaled. For example, petrol fumes, toxic wastes, asbestos, fibre, etc. may be inhaled in working environments.

3.5.10 Ingestion
Although one can choose what to eat, these accidents do occur. For example, one may inadvertently eat or drink contaminated food by eating in a contaminated environment. One may eat while working with, for example, mercury, radioactive materials or salmonella-contaminated food.

3.5.11 Absorption
The absorption through the skin of some toxic agents may result in serious illness. For example, organic phosphate products and some vector and insect sprays handled by farm workers may be absorbed through the skin.

There are other types of accidents not classified here, including accidents not classified for lack of sufficient data.

3.6 Category of injury
There are three basic categories of injuries which the occupational health practitioner may encounter. It is essential that every accident, however small, be recorded since minor accidents or injuries may serve as a warning. With a slight change in circumstances or conditions, minor accidents could result in fatal or serious injuries and property damage. The three categories of injury are:
- Minor injuries that require first aid treatment
- Injuries causing temporary total disablement (one shift or longer)
- Permanent disablement which may be partial, total or fatal.

It is important to remember that the same events that cause injuries also cause damage, disruption, etc. The prevention of these events would therefore be to the benefit of management as they all cost money.

3.7 Factors that may cause accidents
The direct causes of occupational accidents are the end product of unsafe acts and unsafe conditions in the workplace. These unsafe acts and unsafe conditions are controllable and so accidents can be prevented. Accidents do not happen independently, but as a result of a series of events which have taken place. The main factors in an accident are:
- Technical equipment
- Working environment
- Worker.

These three factors in combination are the cause of accidents. The equipment to perform a task, for example, may be inadequate or defective, or safety equipment may have been tampered with or be entirely lacking. There may also have been an omission to inspect equipment.

The working environment may be unpleasant – noise levels may be too high so that it is impossible to hear safety signals; the lighting may be too poor or too bright to see properly; the temperature may be so high or low that workers cannot function well; inadequate ventilation may result in the build-up of toxic fumes and lead to drowsiness.

The worker may also be a contributory factor in that he/she may not have received adequate training, may have little experience of the task, or his/her attitude may not be directed towards safety.

The afore-mentioned causes may lead to the performance of unsafe acts and/or the creation of unsafe conditions because they develop as the result of no or inadequate control.

All occupational accidents are either directly or indirectly attributable to human failings. People are unpredictable and make mistakes. It can be concluded therefore, that most accidents are directly or indirectly attributable to humans.

It is important to realize that the causes of accidents are a complex chain of events and to ascribe the origin of accidents to the carelessness of the worker does nothing to identify the real cause of an accident. Accidents do not just happen, they are caused by definite factors which can all be identified and eliminated. Negligence should never be given as the cause of an accident, as negligence is unacceptable behaviour engendered by some or all of the above-mentioned factors.

Accidents are classified according to their inherent characteristics, but almost every book written and each country has its own classification. The multiple classification system is perhaps one of the most useful. The essential types of accidents may be classified according to the following seven classes (according to the International Labour Organization, Geneva, 1983:13):

- Nature of injury – identifies the injury in terms of its principal physical characteristics
- Part of the body affected – directly affected part of the body is identified
- Source of the injury – the object, substance, exposure or bodily motion which directly produced or inflicted the injury is identified
- Accident type – here the event which directly resulted in the injury is identified
- Hazardous condition – the hazardous physical condition or circumstance which permitted or occasioned the occurrence of the accident is named and identified
- Agency of accident – this identifies the object, substance or premises where a previously identified hazardous condition existed
- Unsafe act – identifies the violation of a commonly accepted safe procedure.

When analysing accidents, the foregoing would give a good indication of some of the causes leading up to an accident. However, more in-depth analyses of accidents are sometimes required to identify tenacious and repetitive causes. Examples are:

- Sections of workplace concerned
- Equipment concerned
- Environmental conditions
- Attitude, training and ability of the worker.

3.7.1 Fatigue and boredom

Fatigue and boredom are important factors to consider when the causes of accidents are to be evaluated. Fatigue does increase the risk of accidents, but the relation between fatigue and accidents is complex. Tiredness may be combined with emotional problems experienced at home and it is then termed 'fatigue'. An extreme state of fatigue is termed 'exhaustion'.

The occupational health practitioner and other health practitioners must be aware of the fact that shift workers may suffer from fatigue due to the disturbance in their biorhythms. These disturbances cause workers to make more mistakes.

Fatigue affects individuals differently. Workers who are interested in their job will give all their attention to it and will not feel fatigue as much as those workers who are bored or do not like their jobs. The latter tend to become inattentive and careless at times.

Accidents are related not only to physical fatigue, but to the mental attitude of workers. By correctly placing a worker and improving the general environment one can create interest and satisfaction among workers. The worker must be recognized as a human being, given responsibility and appreciated by management; he/she should be kept informed of what goes on and be able to make proposals which are listened to; and in general he/she should be well looked after. An enjoyable social setting alleviates boredom, but it is often not recognized nor is it encouraged by management.

There are some people who like to do monotonous work, but some find it intolerable; they could cause accidents as they are intellectually not fitted to do a particularly repetitive job.

This aspect must be considered when selecting a new worker and when placing a worker.

3.7.2 Experience and inexperience

It is difficult to observe a clear-cut correlation between the length of service and experience of a worker and accident rates. There are so many contributory factors leading to accidents. One cannot assume that inexperience leads to accidents, but a new worker who is not familiar with the factory or workplace may be easily distracted and this may lead to a relative frequency of accidents among newcomers.

It is therefore essential that new and inexperienced workers go through a period of training and orientation before being given tasks that may cause accidents. Although experienced workers are not unfamiliar with their surroundings or their jobs, they take greater risks and are less careful.

If no serious accident occurs in a particular type of work for a considerable time, workers tend to become less careful because they think that the danger in what they are doing is not as serious as they have been told. They neglect safety measures until another accident occurs which shows them the importance of safety precautions.

Insufficient skill or attempting a skill beyond a person's ability is often a contributory factor in accidents. Physical limitations, for example size, strength, coordination, age and so on, may also affect performance.

3.7.3 Physiological, psychological and social conditions

Some accidents can be attributed to the worker's physiological, psychological and/or social conditions and occupational health practitioners should give special attention to these cases. If these circumstantial handicaps cannot be eliminated then other more suitable work should be selected for the worker. The importance of giving a handicapped person a chance in life cannot be stressed enough; such handicapped people are as good and loyal as workers without disadvantages.

Physiological factors which are temporary in duration may influence a worker's ability to perform an activity. Reaction time is decreased if a person is dehydrated or has low blood sugar as a result of not eating breakfast.

For the occupational health practitioner the problem is not how to exclude such persons from work, but how to employ them in a useful way despite their physical, psychological and social defects or infirmities.

Physical impairments such as poor eyesight or hearing may cause the worker to miss written or verbal instructions and this may lead to accidents.

One of the most serious social problems that may occur in the workplace is that of alcohol and/or drug abuse and dependency. There are alarming figures of people who are dependent on alcohol or drugs. The occupational health practitioner must recognize an alcohol or drug problem and should become involved in taking steps to rectify it. Early recognition is unquestionably the key to a successful alcoholism or drug control programme and leads to effective accident prevention. The Occupational Health and Safety Act, 1993 (No 85 of 1993) and other occupational legislation make special provision for workers affected by alcohol and drug abuse.

The causes of accidents can be described in terms of the epidemiological triad, as illustrated in Figure 3.3 below.

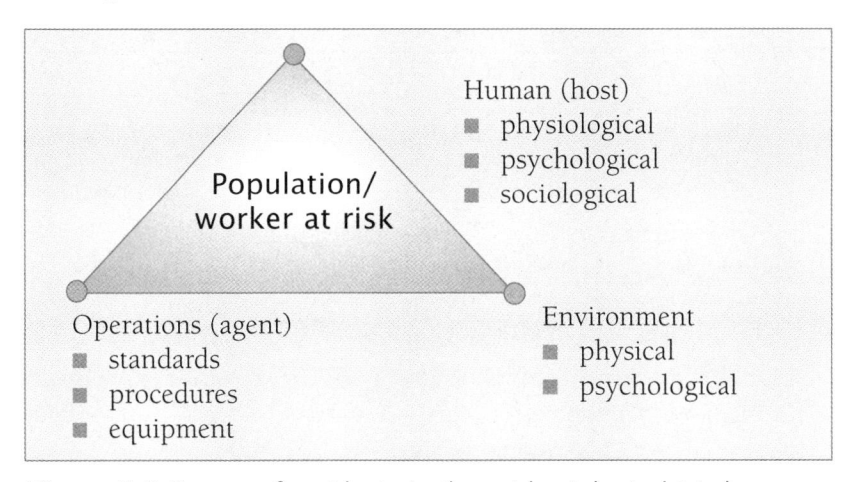

Figure 3.3 Causes of accidents in the epidemiological triad

Attitudes and emotions play an important role in determining and directing people's behaviour. The behaviour of a worker may be positive when his/her attitude is positively directed to safety, but negative if he/she acts in a reckless manner. The supervisor should be assisted in the early identification and subsequent handling of an employee with an alcohol or drug problem. For the occupational health practitioner early identification is valuable because he/she gains knowledge and can assist employees and employer in preventing loss, injury or death through accident.

If the language spoken in the workplace is not understood, safety instructions may be misinterpreted. This may result in negative attitudes and frustration on the job. To assist in this regard the South African Bureau of Standards (SABS) has evolved a system of symbolic safety signs. One of the unique features of this SABS publication is that it contains a training course to teach workers to interpret these signs.

The interaction between the human as host, the operations as agent, and the environment in which the operation takes place, indicates the close relationship between a state of well-being or illness. This also applies to safety. If one of these three factors (host, agent or environment) causes a problem, accidents may occur which may cause serious harm not only to the employees, but also to the community at large. For example, if the human host has a physical problem such as poor eyesight, the agent is affected in such a way that operations cannot be carried out, procedures cannot be followed and the safety of a worker is threatened.

This also applies to the macro-environment. If there is poor lighting, the worker (host) cannot see and procedures cannot be performed effectively, equipment cannot be used according to standards and this may result in accidents.

The identification of the relationship between the agent, environment and the worker is the first step towards a thorough description of the occurrence of injury, accident or disease. This pattern of occurrence permits identification of the population at greatest risk.

The application of sciences such as toxicology, pathology and ergonomics provides the basis for developing theories of causation. Approaches to prevention can then be tested to confirm or disprove these theories.

More recently, in view of the concept of multiple causation, the agent is seen as a part of the environment rather than as a separate factor. This results in an epidemiological dyad consisting of host and environment. In the case of occupational safety, the host is seen as the worker affected by a particular problem, such as a physical, psychological or social problem. The environment comprises all the other factors that affect the safety of the worker. (See Chapter 10 for more detailed information.)

The epidemiological dyad is depicted in Figure 3.4 below.

PERSON (WORKER)

↓ ↑

ENVIRONMENT

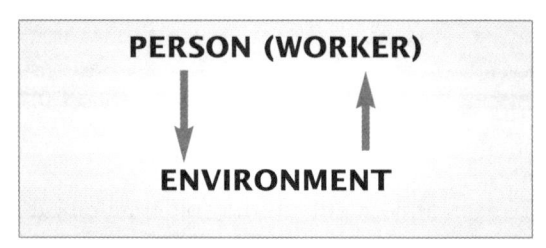

Figure 3.4 The epidemiological dyad

The characteristics of the workforce will determine populations at risk for related occupational injury or illness. It is a well-documented epidemiological fact that, due to genetic aspects, some races are more susceptible to certain diseases.

Classification of groups of employees by characteristics such as age, gender, genetic make-up, type of work and presence or absence of disability provides the healthcare worker with the data necessary for analysis of health risks, for example female assembly-line workers of child-bearing age must be protected from exposure to substances with teratogenic properties.

3.8 The domino cause and control sequence

Researchers who have studied the situational model of accident causation refer to the domino theory. According to this theory six factors are involved in the sequence of events that lead to an accident and its consequences. The injury and the consequences of the injury are the result of the cumulative action of the preceding factors.

An injury is caused by a natural culmination of a series of events or circumstances that is fixed in a logical order. One is dependent on another and one follows because of the other, constituting a sequence of events. The accident itself is one factor in the sequence of events.

Schematically, this can be described in terms of a row of dominoes, as shown in Figure 3.5 below.

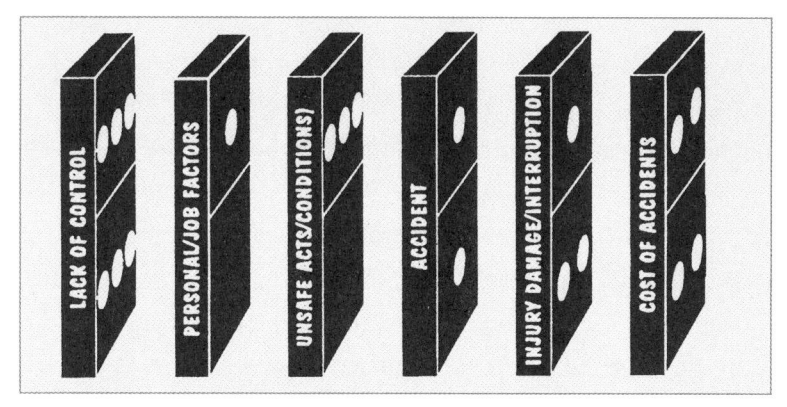

Figure 3.5 The domino sequence of events

3.8.1 Lack of control

Lack of control is defined as 'a lack of an organized system whereby all facets of an operation are subjected to control' (NOSADATA, 1991). These facets include:
- Human beings
- Environment
- Equipment
- Operations.

The problems occurring with a lack of control include the following:
- No programme of work
- No set standards
- No responsibilities or accountability delegated or assigned
- No set measurement of expected performance

- No evaluation of deficiencies
- No organized programme for correcting deficiencies.

All these problems lead to a lack of control – a lack of self-control and/or a lack of supervisory control.

Control is aimed at adhering to strict standards, such as:
- Rigid standards applied in the selection of new workers
- Rigid standards for identifying the needs for upgrading the skills of deficient workers already in employ
- Rigid standards for identifying weaknesses, such as substandard conditions in the environment, equipment, etc.
- Continuous monitoring of conditions and performances by workers
- Corrective action through information gained by audits, inspections, investigations and reports.

Once the programme needs have been identified and the necessary standards or procedures drawn up, supervisors should be appointed as responsible for clearly defined control activities. This appointment is done in terms of the current occupational legislation.

3.8.2 Personal/job factors

Personal and job factors are the human, environmental, mechanical, equipment, procedural and standards inadequacies which directly or indirectly cause the creation of unsafe conditions.

3.8.2.1 Personal factors

Personal factors are seen as anything lacking in a person which could cause him/her to perform an unsafe act or create an unsafe condition. These factors include lack of knowledge and/or skill, physical and/or mental defects and improper attitude. In the modern management system, taking note of these defects is not enough. The question that should be asked is WHY a person with the afore-mentioned defects is selected, placed or allowed to operate without supervision in any work situation. The answer to this question lies in the weaknesses of the management system where there is a lack of specification; either task or job specification and/or worker specification.

Human weaknesses can be controlled through the following measures:
- Proper interviewing of prospective workers
- Checking work records
- Medical examination
- Proper induction training
- Task training with formalized follow-up
- Retraining of older workers who have not kept up with new technology in the workplace
- Regular medical check-ups.

Occupational safety

3.8.2.2 Work or job-related factors
Work or job-related factors may include the following:
- Anything lacking in the environment with regard to machines, equipment, etc. which could cause an unsafe act to be committed or an unsafe condition to be created
- Lack of task or job procedures
- Lack of performance inspections
- Lack of reporting, investigations, training, maintenance, etc.
- Lack of standards in housekeeping, layout, machine safeguarding, personal protective equipment, etc.

In many well-run companies all the essential programmes for upgrading the quality of the workers and the work-related aspects of an operation already exist. All that is needed is to put this into practice through the following measures:
- Setting audits to comply to standards
- Setting up an action plan to introduce controls of the conditions in the environment and the work quality
- Evaluating personal needs through identifying skill requirements, training requirements, and medical and welfare requirements
- Identifying critical areas and/or tasks
- Defining and assigning responsibilities and accountability.

3.8.3 Unsafe acts/conditions
The concept unsafe acts/conditions is defined as any deviation from standards and/or procedures.

Deviations from standards and/or procedures are caused by:
- Lack of training
- Lack of discipline
- Lack of control, such as job observation and spot checks
- No or inadequate procedures or standards
- Ignorance or uninformed workers.

Unsafe conditions develop as a result of:
- Natural deterioration of for example equipment
- Deterioration due to abuse
- Poor design and planning
- No standards relating to physical conditions, machinery, equipment and tools.

The Occupational Health and Safety Act, 1993 is very specific about what standards should be maintained regarding machinery, safeguarding, workplace, etc.

In order to prevent unsafe acts/conditions, the following should be done:
- Training of all workers
- Establishing a standards (steering) committee
- Setting inspecting standards

- Establishing responsibilities and accountability
- Introducing inspection and spot checking
- Liaising between all departments, such as health, operating, engineering, personnel, etc.

3.8.4 Accident
An accident is defined as an undesired event that has caused or has the potential to cause injury, damage and disruption of operations.

Most people associate the term 'accident' with injury. If no serious injury occurs, then they regard it as 'nothing serious'. In the context of loss control, every unplanned event that adversely affects the operation is an accident. Even if the event (accident) does not show a potential to adversely affect an operation, it must be borne in mind that the existence of factors that combine to cause accidents could cause further accidents, which could adversely affect the operation.

The control of accidents includes the following:
- Education of all workers in the interpretation of the concept 'accident'
- Proper reporting of all 'accidents'
- Proper investigation of all 'accidents'
- Proper follow-up to effect remedial action
- A committee to consider all reports and investigations as legally required.

3.8.5 Injury/damage/interruption
Injury, damage or interruption is defined by NOSADATA, 1991 as any adverse effects or potential adverse effects of accidents, which could be minor, serious or catastrophic. Many workers do not report an accident unless it is perceived to be serious. If there are no visible signs of injury (e.g. blood) the accident must still be reported – the psychological or long-term physical effects of an injury that is not serious should be taken into account.

It is important that all injuries, however small, are reported for the following reasons:
- Complications may arise days, months or even years after an accident for which a person could have received timeous treatment or compensation if it was reported at the time of the incident.
- Acceptance of the case in the event of complications, by the Compensation Commissioner, is required for compensation purposes.
- Investigation is required of the incident which could, for example, have led to corrective measures to prevent further injury or accidents from happening.

3.8.6 The costs of accidents – insured/uninsured
Much has been written about the cost of accidents in the workplace, but few attempts have been made to assess them accurately.

Occupational injuries and fatalities should be controlled like all other production costs and are a part of a company's operating costs, for example raw materials, parts and labour.

It is important to calculate the costs arising from compensation for injuries as accurately as possible.

Categories of injuries include:
- *Medical-only cases*, which need first-aid treatment and take the form of cuts, scratches, bruises and minor strains that do not keep the injured worker off the job but for which medical expenses are incurred. It is estimated that these cases account for 67 per cent of all industrial injuries and only for seven per cent of the total cost of industrial injuries.
- *Temporary total disabilities*, which cause the worker to temporarily stay off the job. No permanent disability is incurred but the worker is prevented from performing his/her normal duties. These may be eye injuries, lacerations, strains, broken bones, effects of gas inhalation, skin rashes, and so on.

It is estimated that this category accounts for 25 per cent of all injuries, but for 30 per cent of the total cost.
- *Permanent partial disabilities*, which may result in the worker staying off the job for a while and leaving some permanent damage to the injured worker's body, such as amputation. These cases account for only 6 per cent of all injuries, but for 50 per cent or more of the total costs.
- *Permanent total disability* is an injury that prevents the worker from ever being gainfully employed again, for example loss of sight and limbs or mental disability such as brain damage. These accidents account for an estimated 4 per cent of the total costs.
- *Fatalities*, which result in the death of a worker at any time subsequent to the accident, but as a result of an accident account for an estimated 7 per cent of the total cost.

3.9 Insured and uninsured costs
The costs of an accident may be divided into two parts:
1 Insured costs
2 Uninsured costs.

This can be understood in terms of an 'iceberg' metaphor, as illustrated in Figure 3.6 on page 100.

In Figure 3.6, the insured costs are those above the waterline that are paid out to the company or worker. The uninsured costs are those under the waterline: these are hidden costs and are not covered by insurance. These hidden costs must be carried by the employer or the employee. These costs are up to 50 times greater than insured costs. This is reflected in the accident ratio as given by NOSA.

Out of every one disabling injury there are ten less serious injuries which are mostly not reported as they are seen as unimportant.

Occupational health

The real costs of accidents can be measured and controlled

Insured costs
- Medical
- Compensation

5 TO 50 UNINSURED PROPERTY DAMAGE COSTS

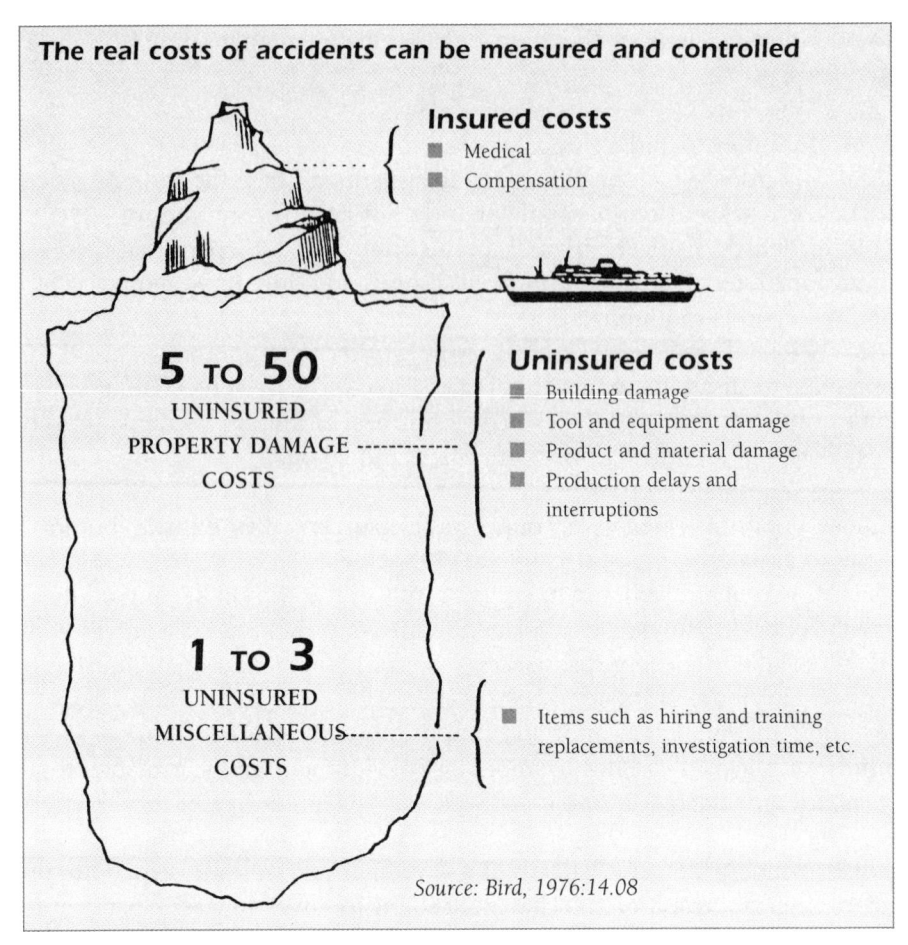

Uninsured costs
- Building damage
- Tool and equipment damage
- Product and material damage
- Production delays and interruptions

1 TO 3 UNINSURED MISCELLANEOUS COSTS

- Items such as hiring and training replacements, investigation time, etc.

Source: Bird, 1976:14.08

Figure 3.6 The 'iceberg' effect

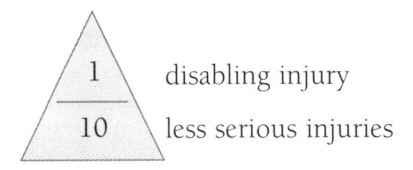

1 disabling injury
10 less serious injuries

It is estimated that out of every one disabling injury, there are 30 cases of property damage. These are hidden costs and not covered by insurance and may cause delays and/or disruptions.

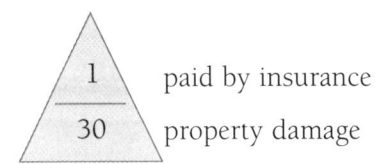

1 paid by insurance
30 property damage

For every one disabling injury, there are 600 accidents or incidents with the potential to damage and/or to disrupt. These potential accidents are also called near-miss accidents.

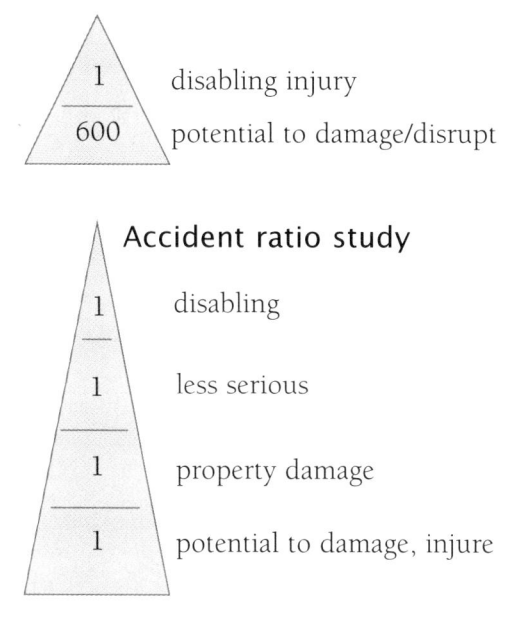

```
    /\
   /1 \      disabling injury
  /----\
 / 600  \    potential to damage/disrupt
/_____\
```

Accident ratio study

```
    /\
   /1 \      disabling
   ----
   /1  \     less serious
   ------
   /  1  \   property damage
   --------
   /   1   \ potential to damage, injure
```

The money paid out by the Compensation Commissioner is only a fraction of the total cost of an accident.

It is essential for the occupational health worker to realize that there are uninsured 'hidden costs' (those under the waterline) which are paid by the employer him-/herself and eventually felt by the community or country as a whole.

These uninsured or 'hidden costs' may take the form of:
- Time lost by workers helping, watching, being curious or sympathizing with the injured worker
- Time lost through injury to the worker
- Time lost by foremen, supervisors and any other team members involved in investigating the accident to assist the injured worker; arranging for the injured employee's production to be continued by another worker
- Time lost to training and selecting a new or other worker to take over the job
- Writing accident reports or other official reports
- Attending meetings or hearings on the case
- Obsolescence of the machine before the accepted depreciated time
- Decreased output when the employee returns to work and cannot continue with his/her activities because of the injury
- Overtime may have to be worked in order to make up for the production loss
- First-aid staff spending time in treating the accident rather than working on accident prevention and other health matters
- Negligence of other work because of time spent on discussion of the accident

- Lowered morale and consequences of the excitement of the workers due to the accident: strikes or unhappiness may occur which may result in further loss
- Making up of salary of the injured worker where the Compensation Commissioner does not pay
- Incidental cost due to interference with production, failure to fulfil orders on time, loss of bonuses, payment of forfeits and other similar results
- Cost to employer under employee welfare and benefit systems
- Cost due to the loss of profit on the injured worker's productivity and on idle machines
- Overhead cost per injured employee – the expense of light, health, rent and other items while the injured worker is non-productive.

These hidden costs are unfortunately not reflected in accounting systems and like all icebergs, the mass below the surface is the most dangerous, especially when we consider what these hidden costs could add up to.

The insured costs constitute only half of the total cost of an accident. The insured costs partly covered by insurance are:
- Transportation to hospital
- Medical care
- Hospitalization
- Rehabilitation
- Compensation.

Medical aids also have their limits, and the worker or employer has to pay the rest. Other insured costs are sometimes covered by commercial insurers and could cover, to a certain extent:
- Damage to property
- Fire losses
- Loss of profits due to some specified factors
- Extra compensation with specified or state benefits.

These insurance premiums are very expensive and cannot cover all the profits lost by the employer. They are a high price to pay for inadequate safety precautions.

Taking all these aspects into account, loss of life is something which cannot be measured or expressed in monetary terms.

3.10 Accident prevention

When an accident occurs the entire plant is affected. An accident involves the workers, machines and materials. For this reason safe working conditions and procedures are of vital importance.

There is always a sequence of events that may lead to an accident. It is the interplay of these events or factors that may produce an accident and any alteration in this sequence or elimination of one of the factors in the accident chain will usually prevent an accident.

If each domino in a series is within striking distance of the next one, all the dominoes will fall if the first one is knocked over. But if one is removed, the subsequent dominoes will remain standing and so the accident will not take place.

This implies that accident prevention is simply the removal of one of these faulty factors.

Accident prevention is not so simple but comprises a complex series of events.

The various means generally used at present to promote industrial safety are, according to the International Labour Organization, Geneva (1983:14–15), the following:

Regulations. These may include mandatory prescriptions concerning matters such as working conditions, maintenance, machine guarding, testing, duties of employers or employees, training, medical supervision and examination, and first aid.

Standardization. This includes laying down official, semi-official or unofficial standards concerning the safe construction of certain types of industrial equipment, safe and hygienic practices, personal protective devices, set practices.

Inspection. Inspection is understood to mean that there may be a certain amount of enforcement of mandatory regulations concerning procedures performed, and the safety of machines or environment.

During a safety inspection the following major categories of conditions and items should be considered:
- Personal protective equipment and clothing, such as eye protection, masks, safety shoes, respirators, and so on, which should be worn at all times and should be clean, well-fitting and of a high quality (personal protective equipment should protect to the maximum and cost should be the least concern when buying this equipment)
- Machinery and parts thereof, such as shields and guards of grinders, chain-saws, pulleys, presses, drills and cutters
- Fire-fighting equipment, such as extinguishers, hoses, hydrants, sprinkler systems and fire alarms
- Vehicles such as motor cars, trucks, forklifts, cranes and railroad equipment
- Structured openings and manholes, such as shafts, pits, floor openings, trenches, drains and storm pipes
- Electrical equipment and conductors: their use, handling and maintenance; lockout systems, cables, wires, switch boxes and lamps
- Hand tools, such as hammers, power tools, screwdrivers, sledges and files
- Pressurized equipment, such as boilers, pots, tanks, pipes and hoses
- Containers, such as gas cylinders, refuse bins and containers, barrels, solvents, acids and fuel tanks
- Hazardous materials, such as flammables, explosives, gases, acids and other toxic materials
- Waste, such as chemical, biological, solid or radiated waste
- Atmospheric conditions, such as presence of dust, gases, fumes, vapours, radiation; also, illumination, noise level and oxygen flow
- Building and construction, such as floors, windows, air-conditioning, stairs, roof, walls, rooms, showers, lockers and bathrooms

- Storage, such as rooms, types of material stored together, ventilation and emergency exits
- Elevators, escalators, lifts, crane cables, controls and safety devices
- Conductors for lightning
- Technical research, which includes matters such as investigation of properties by authorities and the setting of standards for what constitutes harmful materials, the study of machine guards and other safety devices, the testing and inspecting of personal protective equipment, the investigation of methods to prevent fires, explosions, inhalation of gas and fumes and other issues related to prevention
- Medical and nursing research – in the field of occupational health, includes the examination of the physiological and pathological effects of environmental and technology factors on workers and the physical circumstances which are conducive to accidents
- Psychological research is performed to investigate the psychological patterns conducive to accidents, how the physical environment contributes to morale, for instance, and how low morale in turn contributes to accidents occurring in the workplace
- Statistical research, which is done to ascertain what kind of accident occurs, in what numbers and to which departments and people, and in what particular operations, as well as statistics of different diseases that may occur in the specific workplace
- Education and training are an important and integral part of accident prevention, and workers should be instructed in the safe use of tools, materials and equipment
- Safety procedures should be taught in all courses, not only those in which machine use is taught; every person should be educated in safety especially in road safety and home safety
- Safety should be strictly enforced and learned as a daily routine, not only practised at work. It should become a firm habit at home, work or play
- Training – all instructors should instruct workers, and especially new workers, on safety matters
- Persuasion – there are various methods of publicity and there should be appeals to develop 'safety-mindedness'
- Insurance – there should be provision of financial incentives to promote accident prevention in the form of reductions on premiums payable by factories, for example, where safety measures of a high standard are in place.

Each person should take personal responsibility for implementing safety measures. These can also be any measures taken to make sure that no accident will occur which can cause injury or death to fellow workers. The people who should be most conscious and aware of safety include:
- Legislators
- Government bodies, technologists
- Physicians
- Occupational health practitioners

- Hygienists
- Statisticians.

3.11 Accident prevention programmes

The primary aim of any occupational health and safety programme is the prevention of accidents and illness; the principal weapon is knowledge. Only accurate knowledge of the risks and adequate training in handling them can enable workers to adopt appropriate behaviour in a hazardous working environment. Indeed, the identification of the hazards, a knowledge of the technical and procedural means to control them and the capacity to redesign work processes to exclude the dangers through engineering revision are the main tools for creating a safe working environment.

Successful accident prevention programmes depend on three basic principles:
1. Leadership by the employer
2. Safe work habits and practices by employees
3. Safe and healthy working environment and conditions.

An absence of any of these three principles may cause accidents on the job which may result in injuries, property damage, loss of production, escalation of costs, loss of worker morale and even death.

The responsibility for occupational safety and health must be willingly accepted by employers and employees alike and forms an integral part of the job of the occupational health practitioner.

Together, employers and employees should establish safety procedures and policies, stimulate awareness of safety in others and the environment, and show an interest in providing safe and healthy working conditions.

The responsibility for safe working conditions rests on the employer and that for safe work on the worker him-/herself. The worker must develop and follow safe working habits at all times and must use safeguards and protective equipment properly. He/she should always be mindful of his/her fellow workers' safety.

Without the active and positive cooperation, interest and acceptance of responsibility for safety by management, an accident prevention programme will fail.

3.12 Leadership by the employer

Representatives of both line and staff management must have a positive attitude and interest in safety.

The front-line supervisor is the person who deals most directly with the employee and thus bears the greatest responsibility for the implementation of safety and health matters. He/she should be given the appropriate authority, assistance and support to fulfil his/her responsibilities and should be adequately trained in safety procedures.

Top management cannot delegate responsibility in accident prevention and safety as they are the people who must establish safety policies, stimulate awareness of safety and establish measures to promote safe and healthy conditions in the workplace.

Occupational health

Management has certain legal responsibilities towards its employees. The following Acts in particular keep management responsible for its actions:
- The Occupational Health and Safety Act, 1993 (No 85 of 1993)
- Occupational Diseases in Mines and Works Amendment Act, 1993 (No 208 of 1993)
- Compensation for Occupational Injuries and Diseases Act, 1993 (No 130 of 1993)
- The Basic Conditions of Employment Act, 1983 (No 3 of 1983)
- Mine Health and Safety Act, 1997 (No 29 of 1996).

The moral and ethical responsibility of management is directed not only towards the workers, but also towards their families and to the public as a whole.

3.13 Safe work habits and practices by employees

Several factors may play a major role in the safe performance of the worker's activity:
- An understanding of the difficulty of the activity – risks and hazards
- Ability level of a worker – skill and knowledge
- State of mind and physical state of a worker
- Environmental factors.

Understanding the difficulty of the activity – risks and hazards

This is essential to perform any given task. It also involves the understanding of the risks associated with the task. Any task has its risks and benefits but inadequate knowledge may lead to failure to recognize and evaluate the risks or hazards associated with it.

Ability level of a worker – skill and knowledge

Skill is essential for most tasks performed by a worker. Insufficient skill or knowledge or attempts to use a skill beyond one's ken often contribute to accidents.

There are also physical limitations that have to be considered when performing a task. Ergonomic factors must be taken into account. The physically handicapped or the older worker's limitations when performing a task must especially be considered, for example, hearing, vision, mobility, reaction time and so on can limit performances. Without adequate skill and knowledge one cannot perform safely. Fatigue and boredom must be prevented. The environment must be such that an enjoyable social setting can alleviate boredom. Boredom is sometimes the cause of a serious accident and not 'playing with the machine' as the findings of accident investigations sometimes state.

State of mind and physical state of a worker

There is definite proof that physiological, sociological and psychological factors influence the performance and the state of mind of workers. These factors are in constant flux and can be a threat to safety.

Alcohol abuse and social problems go hand in hand with accidents. Often those who are termed 'accident prone' are people whose attitudes, emotions and personal lives are not in order.

Attitude and emotions play an important role in the overall behaviour of a person, and also influence his/her way of thinking about safety. Habits develop because of attitudes, which may be positive or negative, and emotional states change. Bad habits are not easily broken or changed. Strong emotions may sometimes disrupt normal behaviour patterns, causing an individual who normally acts safely to act in a reckless manner, for example not wearing safety attire.

There are some aspects of behaviour to be considered which may also contribute to unsafe acts:

Time and safety. One of the most common reasons for taking risks at work is to save time – time for more leisure, time to enable one to do the job faster, to impress people such as supervisors, to enable one to earn a bonus or more money, to win a competition or to prove something. This wish to save time often results in an unsafe act.

Effort and safety. This means to 'take the easy way out'. The safe way of doing the job may be demanding or seen as an effort either physically or mentally. A negative attitude to safety may result in an unsafe act where the worker takes a short cut.

Group acceptance and safety. Workers are often influenced by the negative attitude of the group and, not wishing to be outcasts, they join the group and ignore their own fears. Sometimes the consequences are dire. Often, therefore, it is new employees who are most at risk.

3.14 Key activities for preventing accidents

3.14.1 Engineering revision

This includes improvements to the guarding of machines and tools in the working environment by qualified and authorized persons only. It also involves revision of work processes and procedures through participation of all concerned and with the consent of management.

3.14.2 Education and training

There should be education and training for all people in the work situation – whether they are management, supervisors or workers.

Proper job description leads to proper job instruction techniques and to the improvement of skills and therefore to the improvement of relationships and attitudes. General safety education should be included in the training and education programme of all employees so as to change or reinforce attitudes to be positively inclined towards safety.

Staff training is an essential part of establishing and maintaining safe working conditions and habits. All employees must, in accordance with the Occupational Health and Safety Act, be informed of the hazards in their working environment and the proper procedures to adopt in order to eliminate or to minimize risk. This can only be achieved with the development of expertise through the support of training institutions, direct in-service training and the integration of training into vocational, supervisory and management training programmes, including the development of appropriate training material and methods for the various target groups. Special attention must be given to the principles defined by the international standards on occupational health.

In many cases, the simple descriptions of safe work habits and health matters are not enough. Procedures need to be demonstrated and practised during training sessions. In many instances, employees must prove that they can master a procedure without making mistakes, before they are allowed to work even under supervision. Some people need to be drilled and 'overlearnt' in order for their actions to become automatic. Management follow-up and reports from supervisors are essential to drive home the message that safety on the job is a shared concern. Properly trained and motivated individuals are less likely to skip security precautions on the job due to haste or indifference. They make a valuable and more positive contribution to the overall productivity of the organization.

Staff training is only effective if it is an ongoing process. Healthcare workers and trainers must keep themselves up to date on safety procedures. Communication channels linking workers, employers and government are becoming a reality in South Africa with computerization. International channels can be reached with the minimum effort and know-how to get information. In many cases, unions and staff representatives convey health and safety information to workers in the various sectors.

3.14.3 Employment practice
The occupational health practitioner's role in the selection of personnel will depend on his/her skill and ability to make an assessment of both the physical and mental ability of the worker and his/her position and attitude as an employee.

Selection of personnel depends on the physical and mental demands of the job, whether it is a new employee or one who has been moved from one job to another and has to be trained to perform a new job.

3.14.4 Setting an example
Safety rules do not exclude anyone – they apply to the occupational practitioner as well. The occupational practitioner must therefore set an example for all to see by obeying safety rules.

3.14.5 Enthusiasm
Enthusiasm, like negativism, is an infectious process – people are affected by it. An enthusiastic leader is one who acknowledges the safety rules and safety achievements of others.

3.14.6 Enforcement
This is the last resort if all else fails in order to enforce discipline on those who break safety rules. This must be applied very carefully, however, and only by those with authority.

Safety posters are an important aspect in accident prevention and should be displayed on the walls at strategic places. These posters remind workers about possible dangers. In this way, the workforce is kept 'safety conscious' at all times.

Surveillance of the workplace allows identification of the factors that could adversely affect the health and safety of the worker. Regular assessment and monitoring of workers' habits, abilities and knowledge, as well as the environment in which the work is conducted, ensures that the workplace is well maintained and properly equipped, that employees use the collective and personal protective equipment provided and that safe work practices are consistently adopted.

Technical and procedural controls can also be reviewed periodically to ensure that they actually provide the necessary protection. Ideally, worksite surveillance should pool the experience, observation and expertise of the workers, technical personnel and trained occupational health and safety personnel, as well as management, so that practical improvements may result.

3.15 Off-the-job safety

Statistics have recently revealed a shocking number of accidents that are not related to the workplace. NOSA states that the ratio of off-the-job accidents can be as high as ten to one compared to those happening in the workplace. This may result in many lost manhours. Off-the-job accident statistics are very difficult to obtain, but by being observant the occupational health practitioner can detect evidence of the occurrence of such accidents.

An analysis of off-the-job accidents cannot be conclusive.

The following areas are the most likely for off-the-job accidents:
- Assaults – these may occur on the way home from work, at work or anywhere else
- Sport – injuries are often a result of unfitness
- Recreation – accidents may take various forms; a person's own self-management should act as a guideline as to whether recreational activities are safe, may lead to injury, and whether they are suited to one's physical build, age and ability
- Entertainment – for example noise levels that may impair hearing
- Home workshop – such accidents happen in the workshop at home and can be in the line of building, metalwork or woodwork, electronic and mechanical work
- Residence, garden – for example tools, pesticides, swimming-pools. The safety measures taken in the workplace should be maintained in the home. All electrical installations in the home should conform to wiring regulations and standards. Only qualified people should modify or repair electrical equipment.

Other potentially hazardous equipment in the home should be handled, stored and treated correctly. The following are potential hazards:
- Lawn-mowers
- Chemicals
- Ladders
- Tools

- Gas cylinders
- Flammables such as petrol, oil, etc.
- Fire arms.

3.16 The health and safety of the healthcare worker

Occupational healthcare and safety personnel are particularly exposed to a variety of hazards in the workplace. Yet health workers are often not seen as workers in need of protection and their health and safety are often disregarded. With their knowledge of hygienic practices, prevention of injury and disease control, they are somehow considered as being safe from harm. The potential health hazards in this sector are in fact numerous and varied. Physically, health and safety workers are exposed to infectious disease, injuries, musculo-skeletal problems, for example, due to bad posture, contact with infectious agents (e.g. bacteria) physical or chemical agents and psychosocial problems, for example those caused by stress.

In hospitals and clinics the design is to protect the patients, not the workers and what is more, existing safety and health legislation excludes certain categories of workers, such as public servants or the self-employed, both of whom are heavily represented in the medical field.

Many industries and other workplaces do give attention to the health and safety of medical and nursing staff and monitor their health on a regular basis, particularly when personnel are exposed to special hazards such as radiation, carcinogens or HIV infection. The World Health Organization publishes extensive documents on the risks faced by medical and related workers. It also issues guidelines and recommends safety procedures to minimize the risks. In collaboration, the International Labour Organization (ILO) publishes the *Employment and conditions of work in health and medical services*, which contains a condensed, but fairly comprehensive study of the risk factors for healthcare workers. Much wider consideration of such international and national information should be encouraged.

Attention must be given to the health and safety of the health and safety personnel with specific attention to the following:
- Immunization of medical workers against infectious diseases (for example hepatitis A and B, typhoid, diphtheria, polio)
- Forbidding pregnant workers to work in areas where they are exposed to ionizing radiation, infectious diseases and certain chemicals
- Working conditions, hours of work and stressful work should be considered and specific measures must be taken to prevent stress and burnout; in many instances it may be necessary to introduce stress counselling, and quality of working-life programmes to help medical and health-related workers to cope with the strain of the job.

3.17 Ergonomics

The application of ergonomic principles has benefits for the worker as well as the industry in a number of ways. Ergonomics is related to health, safety and efficiency and affects all work activities whether simple or complicated. It plays an important and essential role in accident prevention, the promotion of health and the prevention of ill health. The employer as well as the employee must gain a better understanding of the principles of ergonomics. A simple phrase to remember is: whatever is unsafe, is not ergonomic!

3.17.1 Definition

Ergonomics is more than merely fitting the operator to the machine. It is a comprehensive study of the relation between the person, the work and the environment in which this work is done. Ergonomics is concerned with design: work should be designed to match the person and his/her machine and to achieve optimal adjustment between the person and his/her work environment so that the health and ability of the person is enhanced. It is concerned with the detailed study of human attributes, abilities and limitations as applied to the living and working environment. The purpose of ergonomics is to ensure that a person's abilities are utilized efficiently and that the equipment being used will not endanger his/her health or safety.

Ergonomics also refers to the interaction between the workplace, job practices, equipment and the employee's physical, psychological and social well-being. It is closely connected to safety – if the ergonomic design of the workplace is satisfactory, then the worker will work and apply safety measures and safety in the workplace will be maintained. This will lead to work satisfaction among operators, a goal to be achieved by any standards of good management.

Ergonomic interventions in the workplace lead not only to worker satisfaction, but also to increased productivity, minimum work-related morbidity and job turnover. Work stoppages and maintenance problems are also limited if ergonomic factors are considered.

3.17.2 Ergonomics in the practical situation

It is only by a thorough examination and inspection of the work practices, the workplace layout and the environment in which the work is conducted, that a clear understanding of the ergonomic principles can be considered. By applying the key ergonomic principles in a systematic and logical way, accidents and ill health can be prevented and worker morale, productivity, quality of work, worker participation and enthusiasm can be enhanced.

Ergonomic planning begins at the design and planning stage of any industry. By taking ergonomic principles into account, money, time and effort are saved at a later stage when deficiencies would otherwise have to be corrected.

Where a workplace already exists and procedures are already in operation, correction of problems (some of which may be minor modifications but with major positive results) should be implemented.

Ergonomics applies to all work-related activities conducted and planned. Matters for consideration include:

- Good design of work systems, tools, equipment and furniture to lessen the likelihood of accidents and strains
- Taking into account anatomical and physical limitations when designing, building, installing or planning new machinery

- Taking into account the repetitive or static nature of the work and aiming to avoid long sessions
- Proper design of machine interfaces of control rooms and operating procedures to reduce the chance of human error
- Introduction of computers and visual display units in the industry
- Visual abilities and optimal acuity, ventilation provision of articles and machinery that are safe and without health risks
- Avoidance of work arrangements that do not fit the worker's capability and interests
- Surfaces in the work area, for example corridors, doorways, slopes and ramps
- Anthropometric measurements such as weight, height, gender differences and the effect of posture and load size.

Inherent in the consideration of the above issues is the question of fatigue and the effects of stress on the health and safety, not only of a particular worker but on all the other workers. These aspects are addressed in depth by recent research. Examples are:
- Controls and devices – sizes, positions, colours used, placements in relation to the frequency or urgency of use
- Complexity of the operation or work to be conducted – the capacity of the human being to understand, absorb, remember, react and to act safely on multiple sources of information
- Human factors have been found to have adverse effects on the perception and efficiency of the work conducted – and making things easy and comfortable for a worker may also cause boredom and thus carelessness.

It can be seen from the examples given above that ergonomics involves not only the consideration of physical aspects such as overstraining of the musculo-skeletal or cardiovascular systems, but also psychological aspects such as sensory (vision, hearing, touching, smelling) or any other peripheral sensation. Neglecting these issues could result in people taking the wrong decisions and may cause stress in the long run affecting health, sometimes with severe consequences.

Knowledge of shift work times, rest pauses and basic human needs are essential as ignorance of these basic aspects may cause disturbed thinking, fatigue, serious errors and other physical, psychological and social ills.

3.17.3 Anthropometrics
Anthropometrics is concerned with the dimensions of the human body and its variations. The human body differs from person to person and it is therefore not economically possible to take each variation into account whenever machines are designed or related work environments are planned. An acceptable norm is derived from the majority and from that an ergonomic design is developed. To accommodate the exceptions, special arrangements usually have to be made.

3.17.4 Biomechanics
This is the discipline dedicated to the study of the human body as a structure that can function properly only within the confines of both the laws of Newtonian mechanics

and the biological laws of life. Biomechanics relates to push, pull or support powers that can be exerted under varying conditions.

3.17.5 Ergonomics and accidents
The occurrence of accidents is minimized through the application of ergonomic principles already outlined on the person–machine system.

Wherever the prevalence and incidence rates of accidents are high or show signs of increasing, an investigation should be done. Information that should be gathered includes:
- Job descriptions and demands on operators
- Pre-employment data on medical examinations
- Previous medical history
- Epidemiological data on the prevalence of work-related symptoms
- Records of injuries, absence, sick-leave job turnover
- Accident data
- Environmental data
- Productivity data
- Occupational history of workers' qualifications, training and experience
- Workload.

3.17.6 Delayed hazards
The effects of accumulated toxins, chronic radiation overdosage, long-term effects of noise, chronic and long-term visual strain, cumulative musculo-skeletal pathology and other conditions, are not recognized immediately, but may only appear after a number of days, weeks, or years. Some effects are barely distinguishable from the normal aging process. Epidemiological studies have revealed the cumulative effect of physical trauma or stresses.

These include injuries such as vibration, white finger, tendosynovitis, cervical spondylosis, and various forms of back injuries and strain. Repetitive delayed discomfort is associated with a high rate of delayed injury.

Psychological stressors such as noise, highly responsible jobs, dangerous work or tasks such as working in mines, diving, working at high altitude or heights, and working in emergency situations (e.g. police, fire, paramedics), may cause burnout, which in severe cases may lead to post-traumatic stress syndrome.

The question of overcrowding in homes, industries and in society also concerns the ergonomist. With these social factors come exploitation and pollution. Very few studies have been conducted to establish the acceptable levels of tolerance for space limitations, lack of privacy and degree of sophistication, frequency of personal contact, and exposure to disease in what is considered as severe overcrowding.

If the consequences of the physical, psychological and social deficiencies in the workplace and in society are considered, then any contribution in the field of ergonomics, however small, may have major effects on the prevention of chronic illness and disability.

3.17.7 Ergonomic self-assessment by the worker

Workers who evaluate their own workplaces may contribute to valuable ergonomic changes that may benefit both the employee and the employer. If the ergonomic design of the workplace is ergonomically more satisfactory and therefore more comfortable for the worker, he/she can be much more efficient and productive in his/her work. Changes are not always possible for financial reasons, but if a number of options are considered, one can perhaps make changes at no great cost.

Ergonomic improvement should be:
- Cost beneficial
- Practical
- Possible
- Applicable to the majority of workers.

One must be extremely cautious, however, about making changes without prior thorough investigation of all possibilities. Changes in the workplace that recognize an immediate hazard in one area may cause an alteration in the work process, which may result in a new hazard in another area. Ergonomic changes must therefore not concentrate on one aspect only. The full spectrum of the operation must be taken into account, however simple a change has to be made. Complex chain reactions must always be seriously considered, therefore systematic implementation of an all-embracing ergonomic programme can bring employees and employers wide-ranging advantages, but unplanned, sudden changes that are perceived to be an advantage in one area may have serious negative consequences and disadvantages in another. Solutions to ergonomic problems in the workplace must be functional rather than theoretical, and it is here that the workers themselves may contribute to the solution of problems. Changes must, however, be scientifically researched.

Participation is based on mutual orientation and knowledge of the problem. Problem-solving replaces an open-ended preoccupation with methods and concepts and has its own credibility.

3.17.8 Implementation of an ergonomic programme in the workplace

The key to ergonomic change is the implementation of aspects of ergonomics with the active participation of all parties – a positive attitude, long-term commitment and initiative by management are added requirements. If all these factors are not present even though management supports the ideas, any change or programme is bound to fail – support is not enough. The active participation of all employees is essential. They form the backbone of the programme and it is they who have to live and work with the changes. Their participation, inputs and knowledge play an important role in every phase of the programme. To implement such a programme should be part of the vision and the mission of every industry.

Once management approval has been obtained and a policy formulated, a policy document is issued to indicate management's view of a programme and to identify responsible individuals. An orientation programme is initiated by management and employees at all levels. All inputs are carefully scrutinized. Hereafter a workgroup, consisting of managers, specialists of various departments and representatives, is formed. The workgroup may appoint other workers on an ad hoc basis to participate in the debate.

The programme to implement change in the industry will result in the issuing of a document outlining the goals and objectives decided upon. These will depend on the budget, resources available and the limitations of the workplace. It is essential to obtain the expertise of a trained ergonomist to enable the group to achieve the programme goals and objectives.

3.17.9 The occupational healthcare professional's role in ergonomics

Not all industries have trained ergonomists to evaluate the work environment and the procedures in the workplace. Where such a person is available, he/she forms part of the health and safety team, because expert information may be exchanged in the team. Where such a person is not employed on a full-time basis, the health and safety team must give just as much attention to ergonomic aspects as to health and safety. Ergonomics forms an integral part of health and safety and cannot be ignored. The occupational health practitioner is just as important a member of the team as all the others. Unfortunately, the role of the occupational health practitioner is usually rather limited and reduced to that of consultation. Some employers show little interest in encouraging the participation of occupational health practitioners in occupational safety and ergonomics. It is therefore essential that the occupational health practitioner knows and understands all the procedures and the activities on the shop floor. His/her active participation involves various aspects given here. His/her role will be determined by the size of the operation, the type of industry and his/her own enthusiasm, interest and abilities. The occupational health practitioner has a wealth of information and experience to share with a team, for example, injury statistics and all other health-related statistics, disease prevalence rate in certain areas, psychological aspects (e.g. psychosomatic complaints such as headache), the attitude of workers – their motivation and their grievances.

Personal protective clothing and equipment

There are many dangers to health and safety which could be minimized, and in most instances eliminated, by the wearing of personal protective clothing. The excuses of many workers for not wearing PPEs are, among others, that it is uncomfortable, interferes with the performance of their tasks, it's too much trouble to put on and to take off, etc. In fact, many workers are simply too lazy to wear the correct protective equipment. An answer to this behaviour of workers has yet to be found. Allegations of this nature must, however, be viewed in a serious light and investigated. One example of how such an investigation bore fruit was that workers found that it was difficult to wear eye protection (goggles) because of the misting effect, which caused limited vision and considerable discomfort. After thorough research, goggles were designed that could resist misting. A simple procedure but with tremendous positive results – the potential for the misery of serious and often fatal eye injuries was excluded.

Occupational health

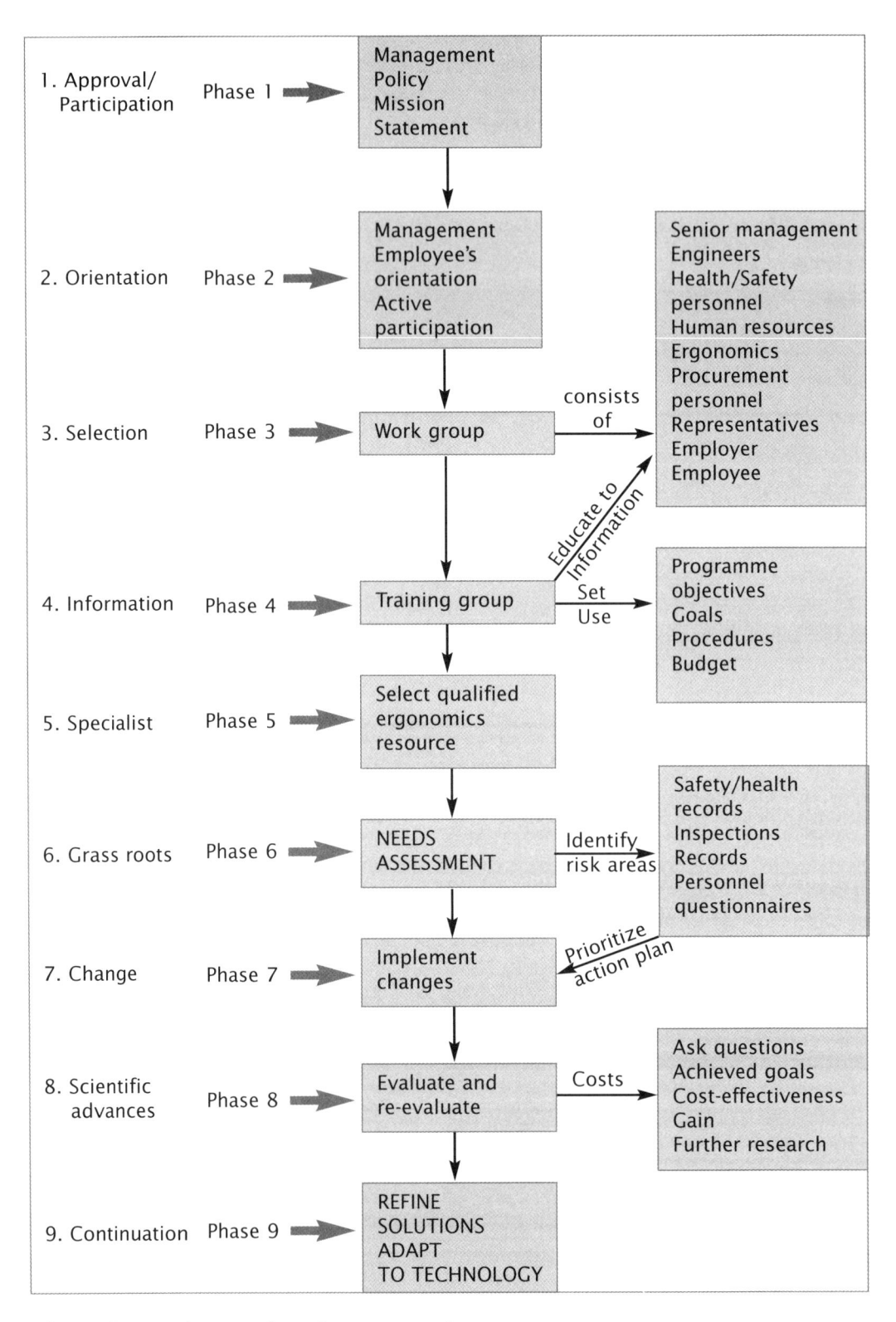

Figure 3.7 Implementation of an ergonomic programme

3.18 The National Occupational Safety Association

The National Occupational Safety Association (NOSA) is an incorporated association not for gain which was established in 1951 through the instigation of the then Minister of Labour, the Honourable Ben Schoeman.

The recommendations of a committee appointed to investigate ways and means of slowing down the ever-increasing injury rate led to the formation of a company. This company, a joint venture of the Workman's Compensation Commissioner and employers, was established through their employer organizations. NOSA claims that this could be considered as one of the very first examples of privatization.

NOSA is partially financed by the State Accident Fund in order to carry out occupational accident and disease prevention work. NOSA is therefore able to give employers a free or subsidized service by virtue of the fact that the employer's money is being fed back into accident prevention work.

The majority of employers fall under the jurisdiction of the Compensation Commissioner, who in terms of the Workman's Compensation Act must contribute towards the State Accident Fund. According to the hazards in industry and claims experienced for each class of injury, the State Accident Fund meets hospitalization, compensation costs, etc. in a case where a worker is injured in the course of employment.

There are, however, certain exempted employers who do not contribute to the State Accident Fund, but run their own insurance companies with the Compensation Commissioner's permission. These employers include certain builders who pay their assessments to the Federated Employers' Mutual Co Ltd; gold mines pay to the Rand Mutual Assurance Co; and some of the larger municipalities and various government departments carry their own insurance.

NOSA involves employers by establishing regional groups in various areas where it has offices in order to supply a service to employers. The regional group serves as a channel of communication between NOSA and employers.

The individual members of the regional group are volunteers who serve their employers and represent their employer organizations or firms within the framework of the objectives of NOSA. These objectives are:
- Guidance
- Education
- Training
- Motivation.

The regional groups are situated in all the major centres of South Africa, and industrial groups that cover mining and aviation have also been established. The regional advisory groups provide a forum where safety and safety-related problems can be discussed, in order to find possible solutions.

They promote safety in general by:
- Talking to others (e.g. engineers, safety advisers)
- Bringing guests to the meetings
- Promoting safety in families, etc.
- Setting an example to strive for safety in the workplace

- Helping to persuade other employers to make use of NOSA training courses
- Selling safety to companies that have no safety programmes
- Giving NOSA feedback on its services in order to make services more effective.

They improve the committee members' own awareness of safety, building up their skills and experience by:
- Assisting with specific safety elements
- Bringing about positive steps in, for example inspection, plant operations
- Previewing the latest video or film material on safety
- Making members aware of training courses or giving feedback on courses on safety and self-development.

3.18.1 NOSA's objectives

The association's objectives are the guidance, education, training and motivation of various levels of management and the workforce alike in the techniques of accident and occupational disease prevention. Through the NOSA MBO system and using the NOSA 5-star objective-setting and recognition system as a framework they will ensure the highest degree of success in the prevention of injuries, damage to property and disruption of business activities.

The modus operandi for achieving these objectives is by means of the NOSA Management by Objectives Safety System, training courses, publicity material and safety promotional activities.

To reach the GET'M-objectives (guidance, education, training and motivation) there are formal and informal activities. The formal activities take place in the classroom where safety training courses are mounted for select candidates. These courses are offered throughout South Africa and after successful completion the candidate is presented with a certificate that licenses him/her to run certain of NOSA's courses. This licensed worker becomes a NOSA 'agent' to train workers. NOSA estimates that over 200 000 persons have been trained over the years.

The informal GETW takes place through the NOSA staff who contact employers. The purpose of the visits to employers is to make them aware and to establish fully fledged safety programmes. This is done by carrying out safety surveys, grading and follow-up audits using the NOSA MBO Safety System as a framework.

3.18.2 NOSA's mission

MISSION STATEMENT

To provide dynamic, proactive and cost-effective consultation services in the fields of Loss Prevention, Occupational Safety and Health in the work environment to all industry and commerce.

CREDO
OUR PROFILE
To provide a comprehensive range of services and products in Occupational Safety and Health Management for all industry and commerce.

OUR PURPOSE
- To provide dynamic, proactive and cost-effective consultation services in the fields of Occupational Safety and Health.
- To strive for excellence in customer service by motivated employees.
- To uplift our employees and ensure the continued growth of our business.

OUR VALUES
We are committed to providing:
- Quality products and services
- Outstanding customer service
- Quality in everything we do

We believe in recognition and reward for our employees who contribute towards the Company's stated objective of providing quality in everything we do.

OUR GOALS
- To be the accepted authoritative consultancy in the field of Loss Prevention and Occupational Safety and Health.
- To guide, educate and train all people in the techniques of Occupational Accident and Disease Prevention.
- To continually strive for service excellence.
- To create a work environment which is conducive to encouraging employees to participate in decisions that directly affect their daily work lives.

3.19 The Occupational Health and Safety Act, 1993 (No 85 of 1993)

3.19.1 The aims of the Act

The Occupational Health and Safety Act, 1993 (No 85 of 1993) replaces the Machinery and Occupational Safety Act, 1983 (No 6 of 1983) and its two Amendments of 1989 and 1991, all of which have been repealed.

The most important aim of this Act is to establish rules and structures for health and safe places of work. Employers who, in accordance with this Act, are found by Inspectors to be negligent, are given heavy fines or prison sentences. This conforms to the common law principle that it is the duty of the employer to ensure that a healthy and safe workplace is provided for every employee. Through this Act the State has taken it upon itself to ensure that the employer performs this duty.

The Act, however, goes further. It includes the responsibility of the employer to ensure the safety and health of the public at large. The employer is responsible for anyone who may be affected by his activities. The Act lays down certain rules in this regard.

Another important principle in the Act is the realization that all efforts to promote health and safety at work will be doomed from the outset if the machinery used in the workplace is defective to begin with. This Act includes many provisions previously contained in the General Administrative Regulations.

The Act also establishes an advisory council for occupational health and safety. One can thus state that this Act was enacted to 'provide for safety and health of persons at work and for the health and safety of persons in connection with the use of plant and machinery; the protection of persons other than persons at work against hazards to health and safety arising out of or in connection with the acitivies of persons at work; to establish an Advisory Council for Occupational Health and Safety and to provide for matter connected therewith'.

3.19.2 The status of the Act
The Occupational Health and Safety Act supersedes all other agreements. This means that there can be no agreement between any party to work or to conduct work in unsafe or unhealthy conditions.

3.19.3 Definitions
Definitions contained in the Act include those of employer and employee, which is the same as in the Labour Relations Act and in the Basic Conditions of Employment Act. The Act does not exclude persons employed in farming operations, domestic workers or the public service. These persons are all covered by this Act.

The Minister of Manpower may by notice declare that a person who belongs to a specific category of persons shall for the purpose of the Act, be deemed an employee and anyone who is in control of and supervises such a person, shall be considered the employer of that person (Miles, 1996:192).

Danger is defined as anything that may cause injury or damage to persons or property.

A hazard is any source of any exposure to danger, and safe is defined as being free from any hazard.

3.19.4 Exclusions
The Act excludes labour brokers as defined under the Labour Relations Act, mines, mining areas or any works defined in terms of the Minerals Act, 1991 (No 50 of 1991) and the Mine Health and Safety Act, as well as any load ship, fishing boat, floating crane, boat or crane in or out of the water in a South African harbour or territorial waters as defined in the Merchant Shipping Act, 1951 (No 57 of 1951), and an employer exempted by the Minister from the application of OHSA.

3.19.5 Advisory Council for Occupational Health and Safety
According to the Act, the Advisory Council for Occupational Health and Safety represents the Department of Labour and serves as an advisory body for the Minister of Labour on the formulation and publication of standards, specifications and other aspects regarding employers and employees with regard to health and safety. The Council may carry out research and conduct investigations when nesessary and may make rules where necessary. The Council consists of 20 members, as specified in the Act.

Technical committees may be established by the Council to advise on any matter. These members are usually specialists in a specified field.

3.20 Safety committees

In terms of the Act, a safety committee must be established wherever two or more safety representatives have been appointed. The Act spells out the appointment of the members and the cooption of advisory members. It is the responsibility and duty of the employer to ensure that a safety committee is established, that regular meetings are held and that the committee is able to perform its duties in accordance with the Act.

A safety committee is established as a practical means to promote safety by cooperation between management and worker. Management often uses safety committees to explain safety policy and workers use the safety committee to bring certain views and suggestions on safety matters to the attention of management.

A safety committee helps to give workers confidence in the safety policy. Management can be confident that workers will appreciate and abide by the safety policy. It is essential that the occupational health practitioner is a member of this committee.

3.20.1 The functions of safety committees

3.20.1.1 Policy

The members of safety committees have the general duty to promote cooperation among all workers in an attempt to improve the safety standards. The committee should make sure that safety standards are set up and followed. The members of the safety committees are chosen from the workers, not necessarily in authority themselves but certainly people who are respected and liked by the workers. Orders then do not carry the stigma of 'authority' or management. The greater the number of workers who can participate in setting safety policy, the more successful the committee will be. The members need not be experts in safety matters but should feel positive and competent to deal with safety issues.

The safety committee should prepare and adopt a constitution and should meet regularly, at least every three months. One item on every agenda should be to discuss any accident that has occurred since the last meeting. It should be clearly stressed that no blame should be put on a person. The discussion should rather be directed at determining the cause of the accident and new measures should be worked out to prevent a recurrence of those circumstances that led to it. Preparation of safety rules and regulations takes place in this safety committee and should be submitted for confirmation to and adoption by the proper authorities. Everything possible must be done to keep the management and members interested in their work. The safety committee must be backed by the employer. Without management's approval, a safety committee cannot function.

The establishment of a safety programme and the evaluation, revision and testing of this programme is an important function of the safety committee. Every worker representative must feel free to express his/her opinion without the fear of criticism from superiors. All proposals for setting up a safety programme should be considered and should have the greatest possible support of both the employer and the workers. All the necessary information, such as statistics, should be available to the committee in order to develop new techniques, or revise those that already exist. The trade unions

Occupational health

are increasingly taking up safety issues at enterprise level. They seek improvements through negotiating health and safety agreements with employers. Participation by trade unions may bring about changes in policy on safety issues.

It is the function of the safety committee to implement and administer the company's statement of policy for a safe plant. This encompasses safety policies and practices, safety standards and industrial hygiene. NOSA emphasizes that no grievances or matters not connected with safety should be discussed by the safety committee.

3.20.1.2 Executive

The safety committee is involved in the investigation of all accidents. In some cases a worker who has had an accident is invited to tell the committee how the accident happened. These cases should be handled tactfully and objective criticism should be given. All accidents are promptly reported to the safety engineer by the committee members. This is done so that hazardous conditions can be immediately removed. Where necessary other specialized members can be coopted to the safety committee or subcommittees or inspection committees can be formed. Another duty of the safety committee is to do plant inspections and self-audits in order to investigate the conditions and procedures that may lead to accidents. It is important that constant auditing of all existing, planned and proposed installations, processes and procedures for unsafe conditions or acts should take place before injury or damage results. The testing and approval of all safety equipment and clothing is done by the committee. Equipment is checked for the necessary safety devices before it is bought.

A specific person or sub-committee is appointed who:
- Records all minor and major accidents in an accident register
- Sees to it that emergency planning has a means, plan and system to keep adequate watch on all sources of danger that can develop in a disaster
- Ensures that proper first aid is provided and, if necessary, further medical treatment to anybody injured
- Does the necessary paper work to notify the authorities concerned
- Forwards the full particulars of an accident to all the members of the committee
- Ensures that all the decisions, instructions and directives of the committee are implemented
- Reports all near-accidents
- Determines the frequency and severity of minor injuries
- Determines the general and specific, actual and potential costs of accidents.

3.20.1.3 Education

It is not sufficient to give workers a booklet on safety instructions – the contents must be explained to them to ensure that they are understood. The safety committee has a responsibility towards workers to inform them of new equipment, policy, procedures or any other changes that have taken place or are planned. This information can reach workers by compiling, editing, publishing and distributing a monthly or bi-weekly safety publication. It must be remembered, however, that not all workers can read or understand the language the publication is written in. This problem can be overcome by lectures, safety talks, demonstrations or by obtaining audiovisual aids.

The introduction of safety competitions, contests, and safety weeks is also a step towards safety but the committee should be alert to the possibility that accidents may not be reported because of fear of being excluded from the competition.

The planning and supervision of the training of all employees or as many as possible should be a priority and should be conducted according to NOSA's training courses. The safety committee promotes safety training by reviewing all audiovisual materials for inclusion in the health and safety training programme for employees, by taking into account the following:
- Nature of work
- Culture of employees
- Level of training
- Age
- Gender
- Attitude
- Relevance to work.

The occupational health practitioner has an important function within the safety committee and can contribute his/her knowledge and skill in health matters making individuals safe and their environment safe to work in. The safety committee also has the important function of establishing appropriate relationships with professional and organizational groups outside the company.

3.20.1.4 Management involvement
Setting up a safety programme without the active interest, participation, involvement and approval of management is useless. The safety committee assists management in developing and operating a programme that will not only protect the worker by preventing accidents, but also by promoting productivity and preventing loss either of money or human life. Management-initiated participation and initiative in setting up a safety programme are essential. The acceptance by various levels of management, both legal and internal, ensures greater management leadership in the programme.

The delegation of responsibilities, both legal and internal, to supervisory and other staff, further helps to ensure good safety performance at all levels. Management involvement further extends to their insistence on the introduction of proper auditing systems.

3.20.1.5 Duties of employers
For a comprehensive discussion of the duties of employees, see the Occupational Health and Safety Act, 1993 (No 85 of 1993).

3.21 The role and functions of the occupational health practitioner in safety and accident prevention
In 1895, Florence Nightingale said: 'Nursing is not only a service to the sick, it is a service also to the well. We have to teach people how to live.'

The role of the occupational health practitioner can never be ignored, nor should it be underestimated or regarded as inferior in any industry or workplace. Most occupational health practitioners working in industry are highly trained professionals who have the necessary skill, knowledge and motivation to participate actively in the safety and accident prevention programme in the workplace. It is important that occupational health practitioners do not take on duties for which they are not prepared. They must be involved and must accept every opportunity to learn more about the work environment and work practices. Occupational health practitioners should not sit in a 'sterile' medical centre, waiting for an accident to happen. The medical facility is much more than a mere clinic, because the services rendered go beyond the therapeutic and prophylactic aspects of illness. The occupational health practitioner is seen as the manager of this department. Medical officers are usually employed on a part-time basis and they see only those cases referred to them by the occupational health practitioner. Where a company employs a full-time medical officer, the managerial duties will have to be shared according to the needs and activities of the company concerned.

It is agreed that prevention is better than cure, and therefore the occupational health worker should and must work with management and other team members involved in safety, towards a safe environment for each worker in order to prevent injury and disease not only in the workplace, but also in their private lives – safety must become a habit.

The functions of the occupational health practitioner and other occupational health practitioners will depend on many factors. The most important are:

- How he/she is regarded by management
- What knowledge, skill, motivation she/he possesses
- What kind of industry he/she is working in
- What the job description is
- What team members are available
- The size of the industry
- The type of industry.

The occupational health worker must have a great awareness of the employee's needs, the legislation pertaining to the employee's welfare, disability, occupational hazards and the health and safety policy of the company.

It is essential that the occupational health practitioner communicates with management and other departments in order to improve and strengthen the welfare of the employee. It is important to have good relationships and open communication channels between management and the workers. Through effective communication the occupational health worker can contribute to the improvement of job satisfaction, a happy and safe environment, loss control and productivity.

It is important to realize that the employee must be seen and treated holistically. The occupational health worker must realize that each employee must be seen as a physical, social and psychological human being with his/her own identity, within a family which is a part of a community.

It is well known that there is interaction between the social, physical and psychological environment of the individual. When the chain between these factors is broken, the individual will become unbalanced. This may cause carelessness, demotivation, and other symptoms that can contribute to unsafe acts.

With extensive training the occupational health worker becomes sensitive to the problems of employees which can be related to social, physical or psychological factors.

The most basic functions of the occupational healthcare team with regard to safety fall under the following main headings:

- Health education and safety teaching to teach workers how they can protect their own health
- Emergency training
- Accident recording and investigation
- Keeping records of claims, minor injuries, reports, statistics
- Being aware of occupational diseases
- Conducting examinations and pre-employment tests to identify physiological, psychological and social problems
- Communication in order to work cooperatively with other team members of the occupational safety and health team
- Coordination with other safety team members
- Personal safeguarding, wearing of protective clothing and other safety attire
- Participation in the development of hazard control programmes geared to the nature and specifics of the workplace. It must be strongly emphasized that the occupational health practitioner, as with all the other safety team members, cannot work on her/his own. It is absolutely essential to perform these functions with the management's approval and together with the other team members, such as safety officers, security officers, loss control officers, hygienists, medical officers, etc.
- Participation in the selection, training and motivation of workers so that they learn how to follow safe work practices
- Provision of primary care so that workers recover from injury and work compatibly with their therapeutic care plans
- Collection and use of data to identify causes and make plans to correct both the situational and the behavioural problems
- Counselling and/or providing crisis intervention and moral support to workers who are experiencing interpersonal, work or family problems that interfere with normal functioning and may be the cause of carelessness
- Participation in environmental control programmes that aim to identify, eliminate and control health and safety hazards.

3.22 Conclusion

Occupational health and safety are a growing concern as workers, managers and governments, nationally and internationally, come to recognize the benefits gained from maintaining safe and healthy working conditions.

An attempt has been made to show the importance of the role of the occupational health worker in accident prevention. An accident occurs as a result of a chain of events of which the occupational health worker should be aware.

Safety concerns EVERYBODY – it cannot be isolated as something that is practised only in the work situation. Safety involves not only the individual, but the whole community, the whole country and even the whole world. One serious accident may harm a whole nation.

It should be remembered that safety should be 'sold', but this is NEVER achieved by the YCNSSBSOYT formula (you cannot sell safety by sitting on your tail). Active involvement and participation by management, health workers and workers are the key factors to the success of accident prevention.

3.23 Bibliography

Bever, D. L. 1984. *Safety: A Personal Focus*. St Louis: Mosby.

Bird, F. J. 1976. *Management Guide to Loss Control*. Atlanta: Institute Press.

Higson, N. 1998. *Risk management – Health and Safety in Primary Care*. Oxford: Butterworth-Heinemann.

Guild, R., Ehrlich, R. I., Johnston, J. R. & Ross, M. H. 2001. *Handbook of Occupational Health Practice in the South African Mining Industry*. Johannesburg: SIMRAC.

Hendrikse, J. 1994. Take a Closer Look at Ergonomics. *Safety Management*, 4(1): 19–21.

Miles, M. 1996. *A Guide to the Industrial Laws of South Africa. Volume I and II*. Johannesburg: Miles.

NOSADATA. 1991. Samtrac Course. Pretoria: NOSA.

World Health Organization in Association with the ILO. 1991. *Statement from the Consultation on Action to be taken after Occupational Exposure of Health Care Workers*. Geneva: WHO.

4 Occupational hygiene

A. J. Kotze and J. Acutt

4.1 Introduction

The working conditions in South African mines have been a cause for concern since the late nineteenth century. In 1902 a commissioner of enquiry into working conditions prescribed dust suppression in an effort to prevent lung diseases (Coetzee, 1995). This was the recognition and control of environmental hazards of occupational hygiene which today includes measurement and evaluation.

Occupational hygiene is the protective and preventive side of occupational health The other equally important side of health promotion and disease detection is addressed in occupational medicine.

4.2 Learning objectives

At the end of this chapter, the reader should be able to:
- Define the concept of occupational hygiene
- Identify the following:
  - basic principles of occupational hygiene
  - procedures in an occupational hygiene programme
- Classify and describe the occupational hazards and how to minimize their effects
- Discuss the role and functions of the occupational health professional in occupational hygiene.

4.3 Definition of occupational hygiene

Occupational or industrial hygiene is an applied science that encompasses the application of information from a variety of sciences such as chemistry, engineering, biology, mathematics, medicine, physics and toxicology.

The American Industrial Hygiene Association defines industrial hygiene as the science and art devoted to:
- The recognition, evaluation and control of those environmental factors or stresses,
- Arising in or from the workplace,
- Which may cause sickness, impaired health and well-being, or
- Significant discomfort and inefficiency among workers or among the citizens of a community (Schoeman & Schröder, 1994:2).

4.4 The rationale of occupational hygiene
Occupational hygiene practice is based upon the following principles:
- Environmental health hazards in the workplace can be measured quantitatively, and expressed in terms related to the degree of stress caused.
- Continuous surveillance of the work environment must be carried out.
- Occupational exposure limits must be adhered to.
- The health effects of hazards in the workplace usually show a dose–response relationship.

The human body has an intricate mechanism for protection against the invasion of hostile stresses into the body and deals with the stress agents when invasion has occurred. Susceptibility to occupational stresses is influenced by genetic factors, health and nutritional status, lifestyle (exercise, excessive use of alcohol and smoking) and psychological factors.

Determinants of occupational diseases include:
- The concentration or intensity of the stress agent
- The duration of exposure
- The frequency of exposure
- Individual susceptibility.

Levels of exposure to specific stress agents should be kept within safe limits as set by the Hazardous Chemical Substances Regulations of 1995 of the Occupational Health and Safety Act, 1993 (No 85 of 1993). Continuous surveillance of the work environment must be carried out to ensure a healthy workplace within the prescribed safe limits.

4.5 Legislative control
The Occupational Health and Safety Act, 1993 (No 85 of 1993) and the Mine Health and Safety Act, 1996 (No 29 of 1996) provide guidelines for the protection of the health and safety of the worker.

Employers have specific responsibilities under these laws, which include:
- Providing and maintaining a working environment that is safe and without risk to the health of the employees
- Establishing the hazards attached to the work performed, the article or substance produced, processed, used, stored, handled or transported
- Instituting precautionary measures and safe work procedures and supplying the means to apply these measures
- Educating and training employees about the hazards and the control of exposure
- Taking reasonably practicable steps to eliminate or mitigate hazards before resorting to personal protective equipment, which must be supplied free of charge to employees
- Evaluating the risks associated with identified hazards, preventing and minimizing

the exposure and carrying out an occupational hygiene programme, biological monitoring and medical surveillance where the Department of Labour has listed work as hazardous
- Designating health and safety representatives for workplaces with more than 20 employees to monitor the work environment and report at health and safety committee meetings
- Reporting hazardous incidents at the workplace to the Department of Labour inspector.

Employees are responsible in terms of the legislation for:
- Accepting responsibility for their own health and safety, as well as for those who may be affected by the work they perform
- Carrying out lawful instructions relating to their work, health and safety
- Reporting any irregularity that may jeopardize their own health and safety or that of their colleagues to their supervisor.

(The above Acts are described in more detail in Chapter 2.)

4.6 The basic principles and procedures of an occupational hygiene programme

4.6.1 The basic principles
The main purpose of any occupational hygiene programme is to ensure a workplace that is safe for the worker. This requires a programme with a multidisciplinary approach involving a team that includes the occupational hygienist, risk manager, occupational health practitioner, and from time to time, the production manager, maintenance engineer, human resources manager, and employee health and safety representatives. It must be designed around the nature of the operations, documented to preserve a sound retrospective record, and executed in a professional manner. The occupational hygienist must be accredited by the Department of Labour in terms of the Occupational Health and Safety Act.

A basic programme should include the following:
- Continuous data collection for identifying and assessing the level of all hazards at the workplace
- Periodic review of worker exposure and health reports to detect new hazards and reassess old ones
- Integration with health and risk management programmes to evaluate current control measures, instituting new ones when necessary
- A data storage system that will permit the retrieval of information to assess the long-term effect of exposure and to assure the relevancy of the data being collected.

4.6.2 Occupational hygiene procedures
The procedure to follow in an occupational hygiene programme is similar to that of a risk assessment programme in the early stages. See 5.6 in Chapter 5.

4.6.2.1 Recognition of all possible hazards
The first step is to recognize that there may be hazards, and to assess the premises and work processes through:
- A 'walk-through' survey of the whole workplace to recognize health hazards
- Consultation with workers at their work stations to elicit actual work procedures and perhaps symptoms of discomfort
- A flow diagram drawn up to show the following:
  - raw materials used, the manufacturing process and the products made
  - all by-products formed during the manufacturing process
  - the general work environment, including noise zones, extractor fans, chemical stores, etc.
  - location of emergency equipment (fire extinguishers, first-aid boxes, etc.) and exits.

4.6.2.2 Identification of hazards
Hazards must be identified by means of:
- Measurement of possible hazards by an occupational hygienist accredited by the Department of Labour
- Identification of all on-the-job health hazards, taking into consideration the following important factors:
  - Occupational Exposure Limits of hazards (OELs) in terms of the Hazardous Chemical Substance Regulations of the Occupational Health and Safety Act (No 85 of 1993)
  - health and well-being effects of exposure to identified hazards on the employees
  - available information on the identified hazards in Material Safety Data Sheets, reference books and the Internet
- All areas and health hazards must be indicated on the flow diagram created during the walk-through survey.

4.6.2.3 Evaluation of hazards
All the collected data must be studied to identify:
- Health risks
- The extent of exposure – level and duration of exposure for each employee
- The number of exposed employees
- The effectiveness of current control measures and personal protective equipment
- The Risk Rating by calculating the likelihood of exposure to the hazard multiplied by the consequence of exposure
- Dangerous work areas that need to be demarcated, enclosed or isolated as a control measure.

4.6.2.4 Control over the effect of the hazard
Control must be achieved by:
- Minimizing hazardous emissions at their source through engineering methods
- Implementing safe work procedures

- Substituting toxic substances with those that are less toxic
- Modifying the process through engineering, enclosure of processes, maintenance of machines to reduce vibration and noise
- Extracting fumes and vapours and improving ventilation
- Educating employees on the effects of the hazard on health and precautions to be taken, including personal hygiene, no eating, drinking or smoking in the work area and the correct use and care of personal protective equipment
- Issuing the correct type of personal protective equipment for the identified hazards after all measures have been taken to reduce the risk of exposure
- Rotating staff in order that one person is not continually exposed to the hazard
- Maintaining 'good housekeeping', which includes a tidy and clean work area with a place for everything and everything in its place
- Monitoring the possible health effects on individuals through a suitable medical surveillance programme.

4.7 The classification and discussion of occupational hazards

An intimate knowledge of the plant and work processes and procedures is essential in any meaningful occupational health programme. The task of recognition, identification, evaluation and the control of hazards in the workplace is the function of the occupational hygienist as a member of the occupational health team, together with the occupational health practitioner and the risk manager.

In order to produce biological or physical harm, a substance must gain access to, or be in contact with the body. The main routes of entry into the body are:

Inhalation. Vapour, gas, fumes, mist, spray or dust enter the body by inhalation.

Ingestion. Poisons are swallowed when people eat or smoke with contaminated hands or swallow particles caught up in the mucus from the back of the nose.

Through the skin. Some chemical substances gain access to the body by absorption through intact or broken skin.

Injection. Hazardous substances can enter the body by injection through the skin as in an injury with a sharp, contaminated instrument.

There are many different kinds of hazards in the workplace and several classification systems are used. Classification of hazards according to their type – chemical, physical, mechanical, biological or psychological is commonly used.

4.7.1 Chemical hazards

Chemical hazards are classified as arising from the following:

Dust, which consists of solid particles, usually arising from processes such as crushing, grinding, detonation, impact, and decrepitation or drying of rock, wood, coal, ore, etc. Inhalation of dust may lead to a variety of lung conditions, or systemic poisoning.

Fumes are finely particulate solids that arise by condensation from a vapour (often after a metal has become molten). The fumes are usually the oxide of a particular metal and are highly toxic.

Gases, which are a formless fluid that can occupy the space of enclosure. Gas can be changed to a liquid or solid by a combination of increased pressure and decreased temperature. Gases are usually irritating to the eyes, nose and mouth, and people will try to escape when exposed. (Carbon monoxide, however, has no smell and leads to loss of consciousness.)

Vapours are the gases given off by a substance. Examples of vapours are solvent or petroleum vapours.

Fluids are liquids that may cause harm to the human body when skin contact or digestion occurs, such as hydrochloric acid or sulphuric acid.

Table 4.1 Classification of occupational hazards

CLASS	HAZARD
CHEMICAL	*Dust* – solid particles arising from disintegration (crushing, grinding, etc) of organic and inorganic substances *Fumes* – arise when a volatilized solid condenses in cool air, as in welding *Smoke* – comes from incomplete burning of carbonaceous material such as coal or oil *Mists* – fine liquid droplets from condensation, from vapour back to liquid, as in spray painting *Vapours* – the gaseous form of substances that are in a solid or liquid state at room temperature and normal pressure as in the evaporation of solvents *Gases* – formless fluids that fill the container and are transformed to the liquid or solid state by increased pressure and decreased temperature
PHYSICAL	*Ergonomics* – optimal adjustment between people and their work environment *Illumination* – suitable level for type of work performed *Noise* – excessive noise in the work environment *Pressure* – abnormal high or low atmospheric pressure *Radiation* – ionizing and non-ionizing *Temperature extremes* – hot or cold work environments *Ventilation* – quality air in the workplace
MECHANICAL	Vibration – vibrating machinery
BIOLOGICAL	Bacterial, viral or fungal exposure
PSYCHOLOGICAL	Stressful work situations

The chemical hazards can also be classified according to their toxicological effects on the human body, for example:
- Irritants, which affect different parts of the respiratory system
- Asphyxiants, which obstruct the oxidation process in the tissues
- Narcotics and analgesics, which affect the central nervous system
- Carcinogenics, which lead to a variety of malignant conditions
- Mutagenics, which affect the genetic structure in the body
- Teratogenics, which may cause abnormalities in the unborn foetus
- Systemic poisons, which may affect the body as a whole
- Dangerous dust particles, which cause fibrosis, allergies and irritations

Table 4.2 Classification of chemical hazards according to their toxicological effects

TYPE	EXAMPLES	EFFECT ON BODY
Asphyxiant	Acetylene Hydrogen cyanide	Dilutes atmospheric oxygen Impedes oxidation process in tissues
Carcinogenic	Aromatic amines Benzene, Coke	Malignancy in healthy cells
Dust	Silica, asbestos	Fibrosis in lung tissue
Irritant	Ammonia Chlorine	Oversecretion by mucous membranes in upper or lower respiratory tract
Mutagenic	Pesticides	Alters genes (chromosomes) of cells
Narcotic	Ethers	Depresses the central nervous system
Systemic poison	Heavy metals	Damage to blood or internal organs
Teratogenic	Lead, selenium	Abnormality in unborn foetus

Today, there are many thousands of types of chemicals and chemical compounds on the market. The principles of dealing with any occupational hazard should be applied when dealing with these.

The Material Safety Data Sheet of all chemicals on site and the manufacturer's literature can be a valuable source of information for the occupational nurse. These should specify the:
- Chemical contents
- Effects of exposure
- Precautions that must be observed when handling the substance
- First-aid treatment, should exposure occur.

4.7.1.1 The absorption of harmful substances into the body

The respiratory system. In the occupational situation, absorption via the respiratory system is probably the most important hazard.

Dust particles affect the airways and can settle in the lung tissue, causing damage. Gases, fumes and vapours, when inhaled, are absorbed into the bloodstream, and spread through the body. The eventual dosage of hazardous substance inhaled, absorbed and accumulated in the body will depend upon:
- The concentration in the air
- The size of the particles and the solubility of the substance
- The duration of exposure
- The respiratory and circulatory tempo
- The biochemical reactivity of the substance.

Substances inhaled via the respiratory system may also be absorbed into the digestive system if particles are swallowed when deposited in the mucus of the nose and throat.
The skin. Solids, liquids and gases may be absorbed through an intact skin. Absorption may take place through the epidermal layer or through the hair follicles. Broken skin provides a direct route for substances to penetrate the body. Special mention is made when determining the Threshold Limit Values (TLV) or Occupational Exposure Limits (OEL) to provide for substances that may be absorbed by inhalation and through the skin.
The digestive system. This method of contamination is not very common. It usually occurs when a substance is accidentally swallowed, or the worker drinks or smokes with contaminated hands. Should he/she cough up contaminated material and swallow it, it will be absorbed through the digestive tract.

4.7.1.2 The result of the absorption of toxic materials into the body

Toxicology is the study of the body's responses to toxic substances. The toxicity of substances can be described as the inherent characteristic of a substance to cause harmful effects when coming into contact with or entering the body.
The toxicity of substances. This can be described as the inherent characteristic of a substance to cause harmful effects when coming into contact with or entering the body.

The toxicity of substances varies considerably, and for this purpose a standardized system was developed to measure and compare toxic levels of substances.

Schoeman and Schröder states the most common rating used is the median lethal (semi-fatal) dose or LID50. This is the statistically calculated dose of a substance which is expected to cause death in 50% of an entire defined experimental animal population, or randomly selected sample of test subjects (Schoeman & Schröder, 1994:25).

The LID50s are usually expressed in weight of toxic substance per unit body mass, e.g. mg/kg. The smaller this value, the higher the toxicity.
The following generally applies to this rating:
- Compounds with an LID of more than 5 000 mg/kg are non-poisonous.
- Compounds with a slight toxicity have an LID of between 1 000 and 2 000 mg/kg.
- A moderately poisonous substance will have an LID of between 100 and 1 000 mg/kg.
- Compounds with a high toxicity have an LID of below 100 mg/kg.

In South Africa, a classification system is used to indicate the potential toxicity of a substance ranging from class I to IV, where class I indicates the highly toxic substances, and class IV those substances with no toxicity. Class I contains pesticides such as DDT, parathion and aldikarb (see The Hazardous Substances Act, 1973 (No 15 of 1973) as amended by Act 53 of 1992).

4.7.1.3 Measurement of chemical hazards

In terms of the Hazardous Chemical Substances Regulations (1995) of the Occupational Health and Safety Act (No 85 of 1993) and the Occupational Hygiene Regulations (2001) of the Mine Health and Safety Act (No 29 of 1996) certain limits are set for all airborne pollutants in industry and mines in South Africa:

- *Occupational Exposure Limit (OEL)* – means a limit value set for a stress factor in the workplace at which there is no significant risk for adverse health effects.
- *Occupational Exposure Limit* – Control limit is the maximum concentration of an airborne substance, to which employees may be exposed by inhalation under any circumstances.
- *Occupational Exposure Limit* – Recommended limit is the concentration of an airborne substance at which there is no evidence that it is likely to be injurious.

The measurement and assessment of chemical contaminants in industry are essential for the evaluation of such hazards. The following are standards used in industry for the evaluation of risks:

- *Threshold Limit Values (TLVs)*. This is the average maximum concentration of substances in air which are normally harmless on prolonged exposure. The TLVs of a large number of industrial materials used in industry are known. The TLV should be regarded as a guide only to the control of risks, and is used as a communication tool between physicians, engineers and hygienists who design control equipment.
- *Time-Weighted Average Threshold Limit (TWA.TLV)*. In practice it is found that the concentration of airborne substances may vary considerably in the course of a working day. The average concentration is calculated and the exposure of the worker determined accordingly. The value to which almost every worker may be exposed repeatedly, constitutes the time-weighted average threshold limit (Schoeman & Schröder, 1994:34).
- *Short-Term Exposure Limits (STEL.TLV)*. These values are used for substances with peak levels which momentarily go beyond the TWA.TLV. This is permissible, provided that the exposure is for a short period only.
- *Ceiling Concentration (C.TLV)*. Certain fast-acting substances such as formaldehyde may have deleterious effects on the human body, even if exposure is only for a short period of time. These substances are controlled by means of a ceiling concentration, which may not be exceeded.
- *Maximum Allowable Concentration (MAC)*. Ceiling values constitute the maximum allowable concentration of these substances.
- *Emergency Exposure Limits (EELs)*. These are used to calculate risks from large-scale accidental air pollution. They are used in two ways:

Occupational health

- To estimate risks to individual rescue workers
- To anticipate the risks to the community in the vicinity of the accident.

Many more standards and measurements are used in the calculation of the exposure, toxicity and effects of substances which cannot be taken up in this publication, because of their specialized nature. The reader is advised to consult additional literature on occupational hygiene if further information is required.

4.7.2 Physical hazards

Physical hazards are sometimes thought to be of less importance than the chemical hazards, but this is not so. Physical hazards can cause severe injuries or disease, sometimes of a less tangible nature, but should not be underrated and overlooked.

The nature of physical hazards is varied, but the examples below are the most common.

4.7.2.1 Radiation

Radiation refers to the process in which energy is emitted by a source, transmitted through a medium and absorbed by another body. Radiation is present in the environment in the form of ionizing radiation from elements of uranium and thorium in rocks and soil, and non-ionizing radiation from the sun, microwaves, radio frequency, lasers, etc. Our concern is the use or production of radiation in industry.

Ionizing radiation. Ionizing radiation is any radiation that produces ions in matter and is produced in industry by:
- Accelerators as used in irradiation processes and for medical applications
- Röntgen rays, or X-rays, are used to screen products for flaws and in humans to detect disease
- Radioactivity where radioactive nuclei emit three kinds of radiation:
  - Alpha particles, which can only penetrate human tissue to the depth of one-tenth of a millimetre. Irradiation is limited to the immediate vicinity of the source.
  - Beta rays exhibit various energies. They penetrate a few millimetres into human tissue before being absorbed.
  - Gamma rays are electromagnetic rays of varying levels of energy. They often have a high penetration potential, and can irradiate all parts of the body uniformly.
- Nuclear reactions – neutrons are uncharged particles with a wide range of energy and power of penetration. They can penetrate the nucleus of an atom, resulting in a nuclear reaction.

Radiation may take place from inside or outside the body. In industry, external radiation may occur, for example, from sealed sources or from X-ray machines and in underground mines, from the rockface. Internal radiation can take place when breathing in or swallowing radioactive material.

The biological effect of exposure to ionizing radiation. The effect of ionizing radiation on the human body is due to the deposition of energy in the tissue cells, the extent of which is characterized by the following reaction phases:
- Ionization occurs instantly
- Physical-chemical reaction between ions and water or molecules, occurs immediately
- Chemical reaction between reaction products and the organic molecules of a cell occurs within seconds
- Biological manifestation of the cell damage can occur within minutes or over many years.

Cell damage may include: destruction of cells, delay in the cell division, and alteration of the inherent cell structure which is seen as radiation burns, hair loss, anaemia, sterility and cancer, depending on:
- The absorbed dose, which is the energy absorbed per unit mass of tissue or organ
- The energy, mass and electrostatic charge of the radiation
- The distribution of the dose within the body (Zenz, et al.,1994).

The norms for the control of radiation exposure. The recommendations of the International Commission on Radiological Protection (ICRP) are accepted in South Africa as the basis for radiation protection. These norms specify that:
- The exposure of individuals to radiation must be justified in terms of the benefits secured when the work is performed.
- When exposure is justified, it must be optimized and in every case kept as low as reasonably achievable in the work situation.
- Prescribed dose limits may not be exceeded.
(Schoeman & Schröder, 1994:183)

In South Africa, the Department of Minerals and Energy administers The Nuclear Energy Act, 1982 (No 92 of 1982) with regard to nuclear installations and nuclear hazard materials and the National Nuclear Regulator Act, 1999 (Act 47 of 1999) for occupational exposure to radiation in mining. The Department of Health administers The Hazardous Substances Act, 1973 (No 15 of 1973), as amended by Act 53 of 1992, and controls electronic products that trigger radiation, issues licences and authorizes the management and handling of radio-nuclides (Guild, et al., 2001).

Units for the measurement of radiation exposure. Schoeman and Schröder describe various terms used in this regard (1994:182):
- Exposure – the amount of ionization caused by ionizing radiation in air. Measurement is made in terms of the electric charge formed as a result of the ionization. Unit of measurement: coulomb/Kg (C/Kg).
- Absorbed dose (D) – the energy transferred to tissue. The unit of measurement used for the absorbed dose is the gray (Gy).
- Various types of radiation each have a different potential to damage tissue. H is used to indicate the harmful dose. By adding a quality factor (Q) which describes the

Occupational health

harmful effect of the radiation, the absorbed dose can be calculated:
H = D x Q.
- The quality factors currently being used are: 1 for beta, gamma and röntgen rays, 20 for alpha rays and other heavy ions, 10 for neutrons.
- Sievert (Sv) – the unit for dose equivalent and effective dose is the sievert (Sv). 1 Sv = Gy x Q (Guild, et al., 2001).

Radiation protection
The measurement of radiation and radiation protection
Levels of radiation must be measured and recorded for individuals potentially exposed to radiation, so that the exposure dose can be compared with the recommended permissible doses. The common method used for recording doses of radiation is by means of individual film badges and dosimeters. These must be worn in an area of the body where most radiation is likely to occur, at all times. The records of radiation of an individual must go with him/her when changing jobs, otherwise his/her cumulative exposure will not be known (Gardner & Taylor, 1975:100).

Control of radiation exposure
As for the control of health risks in general, exposure to radiation is minimized through engineering and administrative control measures and suitable personal protective equipment.
- External radiation can be decreased by shielding the source with suitable substances, such as lead and concrete, keeping a safe distance from the source, reducing the exposure time, and switching machines off when not in use.
- Internal radiation is controlled by preventing the intake through strict zoning and control of working areas; the prevention of the spread of activities to uncontrolled areas; the provision of suitable handling facilities and environmental control; and the use of protective clothing and equipment (Schoeman & Schröder, 1994:185).

Non-ionizing radiation
Many industrial processes make use of or produce relatively intense radiant energy sources. Examples of these are welding, cutting, heating and radio communication (Schilling, 1973:266). Non-ionizing radiation may be considered in four ranges of wavelength:
1 **Ultraviolet radiation and visible light**. This can affect the skin, causing various degrees of sunburn. The incidence of skin cancer in the exposed areas of the skin is higher in people who are continuously exposed to the sun, e.g. farmers and labourers.

   Conjunctivitis can also be caused by ultraviolet light – these conditions are commonly called arc eyes or welder's flash. All visible light sources, such as machines and electronic equipment, produce some infrared emission.
2 **Infrared radiation**. All hot bodies radiate heat. It is felt on the skin as heat, and will activate the normal mechanisms in the body to protect the skin from burning. This is, however, not the case in the eye, where damaging amounts of radiation can be suffered, without feeling the heat. Repeated exposure can cause cataracts,

commonly known as glass blower's cataract. Various other types of eye injuries may also occur in severe and prolonged exposure, e.g. retinal burns.

3 **Laser beams**. The name derives from light amplification by stimulated emission of radiation. It is a beam of light energy of one length, and uniform in phase, which travels together in step and in rhythm. The dangers of laser are inherent in the power or energy density of the beam. Even with a one per cent reflectance from a dark surface, the light can be potentially hazardous to exposed skin or eyes (Schilling, 1973:268).

Protection is based on avoidance of the beam and its reflection, which can be obtained by having non-reflective black surfaces to cut down on the reflection in rooms where these beams are used.

4 **Microwaves and radiofrequency waves**. Microwaves produce heat that is a great deal more penetrating than infrared radiation. An internationally agreed-upon safe exposure limit for microwaves is 10 milliwatts/square cm. Interlocks on oven doors are necessary to ensure that radiation ceases when the door is opened.

Waves shorter than 10 cm are absorbed within the skin (e.g. infrared); 10-30 cm waves are absorbed mostly by subcutaneous fat, whilst the waves of 30 cm and longer penetrate into deeper muscular tissues. For this reason the longer waves provide the main risks as they are absorbed into deeper tissue, without giving the warning sensation of heat.

The cornea and the lens of the eye are again at risk due to the lack of blood supply to these tissues which can dissipate the heat of the waves.

The effects of radiation from video display terminals and similar electronic equipment, cell phones, ultrasound equipment, etc. are suspected of being harmful but confirmed research is not yet documented. General protection principles apply, which include:
- Avoidance of overexposure through curtailing exposure time and personal protection
- Safe work procedures
- Regular measurement of exposure levels and durations of exposure
- Bi-annual medical examination of exposed skin and eyes
- Record-keeping of exposure levels and duration and medical examinations.

4.7.2.2 Noise and hearing conservation

Noise is one of the most prevalent occupational hazards and noise-induced hearing loss a common occupational disease. Noise has auditory and non-auditory effects on the human body which affect safety and productivity in the workplace.

In order to understand the effect of sound/noise on the human body, the occupational health professional should be familiar with the terms listed below.

Sound. Sound is the mechanical vibration of an elastic medium such as air, fluid or resonant objects, resulting in waves of energy being transmitted away from the source. When these sound waves reach the tympanic membrane they are relayed to the brain and perceived as sound. Sound displays various characteristics:
- Sound waves vary in length. Generally, high-pitched sounds have short wavelengths, and low-pitched sounds long wavelengths.

Occupational health

- Sound frequency is the number of vibrations per second in the sound wave. Audible frequencies range between 15 to 20 000 Herz (Hz). Below 20 Hz frequencies are sensed as vibration in solid objects.
- Sound speed is determined by the transfer of momentum in a specific medium. In air, at a temperature of 21 °C, the speed of sound is 344 metre/second.
- Sound pressure is the variation of pressure from the normal ambient pressure in the atmosphere. On the logarithmic decibel scale relative to the normal hearing threshold of zero decibels (0dB), the threshold for hearing loss has been set at 85dB.
- Sound power is emitted by any sound source, and this can be measured in watts. As the sound power is influenced by many external factors, it is a physical characteristic only used to compare sound sources.

Noise in industry. Sound waves usually spread out uniformly through the air. At a reasonable distance from the source, the average noise intensity is proportional to the square of the sound pressure, and inversely proportional to the density of the medium and the speed of the sound in the medium. When applied, this law shows that the pressure in a sound wave reduces by six dB with each doubling of distance from the source to a receiver (Schoeman & Schröder, 1994:200).

The application of various mathematical calculations show that:
- Sound intensity decreases with the inverse square, proportional to the distance from the sound source.
- The sound pressure of a wavelength decreases in direct relation to the distance from the sound source.

This is important in noise control and control of exposure to noise in the work environment.

The measurement of noise. Various instruments and techniques are available to measure noise. Although these devices may provide useful data on whether or not there is a possible risk of annoyance or hearing damage, the definition of hearing risk itself is dependent on a knowledge of how much acoustic energy has entered the ear. The sound level meter is the basic instrument used for measuring noise.

The human ear responds in a non-uniform way to different sound-pressure levels – the perceived intensity/loudness may differ from person to person, and for this purpose a weighting curve has been constructed (A). Sound-pressure levels are then expressed in dB(A), which conforms to the weighting curve, and reflects the perception of that sound emission by the normal human ear (Guild et al., 2000:196).

Types of noise
Din. This is the most common type of noise experienced in everyday life, e.g. the sound of cars, typewriters, music, etc. It consists of a wide variety of frequencies in the audible range between 20–20 000 Hz. We need to hear sound to give us information about our environment, but above a certain din, sound becomes noise.

Ultrasonic sound. This type of sound has frequencies higher than the audible range, and is experienced as vibrations. These can easily be shielded or absorbed and the control of this noise does not really present undue difficulty in industry.

Infrasonic sound. This is the noise below 20 Hz frequencies, and although it loses tonal qualities below 16 Hz, it is now believed that infrasonic noise is audible, and produces physiological effects such as changes in breathing, heart rhythms and disturbances in the functioning of the central nervous system.

Conventional ear protection is ineffective in attenuating infrasonic sound. Because of the physiological effects of this sound, whole body protection should be provided.

Impulse noise. These noises are characterized by a sharp instantaneous rise in sound pressure, such as a gunshot or sudden impact machinery in industry, and may cause instantaneous hearing damage. Other unpleasant physiological reactions such as a rise in blood pressure, increased pulse rate and headaches may also take place as a result of sudden unexpected noise.

Continuous noise. The intensity of noise remains constant for a considerable period of time, e.g. turbines and electric motors.

Fluctuating noise. This is where the intensity of noise varies considerably over a period of time, e.g. an engine running at different speeds, it is described as fluctuating noise.

Interrupted noise. This is when variations in sound level occur due to the switching on and off of equipment, e.g. hand-drills and grinding wheels, it is known as interrupted noise (Schoeman & Schröder, 1994:203).

Auditory effects of exposure to noise
Loss of hearing. Occupational hearing loss is defined as a partial or complete hearing impairment of one or both ears which originates during, and as a result of a person's work. This is a common health risk in industry.

Schoeman and Schröder (1994:74) describe three types of hearing loss as a result of noise-exposure:
1 The loss occurring directly after exposure – a temporary threshold shift (TTS) takes place. The impairment of auditory sensitivity is temporary.
2 The loss occurring after a long-term exposure – a permanent threshold shift (PTS) takes place, and permanent impairment of auditory sensitivity takes place.
3 Acoustic loss – the type of impairment which follows a single intense exposure to noise, e.g. an explosion. This trauma may be reversible.

Non-auditory effects of exposure to noise. The damaging effects of noise are not only limited to hearing, but also present a variety of symptoms such as:
- Emotional effects, e.g. irritability, stress and fatigue
- Physiological effects, e.g. changes in sleeping pattern, increased excretion of

adrenaline, lack of concentration, disturbances of the balance organ leading to dizziness, nausea and sight disturbances.

Controlling exposure to noise. This forms an essential element of any hearing conservation programme. Engineering control of the source of the noise is still the obvious method for silencing machinery which cannot suddenly be replaced without great sacrifice (Schoeman & Schröder, 1994:233).

Four basic ways to effectively control noise are discussed below.
1. *Modification of the noise radiation pattern.* Noise is highly directional, and it is therefore possible to shield and reflect noise so that it can only be heard after it has struck some sound-absorbent surface.

    Movable screens of absorbent material, and an absorbent ceiling covering can do much to reduce personal noise exposure.
2. *Noise suppression.* This may be achieved by introducing noise-absorbing physical barriers and/or enclosing machines that emit noise.
3. *Noise reduction.* Many mechanical processes used in industry produce noise, e.g. cutting, hammering and vibration. For technical reasons these actions cannot be avoided, but with moderate additional costs, they can be made quieter. The fitting of vibration dampers and proper maintenance of machines will greatly reduce the noise emitted.
4. *Noise avoidance.* The changing of equipment in noise-emitting processes for equipment that emits low noise levels can reduce this hazard. Purchasing standards for equipment must include permissible noise emission.

The hearing conservation programme. A well-organized, meaningful hearing conservation programme, accepted and endorsed by management, with a supporting company policy, is an essential element in the control of this health hazard.

An effective programme should contain the following objectives:
- The prevention of noise-induced deafness
- A decrease in noise interference with communication
- Legal compliance
- A decrease in company expenditure for deafness compensation.

Elements of a programme
1. *Organization of programme.* A specific person should be responsible for the coordination of the total programme. This person will make use of the expertise of various specialists, e.g. engineers, architects, health personnel, occupational hygienist, and training and administrative services.

    Each worker should, however, also take responsibility for his/her own health and must be familiar with regulations and the dangers of noise exposure.
2. *Effective policy and legislation.* A hearing conservation policy is drawn up according to policy-making procedure. Legislation makes provision for the protection of the worker against excessive exposure to unacceptable levels of noise in terms of the

Noise Regulations of the Occupational Health and Safety Act (No 85 of 1993). (For further information on legislation, consult Chapter 2.)
3 *Identification of noise areas.* This can be achieved by a noise survey whereby management and health personnel should take part in the identification of noise in the workplace. These areas must be accurately assessed by an accredited occupational hygienist. The nature of the noise and its character, e.g. frequency, type, etc. must be established to design cost-effective measures for reducing the hazard.
4 *Noise control.* Control measures established for a dynamic conservation programme should be based upon the assessment of problem areas, and should include the following:
- Engineering control where engineering departments address the design of plants and machinery to be used in order to reduce noise emissions and isolate the noise
- Standards for purchasing equipment and design specifications
- Maintenance of equipment to reduce vibration and wear and tear
- Effective educational programmes on the long-term danger of noise exposure, self-protection and the wearing and care of hearing protectors
- Administrative control through changes in production programmes, multi-skilling that allows each employee to work with noisy machines for only part of the work day and the rotation of shifts of exposed workers.
- The issuing and wearing of the correct type of hearing protectors for the type of noise exposure is the the last important factor in noise control.
5 *Audiometric testing.* Through the use of audiometric testing the effects of noise on a person's hearing can be measured. In terms of Instruction 171 of the Compensation for Occupational Injuries and Diseases Act, 1993 (No 130 of 1993) the procedure is carried out by a technician who is registered with the Department of Labour as an audiometrist.

The person may not have been exposed to noise for a period of sixteen hours before the test, and the booth and equipment must be calibrated regularly.

The testing procedure is explained to the person to be tested before placing him/her in a soundproof booth and fitting the earphones. Sound is produced in a pure tone, at measurable levels, to one ear at a time. The test commences at 1 000 Hz, which is easy to hear, and the level is reduced until it is inaudible before increasing the level until it is audible again to the person tested. The hearing threshold of the person is established at a particular level. The process is carried on for each ear at various frequencies and graphically recorded. This method provides for a graph screening of a person's hearing.

In terms of Instruction 171 every employee must have a baseline audiogram for determining present and future loss of hearing.
- Pre-placement audiograms. During the pre-placement medical screening process, it is important that a baseline hearing assessment be done and a history of previous exposure to noise be recorded. The person's hearing acuity should be assessed in view of job placement, future hearing conservation and compensation for any hearing loss present.

- Periodic audiometric tests must be done every 6 or 12 months, according to noise level exposure. Every periodic test is compared to the previous and to the baseline audiogram and the results are discussed with the person whose hearing was tested.
- Serial audiometry. Where noise problems do exist, self-recording apparatus may be used for audiometry that is carried out at agreed intervals during the work day.

The role of the occupational health care professional in hearing conservation

Occupational healthcare professionals must be familiar with all aspects of noise and the hearing mechanism to enable them to play a meaningful role in the programme. Although hearing conservation is a team effort that requires management commitment, and participation of all members of the occupational health team, line management and employees, the nurse, for example is the person in the occupational setting who has a direct input when it comes to health matters.

Education and motivation of employers and employees form an integral part of a successful hearing conservation programme and it is also in this area that healthcare professionals play a major role.

Occupational healthcare professionals are active in the following roles:
- Consultant – occupational health nurses act as advisers to both the management and the employees of the company as regards hearing conservation.
- Educator – employees are educated about the dangers of noise exposure and motivated to take part in all activities instituted to protect hearing.
- Administrators – they maintain the necessary documentation so that an accurate record system of workers' health and exposure levels is available.

The functions of occupational healthcare professionals in hearing conservation

Details of their job description may vary from one industry to another, but the following basic functions are usually required from health care professionals in industry:
- Periodic visits to the workplace to consult with managers, and observe procedures applied to protect hearing
- Observation of noisy areas, and comparing noise levels with the legislative requirements
- Noise surveys in the workplace
- Liaison with the occupational health team when reported levels are a health hazard
- Negotiation with management for a control programme if necessary
- Familiarization with actions taken to reduce risks, and actions for the application of hearing protection; and observation as to whether protection is worn
- Health surveillance of the worker; treatment and referral of the affected worker
- Ensuring that audiometric tests are done regularly, that the person and line management are notified of appointments timeously in order that tests may be done before work commences
- Comparing results with the baseline test and discussing them with the person concerned, using the test as an educational tool

- Performing baseline, pre-placement and periodic screening of workers for deterioration of hearing
- Reporting noise-induced hearing loss to the Compensation Commissioner in terms of Regulation 171 of the Compensation for Occupational Injuries and Diseases Act, 1993 (No 130 of 1993).

4.7.2.3 Lighting and vision

Lighting. Light rays of varying lengths are emitted from various sources. Lighting for work purposes is obtained mainly from two sources: natural lighting from the sun, and artificial lighting mainly from electrical sources.

Proper lighting in the workplace will have numerous advantages, such as:
- Preservation of human energy because working under harsh light or poor illumination is tiring
- Prevention of eyestrain, headaches and poor posture as workers strain to see
- Prevention of accidents and poor quality work caused by poor lighting
- Improvement of conditions in the workplace and worker morale
- Increased productivity due to improved accuracy and quality of work
- Promotion of the effective use of human and other resources.

Principles of good lighting. The quality and quantity of lighting in the workplace must be sufficient to enable the worker to see properly, without straining the eyes. The Environmental Regulations for Workplaces, applicable under the Occupational Health and Safety Act, 1993 (No 85 of 1993), lists illumination levels for various places and types of work. Employers must make provision for compliance with these regulations. Where a lack of natural light in the workplace causes dangerous conditions, illumination is required. The installation of windows in order to allow workers to see outside is also prescribed (Schoeman & Schröder, 1994:161).

Good quality light can be obtained from daylight and/or artificial sources, but contrasts and luminance must be adjusted to suit the job required. Glare must be prevented as this may cause discomfort and an inability to distinguish recognizable objects.

Schoeman and Schröder state that glare is probably the greatest enemy of visual performance and thus of productivity and the comfort of the worker. Glare can be described as a kind of unsuitable light caused by any source of excess luminance or brightness in the field of view (1994:162).

Photometers are used to measure illumination. Instruments in different sizes and degree of sensitivity, depending on the type of measuring required, are available.

Sight safety and vision protection. The complex technological developments of the past few decades set visual requirements that necessitate the assessment of the visual abilities of individual workers for specific jobs prior to job placement and also periodically during employment. Vision screening for acuity, near and far vision, depth perception, colour vision and the extent of the vision field is required, bearing in mind that vision can deteriorate with age and can be corrected.

Eye injury due to an occupational accident is common and it is important that hazards be recognized and controlled.

Eye injuries can be classified according to the following causes:
Burns. These can be chemical, thermal or radiation burns. Chemical burns include acid and alkaline burns. Acid burns cause rapid opacification of the corneal epithelium. Alkaline burns are deeply penetrating and the alkalinity may pass into the anterior chamber and cause deep-seated inflammatory conditions.

Thermal burns may cause contracture of the lids, shrinkage of the conjunctiva, and corneal ulceration. These are slow to heal and often lead to permanent scarring of the cornea.

Radiation injuries may be caused by any kind of radiation, e.g. ultraviolet, infrared or emissions from laser sources. Ultraviolet radiation may cause inflammation of the lids, conjunctiva and cornea; infrared rays cause damage to the choroid, iris, ciliary body and retina. Prolonged exposure may cause cataracts. Laser radiation may cause retinal burns and choroidal damage.

Mechanical injuries. Small projectiles (foreign bodies) are the most common cause of mechanical injuries, and may lead to a variety of injuries depending upon the type of injury, nature of projectile and the tissue involved. Foreign bodies may cause subconjunctival haemorrhages, corneal and conjunctival abrasions, as well as extensive trauma, and must be referred to a doctor. See Chapter 9, section 9.14.11.

Penetrating injuries. Penetrating foreign bodies may cause rupture of and displacement of the inner structures of the eyes. If the foreign body is retained in the eye after penetration further complications such as inflammatory conditions may occur. All penetrating injuries must be referred to an ophthalmologist.

Vision protection programmes. As part of the occupational hygiene programme all possible vision risks are identified, eliminated, enclosed and minimized. Employees are educated about the hazards and protective measures, as well as first-aid procedures to be followed in the event of an accident. The use of goggles as eye protection cannot ensure safety, but should form part of a comprehensive protection programme.

Visual welfare programmes. Comprehensive programmes to ensure the visual welfare of employees is an important aspect of occupational health. Such programmes can bring about considerable advantages for both the employer and employee. Aspects that should be considered in these programmes are:
- Visual task analysis, e.g. lighting, distance of task, contrast, movement, colour recognition, duration of task and hazards involved
- Lighting, e.g. minimum levels and type of illumination required for specific tasks
- Working distance from the task to be performed by the worker – this may be described as:
  - teloramic – more than two metres away
  - mesoramic – between 30 cm and two metres

- ancoramic – less than 30 cm
- Size of object involved in the task – very small, small, medium or large
- Contrast between the different light sensations – caused by factors such as brightness, colour and texture
- Mobile objects – make perception of the particular object more difficult
- Definition of the object and legibility
- Job detail analysis – required to determine the visual acuity required to perform the task
- Colour recognition – important in certain jobs where colour coding is important
- Prolonged duration of performance on a specific task – may require some form of visual aid
- Ergonomic factors including correct seating, height of work top, work design, rest periods, and regular change of eye focus play an important role in visual welfare.

Good cooperation between all the parties involved in the planning of the working environment is essential to ensure that the worker has a visual environment in which to perform tasks safely and effectively.

4.7.2.4 Extreme temperatures

Many workers are exposed to very high or very low temperatures in their physical work environment. The effect of these temperatures on the worker is subject to the type of occupation, the duration of exposure, effectiveness of protective clothing and the individual's coping mechanisms.

The human body has a very sensitive temperature control mechanism, which keeps the body temperature at a normal level, even though the skin temperature can vary considerably. Heat is generated in the body by the chemical processes of metabolism.

The transfer of heat in the human body. Temperature should not be considered in isolation, as there are many variables concerned in the transfer of heat, e.g. human and environmental factors.

The following four processes take part in the exchange of heat:
1. *Radiation*. This process accounts for 60 per cent of the total heat exchange during rest. All materials absorb and emit radiant energy, some have a low and others a high emission rate, e.g. matt and polished metal surfaces.
2. *Evaporation*. Twenty-five per cent of the total heat exchange during rest takes place through evaporation. This process can only take place in the presence of a water vapour pressure gradient between the surface of the human body and the environment. A large gradient leads to quick evaporation.
3. *Convection*. Twelve per cent of the heat exchange takes place by convection. Air circulating over the surface of the body transfers heat to and from the body.
4. *Conduction*. This process accounts for 3 per cent of total heat exchange during rest. With the aid of conduction, heat travels from a high temperature to a low temperature area. Under normal conditions the evaporation of perspiration from

Occupational health

the body removes heat and lowers the body temperature, when the environmental temperature is lower than that of the body (Schoeman & Schröder, 1994).

It is said that people can become acclimatized to heat (Schilling, 1981). The body adapts to extreme conditions with the necessary accompanying physiological responses. This will, however, not be applicable in continuous exposure to extreme conditions for prolonged periods of time, as it may still lead to failure of the human body to make the required changes.

Workload. The tempo at which a person performs activities largely determines his/her metabolic rate (energy consumption).

For the purpose of determining energy and oxygen consumption work can be divided into three categories:
1. *Light work*, e.g. sitting or standing to control machines or doing light hand or arm work (energy consumption less than 850 kJ/ hour)
2. *Medium work*, e.g. walking about, medium lifting/shifting equipment (energy consumption 850–1 500 kJ/hour)
3. *Heavy work*, e.g. spade and shovel work (energy consumption more than 1 500 kJ/hour) (Schoeman & Schröder, 1994:131).

This classification of work in terms of energy and oxygen consumption is important to create a healthy workplace for the worker. In the areas of heavy work, suitable workers must be selected and, in order to forestall exhaustion, adequate nutrition and rest periods should be provided during a workshift.

Heat illness/stress. Extreme temperatures in the workplace can cause illness if not properly controlled. The term 'heat illness' is used to describe the failure of the human body to adjust to heat stress. See Chapter 9, section 9.14.12 for additional information. Schoeman and Schröder (1994:141) identify the following manifestations of heat stress in order of seriousness:
- Heat rash – caused by continuous perspiration on the skin
- Heat cramps – caused by factors such as an electrolyte deficiency, dehydration and inadequate blood or oxygen provision.

Heat exhaustion. This is usually caused by physical exertion in a hot humid environment such as underground in mines or when firing up a kiln. The symptoms are:
- Vertigo, headache, fatigue and visual disturbances
- Nausea, vomiting, diarrhoea
- Muscle cramps
- Cool clammy skin
- Shortness of breath, palpitations, fast, weak pulse
- Numbness in arms and legs.

This condition may lead to heat collapse and must be treated as a medical emergency. (See Chapter 9.)

Heat stroke. This occurs when the body fails to adjust to heat stress, owing to:
- *Excessive perspiration* with the resultant loss in body fluids and salt. This may occur when work is done in extremely hot conditions.
- *A rise in body temperature* due to the failure of the normal cooling mechanisms of the body. This is common when working in areas with extremely high temperatures.

The symptoms of heat stress are:
- Hot and dry skin, temperature above 39.5 °C
- Irregular breathing, full bounding pulse
- Pupils dilated
- Convulsions
- Urinary and faecal incontinence.

The patient must be cooled and emergency medical treatment given immediately. (See Chapter 9.)

Prevention of heat illness
- People exposed to such conditions at work should be physically fit and preferably acclimatized.
- An adequate intake of electrolyte solution and water must be maintained.
- Loose-fitting and permeable clothing (cotton) should be worn, but clothing should also be dense enough to protect the person from radiant heat where applicable.
- When exposure to radiant heat also takes place, workers should have resting periods in a cooled area at frequent intervals.
- Physical exertion should be kept to a minimum; this is necessary to reduce internal heat production.

Hypothermia (cold stress). Many workers in outdoor occupations such as the fishing industry and agriculture are exposed to extremely cold conditions in winter, which are aggravated by wind and rain. Indoor occupations, such as working in cold storage areas, also predispose to hypothermia. Exposure to cold conditions increases the metabolic rate of the human body. The general effects of extreme cold conditions occur in the following sequence:
- Excessive heat loss from the body, with a fall in temperature
- Shivering (which is the body's normal reaction to try and increase heat production by muscular activity)
- Extreme exhaustion, pale skin, slow pulse and respiration, incoordination of muscles
- Confusion, unconsciousness and unless treated, death
- Frostbite, which is the freezing of exposed tissue and extremities and is usually only discovered later.

Occupational health

Prevention of hypothermia
- There should be careful selection of workers (people with certain physical characteristics, such as moderate fat and a strong muscular build, seem to do better).
- Protective clothing to insulate the body should be worn.
- Wind and waterproof outer clothing, which is also permeable to allow perspiration to evaporate, should be worn.
- Special protection for extremities, e.g. hands and feet, should be worn.
- If the period of exposure is continuous, time for rest must be allowed in sufficiently heated rooms, with warm refreshments provided to stimulate metabolism.

For the treatment of these conditions, refer to Chapter 9.

4.7.2.5 Abnormal atmospheric pressure

Persons are exposed to high atmospheric pressure in occupations such as underwater operations and compressed air tunnelling and to low atmospheric pressure in aviation and mountaineering.

The barometric pressure at sea level is 760 mmHg or 1 atmosphere. As a person moves higher up into the atmosphere, the barometric pressure decreases (hypobaric), whilst below sea level, the pressure increases (hyperbaric).

An ascent of 5 500 metres into the air is required to halve the atmospheric pressure, but a descent into only 10 metres of water doubles it. Every additional 10 metres adds another 1 kg of pressure per cm.

The change in the pressure of inspired air causes physiological disturbances because the effect of a gas is determined by its partial pressure. At a depth of 30 m the partial pressure of carbon monoxide is four times that at the surface. The major constituents of air, namely oxygen and nitrogen, also present problems in the form of nitrogen narcosis that can incapacitate divers. The increase in air density with depth means that more energy is required for respiration, and as the maximum breathing capacity is reduced, carbon dioxide retention occurs.

The human body reacts to these changes in pressure with physiological adjustments in respiration, blood consistency and circulation depending on the barometric pressure and the person's condition.

High barometric air pressure. This is a condition experienced by people working in areas of compressed air, e.g. in tunnelling, deep-sea diving and in caissons. The effect of high barometric pressure is:
- An increase in the amount of air dissolved in the blood and body fluids
- On rapid return to normal pressure levels, nitrogen gas is released in the form of bubbles. These lodge in the joints and under muscles, causing severe muscular cramps, chest pain, urticaria and decompression sickness (commonly known as 'the bends'). Paralysis and death can occur in severe cases and it is a major problem with underwater accidents where patients need to be brought to the surface urgently. Aseptic necrosis, especially of the hip and shoulder bones, is a delayed complication of decompression sickness. (Zenz, et al., 1994).

The amount of nitrogen dissolving in body tissues is proportional to its partial pressure, solubility coefficient and duration of exposure to pressure.

The reduction of pressure during decompression leads to:
- The expansion of the air in sinuses, ears and lungs
- Trapped excess air in the lung may expand and burst:
  - through the pleura to produce air pneumothorax
  - into the lung to produce emphysema
  - into the vascular system resulting in arterial air embolism.

It is for this reason that persons are subject to stringent medical examination and selection before exposure to abnormal atmospheric pressure.

Low barometric air pressure. Air inhaled at sea level saturates the blood with 97 per cent oxygen. At a level of 10 000 m above sea level, oxygen saturation is only 15 per cent. This leads to a condition of hypoxia in the human body unless the cabin is pressurized or oxygen is supplied.

Lack of oxygen can interfere with concentration and lead to disorientation and blackouts.

At high altitudes mountaineers may suffer from hypoxia (above 4 580 m). Common symptoms are headache, lassitude, dyspnoea on exertion, nausea and vomiting. Adaptation to these conditions can take place, usually after 12–24 hours.

Prevention of barotrauma. Workers must be examined by medical specialists in the fields of aviation and barotrauma before work in compressed air areas commences. Regular medical surveillance is necessary.

Persons with a history of pneumothorax, thoracic surgery, chronic sinusitis, respiratory or ear infection may be excluded from hyperbaric or hypobaric occupations. Applicants with hypertension, diabetes, fractures of long bones in the past five years and migraine sufferers will be carefully scrutinized.

Identification tags should be worn to indicate the area of work and the location of the nearest decompression chamber, for use in the case of decompression sickness.

4.7.2.6 Ventilation

The purpose of a ventilation system is to control the quality of the air in the workplace. The performance of the system must be monitored regularly by ventilation officers to ensure that it serves its purpose.

Temperature, humidity, air distribution and dispersion, and the choice of air filters are important aspects of any ventilation system.

Effective ventilation is required for optimal productivity of the workers for the following reasons:

Health requirements
- Provision of oxygen for breathing
- Prevention of unacceptable carbon dioxide concentrations
- Removal of offensive smells

- Removal of the accumulation of harmful concentrations of organisms
- Removal/dilution of hazardous contaminants
- Aiding in the maintaining of the heat balance of the body.

Thermal comfort
- Removal of excessive heat generated by equipment and the presence of persons
- Heating or cooling the air to acceptable levels as determined by the occupational hygienist.

Engineering requirements. A building requires an effective ventilation system for reasons of safety including:
- Prevention of fire and explosions in hazardous areas
- Ensuring the proper functioning of exhaust systems
- Elimination of pressure differences at doors
- Ensuring complete combustion and so avoiding a build up of carbon monoxide
- Conserving energy that would be required to heat or cool the building if there was no ventilation system.

Legal requirements. The Environmental Regulations for Workplaces applicable under the Occupational Health and Safety Act, 1993 (No 85 of 1993) are in force to ensure that each workplace is properly ventilated so that the health and safety of workers is not endangered (Schoeman & Schröder, 1994:287–291).

4.7.2.7 Ergonomics
Ergonomics is the study of human capabilities, and the interaction of the worker and the job demands. In practice, ergonomics attempts to reduce the physical and mental stress of the job by optimizing the work environment and the design of the work to fit the individual. Grandjean (1980) called it 'fitting the man to the task'.

Human capabilities, both physical and mental, as well as environmental factors, include:
- Physical – body capabilities (size, reach, strength, posture) and workplace design (seating, desk, equipment). An inadequate relationship between the person and the workplace leads to muscle fatigue, back and neck pain, inefficiency, repetitive strain injuries, and accidents.
- Mental – aptitude, adequate training and an efficient work design are required to prevent inefficiency, mental fatigue, lower productivity, muscle tension, stress and low morale.
- Environmental – optimal illumination, ventilation, temperature and pleasant surroundings without vibration, noise, unpleasant smells, etc. If these factors are inadequate, they lead to discomfort, eye strain, headache, irritation, inefficiency and errors.

Ergonomic evaluations are done with a checklist and questionnaire at the work station to assess the:
- Work area – worktop, seat height, workspace, equipment and general environment

- Work design – shifts, work hours, rest breaks, and the arrangement and sequence of processes and methods of work
- Worker in action – body posture, signs of discomfort such as rubbing the eyes or stretching the limbs, restlessness, attitude and morale.

During a workplace walk-through and survey, an investigation of complaints, absenteeism, low productivity and accidents or incidents may also reveal underlying ergonomic problems. (See also Chapter 3, section 3.17.)

4.7.3 Mechanical hazards

The invention of machinery in the eighteenth century brought new hazards to the worker. Many of these machines were dangerous and unguarded, and caused mutilation and deformities.

Today, the dangers of mechanical equipment are well understood, although not always treated with the necessary precautions. The Occupational Health and Safety Act, 1993 (No 85 of 1993) and its Regulations prescribes the specific safety precautions required. The Regulations for General Machinery (1988), Electrical Machinery (1990), Driven Machinery (1992) and Lift, Escalator, and Passenger Conveyor (1994) are applicable. See also Chapter 2 for legislation.

4.7.3.1 Vibration

The increased use of machinery in the occupational environment represents another threat to the health of the worker, in the form of mechanical vibration. Vibration is oscillatory motion about a point and is characterized by frequency and intensity.

Frequency is measured in Hz, and in human exposure the frequencies between 0 and 1 000 Hz are important. The intensity of vibration is the maximum displacement of energy from a central point, and is expressed in centimetres.

Sources of vibration are mainly machines and equipment, e.g. turbines, compressors, electrical pumps and especially truck, tractor and bus drivers usually cause whole-body vibration. Vibrating hand tools, such as chain saws, air pressure drills and jackhammers, cause hand-arm vibration.

The extent of exposure to vibration is determined by factors such as body size, posture and strain.

The effect of exposure is determined by the frequency, intensity, time of exposure, direction of vibration and the isolation effect of clothing.

The physiological effect of vibration on the body. Vibrations do not affect all people in the same way – some people can absorb and/or tolerate more than others.

The human body is most sensitive to vibrations between 0.5 and 20 Hz.

The following symptoms may be experienced in the above range: general feeling of discomfort, muscle contraction, involuntary desire to urinate and defaecate, chest pain, abdominal pain and difficulty in breathing, changes in heart rate and blood-pressure, vertigo and travel sickness. Vibration may also negatively influence achievement – tasks requiring visual acuity and fine motor coordination may be affected.

Hand-arm vibration may give rise to conditions such as:
- Circulatory disorders – Raynaud's phenomenon or Vibration-induced white finger (VWF)
- Bone and joint disorders – osteoarthritis of the bones in the wrist and hand
- Neurological disorders – numbness, tingling and reduced nerve conduction velocity
- Muscle disorders – incoordination of small movements of the fingers.

Vibration-induced white finger can be mild, moderate or severe. At first there are occasional attacks affecting the tip of one finger, then more phalanges and fingers are affected until eventually there are frequent attacks affecting all the phalanges of most fingers.

Preventive measures. Vibration of machinery must be reduced at every level, from:
- The tool and machine manufacturers, who should minimize vibration in the design and improve ergonomic standards of equipment to reduce strain of any group of muscles and tendons
- The company management, who must insist on the best equipment, seek technical advice, replace outdated machines and reduce exposure time through multi-skilling and staff rotation
- The engineers, who need to build vibration absorbers under and around vibrating machines and the handles of tools
- The maintenance staff, who must service machines regularly to ensure smooth running of engines and replace worn parts frequently
- The risk managers, who must assess and keep records of vibration levels regularly and provide suitable protective gear
- The occupational health practitioners, who must do preplacement and periodic medical examinations and recommend no exposure for workers with a predisposition for circulatory problems. They must educate the employees about the effects of vibration and how to prevent excessive exposure
- The employees, who must wear protective gloves, report increased vibration or malfunctioning of equipment, keep hands warm when using hand tools and adopt a good working position. They must avoid excessive exposure to vibration and be aware of early symptoms and report to the occupational health nurse if they do occur.

4.7.4 Biological hazards

Biological agents are defined as 'any micro-organism, cell culture or human endoparasite including any that have been genetically modified, which may cause infection, allergy or toxicity, or otherwise create a hazard to human health'.

These constitute a particular hazard to people who work in laboratories and health institutions as contamination may occur in pursuance of the occupation. Workers who work with animals or animal products are also exposed to these hazards.

The Regulations for Hazardous Biological Agents (2002) of the Occupational Health and Safety Act, 1993 (No 85 of 1993) prescribes protective measures that must be instituted in these work areas including:

- Safe work procedures
- Engineering control measures and good housekeeping practices
- Education about the effects of the agent and personal protective equipment
- High personal hygiene standards
- Medical surveillance and biological monitoring for all workers possibly exposed to biological agents.

In terms of the Compensation for Occupational Injuries and Diseases Act (No 130 of 1993) the following conditions caused by exposure to biological agents at work are compensatable:
- Hepatitis A and B
- Anthrax
- Brucellosis
- Tuberculosis.

4.7.5 Psychological hazards

The mental health of individuals can be influenced positively or negatively by their occupation. Work situations that are very stressful have a negative influence on physical well-being and may lead to mental illness.

It is generally accepted that the following situations may lead to high levels of stress:
- Certain occupations are stressful by nature, e.g. high-powered executive jobs; occupations in the medical and nursing profession; occupations where the worker is exposed to highly dangerous activities, such as mining, flying, diving, etc.
- Poor interpersonal relationships in the work situation may lead to tension and anxiety.
- Job dissatisfaction and uncertainty over job security are stressful.

The list goes on and it must be said that people cope differently with stressful situations and it is in the way that the problem is perceived that the outcome is directed. (Consult Chapter 11 for full details.)

Apart from psychological hazards caused by the work situation, many workers are struggling to overcome personal traumatic experiences, such as criminal violence, domestic and financial problems and Aids. Unhappy people have a negative influence on productivity, work attendance and morale, which is costly to the company. An employee assistance programme where troubled workers are assisted in finding solutions has been proved as cost effective in the workplace.

4.8 The role and functions of the occupational healthcare professional in the control of the environment

The role. Occupational healthcare professionals, such as nurses fulfil several roles in the workplace. With their expertise in occupational health matters they are consultants to management and workers alike – they are educators, clinicians, administrators and professional role models for health.

Occupational healthcare professionals must also be familiar with the work individuals are required to undertake. Knowledge of the workplace and its processes can only be obtained by investigating all aspects that affect or may be harmful to the employees. Continual updating of knowledge on clinical, technical, legal and socio-economic issues is vital for the occupational health nurse. See Chapter 6, section 6.5 for details of the role of the occupational health professional.

These roles, and the contribution healthcare professionals, such as nurses are able to make in the promotion of productivity, may be a new concept to some employers. The contribution healthcare professionals make also depends on the policy of the organization and management's willingness to commit themselves to an environment that contributes to positive health.

The functions. Occupational healthcare professionals, such as nurses in the occupational setting are part of a multidisciplinary team. Their functions therefore cover a wide spectrum of activities that are different from those traditionally ascribed to them in curative health services.

The presence of the healthcare professional (i.e. nurse) in the production areas may initially be viewed with apprehension and suspicion by workers and line managers. Diplomacy and a genuine interest in the work being performed and the well-being of all employees, will lead to acceptance and cooperation.

The functions of healthcare professionals (i.e. nurses) include:
- Managing all aspects of the occupational health service
- Being aware of the potential hazards that appear in the workplace by doing an environmental survey
- Observing the workers to establish the relationship between health problems and the working environment
- Working within an interdisciplinary occupational team and consulting with the risk manager, hygienist, safety professional, engineers, medical team, management and employees
- Developing health policies and strategies
- Assisting in evaluating work procedures to establish their health risk, if any
- Maintaining an efficient record system that will ensure complete and accurate data on all workers
- Planning the occupational health programme to include medical surveillance, health education, clinic times and visits to the plant
- Writing meaningful reports to management on the activities of the occupational health service, giving statistics and making recommendations.

The functions of the occupational healthcare professional are described in Chapters 6 and 7.

4.9 Conclusion

Occupational hygiene is an important cornerstone in the comprehensive occupational health system. The implementation of an environment where the principles of occupational hygiene are adhered to, becomes part of the task of the healthcare professional in this setting.

Other disciplines that contribute to a safe and controlled environment in the workplace are occupational safety and medicine. (See Chapters 3 and 5 for further details.)

4.10 Bibliography

Coetzee, A. M. 1995. *Gesondheidsbestuur waar mense werk.* Johannesburg: Lex Patria.

Gardner, W. & Taylor, P. 1975. *Health at Work.* London: Associated Business Programmes.

Grandjean, E. 1980. *Fitting the Man to the Task.* London: Taylor and Francis.

Guild, R., Ehrlich, R. I., Johnson, J. R., Ross, M. H. 2001. *A Handbook on Occupational Health Practice in the South African Mining Industry.* Johannesburg: SIMRAC.

Rogers, B. 1994. *Occupational Health Nursing.* Philadelphia: WB Saunders.

Rosenstock, L., Cullen, M. R. 1994 *Textbook of Clinical Occupational and Environmental Medicine.* Philadelphia: WB Saunders.

Schilling, R. S. F. (ed) 1973. *Occupational Health Practice.* London: Butterworths.

Schilling, R. S. F. (ed.) 1981. *Occupational Health Practice.* 2nd edition. London: Butterworths.

Schoeman, J. J. & Schröder, H. H. E. 1994. *Occupational Hygiene.* Cape Town: Juta.

Zenz, C., Dickerson, O. B., Horvath, J. R. 1994. *Occupational Medicine.* St Louis: Mosby.

5 Occupational medicine and occupational diseases

J. T. Mets and J. P. Murphy

5.1 Learning objectives

At the end of this chapter, the reader should be able to:
- Define the concepts of occupational medicine and disease
- Identify the main compensatable diseases
- Describe the management of selected occupational diseases.

5.2 Occupational medicine

Occupational medicine is concerned with the potential effect on human health that may be ascribed to factors in the work situation as a whole. As a component of the wider concept of occupational health, it covers the spectrum of prevention, early recognition of disease, treatment and rehabilitation, as well as the promotion of health in the workplace. Because people 'bring their health status from home to work', occupational medicine considers health at work not only in relation to the physical and psychological work environment, but also to the home and community environment from which its clients come.

Occupational hygiene, as the other leg of occupational health, covers environmental and other ergonomic factors and is principally the domain of engineers and safety practitioners, though of course of great interest to health workers. Occupational medicine is practised by doctors, nurses and their assistants after appropriate additional training and is concerned with individuals and groups of people defined by occupational characteristics. Its objectives are the prevention and management of medical problems associated with hazards in the workplace. As a medical speciality it is concerned with 'the appraisal, maintenance, restoration and promotion of the health of workers through the application of the principles of preventive and environmental medicine, emergency medical care, clinical medicine and rehabilitation'.

Clinical medicine, which includes first-contact primary healthcare, remains an integral part of the discipline, not only with regard to occupational diseases and injuries, but also to non-occupational diseases in settings such as prevail in developing countries like South Africa. The discipline rests, for its clinical aspects, on the basic medical sciences of which perhaps the most relevant are physiology and anatomy, pathology (in the sense of deviations of the normal functions and structures of the human body and mind), pharmacology, toxicology and biochemistry, immunology and the supporting discipline of epidemiology. Knowledge of clinical and industrial psychology and social science is of course of great value.

Table 5.1 shows the main elements of occupational medicine as practised in the field and as a component of occupational health. Although occupational medicine is essentially a clinical discipline, of necessity it incorporates a number of related 'non-clinical' elements. Some of the elements listed fall under more than one of the six main categories reflected in the table.

Table 5.1 Elements of occupational medicine

Preventive
1. Pre-placement examinations
2. Screening, periodic health surveillance
3. Monitoring of special and vulnerable groups
4. Monitoring of personal protection methods, including immunization
5. Epidemiological surveillance
6. Health education and training (e.g. first aid)
7. Research (clinical, ergonomic, epidemiological)

Promotive
1. Health education (alcohol, smoking, lifestyle)
2. Health maintenance (general)
3. Rehabilitation and job placement
4. Counselling and referral (employee assistance programmes) and social aspects

Clinical
1. Emergency medical care (acute conditions)
2. Occupational diseases and injuries
3. Primary healthcare
4. Continuing healthcare (chronic conditions)
5. Health surveillance and biological monitoring, e.g. statutory, drivers, 'return to work' examinations, etc.

Environmental
1. Hazard identification, recognition, evaluation and motivation for control
2. Legal requirements, monitoring
3. Extension to 'outside the factory wall' relations

Consultative
1. Placement and transfers on medical grounds
2. Coordination of clinical management of worker/patients
3. Professional to management, workers, unions, industrial relations and safety departments, etc.
4. Coordination of activities of inside with outside health institutions and other agencies
5. Community relations

Administrative
1. Medical, environmental, epidemiological and absenteeism records (not 'control')
2. Statutory records and reports, relevant legislation, e.g. Occupational Health and Safety Act, and Compensation of Occupational Injuries and Diseases Act
3. Policies, procedures, hazard documentation, standing medical directives and protocols
4. Reference library and documentation
5. Applied appropriate research

One of the main aims of the occupational health nurse would be the prevention and early recognition of occupational disease. If prevention has failed, assisting in establishing a diagnosis and in the management of the patient when suffering a work-induced or work-related occupational disease would follow. This would include rehabilitation and follow-up. It deserves emphasis that in the South African context primary healthcare is also very much a component of occupational medicine practice.

As the main subject of this chapter is occupational disease, no further discussion of specific elements of occupational medicine will follow here, except to state that the training of the occupational health nurse should, in order to enable her/him to adequately deal with occupational health problems such as occupational diseases, at least incorporate the following subjects:

1. Toxicology of the substances and pathology of the medical conditions most likely to occur, e.g. dusts causing pneumoconiosis, substances causing asthma, some metals used in industry and mining, organic solvents, toxic gases and vapours, pesticides and also physical agents which may cause harm such as heat, cold, excessive noise and radiation.
2. Relevant legislation pertaining to occupational diseases in the Compensation for Occupational Injuries and Diseases Act, 1993 (No 130 of 1993) (COID); the Occupational Diseases in Mines and Works Act, 1973 (No 78 of 1973) (ODMW) and the ODMW Amendment Act, 1993 (No 208 of 1993) – with sections pertaining to the control of occupational health hazards replaced by the Mine Health and Safety Act, 1996 (No 29 of 1996) (MHSA); the Occupational Health and Safety Act, 1993 (No 85 of 1993) (OHSA) and its Regulations. The latter provide for preventive measures backed by legal requirements and may also serve as a guide to select priorities, e.g. asbestos, lead, noise or any one of the 50 'High Risk Substances' listed in the General Administrative Regulations, or in the Hazardous Chemical Substances Regulations (11995), wherever usage of the substance in question occurs.
3. Clinical training within the scope of occupational health nursing practice in diagnosing and managing occupational disease, as well as primary healthcare.
4. Epidemiological aspects of occupational health with the emphasis on using these as a tool when dealing with groups of workers rather than with individuals only.

5.3 Occupational disease

In general, most so-called occupational diseases are initially indistinguishable from non-occupational diseases in terms of pathological manifestations. Many a case presents with such non-specific symptoms as weakness, insomnia, sweating, malaise, nausea, vomiting, anorexia, dizziness and headache. A list of toxins which may cause headache mentions 168 substances, the best known of which are perhaps carbon monoxide, (ethyl) alcohol and nitroglycerine, to which 'dynamite headache' is ascribed. Or, even more confusing, an occupational disease such as carbon disulphide poisoning presents with coronary artery disease symptoms.

Secondly, there is usually a latent interval between the onset of exposure and the first manifestation of the disease, which may make it difficult to link the two, especially in the case of carcinogens when the latent interval is long, e.g. mesothelioma developing 40 years after the first exposure.

Thirdly, many occupational factors that have an adverse effect on health may act in the same way as non-occupational factors or in concert with such 'outside' factors, e.g. the effect of smoking and of certain dusts on respiratory function.

Fourthly, many substances used in the workplace and that have an adverse effect on health if absorbed, are 'hidden' under a proprietary commercial name, without any indication of the generic, chemical name and thereby of its potential hazardous nature, e.g. 'genklean', which is a chlorinated hydrocarbon solvent.

Fifthly, the effect may well be dose dependent to such an extent that the degree of exposure and absorption determines if and when a noticeable effect occurs, possibly at a time when the relationship between the two is not readily apparent unless one is aware of such a possibility. In the case of zinc fume fever, for example, the delayed effect may mimic an attack of 'flu', which starts many hours after going home from work.

It is therefore very important for the occupational healthcare professional to know not only which potentially toxic substances and hazardous physical factors occur in the working environment of the employees under her/his care, but also to master the skills necessary to make a presumptive diagnosis or even just to suspect that a complaint or adverse effect may be linked to a particular hazard. Taking a detailed and thorough occupational history in addition to a general or specific medical history and ascertaining the quality (type), quantity (degree and duration) of exposure and possible absorption is the most important of these skills. Through a structured inquiry the occupational history should detail all known or suspected exposures to potential hazards, in degree, duration, and periods of time, where these occurred and in what type of job, and in which combinations, if any, with other stresses or hazards. Any effects, complaints, symptoms or signs that have been noticed earlier should also be noted, especially whether these occurred during or after work, were worse on any particular days of the week, or during weekends, at the beginning or at the end of shifts, recurred after periods of holidays or other absences from work and whether other co-workers have had similar complaints or manifestations. All this must of course be complemented by a thorough knowledge of symptoms, signs and laboratory tests which would help at arriving at a presumptive or definitive diagnosis for the particular occupational diseases that may be expected to occur in a particular working environment. In addition to this, a high degree of clinical suspicion, based on such knowledge, and sensitivity to complaints presented by workers and alleged to 'arise out of and in the course of their occupation' would favour early recognition. Good relationships with and an understanding of other departments and their specific expertise, e.g. in the field of engineering controls and personnel relations and close cooperation with other health workers are prerequisites for the nurse to fulfil her/his essential role in this respect: to prevent employees or groups of employees under her/his care from suffering significant adverse effects to their health.

5.3.1 Definitions and compensation aspects

Definitions
- Occupational disease is a disease that is caused solely or principally by factors that are peculiar to the working environment, and therefore arise out of and during work.
- Occupational Disease, according to the COID Act, 1993, 'means any disease mentioned in the first column of Schedule 3 arising out of and contracted in the course of an employee's employment'.

Table 5.2 Schedule 3 of the Compensation for Occupational Injuries and Diseases Act, 1993 (No 130 of 1993)

Schedule 3 of the Compensation for Occupational Injuries and Diseases Act, 1993 (No 130 of 1993)	
Diseases	**Work:**
	a Any work involving the handling of or exposure to any of the following substances emanating from the workplace concerned:
Pneumoconiosis-fibrosis of the parencyma of the lung	Organic or inorganic fibrogenic dust
Pleural thickening causing significant impairment of function	Asbestos or asbestos dust
Bronchopulmonary disease	Metal carbides (hard metals)
Byssinosis	Flax cotton or sisal
Occupational asthma	The sensitizing agents: 1 isocyanates 2 platinum, nickel, cobalt, vanadium or chromium salts 3 hardening agents, including epoxy resins 4 acrylic acids or derived acrylates 5 soldering or welding fumes 6 substances from animals or insects 7 fungi or spores 8 proteolytic enzymes 9 organic dust 10 vapours or fumes of formaldehyde, anhydrides, amines or diamines
Extrinsic allergy alveolotis	Moulds, fungal spores or any other allergenic proteinaceous material, 2.4 tuluene-di-isocyanates

Any disease or pathological manifestations	Beryllium, cadmium, phosphorus, chromium, manganese, arsenic, mercury, lead, fluorine, carbondisulphide, cyanide, halogen derivatives of aliphatic or aromatic hydrocarbons, benzene or its homologues, nitro- and amino-derivatives of benzene or its homologues, nitroglycerine or other nitric acid esters, hydrocarbons, trinitrotoluol, alcohol, glycols or ketones, acrylamide or any compounds of the afore-mentioned substances.
Erosion of the tissues of the oral cavity or nasal cavity	Irritants, alkalis, acids or fumes thereof
Dysbarism, including decompression sickness, barotrauma or osteonecrosis	Abnormal atmospheric or water pressure
Any disease	Ionizing radiation from any source
Allergic or irritant contact dermatitis	Dust, liquids or other external agents or factors
Mesothelioma of the pleura or peritoneum or other malignancy of the lung	Asbestos or asbestos dust
Malignancy of the lung, skin, larynx, mouth cavity or bladder	Coaltar, pitch, asphalt or bitumen or volatiles thereof
Malignancy of the lung, mucous membrane of the nose or associated air sinuses	Nickel or its compounds
Malignancy of the lung	Hexavalant chromium compounds, or bischloromethyl ether
Angiosarcoma of the liver	Vinyl chloride monomer

Schedule 3 of the Compensation for Occupational Injuries and Diseases Act, 1993 (No 130 of 1993)

Diseases	Work
Malignancy of the bladder	4-amino-diphenyl, benzidine, beta naphtylamine. 4-nitro-dipenyl
Leukaemia	Benzene

Occupational health

Melanoma of the skin	Polychlorinated biphenyls
Tuberculosis of the lung	1 Crystalline silica (alpha quartz) 2 Mycobacterium tuberculosis or MOTTS (mycobacterium other than tuberculosis) transmitted to an employee during the performance of healthcare work from a patient suffering from active open tuberculosis
Brucellosis	Brucella abortus, suis or mellitensis transmitted through contact with infected animals or their products
Anthrax	Bacillus anthracis transmitted through contact with infected animals or their products
Q-fever	Coxiella burnetii emanating from infected animals or their products
Bovine tuberculosis	Mycobacterium bovis transmitted through contact with infected animals or their products
Rift Valley Fever	Virus transmitted by infected animals or their products
	b Any work involving the handling of or exposure to any of the following:
Hearing impairment	Excessive noise
Hand-arm vibration syndrome (Raynaud's phenomenon)	Vibrating equipment
Any disease due to overstraining of muscular tendonous insertions	Repetitive movements

The Occupational Diseases in Mines and Works Act of 1973 (replaced by the Mine Health and Safety Act, 1996 (No 29 of 1996)), defines as 'compensatable disease' the conditions listed in Table 5.2. The common factor in these is that the worker must have performed so-called risk work, defined as work involving the risk of incurring a compensatable disease, as declared in a Government Gazette, or deemed to have been so declared under Section 13 of the Act, i.e. where exposure to potentially harmful dust, gases, vapours or chemical substances or factors may occur or where working conditions in the opinion of the Minister are (potentially) harmful.

Table 5.3 Compensatable Diseases (ODMW Act, 1973)

---

a PNEUMOCONIOSIS, a permanent lesion of the cardiorespiratory organs caused by the inhalation of dust in the course of performance of risk work, but excluding a calcified lesion.
b The joint condition of PNEUMOCONIOSIS AND TUBERCULOSIS.
c TUBERCULOSIS, which in the opinion of the certification committee, was contracted while the person concerned was performing risk work, or affected within 12 months immediately following the last exposure to such work.
d PERMANENT OBSTRUCTION of the AIRWAYS, which in the opinion of the certification committee, is attributable to the performance of risk work.
e PROGRESSIVE SYSTEMIC SCLEROSIS, which in the opinion of the certification committee, is attributable to the performance of risk work.
f Any other permanent disease of the cardio-respiratory organs, which in the opinion of the certification committee, is attributable to the performance of risk work.
g Any other disease, which in the opinion of the certification committee, is attributable to the performance of risk work, and which the Minister by notice in the Gazette declared to be a compensatable disease.

Mesothelioma and certain cases of lung cancer have been attributed to risk work in certain mines and have therefore been regarded as compensatable.

It is clear that the certification committee has been given discretion as to what conditions should be compensatable subject to establishing that the condition is closely related to the work situation, i.e. that the patient has performed 'risk work'.

The Occupational Diseases in Mines and Works Amendment Act, 1993 (No 208 of 1993) removed existing discrimination on the basis of gender or 'population group' and created a single system for medical surveillance for all miners in South Africa. It had been under consideration to consolidate all legislation for compensation of occupational diseases and injuries under one Act, covering these conditions irrespective of where they arose, in mines, works or any other workplace or work site. This has not happened, however.

The occupational diseases caused by so-called risk work on mines or in 'works' as defined in the Act, could well be the subject of a separate section of this chapter. These diseases are mostly those affecting the respiratory system. However, they will be incorporated under their general headings and not specified by site (work environment) of origin. It must be emphasized that, under the ODMW Act a legal duty is imposed on all medical practitioners to report any chest disease they diagnose in a living miner and to ensure that the cardiorespiratory organs of any miner or ex-miner who dies when under their care are submitted to the Medical Bureau of Occupational Diseases in Johannesburg for examination. This can be arranged through the District Surgeon service and is necessary to determine whether or not the descendants of such a miner are entitled to compensation, i.e. when significant compensatable occupational disease is diagnosed postmortem.

It should also be noted that some of the occupational diseases are reportable to the Health Authorities under the Health Act, 1977 (No 63 of 1977). These are, among others, anthrax, lead poisoning, poisoning from any agricultural or stock remedy registered in terms of the Fertilizers, Farm Feeds, Agricultural Remedies and Stock Remedies Act of 1947 as amended, and also any primary malignancies of the bronchus, lung and pleura. Under the latter category would fall such occupational cancers as mesothelioma and bronchial carcinoma resulting from occupational asbestos exposure, both compensatable under the Act as mentioned earlier.

However, one should move from the concept of occupational diseases, where well-defined causes are associated with unique disease, to look at possible work-relatedness of all diseases, e.g. ischaemic heart disease, suicide. (See Chapter 2 for more details on legislation.)

The WHO has proposed that there are at least four categories of occupational disease syndromes:
1. Diseases only occupational in origin, e.g. asbestosis and mesothelioma.
2. Diseases in which occupation is one of the causal factors, e.g. bronchial carcinoma.
3. Diseases in which occupation is a contributing factor in complex situations, e.g. chronic bronchitis.
4. Diseases in which occupations may aggravate a pre-existing disease, e.g. asthma.

Occupational hazards that may cause disease

Physical factors
- Noise
- Thermal (hot + cold)
- Radiation
  - ionizing
  - non-ionizing (UV, IR)
- Repetitive motion, lifting

Chemical factors
- Metal and related substances
- Organic compounds
- Dusts, fumes, mists, gases

Biological factors
- Infectious diseases
- Animals
- Plants

Psychological stressors and work organization
- Shift work
- Stress

Remember the multi-causation/associations of diseases, e.g. tuberculosis, is caused by mycobacterium tuberculosis, but associated with exposure to silica, poverty, HIV, alcohol abuse, etc.

Determinants of occupational diseases
- Concentration or intensity of chemical or stressor
- Duration of exposure

- Frequency of exposure
- Individual susceptibility.

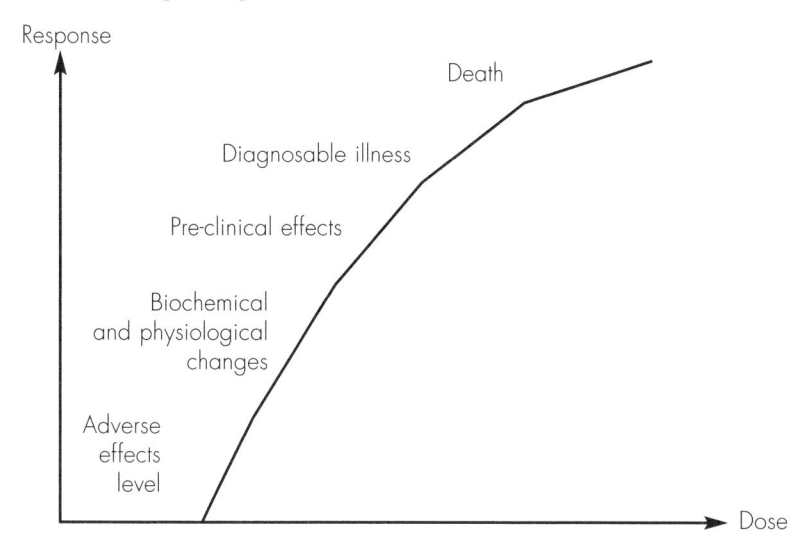

Figure 5.1 The dose-response relationship

Higher doses may cause biochemical or physiological changes, e.g. exposure to a certain concentration of solvents may cause raised liver enzymes, which is reversible when exposure ceases, but no overt clinical disease is evident.

Still higher doses cause overt clinical disease, such as lead poisoning, hearing loss or impaired lung functions.

An extremely high dose may overwhelm the body's defences and cause death.
Many occupational diseases, such as noise-induced hearing loss or silicosis, manifest after 10–20 years of continuous exposure due to 'cumulative dose'.

The primary aim of occupational health programmes is the promotion of well-being among workers and the prevention of occupational injuries and diseases. Medical surveillance and biological monitoring, therefore, have an important role.

Under the OHS Act of 1993 (s 25) a legal obligation is placed on the medical practitioner who examines or treats a person for a disease described in Schedule 3 (or any other disease the medical practitioner believes arose out of his/her patient's employment) to report the case within the prescribed period to the person's employer and to the Chief Inspector of the Department of Labour, as well as to inform his/her patient that he/she has done so. In Chapter VIII (s 74) of the COID Act the legal obligation to furnish a medical report to the employer (or directly to the Commissioner if the patient is unemployed at the time the diagnosis is made) is laid down.

Clearly, it may be expected from occupational healthcare professionals such as the occupational health nurse to support, or even remind, the medical practitioner of these duties, in the interest of their clients. The Act does not, however, exclude compensation for other occupational diseases, provided that it is proved to the satisfaction of the Commissioner that 'such disease has arisen out of and in the course of the person's employment'. For example, a health worker who contracts hepatitis B (which is not a scheduled occupational disease) will receive compensation if it is proven and accepted that the incident of infection had occurred at work and had caused him/her to contract the disease. Occupational asthma had already been incorporated in the schedule of the old Act (Workman's Compensation Act) on 11 December 1992 and is now in Schedule 3 of the present Act. Workers can claim compensation for the following diseases if they are exposed to any one of the substances or work processes listed in Table 5.2.

5.3.2 Epidemiology of occupational diseases

A comparison of diseases reported to the Compensation Commissioner during 1991 and 1998 shows a changing pattern.

Top 5 in 1991 (104 cases)	Top 5 in 1998 (5 716 cases)
■ Pneumoconiosis – 80	■ Noise-induced hearing loss – NIHL 3 175
■ Ankylostomiasis – 12	■ Post-traumatic stress disorder – 734
■ Dermatitis – 7	■ Dermatitis – 678
■ Lead poisoning – 2	■ Tuberculosis – 306
■ Byssinosis – 2	■ Pneumoconiosis – 244

Diseases certified under the Occupational Diseases in Mines and Works Act (ODMWA)

1996/7
- Tuberculosis 4 159
- Pneumoconiosis 3 554
- Obstructive airways disease 343
- Obstructive airways disease and pneumoconiosis 150
- Platinum salt sensitivity 44
- Progressive systemic sclerosis 10
  (Department of Health – Annual Report of the Medical Bureau for Occupational Diseases, 1996/97)

Surveillance of Work-Related and Occupational Respiratory Diseases in South Africa (SORDSA) is a nation-wide programme for reporting such diseases from members of the South African Thoracic Society (SATS), South African Society of Occupational Medicine (SASOM) and South African Society of Occupational Health Nursing Practitioners (SASOHN) to the National Centre for Occupational Health (NCOH). In general, occupational diseases are grossly underreported

5.3.3 Diagnosis of occupational diseases

As with other medical conditions, the diagnosis of an occupational-related condition depends on:
- Taking a good HISTORY
- Doing an EXAMINATION
- Doing SPECIAL INVESTIGATIONS

History
The essentials of an occupational history include:
- What is your occupation?'
  Be specific, i.e.:
  - Describe your work and what you are exposed to.
  - How long have you been doing this job?
  - Do you use protective equipment?

- Other employment, i.e. previous employment in chronological order.
- Symptoms:
  - Timing of symptoms in relation to work.
  - Anyone else with similar problems.

- Other factors
  - Cigarettes – How many per day and for how long?
  - Hobbies

For example, evaluation of pulmonary disease may include:
- A complete history, including questions on chronic cough, sputum, shortness of breath, wheezing, chest pain, and how symptoms relate to the work or non-work environment, and any weight loss.
- A physical examination, with attention to breath sounds.
- Pulmonary function tests, such as spirometry and peak-flow measurements.
- A chest X-ray.

5.3.4 Management of occupational diseases
Summary
- Remove the worker from the hazard.
- Treat the condition where applicable.
- Submit a claim to the Compensation Commissioner and notify the Department of Labour.
- Institute adequate preventive control measures to protect other workers.

Remove the worker from the hazard
The ideal is to remove the worker from the hazard to prevent deterioration of the condition. This must be discussed with the worker and management, as often suitable alternative work may not be available, and possible job loss must be considered.

Treat the condition
This may be possible for conditions such as dermatitis, asthma and musculoskeletal disorders. However, there may be no medical treatment for some disorders, such as hearing loss and pneumoconiosis.

Submit a claim to the Compensation Commissioner and notify the Department of Labour
(Forms differ depending on whether there is an injury or disease)

- Employer reports accident or disease (WCL 1 or 2).
- Doctor completes First Medical Report (WCL 22 or 4) containing:
  - occupational history
  - exposures including recognized causative agents
  - examination and special investigation results.
- The Commissioner's office provides a claim number.
- Progress/Final medical reports (WCL 26 or 5) are sent to the employer or Commissioner.
- WCL 6 is completed by the employer when the employee returns to work.

Institute preventive measures
The aim is to reduce exposure risk to affected and unaffected workers by firstly controlling the SOURCE, which is the most effective, whilst controlling the WORKER with the use of PPE being less successful and which should only be used as a last resort.

Prevention control measures

Source	Path	Worker
■ Eliminate the hazardous agent ■ Substitute the hazardous agent ■ Enclose the process ■ Ensure local exhaust ventilation/extraction	■ Shield the worker ■ Increase the distance	■ Reduce the duration of exposure ■ Enclose the worker ■ Institute education and training

For clarity of presentation, the occupational diseases listed in Schedule 3 may be grouped in six main subdivisions, rather than treated in sequence:
1. Diseases of the respiratory tract
2. Occupational malignancies
3. Chemical elements, substances and groups of compounds injurious to health
4. Allergic or irritant contact dermatitis
5. Diseases and conditions caused by physical agents
6. Diseases of bacterial and viral origin

All these occupational diseases, conditions and manifestations are compensatable and are likely to be the most important or prevalent occupational diseases in South Africa. Where appropriate, the relevant occupational exposure limits, derived from the Regulations for Hazardous Chemical Substances of 1995 (Section 43 of the OHS Act of 1993) will be mentioned. Table 1 of these Regulations lists so-called Control Limits (TWA OEL-CL) that are time-weighted average exposure limits which may not be exceeded. Table 2 lists the so-called Recommended Limits (OEL-RL) which are regarded as reasonably practical to serve as attainable standards to which exposure by inhalation should be reduced (as a maximum allowable).

Table 3 of the Regulations lists Biological Exposure Indices (BEI) which are values for concentration of chemicals in blood or urine (occasionally also in expired air), which should not be exceeded in samples taken at the indicated sampling time.

These BEIs are of great interest to health workers as they represent 'statutory' standards to be observed in biological monitoring (medical or health surveillance) programmes in which they may be involved.

The Hazardous Chemical Substances Regulations are very similar to those used in the United Kingdom. Occasionally, where deemed useful, reference will be made to the annually published recommendations of the ACGIH (American Conference of Governmental Industrial Hygienists), which, in the form of Threshold Limit Values and Biological Exposure Indices have been used as guidelines by occupational healthcare professionals in the United States and many other countries for years.

5.3.5 Health surveillance and biological monitoring

Definitions
- Biological monitoring is the measurement of a substance or its metabolites in various biological media.
- Biological effects monitoring is the measurement and assessment of early biological effects of which health impairment has not yet been established.
- Health surveillance is the medico-physiological examination for early detection of adverse effects and is non-specific.
- Environmental monitoring is the measurement and assessment of agents at the workplace to evaluate ambient exposure and health risk compared to a reference value.

Examples

The measurement of lead concentration in the blood is an example of biological monitoring.

The measurement of the concentration of blood protoporphyrin is an example of biological effects monitoring.

The measurement of nerve conduction velocities is an example of health surveillance.

Biological monitoring aims at PRIMARY prevention, i.e. to limit exposure so that disease processes cannot be initiated.

Health surveillance aims at secondary prevention, i.e. with the pre-clinical or early phase of the disease.

Biological monitoring
- Allows for fluctuation in exposure
- Reflects all routes of exposure
- Measures effectiveness of engineering + PPE
- Takes into account toxokinetic factors, e.g. workload

Occupational health

Sampling
Sampling requires knowledge of:

- Absorption ⎫
- Metabolism ⎬ of substance
- Excretion ⎭

- Possible contamination
- Dietary effects
- Sample type
- Appropriate preservative
- Biological half-life ($t_{1/2}$). The biological half-life ($t_{1/2}$) is defined as the time needed to reduce the absorbed amount in the body by 50 per cent, or to decrease the concentration in plasma by 50 per cent.

For example:
LEAD
90% of lead oxide is absorbed by lungs
5–15% of lead is absorbed by the gastro-intestinal tract
Biological half-life ($t_{1/2}$) of inorganic lead in the blood is 25–28 days.
Lead environmental contamination:
- Heavy traffic (leaded fuel)
- Leaded plumbing
- Cigarette smoking

Dietary effects
- Increased lead absorption with deficiencies of iron and protein, and with milk intake.
- Lead is released from bone with low dietary calcium.

Solvents
- Creatinine correction, to normalize urine results (creatinine must be > 0.5 and < 3)
- Toluene

Biomarker	$t_{1/2}$	Biological Exposure Index (BEI)	Sample
Hippuric acid in urine	2 hrs	2.5 g/g Cr	End of Shift (EOS)
O-cresol U	4–7 hrs	1 mg/g Cr	End of shift (EOS)
Toluene	U, B, EA	Not in general use	

Correct collection of samples
- Half-life   long $t_{1/2}$ Any time
              short $t_{1/2}$ Pre- and post-shift
- Blood or serum
  - Clean area

- Clean clothes + skin (shower)
- Clean venepuncture site
- Appropriate sample container
■ Urine
  - Clean area
  - Shower, clean clothes
  - Appropriate preservative
■ Samples to reach an *accredited* laboratory as soon as possible.

Note:
Medical surveillance and biological monitoring must fulfil a number of criteria:
■ Accuracy and validity
■ Sensitivity and specificity
■ Relevance.

Workers must give consent, i.e. why the test needs to be done and what happens if there are abnormal results, such as compensation and job security.
  Always tell employees their INDIVIDUAL results.
  GROUP results (without names) may be given to management/unions.
  Correlate results with occupational hygiene surveys.
  Atmospheric measurements are more relevant when substances affect site of contact, e.g. respiratory irritants and carcinogens.

5.4 Main subdivisions of occupational diseases
5.4.1 Occupational lung diseases
Classification of occupational lung diseases
1 Pneumoconiosis
  ■ Fibrogenic, e.g. silica, asbestos
  ■ Non-fibrogenic, e.g. tin
2 Chronic obstructive airways disease (COAD)
  ■ Bronchitis
  ■ Emphysema
3 Allergic reactions
  ■ Occupational asthma, e.g. toluene di-isocyanate, platinum salts
  ■ Extrinsic allergic alveolitis, e.g. farmer's lung
4 Malignancies
  ■ Bronchogenic carcinoma, e.g. arsenic, radon, BCME
  ■ Mesothelioma (asbestos)
5 'Acute reactions' to gases + fumes
  ■ Pulmonary oedema
  ■ Pneumonitis
  ■ Metal fume fever

5.4.1.1 Pneumoconiosis-fibrosis of the parenchyma of the lung

Definition
The International Labour Organization (ILO) gives the following definition: 'Pneumoconiosis is the accumulation of dust in the lungs and the tissue reactions to its presence.'

Particle sizes: 0.5–7 μ (microns) are deposited in the alveoli of the lungs, i.e. respirable
7–100 μ may be deposited from the nose to the large bronchi, i.e. inhalable.
    <0.5 μ remain suspended in exhaled air.

They may be classified as either:
- Fibrotic pneumoconiosis, i.e. give rise to lung fibrosis (scarring) with overt clinical signs
- Benign pneumoconiosis, i.e. there is no alteration in lung function.

Diagnosis of pneumoconiosis
- Occupational history
- X-rays.

Radiology. The radiograph is read according to the ILO's International Classification of Pneumoconioses, which describes the capacities according to:
- Size
- Shape
- Profusion.

Rounded opacities	Irregular opacities
p < 1.5 mm	s = fine
q 1.5–3 mm	t = medium
r 3–10 mm	u = coarse

Profusion: 0, 1, 2 or 3.

Large opacities which are greater than 1 cm in diameter are classified as progressive massive fibrosis (PMF).

Differential diagnosis on X-ray
- Miliary TB
- Sarcoidosis
- Histoplasmosis
- Metastases.

'Benign pneumoconioses' include siderosis (caused by iron oxides), stannosis (caused by tin exposure) and baritosis (caused by barium, but rare). All these cause radiographic abnormalities that do not lead to clinical disease and that may disappear again some time after exposure has been discontinued.

Silicosis

Definition

The ILO definition for silicosis is 'a fibrotic pneumoconiosis caused by inhalation of crystalline free silica (quartz) dust, and characterized by discrete nodular lung fibrosis. In advanced cases impaired respiratory function with massive pulmonary fibrosis may occur'.

Silica or quartz is composed of silicon dioxide (SiO_2). It is important to differentiate between free silica (SiO_2) and silicates that are salts formed by the combination of silica and materials such as calcium or magnesium oxides. Non-fibrous silicates usually do not harm the lung. Asbestos is a fibrous silicate that will be dealt with later on.

Sources of exposure to free silica
1. Mining, e.g. quartzites, sandstones on the SA Witwatersrand gold mines.
2. Mining related:
   - Quarrying
   - Ore processing (milling)
3. Foundries: moulding, fettling and sandblasting
4. Ceramics and pottery
5. Abrasive blasting, e.g. sand and shot blasting
6. Glass manufacture
7. Construction.

Pathology

The respirable (0.5–7 µ) silica particles are deposited in the alveoli and engulfed by macrophages. Some are removed by the muco-ciliary escalator and coughed up. The rest move into the interstitial tissues where the inflammatory reaction results in the typical concentric fibrosis of the silicotic nodules. These nodules tend to occur in the upper zones and coalesce, giving rise to progressive massive fibrosis – PMF. Three forms of silicosis have been described – chronic, accelerated and acute.

1 Chronic silicosis
- Most common form of silicosis
- Fibrotic changes occur after 10–30 years inhalation of excessive silica dust
- It is further subdivided into simple and complicated silicosis:

Simple silicosis
- The usual form of chronic silicosis with discrete rounded nodules predominantly in the upper and mid-lung zones on chest X-ray
- Few clinical signs.

Complicated silicosis
- Silicotic nodules increase in size and coalesce into lesions > 1 cm diameter. This is known as progressive massive fibrosis (PMF)
- The patient may have shortness of breath or respiratory failure.

2 Accelerated silicosis
This form of silicosis develops after 5–10 years from inhalation of very high concentrations of silica dust.

3 Acute silicosis
- It develops after inhalation of exceptionally high concentrations of silica over a short period (7 months to 5 years)
- The radiological and pathological changes are similar to 'pulmonary alveolar proteinosis'
- It presents with cough, weight loss and fatigue
- It may rapidly progress to respiratory failure and death.

Associated diseases
The following diseases are often associated with exposure to silica.

1 Tuberculosis
- Silica exposure renders a person more susceptible to pulmonary tuberculosis due to silica particles affecting the pulmonary macrophage. The risk is increased with high silica dust levels, older individuals and established radiological silicosis.
- The risk of developing PTB whilst exposed and after exposure ends, depends on the cumulative silica exposure.
- PTB is increased when there is both HIV and silica exposure.

Tuberculosis is diagnosed by looking for the following:
Suspect TB in:
- An unwell worker: loss of weight, chronic cough, pyrexial, night sweats
- Low levels of dust exposure
- Inappropriate time scale, i.e. radiological changes after a few years of exposure – silicosis can take 10–20 years to develop
- Raised ESR
- Radiological changes not compatible with silicosis, e.g. enlarged hilar nodes, cavitation, effusion and widespread disease.

The diagnosis of active TB depends on the demonstration of acid-fast bacilli, positive culture (sputum, pleural or lymph node aspirate or blood), and responds to treatment.

Reducing the burden of tuberculosis depends on many factors:
- Reducing dust levels and therefore silicosis
- Improving socio-economic conditions with less reliance on single sex hostels
- Reducing the prevalence of HIV through prevention and treatment programmes
- Considering the use of isoniazid prophylaxis in high-risk individuals.

The frequency of radiological surveillance depends on the level of risk:
- Pre-placement – all workers who will be exposed to silica
- Three to four years if low dust exposure, i.e. less than occupational exposure limit

- Yearly if high dust exposure or presence of silicosis
- Exit examination
- Previous exposure but no silicosis, ± 5 yearly.

2 Chronic obstructive lung disease
Silica dust exposure potentiates the damage done by smoking, resulting in emphysema.

3 Lung cancer
The International Agency for Research on Cancer (IARC) has classified crystalline silica as a human carcinogen.

4 Auto-immune diseases
Crystalline silica is linked with scleroderma, rheumatoid arthritis and systemic lupus erythematosus.

Medical surveillance
The frequency depends on level of risk:
- Dust levels and exposure
- Risk of PTB.

History – respiratory questionnaire
Examination
Investigations   – full-sized chest X-ray
                 – spirometry if there is good quality control
                 – chest X-ray
                    (See Figure 5.2.)

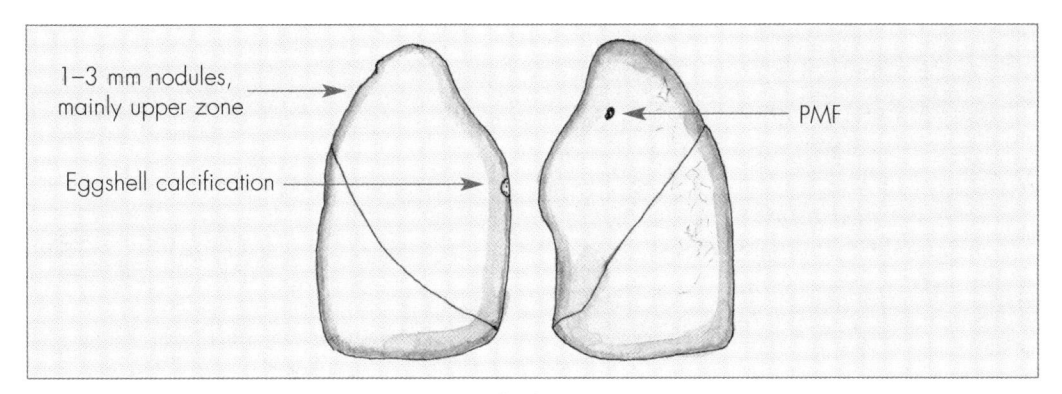

Figure 5.2 Schematic representation of silicosis

The frequency of radiological surveillance depends on the level of risk:
- Pre-placement – all workers who will be exposed to silica
- Three to four years if low dust exposure, i.e. less than occupational exposure limit
- Yearly if high dust exposure or presence of silicosis

- Exit examination
- Previous exposure but no silicosis, ± 5 yearly.

In 1995 a joint ILO/WHO (International Labour Organization/World Health Organization) Committee on Occupational Health proposed a Programme on Global Elimination of Silicosis. Primary prevention measures using appropriate and economically viable methods of dust control will go a long way in reducing silicosis.

Occupational exposure limits for respirable crystalline silica
Department of Labour: TWA OEL-CL (8-hour time weighted average Occupational Exposure Limit – Control Limit) = 0.4 mg/m^3

Department of Minerals and Energy: Use the American Conference of Governmental Industrial Hygienists (ACGIH) Threshold Limit Values (TLVs):

	TLV-TWA
Quartz	0.1 mg/m^3
Cristabalite + Tridymite	0.05 mg/m^3

For quartz-containing dusts the TLV-TWA for respirable particles is calculated as:

$$\frac{10\%}{quartz + 2} \text{ mg/m}^3$$

Remember: A worker exposed for many years at levels of 0.1 mg/m^3 may still develop silicosis due to cumulative exposure.

5 Coal workers' pneumoconiosis (CWP)

Coal workers' pneumoconiosis may develop after 10–20 years of exposure to coal mine dust, and slowly progresses over time and is less fibrotic than silicosis. A minority of individuals may develop progressive massive fibrosis. It is often associated with obstructive airways disease.

5.4.1.2 Asbestos and disease

There are two major varieties of asbestos:
1. Serpentine (wavy configuration) — Chrysotile (white asbestos)
2. Amphibole (straight configuration) — Crocidolite (blue asbestos)
   Amosite (brown asbestos)
   Tremolite
   Actinolite

Asbestos is the collective term to describe fibrous silicates.

Uses of asbestos
Asbestos is very resistant to temperature, pressure and acids, hence it is used for:
- Boiler and pipe lagging
- Asbestos cement board and pipes

- Fireproofing
- Brake shoes
- Gaskets

Asbestos-related diseases
- Pleura   plaques
              thickening
              mesothelioma
- Parenchyma asbestosis
              carcinoma of the bronchus
- Other sites laryngeal carcinoma
              stomach carcinoma

Asbestosis
Asbestosis is a diffuse interstitial fibrosis of the lung (as opposed to silica which forms discrete fibrosis) due to inhalation of asbestos fibres. The size and dimension of the fibres are important with fibres < 1.5 µ in diameter and > 5 µ in length being the culprits.

The fibres interact with macrophages, which set off inflammatory and fibrotic processes.

It affects the lower lobes of the lung first.

Diagnosis
- Exposure history
- Effort dyspnoea
- Basal crepitations
- X-ray changes
- Lung function impairment (restrictive).

Dyspnoea is the first symptom to be noted and the degree of breathlessness may be out of all proportion to the X-ray charges.

Basal crepitations and finger clubbing may be present.

X-ray changes show diffuse interstitial fibrosis with mottling, as well as a cystic or honeycomb appearance, especially in the lower zones. (See Figure 5.3.)

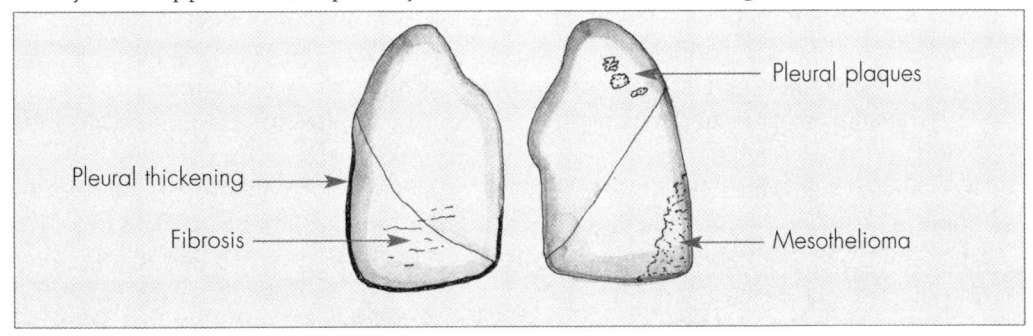

Figure 5.3 Asbestos-related diseases

Lung function tests show a reduced vital capacity.

Mesothelioma
Mesothelioma is a neoplasm of the pleura or peritoneum, caused by occupational or environmental exposure to asbestos. Crocidolite is a more potent cause than chrysotile.
Smoking plays no role, unlike bronchial carcinoma.
It is a notifiable disease.

Clinical features
Chest pain and tiredness are early symptoms, followed by shortness of breath and weight loss.
The chest X-ray may show a pleural effusion or a mass.
The condition is invariably fatal.
There is a synergistic effect between exposure to asbestos and cigarette smoking as the risk of lung cancer is particularly high in asbestos-exposed cigarette smokers.
Recently a 'class-action' suit by former employees for compensation has been made against British-based companies who operated mines in South Africa.

The asbestos regulations have been updated as the Asbestos Regulations, 2001 (published February 2002), which states:
'No employer or self-employed person shall require or permit any person to work in an environment in which he or she would be exposed to asbestos in excess of the prescribed occupational exposure limit' (OEL 0.2 fibres/ml).

The regulations stipulate:
- Ways to minimize asbestos exposure
- Air monitoring
- Medical surveillance
- Disposal of asbestos.

5.4.1.3 Occupational asthma
Definition
Occupational asthma is reversible airways obstruction which is a result of sensitization by a substance in the workplace.
In asthma, the bronchi and bronchioles are affected as a result of muscle construction, inflammation, swelling and oedema, and mucous hypersecretion. This results in airways obstruction.
It should be remembered that many individuals have 'allergic rhinitis'.
The substances listed under Schedule 3 of COID as causing occupational asthma (OA) are:
1. Isocyanates, e.g. TDI, MDI
2. Platinum, nickel, cobalt, vanadium or chromium salts
3. Hardening agents, including epoxy resins
4. Acrylic acids or derived acrylates
5. Soldering or welding fumes
6. Substances from animals or insects
7. Fungi or spores

8 Proteolytic enzymes
9 Organic dust
10 Vapours or fumes of formaldehyde, anhydrides, amines or diamines.

Worldwide, there are at least 200 different substances that may cause occupational asthma.

Three distinct agents are recognized:
1 Large proteins, e.g. grains and latex, IgE mediated or Type 1 hypersensitivity.
2 Small chemical molecules, e.g. isocyanates. Possibly cell mediated reaction. Isocyanates are compounds with a highly reactive -N=C=O group, and appear to be the most common cause of occupational asthma and are used in the production of polyurethanes with applications in foams, electrical insulation and as twin-pack paints and varnishes – spray painters are thus at risk.
Common isocyanates are:
TDI – Toluene di-isocyanate
MDI – Diphenylmethane di-isocyanate
3 Chemical irritants such as chlorine.

Recovery from the acute illness may be followed by persistent bronchial hyperreactivity. This is reactive airways dysfunction syndrome (RADS).

Signs and symptoms
Occupational asthma (OA) should always be considered when asthma first manifests in adults, and particularly if there is exposure to a known causative agent or one of the substances listed in Schedule 3 of the COID Act.
　In many cases patients complain of a chronic cough or slight breathlessness, rather than a wheeze.
　The cardinal feature to look for is symptoms which improve away from work, e.g. over weekends or on holiday.
　Symptoms may come on soon after working with a particular substance, or be delayed for several hours, producing nocturnal asthma.

Investigations
- Two-hourly peak flow measurements (see chart on p 183) to demonstrate work relatedness, including reversibility.

　Diurnal　　　　*Variation*
　Non-asthmatics　< 10%
　Asthmatics　　　> 20%

- Try to identify the causative agent either through a skin-prick test, RAST (Radio-allergosorbent test), which measures antibodies to a specific agent, or specific bronchial challenge test.
　These tests would be conducted by a pulmonologist or at a centre of expertise.

Treatment
- Remove from exposure to offending agent since continued exposure may cause deterioration of symptoms. In the majority of cases the asthma still persists.
- Prescribe appropriate drugs such as inhaled corticosteroids.
- Submit a claim to the Compensation Commissioner.

Prevention
- Minimize exposure through good workplace practices, such as efficient ventilation/extraction.
- Use less allergenic materials.
- Use personal respiratory equipment where exposure to known allergens is unavoidable.
- Carry out periodic medical surveillance with pre- and post-shift peak-flow measurements.

5.4.1.4 Extrinsic allergic alveolitis
The most common clinical condition in this category is 'farmer's lung'. This typically presents with 'flu-like symptoms such as fever, cough, shortness of breath and muscle pains that occur 4 to 8 hours after exposure to mouldy hay. It is a form of hypersensitivity pneumonitis due to the formation of antigen-antibody complexes and inflammation from exposure to spores of 'thermophilic actinomycetes'.

Continued exposure may cause irreversible restrictive or obstructive disease.

Bagassosis is another form of extrinsic allergic alveolitis, caused by the inhalation of fungal spores – thermoactinomyces sacchari – on old mouldy dry bagasse. Bagasse is the fibrous material of sugar cane after the juice has been extracted. There have been no reported cases in the South African sugar milling industry.

5.4.1.5 Byssinosis
Byssinosis is a chronic obstructive airways disease which is regarded as peculiar to the occupation of textile workers. The COID Act, Schedule 3, gives a description of occupation for byssinosis: 'any work involving the handling or exposure to the inhalation of flax, cotton or sisal dust'. The Greek word from which the name is derived refers to fine linen or flax. Byssinosis is a progressive condition which may eventually lead to total disablement if exposure persists long after first symptoms have appeared.

5.4.1.6 Acute reactions to gases and fumes
Pulmonary oedema
Exposure to irritant gases, such as chlorine or nitrous fumes (a mixture of nitric oxide (NO), nitrogen dioxide (NO_2)> and nitrogen trioxide (N_2O_3) may cause a chemical alveolitis with pulmonary oedema.

Nitroux fumes may be generated from the detonation of nitro-explosives or from the fermentation of silage (causing silo-fillers disease).

There may be no symptoms for up to 24 hours, after which bronchospasm, severe pulmonary oedema and death may occur. Hence individuals exposed to these fumes should be observed for 24 hours.

PEAK FLOW MEASUREMENTS

Name _____

Company No. _____

Company _____

Occupation
_____

DATE		MONDAY			TUESDAY			WEDNESDAY			THURSDAY			FRIDAY			SATURDAY			SUNDAY		
		1	2	3	1	2	3	1	2	3	1	2	3	1	2	3	1	2	3	1	2	3
	06h00																					
	08h00																					
	10h00																					
	12h00																					
	14h00																					
	16h00																					
	18h00																					
	20h00																					
	22h00																					
SYMPTONS	Cough Wheezing Shortness of Breath																					
TYPES OF FUMES/ DUST																						
RESPIRATOR	YES/NO																					

5.4.1.7 Platinosis

Platinosis refers to the allergic effects of the various complex platinum salts. Exposed platinum refinery workers may thus experience rhinitis, asthma, urticaria, dermatitis and conjunctivitis.

The only effective management of this disorder is to remove people from exposure.

5.4.2 Occupational cancers

Incidence

Plus-minus 4 per cent of all deaths due to cancer may be due to occupational carcinogens (limits 2–8 per cent). In specific populations located in industrial areas, lung and bladder cancers due to occupational exposures may be as high as 40 per cent.

Occupational health

Tumours of occupational origin generally have no pathological features to distinguish them from other causes, however:
- They tend to appear at an earlier age.
- There is usually a long latent period between the time of first exposure and the appearance of the tumour, e.g. 20 years.
- They arise as a result of repeated exposure.

Known and suspected human carcinogens
The International Agency for Research on Cancer (IARC) has evaluated risks to humans from exposures to chemical, physical and biological agents.

The above agents are classified into one of five groupings:

IARC CLASSIFICATION	
Group 1	Carcinogenic to humans
Group 2A	'Probably' carcinogenic to humans
Group 2Bs	'Possibly' carcinogenic to humans
Group 3	Not classifiable
Group 4	Probably not carcinogenic to humans.

At least 22 chemicals (or groups of chemicals) are established human carcinogens, i.e. IARC Group 1 and Schedule 3 of COID list eight occupational malignancies.

Agents judged to be workplace human carcinogens are as follows:

Substance/Process/Agent	Cancer Sites
■ Asbestos	Lung, pleura, larynx, peritoneum
■ Alkylating agents, e.g. bischloromethyl ether	Bronchus
■ Benzene	Bone marrow (leukaemia)
■ Benzidine, betanapthylamine (aromatic amines)	Urinary bladder Urinary bladder
■ Chromates (hexavalent) – pigment chromate production – electroplating	Lung, nasal sinus
■ Ionizing radiation Gamma rays	Skin, thyroid, bronchus, bone marrow
■ Mining + smelting – arsenic mining – uranium mining – nickel refining	Lung, skin Lung Lung, nasal sinus
■ Polycyclic aromatic hydrocarbons (PAHs) (from coal tar, coke, mineral oils)	Bronchus, skin, scrotum
■ Sulphuric acid mist	Nasal cavity, lung
■ Vinyl chloride monomer	Liver

General comments
- Cancer caused by chemicals involves two processes – initiation and promotion. Most initiators are mutagens, i.e. change the DNA structure, and the process is not dose dependent.
- The first recognized association between cancer and occupation was by Percival Pott in the 1770s when he observed an increased incidence of scrotal cancer in chimney sweeps. Polycyclic aromatic hydrocarbons were later implicated in causing these tumours.
- Polycyclic aromatic hydrocarbons (PAHs) result from incomplete combustion of organic materials that contain carbon and hydrogen.

Occupational skin cancer has been found to occur on exposed skin surfaces with individuals who worked with pitch, tar and mineral oils, with polycyclic aromatic hydrocarbons being the causative agent. Wart-like papillomas may develop on damaged skin, which may later develop into squamous cell or basal cell carcinomas. Arsenic and exposure to UV radiation may also cause skin cancers. Regular medical inspections may help in the early detection of growths.

Malignancies of the lung. Lung cancer is the most common fatal cancer among males in South Africa, with smoking the major cause.

Occupational agents include:
- Arsenic
- Asbestos – all types
- Beryllium and its compounds (used in aerospace industry)
- Bischloromethyl ether (BCME): chemical intermaliate.

Polycyclic aromatic hydrocarbons such as benzo(a)pyrene are thought to be the carcinogens in coal-tars, coal-tar pitches and bitumens that are distillation products from coal or crude oil. Cancers that have been associated with these compounds include lung and skin tumours.

The increased risk of lung cancers in individuals exposed to diesel exhaust fumes can also be explained by PAHs, as can the lung and bladder cancers in aluminium production when coal-tar pitch is used.

For occupational malignancies, perhaps even more than for any other irreversible occupational disease, prevention equates cure.

Prevention involves:
- Eliminating or substituting known carcinogens
- Ensuring any exposures are kept as low as possible below the occupational exposure limit – ceiling value by good engineering and hygienic practices. Personal protective equipment must be used as a last resort, and be suitable for the purpose
- Performing health surveillance, e.g. skin – look for lesions such as papillomas that may be pre-cancerous/cancerous

Occupational health

- Examining the bladder – cytological examination of urinary sediment for malignant cells
- Examining the lungs – tumours are generally detected too late by chest X-rays.

The use of tumour markers and DNA adducts (molecular biomarkers of carcinogenic exposure) will only be used more frequently in the future once the complex issues of sensitivity, specifically, ethical and legal concerns are addressed.

5.4.3 Chemical elements, substances and groups of compounds injurious to health

An enormous number of potentially toxic materials are used in industry, and therefore only a few important ones will be described.

5.4.3.1 Lead
Lead was one of the earliest metals used.
    The Factories Act in Britain was passed in 1883 on account of the incidence of lead poisoning, especially among women and children.

Exposure to inorganic lead
Mining and processing of lead-containing ore
Metallurgical assay laboratories
Manufacture of car batteries
Manufacture of ceramic and glass articles
Paint manufacture

Exposure to organic lead
Alkyl lead compounds are used as anti-knock additives in petrol, but their use should decline with the use of unleaded fuel.

Absorption
Industry: Inhalation of dust and fume.
Organic compounds may also be absorbed through the skin.
General environment: Ingestion is the predominant route.

Ninety per cent of the total body burden of lead is in the bones.
Inorganic lead does not normally cross the blood brain barrier.

Classical symptoms and signs of lead poisoning:
- Anaemia
- Blue line on the gums
- Abdominal colic
- Palsy – wrist and foot drop
- Encephalopathy

The classical symptoms are rarely found in industry, but the following vague symptoms are observed:
- General fatigue
- Muscular pains
- Constipation
- Abdominal pain.

Long-term effects of lead
- Hypertension
- Nephritis
- Paralysis.

Lead affects many enzyme systems in the body, particularly those containing sulphydryl (-SH) groups.

Organic lead effects relate mainly to the central nervous system.

Haemopoietic system
Anaemia occurs only in inorganic poisoning and usually late in the disease. However, disturbances in haemsynthesis can be detected early, as a number of enzymes are inhibited.

Nervous system
Lead interferes with neurotransmitters.

Symptoms may be non-specific, e.g. headache, sleep disturbance, increased irritability, or severe with convulsions, delirium and coma.

Children are more sensitive to the effects of lead, e.g. in young children there is a 2–8 points decline of the developmental index for every 10 μg increase in blood lead levels.

Pregnant women should not be exposed to lead because of the effects on the brain of the foetus.

Lead Regulations 2001
The regulations require:
1. Risk assessment whenever lead may be inhaled, ingested or absorbed by any person in the workplace:
   - Assessment of potential exposure in conjunction with health and safety committee
   - Air monitoring by an approved inspection authority.
2. Workplace practices. Lead exposure must be prevented or where this is not reasonably practicable, adequately controlled. This implies that the level of airborne lead is below the OEL (0.15 mg/m^3 for inorganic lead), or if above the OEL, reasonably practicable steps are taken to lower levels OR for ingestible lead, the blood lead level is less than 20 μg/100 ml or for lead alkyls, the urinary lead level is less than 120 μg/l.

   Control measures include substituting lead, limiting the number of people and period of exposure to lead, automation or enclosure, local extraction ventilation, and the use of wet methods where appropriate.

All workplaces are to be kept in a clean state, with vacuum-cleaning equipment of at least 99 per cent efficiency. There are prohibitions on the use of compressed air as well as smoking, eating or drinking in lead areas.

Suitable protective clothing and equipment must be provided to prevent inhalation, ingestion or skin absorption of lead.

Adequate washing facilities, and two separate lockers for 'protective clothing' and 'personal clothing', located in both the 'dirty' and 'clean' change rooms, must be provided.
3 Employee information. Employees must be adequately and comprehensively informed of the hazards and precautions to be taken.
4 Medical surveillance by an occupational medicine practitioner (doctor with an occupational health qualification) is required if:
  - Airborne lead concentrations exceed the OEL, or
  - Tetra-alkyl lead exposure, or
  - On recommendation of the occupational medicine practitioner.

The frequency of biological monitoring depends on previous results:

Blood lead µg/100 ml	Maximum intervals between blood lead measurements
Under 20	12 months
20 – 39	6 months
40 – 59	3 months
60 and over	

The employee is certified to be unfit to work in a lead area when the blood lead concentration is greater than 60 µg/100 ml. (There is a phasing-in period for this limit.)

For organic lead adsorption, urinary lead estimation should be used, and the employee should be certified unfit for work when the urinary lead concentration exceeds 150 µg/litre.

It should be remembered that the trend in blood lead levels (increase or decrease) may be just as important as a single value. A proper medical surveillance includes history, examination and measurement of lead level, haemoglobin and zinc protoporphyrin (ZPP) concentration. Increased ZPP is an early warning sign of the effects of lead exposure, and is quick and convenient to do (only a drop of blood is required). Anaemia would be caused by the inhibition of haemoglobin synthesis and shortened lifespan of red blood cells.

Treatment
Lead colic – IV calcium gluconate. Removal of lead from circulation – chelation therapy, e.g. calcium EDTA.

5.4.3.2 Mercury
Exposure to mercury
- Chloralkali plants
- Amalgamation of gold
- Mercury vapour lamps and incandescent electric lamps
- Dental amalgams (no longer used)
- Depigmentation creams.

Absorption
- Inhalation: Mercury vapour is readily absorbed through the respiratory tract.
- Ingestion: Metallic mercury is poorly absorbed from the gut, but water-soluble mercury compounds are readily absorbed.
- Skin.

Mercury is able to cross the blood/brain barrier.

Signs and symptoms of mercury poisoning
- Stomatitis – inflammation of the mouth, even leading to loss of teeth
- Tremor
- Erethism
- Kidney disease: proteinuria and chronic renal failure.

Symptoms of mercurial erethism
- Irritability
- Irrational outbursts of temper
- Shyness – avoidance of friends
- Excitability
- Tendency to blush easily
- Depression/anxiety.

The personality change can cause untold suffering, e.g. divorce.

Neurological signs
- Tremor – disturbs handwriting
- Cerebellar ataxia
- Spastic gait
- Sensory disturbance: paraesthesia, alteration in taste and smell, loss of propioception.

Medical examinations
Pre-placement: pay special attention to oral cavity, nervous system and mental health. Take a sample of handwriting.
    Periodic: as the pre-placement examination.

Occupational health

Exposure limits
WHO: Air: 25 µ g/m^3
Urine: 50 µ g creatinine.

Environmental disasters
In Minamata Bay, Japan, a factory manufacturing vinyl chloride and using a mercuric chloride catalyst discharged its effluent into the bay, where methyl mercury was formed and entered the food chain and fish supply of the local population. From 1953 to 1961 over 111 cases of poisoning, with 41 deaths, occurred. Minamata disease manifested with cerebral ataxia, dysanthria and constriction of visual fields. Over 10 per cent of children born of exposed women had central nervous system damage. For the first time in the history of occupational health, company directors were charged with culpable homicide.

5.4.3.3 Chromium
Chromium is used in stainless steel, electroplating, pigments and leather tanning.

Health effects
Chromium is an essential trace element involved in glucose metabolism.
   The valency of chromium and its compounds is: zero – Cr, trivalent – Cr^{3+}, and hexavalent – Cr^{6+}. Certain hexavalent chromium compounds may be irritant, corrosive, allergic or potentially carcinogenic, resulting in:
Skin – irritation resulting in chrome ulcer or hole and allergic contact dermatitis.
Mucous membranes – nasal septum ulcers or even perforations.
Respiratory tract – bronchoconstriction from irritation and allergic asthma. Slightly soluble hexavalent chromate compounds are associated with an increased risk of lung cancer, e.g. in electroplating.
Kidneys – renal tubular dysfunction.

Health surveillance
The examination should focus on the skin, nasal membranes, lungs and urine.
Urinary chromium post-shift may indicate exposure levels, but may be poorly correlated with toxicity.

5.4.3.4 Solvents
Definition
A solvent is a substance used to dissolve another substance (solute) into solution.

Uses
- Paints and inks
- Degreasers
- Drycleaning agent
- Reactants and intermediates in the manufacture of other chemicals
- Extraction of edible fats and oils
- Components of motor and aviation fuel.

Classification
- Aliphatic hydrocarbons. These are open carbon compounds, e.g.: Stoddard solvent – C_9 to C_{11}, and Hexane – C_6H_{14}
- Aromatic hydrocarbons. These have at least 1 or more Benzene (C_6H_6) ring, e.g. benzene, toluene, xylene.
- Halogenated hydrocarbons. They have at least one or more halogen (e.g. chlorine, bromine) atom in the molecule, e.g. carbon tetrachloride, trichlorethylene.
- Alcohols and glycols. These contain at least one OH group, e.g. ethanol.
- Ketones (R-CO-R), e.g. acetone, methyl-butyl ketone.
- Ethers
- Esters, e.g. ethyl acetate.
- Miscellaneous.

Health effects
These depend on:
- Route of exposure: Inhalation of vapours, skin contact
- Airborne concentration
- Duration of exposure
- Number of solvents present.

Central nervous system (CNS)
Virtually all organic solvents depress the CNS. Effects can range from headache, inebriation, and in high concentrations, to coma and death. (One has only to look at the effects of alcohol and anaesthetics such as ether and trichlorethylene.)

Solvent neurotoxicity
The results of numerous epidemiological studies have suggested that long-term occupational exposure to organic solvents may result in damage to the CNS. In many cases these effects are subtle, occurring in the absence of overt clinical signs and only measurable by the use of psychological test procedures.

Exposure may affect:
- Short/long-term memory
- Psychomotor function, e.g. coordination, dexterity
- Mood
- Reasoning ability.

Potential confounding variables include age, intelligence, alcohol ingestion, exposure to other neurotoxins, e.g. lead.

Peripheral nervous system
Peripheral neuropathy (e.g. reduced nerve conduction velocity, wrist and foot drop) may be caused by:
- hexane

Occupational health

- methyl-butyl ketone (MBK)
- carbon disulphide (CS$_2$).

Liver
- Carbon tetrachloride (CC$_{14}$) and other chlorinated solvents may cause acute liver necrosis.
- Toluene may cause elevated transaminases.

Kidneys
Glomerular nephropathy may be caused by carbon tetrachloride (CC$_{l4}$), methylene chloride, trichlorethyle and ethylene glycol.

Cardiovascular system (CVS)
- Carbon disulphide – CS$_2$ can cause sclerotic changes in arteries thus leading to ischaemic heart disease – IHD.
- Some halogenated hydrocarbons in high concentrations have been associated with sudden death due to arrhythmias and reduce myocardial contractility.
- Metabolism of methylene chloride produces significant levels of carbon monoxide (CO).

Blood
Benzene may cause:
- Anaemia, lowered white blood cells (WBCs), lowered platelets
- Aplastic anaemia
- Acute leukaemia, e.g. acute myelogenous leukaemia (AML).

Reproductive system
- Reduced male fertility may be caused by: Ethylene glycol ethers and carbon disulphide
- In females, an increased risk of spontaneous abortion with ethylene glycol ethers.

Skin
- Dermatitis due to degreasing effects.

Fire and explosion hazards
Flash point, boiling points, upper and lower explosive limits and evaporation rate are useful parameters in assessing fire and explosion hazards.

Benzene – C$_6$H$_6$
(an example of a solvent)
Clear, colourless, highly flammable liquid.

Absorption of benzene
Benzine is absorbed by inhalation, ingestion, or through the skin.

Acute toxicity
- Irritation of mucous membranes
- Central nervous system depression: headache, dizziness, convulsions, coma and death.

Chronic toxicity
- Bone marrow depression – anaemia, leucopaenia, thrombocytopaenia
- Aplastic anaemia (treatment involves a bone marrow transplant)
- Acute leukaemia
- Acute myelocytic leukaemia (AML).

Metabolism
- Sixty per cent of absorbed benzene is metabolized.
- The measurement of total urinary phenols gives an indication of benzene exposure.

5.4.4 Occupational skin diseases
Categories
- Chemical – irritant, allergic, occupational acne
- Mechanical and physical
- Biological
- Occupational skin cancer

Chemical hazards
Occupational dermatitis

Frequency of occupational dermatitis
Occupational dermitits most often involves the hands, wrists and forearms. It is very common, but under-diagnosed and under-reported.

Irritant contact dermatitis (ICD)
- Irritant contact dermatitis is the most common form (+ 70 per cent) of occupational contact dermatitis.
- In the acute form the severity depends on the dose and reactivity of the agent, e.g. strong acids or alkalis. It usually resolves spontaneously once the irritant factor is removed.
- The more common chronic form results from cumulative damage from repeated exposures. The inflammatory reaction may persist even after exposure has ceased. Flare-ups may happen with re-exposure even to minor irritants.
- Trauma and dryness aggravate the problem.
- Common irritants include solvents (degreasing effect), detergents (also degreasing), wet cement.
- Clinically it often presents in web spaces, back of hand, forearms, but vesicles are uncommon.

Treatment
- Remove irritant.
- Use topical steroids.
- Use protective garments/gloves.

Allergic contact dermatitis
- Hypersensitivity reaction in sensitive individuals
- Latent period with gradual onset (can be many years)

Examples of substances that cause allergic contact dermatitis are:
- Metals: nickel, chromates (hexavalent)
- Epoxy
- Rubber accelerators and anti-oxidants
- Latex
- Oils, e.g. cutting oils
- Dyes and their intermediates.

The chemical combines with an epidermal or dermal protein to form an antigen against which antibodies or lymphocyte reactions occur.

Immune response
Type 1 Immediate (3–30 minutes). IgE antibodies interact with mast cells with release of histamine.
Type 4 24–48 hours after contact, mediated by lymphocytes.
Over 3 500 chemicals are listed as sensitizers.

Clinically, the disease presents as acute/subacute eczema at site of contact, vesicles, swelling, oedema.

Investigation
Patch testing is necessary to identify the cause of ALLERGIC contact dermatitis. It must be performed by a person familiar with the technique. The test is read after 48–72 hours.

Treatment
- Remove worker from exposure.
- Prescribe corticosteroids.

Occupational acne
Occupational acne may arise from exposure to oils, coal-tars or certain halogenated substances.
  Oil acne may occur from exposure to petroleum-based cutting oils.

Dermatitis from rubber chemicals/products
Causes of this dermatitis include accelerators and anti-oxidants. Latex allergies (due to impurities) have recently come to the fore.

Cement dermatitis
- Irritant effect: alkalinity, abrasiveness.
- Allergic effect: hexavalent chromium, cobalt.

Mechanical and physical hazards
Mechanical hazards include trauma, abrasions and friction. Acute damage may cause blisters or burns. Chronic reaction leads to skin thickening with corns or calluses. Extremes of temperature can cause frostbite, miliaria or heat rash.

Skin cancer
Skin cancer is caused by long-term exposure to a number of workplace agents:
- Sunlight/UV radiation
- Ionizing radiation
- Arsenic
- Coal-tar, pitch.

Biological hazards
Working in a hot, humid environment may encourage the growth of fungal and yeast infections. Skin conditions are extremely common in people living with HIV/Aids.

Prevention of occupational skin disease
The thin outer horny layer (stratum corneum) of the skin, combined with a lipid layer, form an important barrier. As mentioned previously, solvents, soaps and chemical can remove the fatty layer.
- Engineering controls:
  - Substitution of offending substance
  - Enclosed systems
  - Mechanical devices, e.g. splash shields.

  In other words, try to control the PROCESS, not the PERSON.
- Personal protective equipment is important, e.g. the right glove is an intact glove, clean glove, clean hands used in accordance with defined working practice. Use cotton or leather gloves for friction or dusts and rubber gloves for acids and alkalis. Neoprene-dipped cotton gloves will protect against most liquid irritants. Viton gloves are more expensive, however, they give the best protection against xylene, trichlorethylene. Gloves may need cotton liners.

  Barrier creams are probably not effective.
- Personal hygiene is important. Remove soiling frequently. Use the correct cleanser (not solvents). Rinse hands or skin in running water at correct temperature (not hot water as it destroys lipid layer). Dry skin properly. Use an emollient cream.

Occupational health

Occupational dermatitis and compensation
Reporting forms:
- W.Cl.1 – Employer's report of an occupational disease
- W.Cl.22 – First medical report
- W.Cl.14 – Notice of an Occupational Disease and Claim for Compensation
- W.Cl.110 – Industrial history or an appropriate employment history
- W.Cl.26 – Progress/Final medical report
- Medical report detailing the employee's symptoms and clinical features, and results of special medical tests or investigations carried out by a dermatologist.

5.4.5 Latex allergy
Clinical manifestations of latex allergy include urticaria, rhinitis, asthma and in severe cases, anaphylaxis – all due to immediate IgE type 1 allergy.

People at risk
- Healthcare workers – the biggest single group at risk
- Workers in latex industry
- Patients with multiple hospitalizations
- Atopic individuals (tendency to many allergies)
- People who are allergic to avocado, banana, tomato, etc.

Sources of latex exposure
- Gloves
- Anaesthetic apparatus
- Balloons
- Chewing gum
- Condoms
- Drip sets
- Shoes
- Syringes

Diagnosis
- History: Skin rash, hives, asthma and predisposing factors, e.g. atopy, food allergies.
- Examination: Distribution of affected areas.
- Investigations: RAST (radio-allergosorbent test) has 80–90 per cent sensitivity; skin-prick tests with latex extract should only be done in a hospital setting.

Prevention of latex allergy
- Healthcare workers should purchase high-quality, low latex, powder-free gloves, as well as latex-free gloves.
- Latex-sensitive people should wear Medic alert bracelet and travel with non-latex gloves, antihistamine and adrenalin.

5.4.6 Diseases and conditions caused by physical agents

In Schedule 3 of the COID Act, five occupational diseases due to exposure to physical agents are listed as compensatable. These are:
1. Hearing impairment
2. Hand-arm vibration syndrome (Raynaud's phenomenon)
3. Any diseases due to overstraining of musculo-tendonous insertions
4. Dysbarism, including decompression sickness or osteonecrosis
5. Any disease due to ionizing radiation from any source.

Hearing impairment due to excessive noise, at present the most prevalent condition, and the syndrome resulting from excessive vibration are discussed at some length, the others in a shorter summary form. In 1995 the Compensation Commissioner received 1 447 claims for hearing loss, many more than in earlier years before the COID Act came into force on 1 March 1994.

5.4.6.1 Occupational hearing loss

There are many causes of deafness, which can essentially be divided into two main types:
- Conductive
- Sensoneuronal.

Conductive hearing loss occurs when the transmission of sound to the inner ear is affected, e.g. performation of the eardrum or damage to the ossicles.

Sensoneuronal hearing loss results from damage to the inner ear – sensory loss, e.g. from noise or damage to the auditory nerve – neuronal loss.

Clinical effects of noise
Noise can affect hearing in three ways:
- Acoustic trauma
- Temporary threshold shift (TTS)
- Permanent threshold shift (PTS).

Occupational hearing loss due to exposure at 'work' to excessive noise, as it is specified in the second column of the Schedule, is a risk to a large proportion of the workforce in South Africa. In many places of the working environment employees are exposed to noise levels of 85 dB or higher, which is regarded as excessive noise. It is well established that, at these levels, exposed unprotected employees will experience a gradual hearing loss in excess of what would be expected due to natural ageing in the general population.

Occurrence
In mining, open-air work like agriculture, road building, the construction industry and transportation, in the textile industry, in stone crushers and all sorts of mills, foundries, the metal industry, certain workplaces in the chemical industry, boiler rooms, power stations and engine rooms, as well as in many isolated operations,

employees are at risk. Excessive continuous noise, especially if exacerbated by intermittent impulse noise, will cause irreversible damage to hearing, the degree of which would depend on level of the noise, duration of exposure (per shift and over a working lifetime) and personal protective measures taken. Susceptibility is variable but every worker must be regarded as susceptible where and when the exposure limit of 85 dB is exceeded.

Acoustic trauma
- Instantaneous painful hearing loss
- Mechanical destruction with ruptured tympanic membrane and damaged ossicles.

Temporary threshold shift
There is a temporary decrease in hearing following noise exposure and this may include tinnitus and sensation of muffled hearing, that resolves after removal from noise.

Permanent threshold shift
This is a persistent and irreversible hearing loss following repeated noise exposure.

Characteristics of noise-induced hearing loss
- Sensineuronal hearing loss with damage to the cochlea hair cells occurs in the second quadrant of the basal turn of the cochlea. The hair cells in this area are sensitive to between 3 000 and 6 000 Hz sound.
    Initial damage is due to metabolic injury. More severe noise exposure leads to ischaemia and later death of the hair cells.
- Some speech effects are noticed with the 3 000 to 4 000 Hz drop. It becomes more noticeable once the 2 000 Hz frequencies are lost as consonants are affected. (See Figure 5.4)

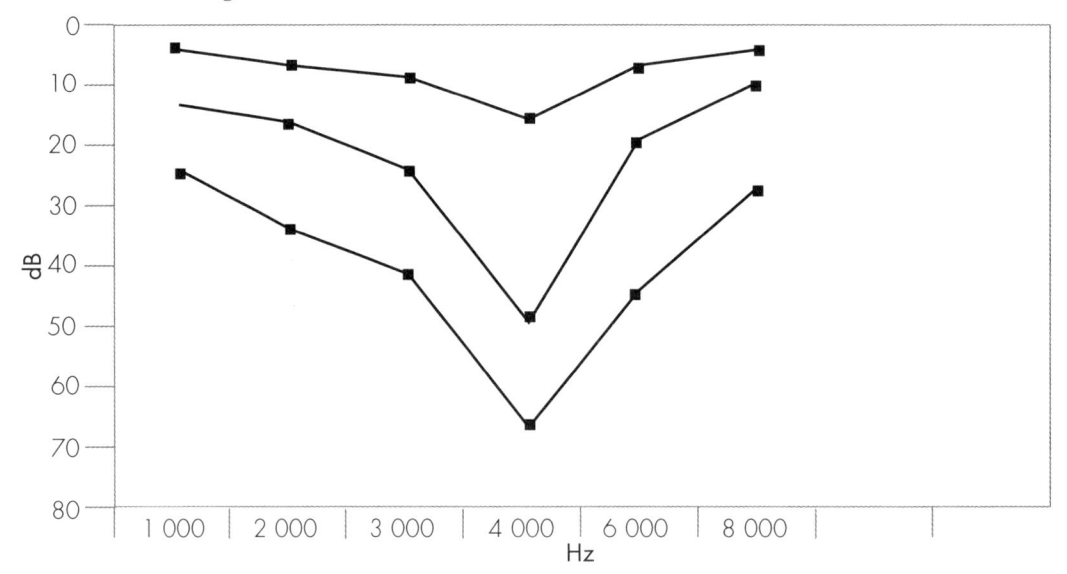

Figure 5.4 Audiogram showing the progression of NIHL and 4 000 Hz dip

Occupational medicine and occupational diseases

Prevention of noise-induced hearing loss
For every 3 dB reduction in noise, sound exposure is halved. For example, if noise levels are changed from 91 to 85 dB, noise exposure is four times less a quarter [?of ...?]. Controlling noise may involve the SOURCE, TRANSMISSION path or the WORKER.

1 Reduction at source:
- Improved design
- Better maintenance
- Silencers on air-drills
- Change process, e.g. welding not riveting.

2 Transmission:
- Enclose process
- Use absorbent material for reflected noise.

3 Worker:
- Reduce duration of exposure
- Use personal protective equipment – plugs, muffs.

Determination of permanent disablement for occupational noise-induced hearing loss – Instruction 171 COID Act

Baseline audiogram
- Use better of two initial screening audiograms performed prior to employment or within 30 days (can be performed on same day).
- Perform the test after the person has been at least 16 hours away from noise.

Percentage loss of hearing (PLH) definition

The percentage loss of hearing is the sum of hearing loss calculated at 0.5 kHz, 1 kHz, 2 kHz, 3 kHz and 4 kHz from an audiogram, and using the frequency specific tables supplied as part of Instruction 171. 1 kHz is weighted more than 0.5 kHz and 2 kHz. Permanent loss of hearing (PLH) greater than 10 per cent is compensatable.

Example:
- At baseline

Frequency (kHz)	Db L	Db R	Hearing Loss (from Tables)
0.5	15	15	0,2
1	20	20	1,2
2	20	25	1,1
3	25	25	0,7
4	25	30	0,5
			3,7% PLH

Occupational health

- Some years later

Frequency (kHz)	Db		Hearing Loss (from Tables)
	L	R	
0.5	25	30	2,0
1	30	35	6,3
2	35	35	5,1
3	40	40	3,2
4	40	45	2,7
			19,3% PLH

Deterioration = 19,3 – 3,7 = 15,6 PLH

According to COIDA Instruction 171, a person may be considered for compensation if Permanent Loss of Hearing (PLH) is greater than 10 per cent.
- 100 per cent deafness is 50 per cent Permanent Disability (PD)
- Here PD = = 7.8 OR 8 per cent Permanent Disability
- Medical opinion must be given by either an occupational medicine practitioner in uncomplicated cases and where permanent loss of hearing (PLH) is less 30 per cent from the baseline, or an ENT specialist in complicated cases or where permanent loss of hearing (PLH) exceeds 30 per cent from the baseline.
- Documents to accompany NIHL claim:
  - claimant's service record, and in particular noise levels greater than 85 dB(A) and duration of exposure
  - two diagnostic audiograms performed by a diagnostic audiologist
  - copy of the baseline audiogram (the hearing will be assumed to be normal if the baseline audiogram is unavailable).
- A medical opinion stating that the hearing loss is compatible with noise-induced hearing loss (NIHL).

Advantages of baseline approach
- The focus is on PREVENTION. Employers are responsible for hearing loss they cause.
- There is no discrimination against the employment of workers with pre-existing hearing loss.

5.4.6.2 Occupational vibration
Vibration is oscillatory motion about a point. There are two types to which workers may be exposed:
- Hand-arm vibration (HAV)
- Whole-body vibration

Hand-arm vibration (HAV)
Workers are exposed when using vibrating hand tools such as jackhammers, pneumatic chipping hammers or chainsaws.

Types of HAVs
- Vascular – 'vibration white finger' (VWF)
- Sensineuronal
- Combined vascular and sensineuronal.

The vascular effects may start with occasional blanching of the tips of fingers. These blanching attacks are precipitated by cold after vibrating tools have been used. The blanching attacks continue until the fingers are rewarmed. In severe cases, there are frequent attacks affecting all phalanges of most fingers or even skin changes in the fingertips, including gangrene.

The neurological effects have sensory and motor components and are the most unpleasant for the individual:
- Numbness, tingling
- Reduced sensory perception (vibration, temperature)
- Reduced manipulative dexterity with inability to perform intricate tasks.

The Stockholm Workshop Scale is used to classify the severity of both the vascular and 'sensineuronal' components.

The latent period for the condition can vary from six months to over 20 years. The vascular component of the condition would appear to be less than expected because of the warm climate.

Hand-arm vibration syndrome may be suspected in individuals who have tingling, numbness or blanching when operating vibrating tools. A number of tests, such as grip strength, measuring the vibrotactile threshold and performing a cold provocation test would help confirm the diagnosis.

It should, however, be remembered that other conditions can mimic HAVs, e.g. Raynaud's disease, and HIV, diabetes and drugs such as isoniazid may cause a peripheral neuropathy.

Preventive measures include:
- Ergonomic design to reduce grip force and vibration
- Keeping warm
- Minimizing/stopping smoking.

5.4.6.3 Work-related musculoskeletal disorders
There is a high incidence of musculoskeletal disorders among workers exposed to:
- Manual handling
- Repetitive and static work
- Poor psychological and social conditions.

The risk factors for the development of musculoskeletal disorders are all those that relate to poor ergonomics:
- Force required
- Repetition
- Duration

Occupational health

- Awkward posture.

Force required. The greater the force required by the individual to complete a task, the greater the load on the muscles and tendons, and the greater the chance of injury. Awkward postures often require greater forces.

Repetition. Fatigue and muscle strain can occur with increased repetition of a task, especially if combined with the other risk factors.

Duration. The longer the period of muscle contraction, the longer the recovery time required to prevent fatigue.

Awkward postures. The following are examples of awkward posture:
- Working at a computer screen with the neck excessively extended backward, flexed forward or turned to the side
- Shrugging the shoulders when the work station is too high causes fatigue as there is increased contraction of the trapezius muscles.
- Working above shoulder height is extremely tiring, and the 'rotator cuff syndrome' is more prevalent in employees involved in overhead assembly.
- Severe forward bending predisposes to backache.

Figure 5.5 illustrates the damaging effects of poor ergonomics on both the individual and the organization.

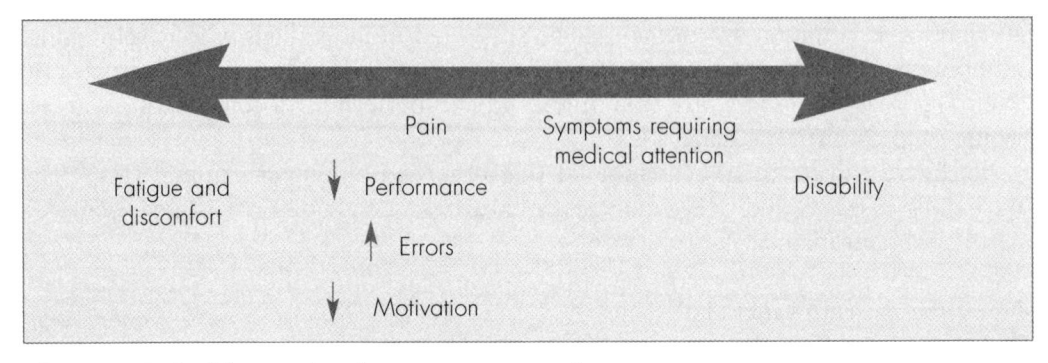

Figure 5.5 Problems related to poor ergonomics

The cumulative effects can be:
1 Physical
- Discomfort, fatigue
- Obvious pain and tenderness
- Damage to musculoskeletal system

and

2 Psychological
- Stress
- Reduced motivation and performance
- Increased errors
- Increased absenteeism.

Work-Related Upper Limb Disorders (WRULDS). The Compensation Commissioner has issued Draft Guidelines on Work-Related Upper Limb Disorders – draft circular instruction 180.

WRULDs may be defined as musculoskeletal overstraining and contiguous soft tissue disorders of the upper limb as a result of work-related cumulative, repetitive and/or forceful movements, and static loading and/or sustained postures.

These overuse disorders arise from repeated actions that are not injurious – they happen as a single event or on a few occasions, but the cumulative effects can cause injury – hence the alternative names of 'Cumulative Trauma Disorder' (CTD) or 'Repetitive Strain Injury' (RSI).

Work Related Upper Limd Disorders may include:
- Inflammation of tendons (tendonitis and tenosynovitis); examples include rotator cuff syndrome at the shoulder or epicondylitis at the elbow
- Myalgias – pain and impairment of muscles
- Nerve compression/entrapment, an example is the 'carpal tunnel syndrome' with compression of the median nerve at the wrist, resulting from highly repetitive movements and abnormal positions.

Diagnosis

According to a survey report from England the occupations from which most of the cases of repetitive strain disorder originated were assembly workers, garment workers, typists, computer operators, bank clerks and musicians. Diagnostic criteria used by orthopaedic surgeons, occupational health physicians and other experts were: a history of repetitive actions performed at work, with a frequency of between one per second to one per minute, onset of symptoms while at work, amelioration of symptoms away from work during time off, but not a history of one single event (injury), which would seem rather obvious in this context. The two obligatory symptoms reported were pain and tenderness on pressure. Symptoms and signs not regarded as essential for the diagnosis were: visible swelling of parts of the body, skin colour changes (blanching or hyperaemia), numbness, pins and needles, while some doctors regarded crepitations either audible or perceived by touch on examination as indicative (of tenosynovitis). Any syndrome resulting from repetitive overstrain movements develops only after some time. Elements of importance in causing overstrain by repetitive movements are: temperature (no cold air should blow over the hands while working), position of the wrist (no continuous flexion, extension or lateral deviation of the hand, forearm or even of the upper arm such as may occur during working overhead), wringing action or overwide 'spanning' of the fingers, overreaching, one-handed repetitive action in lieu of alternating hands, lack of adequate recovery time between movements (allowing relaxation of muscles between acts involving gripping, holding, squeezing in particular), the need for excessively tight grip, inappropriate ergonomic design of tools and of work procedures. Muscles and tendons, including insertions, can best withstand fatigue and will recover better if they are given a variety of demands to meet (tasks) and also provided with regular relaxation breaks between actions. If these breaks are deficient, overstrain will occur. A list of conditions which may be regarded as caused or aggravated by overstraining repetitive movements reads: Tendonitis, tenosynovitis, De Quervain's stenosing tenosynovitis, trigger finger, carpal tunnel syndrome, golfer's elbow (medial epicondylitis), tennis and pitcher's elbow (lateral epicondylitis), rotator cuff syndrome, frozen shoulder and Dupuytren's contracture. It must be emphasized, however, that these conditions do occur anyhow and are certainly not exclusively caused by repetitive movements at work!

Prevention

All the above elements and a few more, such as the anthropological characteristics of operators, are to be taken into account for the purpose of prevention. General and specific checklists should be developed (some are available) to devise a prevention programme guided by ergonomic principles. The participation and cooperation of the employees should be sought at an early stage, as they are likely to know the problems at hand. A most important feature is to train operators in intermittent relaxation techniques and to observe appropriate breaks between operational actions. The reader is referred to the Bibliography for an excellent source of information on cumulative trauma disorders, a NIOSH publication edited by Vern Putz-Anderson.

5.4.6.4 Ionizing radiation

Ionizing radiation may be classified into two varieties, i.e. particulate radiation which includes alpha particles, beta particles, neutrons and protons and secondly, electromagnetic radiation which includes gamma rays and X-rays. The several types of radiation vary not only in their power of penetration but also in relation to the number of electrically charged ions that they leave in their tracks when they pass through tissues. It is these electrically charged particles or ions that are mainly responsible for damage and injury to human tissues.

Alpha particles are nuclei of helium atoms, which travel only a few centimetres in air and less than 100 microns through tissues. They do not penetrate the skin and are therefore not much of an external hazard. However, alpha-emitting substances when taken into the body are dangerous. Examples of such elements are radium, thorium and polonium.

Beta particles are emitted by heavy and light radioactive elements and travel up to a few centimetres in tissue or more than a metre in air. Exposure to external sources is potentially hazardous and if taken into the body beta particles are dangerous. They are produced by accelerators and by radioactive decay. Most of the known radioisotopes emit alpha and beta particles. Protons are only produced by high energy accelerators as for instance in the National Accelerator Centre of the CSIR outside Cape Town. Neutrons are neutral particles that may interact with matter by collision with nuclei, which may then ionize surrounding atoms. Neutrons have considerable power of penetration. Gamma rays and X-rays have similar properties, but X-rays have longer wavelengths and lower energies. Both types of electromagnetic radiation are very penetrating and pose an external hazard to the human body. Examples of gamma-ray emitters used in industry are cobalt-60 and iridium.

Occurrence of occupational exposure
The greatest exposure to artificial sources of ionizing radiation is from medical radiography, radiotherapy and nuclear medicine procedures. X-rays and radioactive sources are increasingly used in industry and science, e.g. for radiographic or crystallographic examinations of castings and welding, and in electron microscopy. Radium, thorium and other radioactive substances are used as constituents of self-luminous paints and for petroleum pressure lighting equipment. Radioactive isotopes are used in medical examination and research but also for industrial purposes, as are beta emissions in the petroleum and printing industries. Examples of worker populations at risk are therefore: medical radiographers and radio therapists, nurses and dental care personnel, atomic energy plant and electronic industry employees, radium refinery and laboratory employees, uranium and thorium miners and employees of refining plants and thickness gauge (betarays) operators and industrial radiographers.

Adverse effects
It is generally accepted that ionizing radiation may induce mutations, is teratogenic and carcinogenic, and that exposure at any rate or level may result in damage to the human body. Adverse effects of ionizing radiation on the skin include burns and inflammation, necrosis and ulceration, chronic dermatitis with hyperkeratosis and degenerative changes of deeper tissues and malignant disease, usually starting as epitheliomatous warts in areas of chronic dermatitis or in normal skin and alopecia, which is a common occurrence when patients are treated with radiotherapy. Aplastic anaemia resulting from gamma rays or X-rays is a recognized hazard. The prognosis of aplastic anaemia is not good and treatment difficult. In the case of overexposure to X-rays the earliest change is usually a decrease in polymorph leukocytes, sometimes also of the lymphocytes, but occasionally a relative lymphocytosis occurs. With radium irradiation or when it is taken into the body, the first sign may be over-stimulation of the formation of all blood cells, in particular lymphocytes that show high numbers of immature or abnormal cells in peripheral blood smears. Other blood dyscrasias caused by ionizing radiation are leukaemia of all types except perhaps chronic lymphocytic leukaemia. Cataracts may be produced as a result of exposure to X-rays, gamma rays and to neutrons with a latent period of between six months and many years, depending on the dose received. Bone lesions also may result from ionizing radiation, in particular when due to radium accumulated in bone after inhalation or ingestion. The lesions may either be necrotic with features of rarefaction, leading to spontaneous fractures, or worse, malignancies, usually osteosarcomata. Lung carcinoma has been found in excess among uranium miners and this has been ascribed to radon and its daughter products as causative agent.

Prevention
Guidelines or monitoring exposure for occupations exposed to risk by personal dosimeters and other methods and for reducing the risk by engineering methods (shielding, isolation, wearing lead-containing protective aprons, gloves and special goggles) are available. Specific legislation prescribing how such protection must be

given exists worldwide and also in South Africa where a governmental body, the Atomic Energy Board, in cooperation with the Department of Health and of Labour, is charged with the task to supervise and monitor all aspects of radiation control. Exposure limits for ionizing radiation have been recommended by the ILO and WHO in cooperation with other international bodies. For the control of so-called stochastic effects (effects caused by any exposure at all and for which there is no threshold limit of exposure) the annual effective dose equivalent is recommended as not to exceed 5 rem (50 mSv). Potentially exposed employees are required to wear personal dosimeters that are monitored by an independent authority. Pregnant women should not be exposed to radiation at all but 30 per cent of the annual dose-equivalent limit is regarded as acceptable by some.

5.4.7 Tuberculosis

As presumptive clause the stipulation is made for this disease in column two that (1) exposure to crystalline silica (alpha quartz) is a requirement to accept tuberculosis of the lung as an occupational disease, or (2) that 'mycobacterium tuberculosis or MOTTS (mycobacterium other than tuberculosis) (has been) transmitted to an employee during the performance of healthcare work from a patient suffering from active open tuberculosis'. The presumption with regard to the second causation is therefore that exposure to a patient with active open tuberculosis (positive sputum in case the patient suffers from lung tuberculosis) in the performance of healthcare work implies transmission of the disease to the employee if he contracted pulmonary tuberculosis at that time.

Tuberculosis is a notifiable medical condition under the Health Act, as are anthrax, brucellosis and rift valley fever, while all these, when diagnosed as an occupational disease, must be reported by the medical practitioner to the employer and to the Department of Labour (Compensation Commissioner). Tuberculosis is the most common disease in the general population and the workforce in South Africa. Association with exposure to silica, which does not only occur in mines but also in many other workplaces, e.g. in foundries, would classify newly contracted tuberculosis in an employee who has been or is being exposed to alpha quartz as occupational disease without argument. It is expected that an occupational health worker, especially in the Cape Provinces, may find one or two cases of active lung tuberculosis per 100 employees under her/his care per month. It is incumbent on health workers to determine whether or not any exposure to silica has taken place in the work history of such employees. Apart from these only those employees who work in the healthcare sector looking after patients with open tuberculosis would qualify for classifying contracted lung tuberculosis as 'occupational disease' under this Act. Of course laboratory workers who examine sputum of such patients would fall under the presumptive clause too. During 1995 the Office of the Commissioner received 348 claims for tuberculosis as an occupational disease. Persons infected with the Human Immuno-Deficiency Virus (HIV) are at higher risk of developing active tuberculosis and there is an epidemiological association with multiple drug resistance in these patients. This poses an additional risk to health workers of which they should be aware. Under certain conditions contracting Aids (due to HIV infection) may be regarded as an occupational, compensatable disease. Prophylactic medication with INH has been advocated for HIV-positive healthcare workers who may come into contact with tuberculosis patients.

Prevention
Avoiding being infected by inhalation of the responsible micro-organism in aerosol form is, as in many other situations, an essential element. For this particular occupational disease avoidance of inhaling silica is an equally relevant factor. Hospital employees and other persons infected with the human immunodeficiency virus (HIV) have a higher risk of contracting active lung tuberculosis than others when they provide healthcare to patients with open lung tuberculosis. In some hospitals such employees are given prophylactic INH medication. Under certain conditions of course, contracting Aids may be accepted as catching an occupational disease in its own right.

Bovine tuberculosis
Bovine tuberculosis refers to human infection by *Mycobacterium bovis*, transmitted through contact with infected animals or their products and causing disease of the employee. Historically, bovine tuberculosis used to be transmitted to humans mainly by ingestion of infected milk, rarely by inhalation causing tuberculosis of the lung due to *M bovis*. Generally speaking, infection with this organism is expected to cause abdominal tuberculosis, with ulceration of the bowel, lymph gland involvement, formation of granulomata, caseation, low-grade peritonitis with widespread miliary tubercle formation, haemorrhagic exudate, ascites, adhesions and possibly formation of fistulae. Children were affected to a much greater extent than adults in times when widespread consumption of unpasteurized infected milk was rife. Employees at risk would be found in abattoirs and on cattle and dairy farms where cattle herds are not kept tuberculosis free.

Anthrax
Anthrax is caused by 'bacillus anthracis' and is now newsworthy as a biological weapon of mass destruction or, more correctly, 'mass fear'.
- *Bacillus anthracis* spores are extremely resistant and can survive for long periods in soil and animal products
- Occupations at risk include hide processors, butchers, agricultural workers and veterinarians
- Cutaneous anthrax occurs when spores from infected material gain entry through cuts or abrasions on the skin. It forms a so-called malignant pustule where the lesion has a thick black crust.
- Pulmonary anthrax used to be common among wool industry workers, giving rise to 'wool-sorters' disease. Death is very common in this form of the disease due to septicaemia.
- Treatment: penicillin or ciprofloxacin.

Legionella

Legionnaires' disease is caused by 'legionella pneumophila' and was first identified by the Centre for Disease Control (CDC) in 1977 after an outbreak of pneumonia in 1976 at an American Legion convention in Philadelphia. Over 200 individuals developed pneumonia, with 34 deaths.

The incubation period is between two and ten days. The symptoms are are follows:
- 'Flu-like symptoms
- Pneumonia-like symptoms: high tempature 39–41 °C, cough and chest pain
- Gastrointestinal (GIT) symptoms: vomiting and diarrhoea.

Treatment is with erythromycin. The fatality rate is 15 per cent.
Conditions that promote growth of Legionella are:
- Stagnant water
- Water temperature between 20 and 50 °C
- Ph between 5–8
- Sediment that tends to promote growth
- Presence of micro-organisms, e.g. pseudomonas.

Common sources of contaminated water are:
- HVAC – heating ventilation air conditions, cooling towers
- Humidifiers and decorative fountains
- Domestic water system with water heaters < 60 °C
- Warm water for eye washes and safety showers.

Putting biocides into drain pans will have no effect on Legionella if a biofilm is present.

Rift valley fever

Rift valley fever is caused by exposure to a virus that is transmitted by infected animals or their products. This is one of the haemorrhagic fevers of Africa. Others are Congo, Ebola, Marburg and Lassa fever, transmitted usually by arthropods (arbo viruses) but which are not incorporated in the Schedule. Rift valley fever is caused by a Bunya virus, transmitted in nature by certain mosquitoes. Epizootics, epidemics among animals, have occurred in the 1950s and 1970s when farmers, veterinarians and others were also infected, mainly through handling of carcasses of infected domestic animals. At risk are farmers, veterinarians and certain laboratory employees and wildlife park workers handling infected animals or their remains.

Adverse effects. An acute phase of illness, fever, headache, and general ill feeling is followed by a silent, symptomless phase which may also be a prolonged reconvalescence stage. One of the most frequent complications is inflammation of the retina around the macula which causes defective vision; a rare one is encephalitis, although fatal outcome is not infrequent during massive epizootics when animals die by the thousands.

Neither the other haernorrhagic fevers nor other infectious diseases which might originate in the working environment are listed as compensatable occupational diseases in the Schedule. However, as was stated earlier, the COID Act makes provision for an infectious disease to be accepted as an occupational disease under the Act if it is proven to the satisfaction of the Commissioner that the disease 'has arisen out of and in the course of employment' of the employee concerned (section 65). Healthcare workers could be regarded as at risk to contract such a disease, by virtue of providing healthcare (work) for infected patients who are capable of transmitting the disease. Infectious diseases presenting a risk are, e.g. viral hepatitis (B) (handling infected blood), Aids (HIV transmission by needle-stick injury), typhoid (salmonella), bacillary dysentery (shigella), amoebiasis (*Entamoeba histolytica*). The first two mentioned are of considerable concern because of the impact that contracting the disease, in particular Aids, has on the individual. Other occupations may put employees at risk to contract a wide range of infectious diseases such as leptospirosis (which is a 'prescribed disease' in the United Kingdom), rabies, cat-scratch disease, Newcastle disease (*Myxovirus multiforme*), ornithosis (Chlamydiae), tularaemia (*F tularensis*) and fungal diseases such as aspergillosis, coccidioidomycosis and histoplasmosis. For all these diseases, alleged occupational origin would be the deciding factor whether they should be regarded as occupational disease in a particular case. It is outside the scope of this chapter to discuss them all; information is readily available from textbooks and other publications in medical libraries.

5.4.8 Psychological factors
5.4.8.1 Stress
Psychological stress may occur when an individual has an imbalance between the demands made and the perceived ability to meet them. Some stress is, however, necessary in order to perform and produce excellence (e.g. during exams).

Occupational stress is on the increase due to people having to deliver a greater quality and quantity of work in less time. In some countries up to 20 per cent of workers reported very high or extremely high stress levels.

The effects of stress on the individual and the organization are given below.

1 The individual
- Lack of concentration
- A lack of interest and unhappiness with one's job
- Lack of confidence
- Irritable and aggressive behaviour
- Non-specific symptoms such as headache, dizziness and palpitations
- Anxiety and depression
- Increase in cardiovascular diseases, such as myocardial infarct and stroke
- Social breakdown with increase in divorce.

2 The organization
- Production loss due to lower productivity levels
- Increased absenteeism

Occupational health

- Increased healthcare costs with spiralling medical aid costs
- Increased accidents and injuries.

Causes of stress
- On the home and extraorganizational, i.e. the family, the economy and on quality of life
- On the workplace, i.e. job content (work overload or underload) and role ambiguity
- On the organization: i.e. climate, management styles, communication and feedback, poor working relationships.

Recognition and management of occupational stress
The causes and levels of stress in an organization may be assessed by a climate survey, and in individuals by interviews.
1. The workplace. Apply reasonably practical steps to change organizational factors such as control, social support and rewards. The results of such interventions must be quantified, i.e. is there improved productivity, reduced absenteeism, improved morale.
2. The individual. The individual should follow a holistic wellness approach with regard to physical, mental and social well-being, that encompasses:
   - Taking responsibility, being proactive
   - Undertaking personal development
   - Reducing smoking and alcohol intake
   - Showing environmental sensitivity
   - Identifying and reducing stressors
   - Cultivating social support among family, friends and colleagues
   - Practising good nutrition and physical fitness: employee fitness programmes can be cost-effective in reducing medical costs and absenteeism and are positively linked with job performance
   - Practising stress reduction techniques such as meditation.

5.4.8.2 Post-traumatic stress disorder (PTSD)
The Compensation Commissioner's Circular 171 is a set of guidelines to be followed in the handling of post-traumatic stress disorder.

The definition of PTSD is:
- A mental disorder that follows an exposure to extreme trauma or unusual stressor
- The event was outside the individual's usual psychological defences
- The incident was unexpected, sudden and non-routine, e.g. armed robbery, hijacking, rape.

Signs and symptoms of PTSD are:
- Flashbacks or recollections of the incident
- Avoidance of anything associated with the incident
- Social withdrawal, hyper-alertness, insomnia, anxiety or depression.

The treatment of PTSD is as follows:
Refer for:
- Behavioural desensitization
- Antidepressants where indicated.

For compensation to be considered, the condition must have arisen out of and in the course of employment, and must have been referred to a psychiatrist for assessment.

5.5 Shiftwork

In many countries, including South Africa, ± 20 per cent of the workforce is involved in shifts that cut across the day-night work-sleep pattern. The reasons for shiftwork are:
- Emergency services
- The 24-hour global society
- Making maximum use of machinery.

Shiftwork can disrupt the body's circadian ('about a day') rhythm, which includes body temperature, metabolic activities, hormone production and sleep.

The health effects of shiftwork are:
- Disturbed sleep. Shift workers tend to sleep less with disturbance of REM (rapid eye movement) sleep which is important for an individual's well-being.
- Malaise and fatigue
- Gastrointestinal problems – may be due to altered dietary habits or increased use of tobacco and caffeine
- Cardiovascular disease – this increase in cardiovascular risk may be due to altered eating habits, and sedentary lifestyle
- Substance abuse – some individuals may use alcohol and sleeping pills as coping mechanisms
- Divorce – disruption of family life
- Safety – accidents and errors may be caused by the malaise and fatigue.

Contraindications to shiftwork – the following conditions would be aggravated by shiftwork:
- Insulin-dependent diabetes
- Ischaemic heart disease
- Severe gastrointestinal disease
- Depression and psychosis
- Epilepsy
- Pregnancy.

The Basic Conditions of Employment Act (BCEA) (No 75 of 1997) has a Code of Good Practice on the Arrangement of Working Time that covers:
- Employers informing employees of the health and safety hazards associated with shiftwork

Occupational health

- Design and evaluation of shift system and rosters
- Performance of safety – critical tasks
- Health assessment and counselling.

This includes pre-placement and routine health examinations and advice on coping strategies.

Coping strategies are as follows:
- Try to maintain a regular sleep routine
- Block out noise and light when sleeping during the day
- Keep to a healthy diet
- Exercise (not before bedtime, as this can disrupt sleep)
- Allow time each day to be with family, including mealtimes
- Do not take sleeping pills, as they are addictive and affect REM sleep.

5.6 Practical exercise
This case study pulls together many of the topics covered in this book.

THEORETICAL CASE STUDY

You have been appointed as the occupational healthcare professional at a heavy engineering company that manufactures and assembles large trucks and trailers. The firm employs 800 employees, many of whom are involved in welding, assembly work and spray painting. Little attention was paid to occupational health in the past, but the company wishes to rectify this and has appointed you on account of your occupational health qualification.

After a few days at work and a walk through the factory, you find:
- There appears to be a lot of welding fumes and noise. PPE is used on an ad hoc basis.
- Some of the employees complain that the fumes are affecting their health, e.g. tight chest. When they complained, they were given milk as prophylaxis.
- The production manager asks you for the medical records of those who are alleging ill-health effects due to workplace exposure. He tells you that you cannot refuse as the company pays your salary and the records belong to the company.
- Some employees also complain of backache and shoulder pain and there have been a number of hand injuries and arc-eye cases in one week. The supervisor asks you for anaesthetic eye drops for the welders as they need to complete an urgent order.

Questions:
1. What are the hazards that employees may be exposed to in this factory, and how would you assess these hazards, and minimize their impact?

2. How could safety be improved?
3. Would you
   - Give the medical records to the manager?
   - Continue with the milk for those exposed to fumes?
   - Give the welders anaesthetic eye drops?
4. What are the characteristics of health professionals that enjoy credibility with both workers and management? (I assume you wish to be one of them!)

Answers:
(For brevity, some of the main points only will be outlined)

1 Hazards in a heavy engineering plant
Occupational health hazards in any setting can be divided into four main categories:
- Chemical
- Physical
- Biological
- Psychosocial

Ergonomic hazards overlap with physical and psychosocial.

Chemical hazards
Welding fumes – constituents may include iron, hexavalent chromium, nickel, manganese, ozone, carbon monoxide/dioxide and nitrous fumes.
Chromium – excessive chronic exposure to hexavalent chromium has been associated with increased risk of lung cancer and skin irritation.
Manganese – chronic manganese exposure may cause central nervous system problems, psychiatric symptoms, muscular weakness, Parkinson-like disease.
Iron – acute symptoms include irritation of the nose, throat and lungs. The major chronic condition is siderosis.
Ozone – this is formed by the action of UV light on oxygen in the air. Acute effects include irritation of mucous membranes to pulmonary oedema. Chronic effects include changes in lung function.
Nitrous fumes – like ozone, formed in the arc by UV radiation, and have similar health effects.
Carbon monoxide – can be formed by the burning of the flux.
Welders may have symptoms of chronic bronchitis, asthma or 'metal fume fever' – 'flu-like illness that may occur on re-exposure to metal fumes after a few days lay-off.

Physical hazards
- Noise. Noise levels can vary between 90 and 120 dB(A) in welding workplaces because of gouging, pneumatic chisels, grinders, etc.
- Hand-arm vibration. This may arise from the use of hand-held grinders.
- Radiation. The welding arc produces intensely bright light in the visible, ultraviolet, infrared wavelengths.

Ultraviolet light may cause 'arc-eye' or keratoconjunctivitis. Onset may be delayed. UV light can also cause 'sunburn'. Visible radiation can damage the retina if too intense. The lens of the eye can be clouded by IR radiation and cause cataract. Therefore adequate protection for the eye and skin areas is necessary.
- Burns. These may be thermal (from hot metal or slag) and radiant.

Spray painting may include:
- Polyurethane paint, which uses isocyanates as catalysts, as well as epoxy paints, may both cause occupational asthma.
- Solvent exposure may depress the central nervous system.

Ergonomic hazards may include:
- Lifting and lowering of heavy loads such as metal sheeting.
- Welding in the bending, stooping, squatting or overhead positions.

Biological hazards are not applicable.

Psychosocial hazards, e.g. stress, may be due to:
- Shiftwork
- High demand for work output but low control over the pace of work
- Less than ideal working conditions
- Conflict with colleagues.

Risk assessment. A team approach is best adopted comprising the health and safety representatives, manager of the area, occupational health nurse and doctor, risk manager, engineer and, where indicated, occupational hygienist and ergonomist. Various members of the team may:
- Do a 'walk-through' survey, i.e. see what people do and how they do it.
- Take occupational hygiene measurements, i.e. quantify levels of noise, welding and paint fumes compared to the occupational limit.

  Whilst welding fumes per se are not listed in the Hazardous Chemical Substances Regulations of 1995, a number of constituents are. The additive action should therefore be taken into account by the fractional exposures:

$$\frac{C_1}{T_1} + \frac{C_2}{T_2} + \frac{C_n}{T} > 1$$

C = concentration of contaminant
T = Threshold Limit Value/Occupational Exposure Limit of contaminant.

If this sum exceeds unity (1), the combined concentrations of the contaminants have exceeded the exposure limit.
- A history of occupational injuries and diseases such as noise-induced hearing loss, occupational asthma, dermatitis, musculoskeletal-related disorders would be relevant.

Quantifying occupational risk. There are numerous scoring systems in place to quantify the risk, e.g. Risk (1-100) = Probability of Occurrence (1-10) x Severity of Consequence.

Probability of occurrence depends on:
- Level of exposure compared to occupational exposure limit
- Frequency of exposure
- Duration of exposure
- Quality of control measures.

The severity of consequence could be as follows:
Very high consequences would include cancer, allergies, or the development of a condition which would result in an employee having to be removed from current job, or being placed on ill-health retirement or could result in injury or death, e.g. if welding fumes were measured at 4 times the occupational exposure limit, and welders are exposed 7 hours a day, 5 days a week, control measures are poor, and some have been diagnosed with occupational asthma requiring them to be relocated to other areas where they are not exposed to fumes, then:

Probability of Occurrence = 7/10
Severity of Consequence = 8/10
Therefore Risk = 56/100 (medium to high).
All other risks such as noise, solvents, ergonomic, stress can similarly be scored.

Hazard control involves dealing with the SOURCE, TRANSMISSION PATH and WORKER.

Where fume levels exceed the action level, the best solution is to remove the fumes by means of a suitable extraction system where possible. Fumes should be collected as close to the point of origin as possible.

Respiratory protection includes a disposable welding mask (protection factor up to 10) or an airline-fed respirator.

For all arc-welding work, either a helmet or hand-held face shield is necessary for protection from radiation, spatter and hot clay.

Leather gauntlet-type gloves, aprons, capes are necessary for protection from heat, burns and radiation.

The services of an ergonomist should be considered for recommendations regarding manual lifting, lowering or moving heavy items or materials, as well as the correct height at which work is carried out.

Health surveillance
History. Any complaints such as chronic cough, shortness of breath, irritation of eyes or throat, skin problems, muscle or joint pains.

Physical examination. Special reference to skin, nasal membranes, lungs and eyes, and musculoskeletal system.

Special investigations
- Audiograms
- Spirometry or two-hourly peak flow if asthma is suspected
- Chest X-ray, when considered necessary
- Perhaps biological monitoring, e.g. urinary pre- and post-shift chromium and manganese in a random sample of welders.

Any cases of occupational asthma and noise-induced hearing loss would need to be submitted to the Compensation Commissioner. Relocation of workers with occupational asthma to areas where they would not be exposed to fumes must be considered.

2 Improve safety
A thorough investigation must be done to get to identify and rectify the root causes, which may be:
- Poor engineering
- Poor maintenance
- Poor training
- Fatigue from stress, overtime
- Poor supervision.

3 Access to medical records, prophylactic use of milk and anaesthetic eye drops
The answer to all three is NO!
- Confidentiality of clinical information
  Disclosure of clinical information about a worker may not be divulged to third parties (e.g. management, co-workers) without written informed consent. Informed consent must be made without coercion or fear and the worker must understand why the information must be divulged, what information will be supplied and to whom, and what consequences may follow.
  Disclosure to a third party without consent may only take place if a person is placing himself or others at risk of death or serious injury, and the individual must be informed that you intend breaking confidentiality.
  You can tell the manager that breaking confidentiality without consent:
- Is against the rules of the Nursing or Health Professions Council
- Would lead to loss of credibility.
- The prophylactic use of milk to prevent adverse ill-health effects from fumes has absolutely no benefit and should be discouraged. It may, however, be used as a beverage.
- Painful eyes signify damage. Anaesthetizing the eyes would cause further damage from excessive exposure to UV light.

4 Habits of effective individuals who enjoy credibility with the workers and management
- Be caring – you will soon be asked to leave if you are perceived to be uncaring

- Practise according to the highest professional standards and competence – you will be expected to be trustworthy and to keep up to date
- Focus on important health issues
- Be proactive
- Be a team player
- Focus on prevention
- Communicate what you do and what you have achieved, e.g. improved health of workforce to stakeholders.

You may wish to add other habits and characteristics.

5.7 Bibliography

Textbooks

Dixon, W. M. & Price, S. M. G. (eds.) 1984. *Aspects of Occupational Health*. London: Faber & Faber.

Guild, R., Ehrlich, R. I., Johnston, J. R., Ross, M. H. (eds.) 2001. *Occupational Health Practice in the South African Mining Industry*. SIMRAC.

Kroemer, K., Kroemer, H., Kroemer-Elbert, K. 1999. *Ergonomics: How to Design for Ease and Efficiency*. New York: Prentice Hall.

Lauwerys, R. L. 1983. *Industrial Chemical Exposure: Guidelines for Biological Monitoring*. Davis, California: Biomedical Publication.

Levy, B. W. & Wegman, D. H. (eds.) 1983. *Occupational Health, Recognising and Preventing Work-related Disease*. Boston: Little, Brown & Co.

McCunney, R. J. (ed.) 1988. *Handbook of Occupational Medicine*. Boston: Little, Brown & Co.

Plunkett, E. R. 1977. *Occupational Diseases: A Syllabus of Signs and Symptoms*. Stamford, Connecticut: Barrett Book Company.

Rom, W. N. (ed.) 1990. *Environmental and Occupational Medicine*. 2nd edition. Boston: Little, Brown & Co.

Rosenstock, L. & Cullen, M. R. 1986. *Clinical Occupational Medicine*. Philadelphia: WB Saunders.

Schilling, R. (ed.) 1981. *Occupational Health Practice*. 2nd edition. London: Butterworths.

Stellman, J. M. & Permeggiani, I. (eds.) 1983. *ILO Encyclopaedia of Occupational Health and Safety*. 3rd revised, 4th edition. Vol 1–4. Geneva: ILO.

Waldron, H. A. 1985/1989. *Lecture Notes on Occupational Medicine* 4th edition. Blackwell Scientific Publications.

Zens, C (ed.) 1994. *Occupational Medicine, Principles and Practical Applications*. 3rd edition. St Louis: Mosby.

Further reading
Specific texts on recognition of occupational disease

Key, M. M. 9ed.) *Occupational diseases, A guide to their recognition*. NIOSH Publication. no 77–181.

Early detection of chronic lung diseases. WHO Euro Reports and Studies no 24, Copenhagen.
Health promotion for working populations. WHO Technical Report Series 765, Geneva 1988.
Notes on the diagnosis of occupational diseases. Dept of Health and Social Security, London UK. Her Majesty's Stationery Office, Revised edition 1983.
Rapid revision in respiratory disease. F. Wiles, S. Zwi & E. Baskind. *Medical News Tribune* (SA) (Pty) Ltd, Rivonia.
Occupational cancer: Prevention and control. ILO Occupational Safety and Health Series no 39, Geneva 1988.
WHO. 1986. *Early detection of occupational diseases.* Geneva: WHO.
WHO. 1985. Identification and control of work-related diseases. Geneva: 1985.

Epidemiology
M. Karvonen & M. I. Mikheev (eds.) *Epidemiology of Occupational Health.* WHO Regional Office for Europe. European Series no 20, Copenhagen 1986.

Environmental aspects
Rapid Guide to Hazardous Chemicals in the Workplace. Eds. N. 1. Sax and R. J. Lewis. 1986 Van Nostrand Reinhold Company, New York.
The Hazards of Work: How to fight them. Patrick Kinnersly. PLUTO's Press Ltd, London (Workers Handbook no 1, 19731980).
International Labour Standards. A worker's education manual, 2nd edition. ILO, Geneva 1982.
HEALTH AND SAFETY (COSH) REGULATIONS. 1988. The control of substances hazardous to health. (HMSO) Her Majesty's Stationery Office, London, UK.
Guidance Note EH 40/94 annually revised by the Health and Safety Executive UK (HMSO).
Threshold Limit Values for Chemical Substances and Physical Agents in the Work Environment and Biological Exposure Indices. Published annually by the ACGIH, 6500 Glenway Avenue, Cincinnati, OH 45211–4438 USA.
Recommended health-based limits in occupational exposure to heavy metals. WHO Technical Report Series 647, Geneva 1980.
Recommended health-based limits in occupational exposure to selected mineral dusts (silica, coal). WHO Technical Reports Series 734, Geneva 1986.

Recommended papers published in journals or as monographs
Occupational Health Nursing in *Nursing SA.* May 1987 vol 2, no 5, pp. 5–47.
Occupational Medicine in *SA Journal of Continuing Medical Education.* April 1986 vol 4 pp. 5–128.
Proceedings of the International Symposium on Research on Work-related Diseases. Espoo Finland 1984 in the *Scandinavian Journal of Work, Environment and Health.* December 1984, vol 10, no 6 (special issue).
The ALLSA Handbook of Practical Allergy. Janssen Pharmaceutica 1994. Creda Press: Eppindust.

Poisoning by Chemicals in Agriculture and Public health. H. 0. Fourie. 1984. Sigma Press, Pretoria.
Biological Monitoring of Workers Exposed to Pesticides. Guidelines for Field Application 1995. Available from: Occupational Health Research Unit, Dept of Community Health, UCT Medical School, Observatory 7925.
Tuberculosis. A Century of Tuberculosis, South African Perspectives. Eds: Coovadia, H. M. & Benatar, S. R Cape Town: Oxford University Press 1991.
Cumulative Trauma Disorders. A Manual for Musculoskeletal Diseases of the Upper Limbs. Ed: Vern Putz-Anderson. NIOSH, Cincinnati, Ohio, USA. 1988. London and New York. Taylor & Francis.
Occupational Health. *Continuing Medical Education Journal.* CME. Sept 1996. SAMA
Compensation for Occupational Injuries and Diseases Act, 1993 – The Determination of Permanent Disablement Resulting from Hearing Loss caused by Exposure to Excessive Noise and Trauma. Circular Instruction No. 171. GN No. 422 (16 May 2001).
– Circular Instruction 176 Regarding Compensation for Occupational Asthma. GN No. 82 (10 Jan 2003).
– Circular Instruction 178 Regarding Compensation for Pulmonary Tuberculosis in Health Care Workers. GN No. 81 (10 Jan 2003)

Legislation

Occupational Health and Safety Act, 1993 (No 85 of 1993), Government Gazette Vol 337, No 14918 (2 July 1993), Dept of Labour.
   a Asbestos Regulations GN No R773 (1987) R155 (2002)
   b Lead Regulations GN No R586 (1991) R236 (2002)
   c Regulations for Hazardous Chemical Substances GN No R1179 (1995)
Compensation for Occupational Injuries and Diseases Act, 1993 (No 130 of 1993) Government Gazette Vol 337, No 14918 (2 July 1993).
Occupational Diseases in Mines and Works Act, 1973 (No 78 of 1973).
Occupational Diseases in Mines and Works Amendment Act, 1993 (No 208 of 1993) Government Gazette Vol 343, No 15449 (1994).
Mine Health and Safety Act, 1996 (No 29 of 1996) Government Gazette Vol 372, No 17242 (14 June 1996).

6 Occupational health service management

J. Acutt

6.1 Introduction

Occupational health nursing is a speciality nursing practice that makes provision for and delivers varied healthcare services for companies and their employees. In terms of the World Health Organization definition of occupational health, this practice is aimed at promotion, protection and restoration of the health of all employees in a safe and healthy work environment.

This chapter presents the management framework for a programme to protect and promote the health of all employees by correct placement of employees in a work environment suited to their physical and psychological capabilities, medical surveillance, health education, and the prevention and treatment of illness and injury.

6.2 Learning objectives

At the end of this chapter the reader should be able to:
- Define occupational health nursing
- Describe the role and responsibilities of the occupational health nurse
- Design a job description for an occupational health nurse in a specific type of industry
- Identify the elements of the management process
- Plan and establish an effective occupational health programme
- Develop an occupational health policy, and a policy and procedure manual
- Design an annual health promotion programme for a specific company
- Plan for and control financial resources in the occupational health service
- Evaluate the quality and effectiveness of the occupational health service
- Apply the nursing process in occupational health nursing.

6.3 The occupational health nurse

The occupational health nurse is a registered professional nurse with specialized knowledge and skills to identify health risks at the workplace, create a safe and healthy work environment, and prevent injuries and deviation from health in the workforce.

The occupational health nurse functions independently, making autonomous decisions using his/her professional judgement in analysing data gathered from clients, the work environment, and members of the occupational health team. As a professional, responsible and reliable person who strictly observes the provisions of the Nursing Act, 1978 (No 50 of 1978 as amended), he/she is trusted and respected by management and employees alike.

6.3.1 Knowledge and experience
Occupational health nursing is a highly specialized field and in order to provide an effective health service that benefits the employees and the company, knowledge and experience are required of the following:
- General and occupational health nursing
- Ethical and legal compliance
- Emergency and trauma care
- Primary healthcare
- Health promotion and health education for adults
- Toxicology and medicine
- Pharmacology
- Social and behavioural sciences
- Management of a health service
- Environmental hygiene, risk management and safety.

Occupational health nursing is diverse and in any one day the nurse may:
- Start the day with audiometric testing of workers exposed to high noise levels and medical surveillance, according to the annual programme
- Attend to a steady stream of employees with day-to-day ailments, minor injuries or chronic diseases during a primary healthcare clinic
- Attend to a victim of a workplace accident
- Give a health promotion presentation
- Counsel a young drug addict
- Investigate a health hazard
- Attend a health and safety meeting
- Present a motivation to management for a new programme
- Record all the above in the daily activities file, personal medical files, the medicine register, the accident register, in memorandums, reports and correspondence.

In keeping with the provisions of the Nursing Act, 1978 (No 50 of 1978, as amended), occupational health nurses will identify their own shortcomings and address their training needs on an ongoing basis.

6.3.2 Principles of ethics for the occupational health professional
The International Commission on Occupational Health (ICOH) has prepared a code of ethics that states:

> Occupational health practice must be performed according to the highest professional standards and ethical principles. Occupational health professionals must serve the health and social well-being of the workers, individually and collectively. They also contribute to environmental and community health
> (ICOH, 1996).

The occupational health professional has an obligation to:
- Protect the life and health of the worker
- Respect human dignity
- Promote the highest ethical principles in occupational health policies and programmes
- Act with integrity and impartiality
- Protect the confidentiality of health data and the privacy of individuals

The occupational health professional is an expert who must be given full professional independence in carrying out his/her tasks and the means to do this according to good practice and professional ethics.

The occupational health professional must acquire and maintain the competence required to execute his/her functions.

It is the responsibility of the occupational health nurse to coordinate the service to the benefit of the employee and employer. He/she has a duty towards:

The employee. As in all nursing, the occupational health nurse's first obligation is towards the patient or client (the employee) or even the whole workforce and his/her primary responsibility is to protect the well-being of the employee.

The employer. The occupational health nurse is loyal towards his/her employer and protects the company from the adverse effects of hazardous substances, dangerous work processes, injuries and disease. It is his/her duty to know the risks on site and how to deal with them.

Colleagues. As a team member the occupational health nurse liaises closely with the company physician, the risk manager, occupational hygienist, safety officer, the client and his general practitioner.

6.3.3 The dependent, interdependent, and independent nature of the functions of the occupational health nurse

1. **The dependent function**. Occupational health nurses are dependent upon the law that authorizes them to practise, as well as common and relevant statutory laws. They must ensure that they are and remain registered with the organization that regulates nursing practice in the country, as well as being members of a professional society that offers assistance under a professional indemnity scheme.
2. **The interdependent function**. Occupational health nurses provide a healthcare service to the employee and the company in cooperation with persons registered under:
   - The Nursing Act, 1978 (No 50 of 1978) as amended
   - The South African Health Professions Act, 1974 (No 5 of 1974)
   - The Pharmacy Act, 1974 (No 53 of 1974)

   and other members of the occupational health team in the company they work for.

   Nursing practitioners accept responsibility for the manner in which they execute instructions or requests and for keeping their knowledge up to date in order to contribute positively to the occupational health programme of the company.

3 **The independent function**. Occupational health nurses, as professional practitioners, are totally responsible and accountable for their own actions and omissions and are aware of the extent of their knowledge, skills, abilities and limitations in the performance of occupational healthcare duties. The employee, employer and the members of the occupational health team can expect an occupational health nurse to be competent and reliable, carrying out his/her duty with accuracy and skill.

However, an occupational health nurse may refuse to carry out instructions in the case of an illegal act, over-prescription, inaccurate prescription, contravention of the policy of the organization or of the employees' wishes, or anything beyond his/her competence.

6.4 The appointment of an occupational health nurse in an organization

The aim of all business organizations is to be productive, cost-effective and profitable. The task of the occupational health service is to contribute to these aims by ensuring that:
- Individuals are fit to do a specific job
- Their health is not adversely affected by their work and vice versa
- Employees who are incapacitated for any reason are returned to work as soon as possible.

This opens up broad new avenues of service and offers a grand challenge to the professional capabilities of the nurse who must understand that he/she is a health consultant to the organization and all persons employed there.

The time to establish a correct professional understanding and working relationship with the employer is during the interview for the post and prior to acceptance of a contract of employment and the position charter or job description.

6.4.1 The employment interview

The interview provides the nurse with the opportunity to establish the scope and responsibilities of the post, the functions to be undertaken and the status, remuneration and conditions of work under which he/she will be expected to operate. The interview may not always provide clarity about the proper role and function of an occupational health service. If duties and responsibilities are suggested that have no bearing on this, the nurse should not accept the post, unless changes can be negotiated that will allow him/her to contribute his/her knowledge and skills in an appropriate manner, for the maximum benefit of the organization and all the employees.

The occupational health department, whether it is staffed by one nurse or a team of nurses and doctors, is a separate specialized functional department within the organization.

The senior occupational health nurse will assume managerial control and responsibility for the smooth running of the department. Accountability for administrative aspects should be to a senior member of the organization's management and for clinical aspects, to the company's medical officer.

The success of an occupational health service depends on the establishment of effective relationships with members of the various departments within the organization. These relationships can be hindered by the lack of understanding of one another's role and a breakdown in effective communication.

6.4.2 The position charter and appointment

The position charter is the most important document the occupational health nurse will have. Duties, responsibilities and functions should be clearly stated but be flexible enough to accommodate the nurse's changing and expanding role as the organization grows.

The position charter or job description should include the following aspects:
- Academic qualifications and experience required for the position
- Reporting relationships for medical and administrative direction
- Nursing ethics – it should be stated that the occupational health nurse will uphold these at all times

The broad functions of the position should be stated, for example:
- Development and administration of the occupational health programme
- Health assessment and medical surveillance with the appropriate action
- Health promotion through health education, primary health and counselling
- Emergency preparedness and first-aid training.

The appointment letter must be accepted by the applicant for an occupational health nursing position and should state the company service conditions including:
- Employment benefits, which would be the same as for other professional employees within the company
- Hours of work, shift differential and number of statutory holidays
- Remuneration including starting salary, increments, overtime pay
- Leave of absence, sick leave
- Group insurance, medical scheme, retirement plan, etc.

These conditions should be confirmed in writing and understood before the position is accepted.

Professional recognition as a member of a team within the company to promote health and provide a safe working environment must be afforded the occupational health nurse.

Provision of in-service training and ongoing education in order to maintain his/her skills and professional knowledge must be agreed. This includes the attendance of refresher courses and conferences and the provision of reference material by the employer. Internet access, books and professional journals on occupational health nursing and subjects related to the industry are required to keep up to date with changes in legislation, medical techniques, technology and socio-economic development.

6.4.3 The basic job description

A job description for an occupational health nursing practitioner is adjusted to different company climates and to their workforce health needs. The size of the workforce and the health risks at work dictate the size and type of occupational health team and the health service required.

The job description is a management tool used by the human resource department. It is drawn up after a job analysis has been done and the job output requirements have been discussed with the company medical officer.

Occupational health nurses must evaluate their job description in the light of their responsibility to provide quality and effective occupational healthcare to the company and the employees. They alone can reveal excellent work when their superior evaluates their job performance.

The duties of the occupational health nurse include the following:
- Development and management of the occupational health programme including the setting of objectives, budgeting, administration, medicine control, report writing and the evaluation and adaptation of the service to address changing needs
- Health assessment, diagnosis, treatment or referral with a view to addressing the employee's health needs and to make recommendations regarding the placement of employees in employment suited to their work capabilities
- Medical surveillance as required for exposure to hazardous procedures
- Health promotion through health education, medical surveillance, counselling of employees with individual problems, and rehabilitation
- Emergency preparedness and first-aid training
- Liaison with outside agencies (doctors, healthcare agencies, support groups and occupational health specialists)
- Environmental monitoring and safety aspects in collaboration with the occupational hygiene and safety team in order to assess the effects of the work environment on health.

6.5 The role of the occupational health nurse

Role refers to a set of prescriptions defining behaviour in terms of professional practice. The occupational health nurse has a duty to take care of the company and its employees and is committed to:
- The wellness of employees, employers and the community if affected by the organization's activity
- Quality care and standards of practice
- Education and research
- Personal and professional accountability.

The role of the occupational health nurse is complex due to the variety of functions within the position and includes the aspects discussed below.

6.5.1 Professional
As a professional person the occupational health nurse adheres to the professional code of ethics and of practice which dictates that nurses are responsible and accountable for professional behaviour. This includes the application of the nursing process and cooperation with appropriate others within current legislation affecting nursing practice and health.

The occupational health nurse acts within the context of the policies and practices of the employer and within the values and culture of the society served.

The nurse respects all confidences and protects the interests of clients. In the event of a dispute the role of an impartial adviser to both parties is assumed.

6.5.2 Clinician
In the provision of quality nursing care, including emergency care, accurate medical surveillance, biological and environmental monitoring, the nurse fulfils the role of the clinician. The occupational health nurse keeps up to date with the latest information and clinical techniques.

6.5.3 Administrator
The administrative role encompasses the provision of structure and direction for the development, implementation, evaluation and control of the occupational health programme. The administrator is a goal setter, policy maker, record keeper, report writer, programme evaluator, budget controller and researcher, as described in relevant sections of this chapter.

6.5.4 Educator
Apart from being a health promoter to the employer and employees, a trainer to first-aiders and health and safety representatives, an educator to students and colleagues, the occupational health nurse constantly updates his/her own knowledge

6.5.5 Consultant
As a consultant, the occupational health nurse has the expertise to advise management and occupational health team members on occupational health aspects, including legislative requirements. The nurse as the company consultant on health matters is the coordinator of treatment programmes with external agencies including local hospitals, clinics and general practitioners.

6.6 Management principles in occupational health
Management is a process of getting things done or achieving objectives. It involves activities that are generally defined as:

Assessment – gathering information about the company, the employees and all health risks

Planning – evaluating the information, prioritizing and deciding what needs to be done and setting objectives

Organizing – implementing plans and directing the proceedings to achieve the objectives
Control – evaluation of what has been achieved and if it is of acceptable standard.

The management process is implemented when planning commences before establishing an occupational health programme and is ongoing as the programme continues. It needs to be dynamic and proactive, as the occupational health programme is never static. Developments in legislation, technology, health and socio-economics influence the occupational health programme and must be accommodated (Booyens, 1996; Guild, et al., 2001).

6.6.1 The philosophy, objectives and policy of an occupational health programme

The occupational health service requires a philosophy of healthcare as a framework for action. This philosophy reflects the values and beliefs of the occupational health nurse and addresses the workers, the nurse, nursing practice and the work environment. It needs to be written out and displayed in the occupational health centre, and in the policy and procedure manual.

The philosophy is kept in mind when setting objectives for the occupational health service. Objectives are the basis for the programme and the standards against which performance is measured. They are set when commencing a service or when planning a new programme and must be functional and achievable within a specific time period. Short-term objectives are set to be achieved within a year and long-term objectives are set for new programmes or equipment in the future.

An effective occupational health policy must be established by top management in consultation with the occupational health team and the employees. The policy must be:

- A brief, clearly written statement that is signed by the company executive officer and dated
- A statement that includes a commitment to ongoing improvement in the prevention of health and safety risks in keeping with legislative requirements
- Communicated to all employees and displayed
- Reviewed regularly, especially when changes occur in legislation, management, work processes, etc.

(See Appendix 6.1 An example of a company policy for a special health issue.)

6.6.2 Assessment for an occupational health programme

A complete assessment of the health risks, be they hazards in the work environment or ill health for whatever reasons, and of the company structure and its policy must be made in order to collect data that will determine the company's requirements and the health needs of the employees.

6.6.2.1 Health risk assessment and management

Risk is a measure of the likelihood that a hazard may occur. A hazard is anything that has the potential to cause harm.

Occupational health

To assess health risks, the following steps need to be planned in order to ensure that all forms of hazards are considered during the assessment:
- Consider all activities – routine, non-routine and emergency situations
- Identify the hazards
- Identify all individuals or groups that may be exposed to hazards
- Identify the control measures and determine whether they are adequate
- Determine and assess the risks to health.

Risks need to be quantified in terms of the likelihood of occurrence and the severity of consequence if they are not controlled.

Risk = likelihood of occurrence X severity of consequence

The likelihood of occurrence is evaluated according to the actual level of exposure compared with the occupational exposure limit as laid down by law, and the frequency and duration of exposure. The severity of consequence is rated high if the person could be injured or develop an occupational disease. See Table 6.1 for the calculation of the risk rating of exposure to noise at the level of 85 dB for an hour a day. There is a low risk of noise-induced hearing loss as the level of noise is 85 dB, the duration is one hour a day and the worker wears suitable hearing protectors, thus the value of 4 is allocated to the likelihood column. However, the consequence of exposure should any of the mitigating measures not be in place would be high and the value of 8 is allocated to the consequence column.

The resultant risk rating (4 x 8 = 32) indicates that a moderate occupational risk is present in the work process.

Table 6.1 Quantifying occupational risk for noise-induced hearing loss at a machine used for one hour a day at noise level 85 dB

Risk exposure	Value	Occurrence likelihood	Consequence severity	Occupational risk rating
Very high	10			
High	8		8	32
Moderate	6			
Low	4	4		
Very low	2			
None	0			
Evaluation:	Serious occupation risk	> 50		
	Moderate occupational risk	30–49		
	Minor occupational risk	0–29		

Health needs and priorities are identified by analysing data collected from inspecting the entire worksite. Visiting the safety, human resource, finance, production and buying departments provides information on factors that impact on the planning of the service. These factors include:

- The nature of the employer business, that required specific health programmes, for example food handlers need early care of minor infectious ailments and injuries, and in dangerous work a full paramedic team may need to be on standby.
- The number of employees have an influence, for example a larger workforce will make greater demands on the health service.
- The age and gender of employees will influence the type of service required, for example women of childbearing age require more clinic time for family planning, antenatal and postnatal services. Older workers may require clinic for chronic diseases.
- Disabled persons require specific healthcare and facilities such as ramps or larger toilets for wheelchairs.
- The hours of work, including shift work and overtime, may necessitate the clinic being operational after hours and require extra health personnel.
- Previous sick leave and injury-on-duty records will indicate the type of illnesses and injuries that will need to be addressed.
- Environmental factors, such as hazards, air or water pollution, the climate, prevailing endemic diseases, etc. will have a bearing on the occupational health service required.
- Raw materials and specific hazards will dictate types of health screening, education and health protection required.
- The legislation applicable to general health and to occupational health and safety prescribes minimum standards to be attained, precautions to be taken, biological monitoring and medical surveillance to be executed and recorded; certain medical conditions must be reported to the authorities.
- Trade union and employee representatives should be approached to elicit their views on the health needs of the workers.
- The location of the occupational health centre needs to be assessed for cost-effectiveness and future expansion as the company grows.
- Access to local health facilities, such as doctors, hospitals, ambulance and specialist services, will influence the level of care to be rendered on site; the more remote these supporting services are the greater the extent of the occupational health service needs to be.
- The appointment of a company doctor (either full-time or on a part-time basis) and personnel for the occupational health service will be evaluated once the health needs of the company have been assessed.
- The presence of other members of the occupational health team, including a safety officer and an occupational hygienist, influences the planning of the occupational health service.

The identified priorities are discussed with management and the risk control officer, production manager, human resources manager and trade union representatives and, should an existing medical centre need to be altered or a new one built, the site manager and architect.

The relative importance of each of these factors will vary in differing situations. For example, the occupational health requirements of a mine will differ greatly from those of a supermarket.

Once the above data has been evaluated, the occupational health service must be planned systematically in order to be efficient and cost-effective. The first step is to define the aims and objectives of the service, then a philosophy must be established and a health policy drawn up.

The medical centre is planned for easy access for workers and emergency services with wide doors, a ramp for wheelchairs, a waiting-room, treatment rooms, offices, toilets, a secure dispensary and a store-room. Special facilities for audiometry, lung function tests, vision screening or for training and education must be considered. Practical aspects, which include the layout for convenient flow of traffic, washable walls, worktops and floors and double-glazed windows to keep out noise and dust, are best seen in established occupational health centres of major companies. Guidelines and advice are available from societies for occupational health practitioners.

Equipment, stocks and stationery can only be acquired once quotations and the available budget have been studied.

6.6.2.3 Selected criteria for the planning and establishment of an occupational health service

Several factors influence the level of occupational healthcare required by a company, which includes the commitment of the company's management, the industry size and nature, and accessibility and level of local health services. Occupational healthcare is available at three levels:

1 Legal compliance. The Occupational Health and Safety Act, 1993 (No 85 of 1993), the Mine Health and Safety Act, 1996 (No 29 of 1996) and other applicable legislation require:
- Environmental monitoring of listed hazards
- Biological monitoring and medical surveillance
- Provision of personal protective equipment and information on hazardous procedures
- First-aid training.

This can be done annually by a suitably accredited agency and protects the employer from legal risks, and the employees from the effects of hazardous substances.

2 Basic occupational healthcare. This level of care provides for legal compliance and basic healthcare by a part-time medical service through:
- Environmental monitoring for control
- General and specific health assessment and biological monitoring before placement of an employee and periodically thereafter
- Education about hazardous procedures and the need for protection

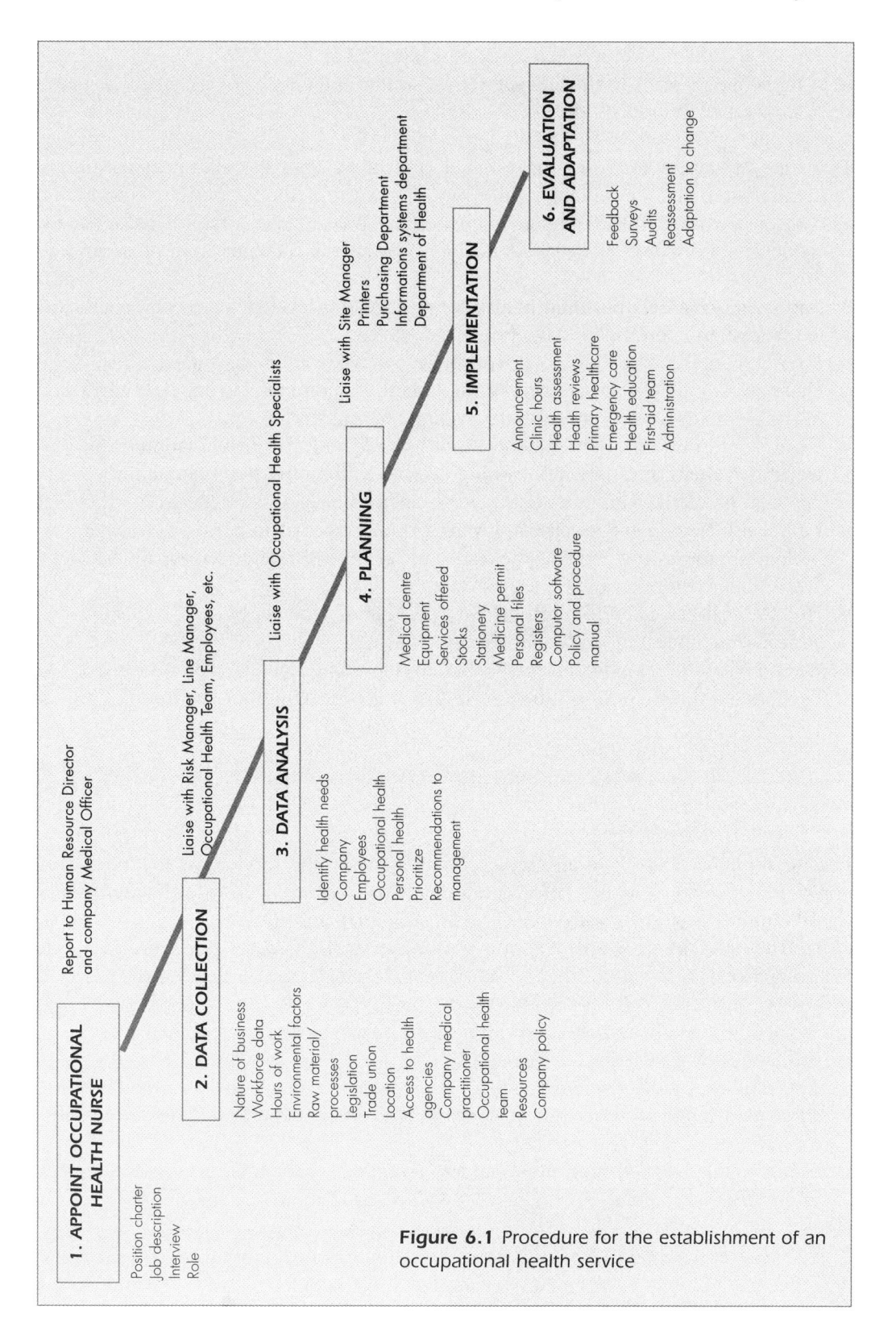

Occupational health service management

1. APPOINT OCCUPATIONAL HEALTH NURSE

Position charter
Job description
Interview
Role

Report to Human Resource Director and company Medical Officer

2. DATA COLLECTION

Liaise with Risk Manager, Line Manager, Occupational Health Team, Employees, etc.

Nature of business
Workforce data
Hours of work
Environmental factors
Raw material/processes
Legislation
Trade union
Location
Access to health agencies
Company medical practitioner
Occupational health team
Resources
Company policy

3. DATA ANALYSIS

Liaise with Occupational Health Specialists

Identify health needs
Company
Employees
Occupational health
Personal health
Prioritize
Recommendations to management

4. PLANNING

Liaise with Site Manager
Printers
Purchasing Department
Informations systems department
Department of Health

Medical centre
Equipment
Services offered
Stocks
Stationery
Medicine permit
Personal files
Registers
Computor software
Policy and procedure manual

5. IMPLEMENTATION

Announcement
Clinic hours
Health assessment
Health reviews
Primary healthcare
Emergency care
Health education
First-aid team
Administration

6. EVALUATION AND ADAPTATION

Feedback
Surveys
Audits
Reassessment
Adaptation to change

Figure 6.1 Procedure for the establishment of an occupational health service

- Advice about suitable personal protective equipment
- A part-time primary healthcare service for minor ailments
- Follow-up of injuries on duty.

This type of service increases the level of protection from the effects of hazardous procedures and saves production time by following up injuries and treating minor ailments. Depending on the company requirements, the service may be offered for a few hours once or twice a week. Legal compliance protects the company from prosecution.

3 Comprehensive occupational health service. At this level all aspects of healthcare are addressed and controlled, namely:
- Environmental monitoring of all workplace conditions including noise, dust, chemicals, lighting, temperature, ventilation and ergonomic factors and the effects of the company activity on the surrounding community
- Elimination, minimization and control of hazards with full participation of the workforce after education and training, as well as the provision of suitable personal protective equipment and enforcement of use
- Full health assessments of all employees, pre-placement and periodic, with biological monitoring and specific tests and reassessment after serious illnesses or accidents or before termination of service
- Holistic healthcare service with primary healthcare, emergency care, health education, counselling and rehabilitation
- Accurate record-keeping and reconciliation, including sick leave monitoring
- Rehabilitation after serious illness or injury and counselling for the troubled employee
- Research and epidemiological studies.

6.7 The implementation of the occupational health programme

A general announcement to all employees introducing the service, its functions and clinic times should be issued before the service commences. Basic health assessments for all employees starting with those at risk is the first priority.

In 1959 the International Labour Organization (ILO) defined an occupational health service as being established '... in or near a place of employment for the purpose of:
- Protecting workers against any health hazard that may arise out of their work or the conditions in which it is carried on
- Contributing towards workers' physical and mental adjustment in particular by adaptation of the work to the workers and their assignment to the jobs for which they are suited
- Contributing to the establishment and maintenance of the highest possible degree of physical and mental well-being of the workers' (Rantanen, 1990).

There are several ways in which the occupational health nurse can achieve these aims, and the clinical functions are discussed in detail in Chapter 7. Health promotion and health education programmes would be planned as a management function and are discussed in Chapter 8.

6.8 Control through administration and management

The occupational health nurse is fully responsible and accountable for the administration and management of the occupational health service. Medicolegal risks can be readily inferred from written records that are not clearly and accurately presented.

6.8.1 The policy and procedure manual

The policy and procedure manual is a valuable legal document. It is a management instrument which contains the scope of departmental responsibilities and a framework within which the health service objectives are implemented.

The policy and procedure manual aims to:
- Serve as a guide in decision-making
- Safeguard employees and health workers
- Direct, coordinate and 'articulate' the functions of the occupational health service
- Assure standardization and continuity of care and administration during staff changes.

Basic principles for the development of policies and procedures encompass the following:
- Policies must be in line with the philosophies, policies and nature of the specific company.
- Policies and procedures must be:
  - unambiguous, broad and durable for different circumstances
  - general enough not to need continual updating but only when changes are required
  - thought through very carefully by a policy committee who reviews all policies and develops new ones as changes in legislation or occupational health occur.
- All changes in policy must be communicated to the staff.
- Policies should guide the coordinators of the occupational health service for effective administration, uniformity and continuity of healthcare and standardization of methods.

The content of the manual is often on computer but the manual must also be physically available as a loose-leaf file in the occupational health centre for ease of use when a client, colleague or relief nurse requires information.

The policy and procedure contains the following:
  Title page with name of company and occupational health service set out neatly to attract the reader
  Foreword – an introduction to the company and its mission statement
  Table of contents arranged in sections with numbering that can accommodate

Occupational health

changes and additions and still allow for ease of reference
Introduction to the manual
Occupational health service philosophy statement
Company health policy and other company or specifically occupational health centre policies, e.g. the management of alcohol misuse, disability, HIV/Aids or life-threatening diseases, ethics policy, sexual harassment policy, etc.
Occupational health service objectives
Company organigram, including the occupational health team
Occupational health programme for current year
Sections, usually in alphabetical order to include, for example:
- Administration
- Budget and financial plan and control
- Community resources
- Conditions of service
- Disaster plan/evacuation
- Emergency procedures
- Employee assistance programme, counselling, rehabilitation
- Environmental monitoring and occupational hygiene
- First-aid teams, training, equipment
- Hazardous substances
- Health education/promotion
- Injuries on duty; job descriptions; legislation; medical protocol; medicine control; legislation
- Medical surveillance; biological monitoring; exit medical examination; periodic health reviews; pre-placement medical examination; special or transfer health reviews
- Nursing procedures
- Occupational diseases
- Research
- Safety and so on.

6.8.2 Administration of the occupational health service

The administration of the occupational health service needs to be kept up to date daily when information is fresh in the mind. Omissions occur when paperwork accumulates.

6.8.2.1 Occupational health records

Records and registers are legal documents. The information in these written accounts must be accurate, complete but concise, in chronological order and signed by the attending occupational health practitioner. Personal files are confidential and must be stored securely with the occupational health nurse and doctor having sole access.

Records are classified under the following headings:
Personal files. A file is opened for each employee on his/her appointment and contains all the health information under the following headings:

- Consultations are entered on a daily basis with the date, exact time, full details of the nature of the problem, findings and recommendations, signed by the attending person
- Health assessments from the first basic assessment, all periodic assessments are filed for comparison and detection of changes in the health status which will be followed up
- Injuries on duty and incidents are recorded with full details and all reports and correspondence with the Compensation Commissioner
- Laboratory and medical reports are kept in chronological order
- Sick leave records and certificates are kept for monitoring the person's health profile.

Statutory records. All registers, records and reports required by the different acts of legislation for medicine control, injuries on duty, calibration of equipment, inspection and environmental monitoring, etc. may be inspected at any time by officials from the Departments of Health, Labour or Mineral and Energy Affairs.

Service management. Files must be kept in the medical centre for:
- Policies, procedures and written protocol for diagnosis and treatment and emergency procedures
- Year plan and occupational health programmes for medical surveillance, health education, etc.
- Daily attendance in the clinic
- Monthly and annual reports, as well as special reports and memoranda
- Statistics of clinic attendance, medical surveillance tests, injuries, sickness absence rates, etc. are kept for inclusion in reports and research
- Medicine control, including purchasing orders, invoices, receipts and issue records and registers
- Injury on duty and occupational diseases register
- Financial planning and control of budget and expenditure
- Occupational health audits, quality control and programme evaluation reports
- Minutes of health and safety, occupational health team and departmental meetings
- Inventory of assets, equipment and stock
- Hazardous substances in use in the company and material safety data sheets and other relevant documents.

6.8.2.2 Computerization of records

Computer software for the administration of occupational health programmes is commercially available. Many companies with information systems developers have developed their own programmes. These programmes can store a vast amount of data and it is time saving and accurate to be able to extract statistics on clinic attendance, types of illnesses or injuries treated, number of referrals, costs, etc. for reports, epidemiological studies and research.

Programmes exist for health assessments, biological and environmental monitoring, audiometric, spirometric and vision screening, compensation commissioner reporting, etc. A reliable anti-viral computer program and a back-up system to secure information in the event of power failure or theft is required.

Information can be secured with a password and be rendered 'read only' and thus cannot be altered once entered.

Despite security measures it remains questionable whether these reports will be accepted as legal documents in any dispute and it is recommended that physical personal medical files containing original signed documents are available as a measure to control medicolegal risks. All records are stored for 40 years.

6.8.2.3 Statistics and reports

Meaningful statistics should be prepared from the clinic activities and presented at regular intervals to the company doctor and to management to inform them of the service activities, prevailing conditions, sick leave, absence rate, etc.

Daily reports are kept in the occupational health centre from which information for monthly reports can be drawn for the company doctor and management. Concise, meaningful facts, graphs and statistics are given but no confidential information. Special reports may be required on specific issues from time to time.

See Appendix 6.2. An example of a monthly or annual occupational health service report for the facts to be included in a monthly or an annual report on the activities of the Occupational Health Service.

6.8.2.4 Legislation

Applicable acts of legislation as described in Chapter 2 must be on hand in the occupational health centre and the nurse must know what applies to the service, and have a system whereby he/she keeps up to date with changes in legislation and new regulations.

6.8.2.5 Medicine control

The Medicines and Related Substances Control Act, 1965 (No 101 of 1965) makes provision for Companies to buy, store or dispense medicines in their occupational health centres subject to certain conditions set out in section 22 A (12) of the Act (at the time of publication).

In order to buy, store or dispense any medicines in an occupational health centre, the company must apply for and be in possession of a valid medicine permit which is displayed in the centre.

The occupational health nurse may initiate the process and obtain the necessary application forms from the Pharmaceutical Services department at the Department of Health. The manager of the company and the company doctor sign the application.
A permit can only be issued once the Pharmaceutical Services department has inspected the service. The permit number must be quoted on all orders for medicines. Strict adherence to the regulations is required:
- The company must appoint a doctor who visits the clinic regularly, provides effective supervision and takes full responsibility.
- The company must employ a registered nurse who is responsible for the clinic service rendered and has completed a pharmacology course.

- The company must inform the department of any changes in the particulars given in the original application. The names of health professionals, the company and its address must be correct for the permit to be valid.
- Medicines must be securely stored under the correct conditions and strictly controlled.
- Pharmaceutical regulations apply to the ordering and storing of medicine, issuing with correct labels and control. Medicines must be issued free of charge.
- Only medicines on the prescribed essential drug list may be used unless specific motivation from the company doctor for an unlisted item is approved.

The occupational health nurse requires pharmacology training for nurses in order to understand drug interaction and reactions, safe storage and dispensing of medicines.

6.8.2.6 Sickness absence monitoring

All doctor's certificates and sickness absence forms should be routed to the occupational health centre where the occupational health nurse integrates the information with clinic records so that a health profile can be built up for each employee. Serious illness, major surgery and irregularities are discussed with the employee concerned.

Sickness absence trends can be followed for the individual, a department or the company as a whole.

$$\text{Sickness absence rate} = \frac{\text{Number of sickness absence days} \times 100}{\text{No of employees} \times \text{No of working days}}$$

6.8.2.7 Financial costs management

The budget is a financial control system and can be defined as a tool for planning, monitoring and controlling costs. It includes two types of expenditure:

1 Operating expenditure. This is expenditure as in monthly operating expenditure which includes salaries, medicines, medical stock, education, injuries-on-duty costs, stationery and printing, and in some companies rent, telephone, electricity, etc.

2 Capital for major purchases of assets, equipment or building alterations, etc. The source of the finance is usually the company budget and it needs to be planned for and strictly controlled as a short-term plan for the next financial year or as a long-term (2–5 years) plan.

The occupational health nurse will need to plan ahead carefully and motivate enthusiastically for the financial resources required to render quality occupational healthcare. It is advised that the new occupational health practitioner consults with the financial manager at an early stage to discuss the costs of quality healthcare.

6.8.2.8 Quality assurance in the occupational health service

Quality assurance is the monitoring of the activities of client care to determine the degree of excellence attained, and the effectiveness and efficiency of the occupational health service. Quality assurance activities assist the professional nurse in self-regulation and accountability for the nursing practice.

Practical changes to the service are essential as it grows and expands or when critical reviews identify a shortcoming.

The occupational health service should be audited annually for quality care, cost-effectiveness and legal compliance. Quality assurance programmes include standards and criteria against which the service is evaluated, and improvement or adaptation to address identified shortcomings is vital.

Objective and systematic evaluation of the occupational health service and adaptation to address developments in technology, medicine, knowledge, legislation, the company and the healthcare needs of the clients is the main process in quality assurance.

The quality assurance programme commences with the planning of the occupational health service and the drawing up of a healthcare philosophy and a health policy to address the health needs of both the company and its employees. The Policy and Procedure Manual for the Service is a framework containing the goals and objectives for the service and the standards and evaluating elements such as structural, process and outcome elements.

Structural elements include the available resources or structures:
- The physical setting of the medical centre
- The philosophy of health by management, the employees and the healthcare professionals
- The organizational structure and its mission
- The occupational health service goals and objectives
- Resources – human, financial, facilities and operational resources.

Process elements include the actions that are taken, such as:
- The management of the health service
- Decision-making processes and collaboration with occupational health team
- Nursing intervention and medical surveillance
- Other programmes, such as health education, health and safety inspections
- Written reports and updated records.

Outcome elements are the results of the process:
- Legal compliance by the company and health service
- Improved health, well-being and morale of the employees
- Reduced sick leave, morbidity, injuries and deviations from health
- Greater responsibility for own health and safety accepted by employees
- Feedback from management, employees and other health agencies.

The quality assurance process includes:
- Identifying values that are required in quality programmes
- Identifying standards and criteria that indicate quality
- Setting measurements for evaluation
- Measuring each standard and allocating points
- Deciding on the course of action/correction to be taken or adaptation to be made.

The advantages of quality management in the occupational health service include:
- Increased quality of care and of management in the occupational health service
- Ownership of the effectiveness and efficiency of the service
- Increased productivity and time-saving
- Improved cost-effectiveness
- Improved morale and confidence
- Management approval and respect.

The various strategies and methods of monitoring the quality of the service include:
- Self-evaluation of compliance with standards for each aspect of the service
- Self-judgement to evaluate own level of competence and whether set goals and objectives are achieved
- Peer evaluation where colleagues with the same knowledge and competence evaluate the work performance of another
- Feedback from management and clients
- Document (policy and procedure manual, client files) evaluation for accuracy and completeness
- Internal or external audits
- Risk identification and management where health risks are identified, evaluated and addressed through mitigation and safe work procedures and monitored through medical surveillance.

Setting and maintaining high standards in occupational health nursing in general is being addressed through professional bodies and credentialling and the setting of standard procedures is in the process of being developed.

See Appendix 6.3. An example of an Occupational Health Service Audit Document – it is not the same as an Occupational Health Programme Audit.

6.9 Epidemiology and research orientation

Epidemiology is defined as the study of the distribution and determinants of diseases and injuries in human populations (Mausner & Kramer, 1985:1). The occupational health nurse is well positioned to study the records and identify employee populations with similar health deviations.

Research can be done to find links between health factors and occupational exposure or population groups. Screening for evidence of non-occupational disease gives the occupational health nurse the opportunity to do meaningful surveys. Refer to Chapter 10 for details of this important element.

6.10 Benefits of an occupational health service
A comprehensive occupational health programme pays dividends by:
- Ensuring a safe work environment, thereby reducing risks to health and production and profits
- Monitoring staff health on an ongoing basis – a healthy employee is a productive employee
- Promoting and maintaining the health of all employees and improving quality of life and reducing days lost due to illness
- Facilitating pre-placement health assessments in order that prospective employees are placed in positions suited to their physical capabilities
- Offering specialized health education
- Communicating to motivate the promotion of health to all role players
- Monitoring sick leave to benefit both the employer and the employee.

6.11 Practical assignment
As a qualified occupational health practitioner you have been invited to develop an occupational health programme for a new milk products factory employing 200 unskilled workers in a remote area. Key points to address would be:
- Workplace walk-through and health-risk identification in a food industry – chemicals, machines, noise, biological, etc.
- Applicable legislation
- Workforce size, gender, age, range, educational level, healthcare needs
- Development of a health policy, medical surveillance, induction, health education and health promotion programmes
- Assessment of the safety, risk and occupational health personnel required or available
- Design and budget for a medical centre, equipment and services in a remote area – short term and long term
- Planning for the training of first-aiders, health and safety representatives and meetings.

6.12 Conclusion
The ultimate aim or goal of a successful occupational health service is to address all aspects of occupational health, but the establishment of a comprehensive service takes time. Familiarity with the aims and functions of the employing organization and with the people employed is essential basic knowledge which every occupational health nurse requires. It is unwise to implement rapid changes before the nurse is accepted as part of the organization by management and the workforce.

6.13 Bibliography
Acutt, J. 1996. The policy and procedure manual in an occupational health service. *Occupational Health Southern Africa*, 2 (4), 22–23.

Booyens, S. W. (ed.) 1996. *Introduction to Health Services Management.* Cape Town: Juta.
Guild, R., Ehrlich, R. I., Johnston, J. R., Ross, M. H. 2001. *Handbook of Occupational Health Practice in the South African Mining Industry.* Johannesburg: SIMRAC.
International Commission on Occupational Health. 1996. International Code of Ethics for Occupational Health Professionals. Singapore: I.C.O.H.
Mausner, J. S. & Kramer, S. 1985. *Epidemiology. An Introductory Text.* Philadelphia: WB Saunders.
Muller, M. M. 2002. *Nursing Dynamics.* 3rd edition. Johannesburg: Heinemann Publishers.
Rantanen, J. (ed.) 1990. Occupational Health Services – An overview. European Series No.26. Geneva: WHO.
Rogers, B. 1994. *Occupational Health Nursing. Concepts and Practice.* Philadelphia: WB Saunders.
Searle, C. & Pera, S. A. 1995. *Professional Practice. A South African Nursing Perspective.* 3rd edition. Durban: Butterworths.
Yoder Wise, P. S. 1995. *Leading and Managing in Nursing.* St Louis: Mosby.

7 Clinical occupational healthcare

J. Acutt

7.1 Introduction

The Nursing Act, 1978 (No 50 of 1978), as amended, governs nursing practice in South Africa. In terms of this Act a professional nurse must register with the South African Nursing Council in order to practise within the scope as laid down. The Act also states that the knowledge and skills required to practise must be kept up to date. Clinical skills are those of observation and treatment of patients. Many occupational health practitioners work alone and as the sole provider of healthcare at the workplace need to evaluate their own clinical performance objectively and arrange for continuous up-dating of knowledge and skills.

Occupational health nursing is a specialty practice that makes provision for and delivers varied healthcare services to companies and their employees. In terms of the World Health Organization definition of occupational health, this practice focuses on promotion, protection and restoration of health of all employees in a safe and healthy work environment.

The term occupational health practitioner implies a person qualified in medicine or nursing who holds an additional qualification in occupational health as recognized by the South African Medical Council or the South African Nursing Council. Occupational health professional has the same meaning.

This chapter presents a framework for the clinical occupational care required to protect and promote the health of all employees through prevention and treatment of illness and injury, medical surveillance, education and counselling.

7.2 Learning objectives

> At the end of this chapter, the reader should be able to:
> - At the end of this chapter, the reader should be able to:
> - Define clinical occupational health nursing
> - Describe the health assessment process
> - Describe the special tests required in medical surveillance
> - Describe primary healthcare in industry
> - Describe protocol required for acute and chronic illnesses and injury
> - Identify vulnerable employees and address their needs
> - Apply the nursing process in occupational health nursing.

7.3 The occupational health nursing practitioner

In 1959 the International Labour Organization (ILO) defined an occupational health service as being established '... in or near a place of employment for the purpose of:
- Protecting workers against any health hazard that may arise out of their work or the conditions in which it is carried out
- Contributing towards workers' physical and mental adjustment, in particular by adaptation of the work to the workers and their assignment to the jobs for which they are suited
- Contributing to the establishment and maintenance of the highest possible degree of physical and mental well-being of the workers' (ILO, 1959).

A registered professional nurse with the postgraduate qualification in occupational health nursing has specialized knowledge and skills to carry out these aims of protecting and promoting the health of employees at the workplace.

The occupational health nurse functions independently, making autonomous decisions after analysing data gathered from clients, the work environment, and members of the occupational health team. He/she is professional, responsible and reliable – trusted by the employees and management to provide quality nursing care.

7.3.1 Basic nursing training and experience

This highly specialized field requires experience in general nursing, primary healthcare, occupational health nursing, emergency and trauma care, toxicology, pharmacology, social and behavioural sciences, environmental hygiene, ethical conduct and legal compliance, for effective healthcare at the workplace.

7.3.2 Responsibilities of the occupational health nursing practitioner

The occupational health nursing practitioner has a responsibility towards the employees, the employer and the members of the occupation health team to provide quality clinical care according to the requirements set out in a company's health policy. The health risks on site must be addressed in the nursing practitioner's job description as a guide towards quality care.

To achieve this requirement the company must provide the means to address quality clinical care, including:
- A suitable venue – secure, clean, in good repair, affording privacy and free of health risks
- The necessary equipment to perform health assessment and special tests
- Furniture, secure cabinets for files, medicines and stocks
- Electricity, telephone, Internet connection, running water, toilets, etc.

The occupational health practitioner is dependent upon the law that authorizes him/her to practise and acts interdependently with other members of the occupational health team.

Nursing practitioners accept responsibility for the manner in which they execute their duties, are totally responsible and accountable for their own actions and are aware of the extent of their knowledge, skills, abilities and limitations in the performance of occupational healthcare duties. The employee, employer and the members of the occupational health team can expect the occupational health nurse to be competent and reliable, carrying out his/her duties with accuracy and skill.

However, an occupational health nurse may refuse to carry out instructions in the case of an illegal act, over-prescription, inaccurate prescription, contravention of the policy of the organization or of the employees' wishes, or anything beyond his/her competence (Rogers, 1994).

7.4 Clinical functions of an occupational health nurse

The clinical function of the occupational health nurse includes all interaction with the patient as in interviewing, assessing, examining, testing of functions, treating, communication, teaching, counselling, decision-making and implementation of health interventions and recording of all these actions.

7.4.1 Clinical nursing guidelines and protocols

Healthcare must be standardized for quality and consistency to achieve a goal-directed outcome. Occupational health nurses will refer to the prescribed protocol and as independent practitioners, make their own observations of each individual client's response during medical surveillance or nursing care. These observations must be accurately documented in the client's file.

7.4.2 Health assessments and medical surveillance

Medical surveillance is the periodic health examination and special tests performed by a qualified occupational health practitioner as defined in the Occupational Health and Safety Act, 1993 (No 85 of 1993). It is a control mechanism in the programme to protect a worker's health and prevent deviations from health due to workplace hazards. Health assessments are not only performed to exclude disease but also to ascertain the ability of each person to perform their jobs and meet their obligations in life.

To ensure that all employees are both healthy and suitable for the work that they are required to perform, the examiner must have a comprehensive knowledge of the work process, the various hazards that they will be exposed to and their effects, as well as the statutory requirements for control of the hazards and the company policy. The following has a bearing on the health assessment:

Legal requirement. A medical surveillance programme is a legal requirement whenever an individual is exposed to health risks at work, in terms of the Occupational Health and Safety Act, 1993 (No 85 of 1993) and the Mine Health and Safety Act, 1996 (No 29 of 1996). However, it must be remembered that it is an offence to discriminate against an employee, or a prospective employee, on the basis of health in terms of the Employment Equity Act, 1998 (No 55 of 1998). This act specifically states in section 8, 'Psychological testing and other similar assessments of an employee are prohibited unless the test or assessment being used –

(a) has been scientifically shown to be valid and reliable;
(b) can be applied fairly to all employees; and
(c) is not biased against any employee or group.'

It is therefore imperative that the occupational health practitioner explains the medical surveillance procedure in relation to the nature of the work and the possible effects of hazard exposure.

Man–job specification. The man–job specification is a guiding document for the physical attributes required to prevent risks to health in a specific job. The specification may be in the form of a check-list, which includes working environment factors, physical requirements, protective equipment requirements and conditions excluded from the task. (See Appendix 7.1.) It is drawn up by human resources and line management with input from the occupational health risk assessment team for each task that exists in the company, to match each incumbent with the physical requirements for the job.

The placement of an employee in a specific job depends on the results of the health assessment and recommendation made by the occupational health practitioner in terms of the man–job specification. (See Table 7.1.).

Establishing rapport. A relaxed, secure approach by the health professional generates similar feelings in the client and influences the quality of the relationship between the health professional and the client, whose cooperation is required in the medical surveillance programme for years to come. The nurse builds a positive relationship with tact and diplomacy. The reason for the assessment and an explanation of all procedures and the results are human rights, as well as a legal requirement in terms of the Occupational Health and Safety Act, 1993 (No 85 of 1993) and the Mine Health and Safety Act, 1996 (No 29 of 1996).

Observation and communication. The assessment starts when the nurse approaches the client and observes his/her attitude and response to the greeting. Communication is at adult level and verbal and non-verbal responses are noted. Note is taken of personal hygiene, nutritional state, scars, gait or limp and anything unusual, especially in the reply to an enquiry after the client's well-being.

History-taking. An accurate and complete medical, family, social habits, occupational and hazard exposure history is taken at the baseline interview. It is most important that this is truthful and complete and time must be taken to be accurate in recording the facts. The medical history form is a legal document and signed by the client and the nurse. Facts may be required at a later stage when investigating an accident or illness – especially as it may be work related.

General health assessment. The clinical assessment follows the history-taking and a specific routine is followed in order that no aspect is overlooked:
- Blood pressure is taken when the client is at rest.

- Temperature is taken and recorded.
- Respirations are counted and recorded.
- Pulse is counted at rest and again after ten brisk genu-flexions and two minutes later at rest to ascertain a degree of cardiovascular fitness – note is made of the number of beats per minute, the volume, rate and rhythm of the pulse and any discomfort experienced by the client.
- Urine is tested for protein, glucose, ketones and pH and whatever else may be important.
- A basic health examination from head to toe is undertaken, taking special note of skin, scars and chest/lung conditions.
- Special attention is paid to bodily systems that may be affected by workplace hazards, e.g. chrome may cause ulceration of the nasal septum and epistaxis or mercury may cause stomatitis, tremor and erethism.
- All findings are recorded accurately and not just as 'normal' or 'no appreciable disease' (NAD). Thus the temperature is recorded as 37 degrees Centigrade and not as 'normal'.
- Findings are communicated to the client and the implications explained if necessary.

Special tests, such as spirometric, audiometric, vision screening and biological monitoring are discussed in detail in section 7.5 below.

Pre-placement medical examinations. These examinations are also known as the baseline medical examination. It is of the utmost importance that the examination is accurate and complete as all future assessments are compared with or measured against the 'baseline' to detect deterioration and deviations.

This examination should be performed before an applicant is appointed and placed in a job, in order to prevent costly, time-consuming and often unpleasant consequences if the person is found to be unsuitable after commencing work and needs to be moved.

All information is confidential and the occupational health nurse keeps the record. An indication of an applicant's suitability for the specific job is the only information passed on to the employing officer, in the form of an employment category. See Table 7.1. for an example of a form that may be used. Category C is allocated when the applicant may be reconsidered after undergoing treatment to stabilize a health problem and it is for the employing officer to decide whether the position needs to be filled urgently or can wait a month. No further details are given and the occupational health practitioner's professional opinion must be respected.

Periodic and additional medical examinations. The periodic medical examination is a full medical examination performed every six to twelve months according to a medical surveillance programme for the specific health risks the employee is exposed to. Should exposure limits or exposure duration increase or the test results show deterioration, the periodic medical examination will be repeated more frequently. Additional medical examinations are required:
- After a serious illness or injury
- After chemical spills and accidental exposure

Table 7.1 Example of employment category based on health assessment

Description of employability	Category	Result
Fit for any position	A	
Fit only for position applied for	B	
For re-assessment in one month	C	
Unfit for work	D	
Examiner:	Date:	

- When the production process increases, changing the level or duration of exposure
- When a person is to be transferred to another department with different hazards or exposure levels.

Ideally, all employees will be screened periodically to detect early signs of disease or defects. The procedure, its reasons and results should be discussed with each individual and should be confidential unless the employee gives written consent for the information to be passed on to management, when a less strenuous job is required for a medical reason, for instance. Any adverse findings must be acted on in the appropriate manner.

By law, employees exposed to hazards such as noise, lead or radiation must be screened regularly, using specific tests and biological monitoring to protect their health. Apprentices, public vehicle drivers, airline pilots and food handlers require health assessments in terms of different acts of legislation.

The occupational health nurse has first-hand knowledge of the state of health of each employee and should be consulted when promotions of transfers are being considered. This would help avoid potential risks, e.g. an employee with a cardiac condition or a psychological problem being placed in a stressful work environment. It is not for the occupational health nurse to interfere with promotion or transfers but to advise the employee and management if there are health risks, whilst maintaining confidentiality of health information. A full medical examination should be done and the results explained to the employee in terms of the man–job specification for the post.

Whenever deviations are found the tests are repeated a few days later and if they show a deterioration, the person may need to be removed from exposure to hazards in his/her work area. There must be a company policy in place for this recommendation from the occupational health practitioner – an employee may resent the transfer as it may influence his/her earnings or perceived status and be stressful to adjust to new duties, colleagues and surroundings. Like all policies, this policy is drawn up with worker representatives in the interest of health for all employees. Multiskilling is an advantage for the employee and the company to cope with this kind of situation.

Exit medical examinations. These examinations are a legal requirement in the mining industry in terms of the Mine Health and Safety Act, 1996 (No 29 of 1996). It makes good business sense to perform this final medical examination and special tests before an employee leaves the company. Employees are given a written medical report of their health status which they may want to show to their next employer. The medical examination is documented to safeguard the company against future claims and is stored for 40 years. (See Appendix 7.2. An example of an exit medical examination form.)

Statutory medical examinations. Apart from the Occupational Health and Safety Act, 1993 (No 85 of 1993) and the Mine Health and Safety Act, 1996 (No 29 of 1996) which prescribe medical surveillance to protect the worker, there are several other Acts of legislation that require medical examinations for certain categories of personnel to protect the public and the employee. These include:

- The National Road Traffic Act, 1996 (No 93 of 1996) for heavy-duty vehicle and public transport drivers
- The Civil Aviation Authority Act, 1998 (No 40 of 1998) for air pilots
- The Manpower Training Act, 1981 (No 56 of 1981) for apprentices
- The Nuclear Energy Act, 1999 (No 46 of 1999) for persons exposed to radiation, and various local government regulations for food handlers.

7.5 Specific occupational health screening tests

7.5.1 Biological monitoring

The Occupational Health and Safety Act, 1993 (No 85 of 1993), defines biological monitoring as 'a planned programme of periodic collection and analysis of body fluid, tissues, excreta or exhaled air to detect and quantify the exposure to, or absorption of, any substance or organism by persons'. It follows then that the health risks of potentially toxic substances can be defined before measures are taken to minimize them in terms of occupational hygiene measures.

Biological monitoring has as its primary objective the prevention of human exposure to potentially toxic chemical substances used in industrial processes. It measures the toxic substance in blood or urine or the biological markers of disease in blood or urine to give an indication of damage to organs in the body.

Sample collection is specific in respect of the timing (before, during and after a shift), precautions that need to be taken during the collection and with storage and transport, and is done after consultation with the pathological laboratory concerned. The pathological laboratories often prefer to come on site at regular intervals to collect the samples from the employees.

The occupational health practitioner plans the programme, explains the procedure to the employee and obtains his/her written consent to the test. The results from the laboratory are discussed with the employee and recorded on the client's file before referring him/her to the company doctor for his/her medical examination. Results are not given to anyone without the employee's written consent. Only statistics may be reported to the occupational health team and management.

7.5.2 Spirometric testing

This test is also known as lung function testing to assess the effect of airborne pollutants such as dust, fumes, vapours, smoke and gases on the lungs. The test consists of maximum inhalational and expirational manoeuvres for the measurement of Forced Vital Capacity (FVC), Peak Expiratory Flow (PEF) and Forced Expiratory Volume in one second (FEV1) and is performed on a spirometer.

Quality control of spirometry is essential to produce valid, meaningful results. Accuracy and repeatability of the curves are of the utmost importance and are affected by the equipment used, the tester and the action of the person being tested:

- The equipment – several spirometers are available commercially and it is imperative to use one that is set according to American Thoracic Society (ATS) standards. The spirometer needs to be calibrated with a 3-litre syringe at different rates daily, on relocation of mobile equipment or 4-hourly should several tests be performed on the same day.
- The tester requires an accredited course in spirometry to ensure competency. Instructions from the supplier will not suffice.
- The person being tested needs to understand the test and cooperate with the instructions given.

The following procedure must be followed when performing the spirometric test:
- Check the spirometer for correct assembly and calibrate.
- Explain the test to the person and reassure him/her.
- Instruct and demonstrate the test by:
  - standing or sitting upright with the neck straight and looking ahead
  - inhaling completely
  - attaching the nose clip, positioning mouthpiece and closing the lips around it
  - exhaling with maximum force and continuing until the lungs are empty.
- Demonstrate and coach the person while he/she is performing the manoeuvre.
- The person being tested must repeat the manoeuvres at least three times and maximally eight times.
- The test is acceptable only if volume-time and corresponding flow curve meets prescribed criteria. (See the next section on spirometric test acceptability and reproducibility.)
- The whole procedure is repeated at a later stage if the tests were not acceptable.

Spirometric test acceptability and reproducibility. It is critical that spirometric tests comply with international standards as the results are referred to every year when deviation from the previous tests are looked for. The occupational health practitioner must be qualified to obtain acceptable and reproducible curves from the employee who cooperates with enthusiasm.

1 **Acceptability**. The criteria for an acceptable spirogram or curve includes:
  - A satisfactory start of test is necessary with an extrapolated volume of less than 5 per cent of the Forced Vital Capacity (FVC) or 0.15 litre, whichever is greater on the curve.

Occupational health

- Peak expiratory flow (PEF) should be reached within the first 15 per cent of the FVC.
- The spirogram (curve) must be free from artifacts such as a cough, glottis closure, a hesitation in expiration or early termination of exhalation.
- The technician must observe for air leaks around the mouthpiece or an obstructed mouthpiece.
- The minimum Forced Vital Capacity (FVC) exhalation time of six seconds is shown on the curve.
- The curve meets the zero axis showing complete exhalation at the end of the test.

These are some of the more obvious criteria that one can identify on a spirogram or curve as the employee performs the test. Spirograms that do not meet the criteria are rejected and the acceptable curves are stored for reproducibility evaluation at the end of the session.

2 Reproducibility. The reproducibility of spirograms indicates that at least three of the individual tests in one session are similar, according to the following criteria:
- Check for three acceptable curves and check if the two largest Forced Vital Capacities (FVC) readings are less than 0.2 litres (200 millilitres) apart.
- Check also if the two largest Forced Expiratory Volumes in one second (FEV1) are less than 0.2 litres (200 millilitres) apart.
- If above criteria are met, i.e. three acceptable curves; FVC curves less than 0.2 litres apart; FEV1 curves less than 0.2 litres apart, conclude the test session.
- If the criteria are not met, continue testing until the criteria are met. The session is concluded after eight spirogram attempts maximum or if the person is tired. Another session must be arranged for a week later.
- Save a minimum of the three best manoeuvres.

7.5.3 Audiometric testing

Audiometric testing for the hearing acuity of employees exposed to noise levels above 85 decibels are screening tests. A five-day course at a training centre accredited with the Department of Labour must be attended before successful candidates may apply for registration as audiometric screening technicians.

Quality control in audiometry is crucial to detect early signs of noise-induced hearing loss. All tests are compared with the baseline or first test performed for an employee to detect deterioration. The quality of tests is controlled through the Code of Practice for the measurement and assessment of occupational noise for hearing conservation purposes as set out in the South African Bureau of Standards Code 083 of 1996 (SABS 083). This document also sets out standards for the calibration of equipment, test conditions and audiometry:
- Calibration of the soundproof booth and the audiometer must be done at least annually or whenever it has been moved, by a technician who is accredited by the Department of Labour.
- Biological calibration of the audiometer by the tester using him-/herself as the subject at least once a week.
- Test conditions require that the subject has not been exposed to noise above

80 decibels for at least 16 hours prior to the test. Another condition is a quiet area with no distractions such as people walking past the audiometric booth window.
- Before placing the employee in the soundproof booth the occupational health nurse would enquire about possible ear problems, upper respiratory tract conditions and working conditions that may influence the outcome of the test. A thorough otoscopic examination of both ears is done to exclude conditions, such as excessive cerumen or scar tissue, that may influence hearing.
- The occupational health nurse will explain the procedure and give careful instructions to the person as to what to listen for and how to indicate that the tone is heard.
- If satisfied that the employee understands the procedure, the nurse positions the ear phones correctly.
- The test is commenced and the nurse subtly observes the test performance without distracting the employee. Body language displayed may indicate hesitation and loss of concentration.
- The test is interrupted and tactful instruction is reinforced should inconsistencies occur during the test.
- On completion of the test the results are printed and discussed with the employee.

The results are explained and compared with previous results together with the employee and if accepted he/she and the occupational health nurse sign on the form. Results are filed in the person's medical file and only revealed to the company physician if the employee has given written consent to inform his/her supervisor. It is necessary to discuss hearing deterioration due to high noise levels with the supervisor before an investigation of noise levels in the area where the employee is exposed can take place. Consent to reveal test results is also required where the employee needs to be removed from the noise. It is the occupational health nurse's duty to persuade the employee that it is in his/her own best interest to be moved.

Hearing loss is calculated in terms of Regulation 171 of the Compensation for Occupational Injuries and Diseases Act, 1993 (No 130 of 1993) and the employee is referred to an Audiologist for diagnostic audiometry. If noise-induced hearing loss is diagnosed a claim for compensation is lodged with the Compensation Commissioner. See also Chapter 4.

7.5.4 Vision screening

Vision is one of the senses that deteriorate in many cases as a person ages. Advanced equipment is readily available to test vision accurately. It is the occupational health practitioner's responsibility to learn to use the equipment to get quality tests, and to explain the tests and the implication of the results to the employee.

Certain categories of workers require acuity, perception, distance, colour and vision field screening to be able to perform their duties without endangering themselves, their clients and the public at large. Others require vision tests to determine negative effects of exposure to damaging light or rays. There needs to be a company policy as regards vision correction and the costs involved.

7.6 Primary monitoring to identify unrecognized hazards

Conventionally, this term includes the discovery of new hazards by chemical analogy, evaluation of routine measurements or by epidemiological survey. Occupational health nurses render primary healthcare and have a vital role to play in primary monitoring. They are in close contact with the workers and therefore have the ideal opportunity to observe, record and interpret health changes. By referring to records, an unusual prevalence of certain conditions or injuries in specific work areas can be ascertained and must be investigated.

Regular visits to the work areas enable a nurse to establish a correlation between the environment, the worker and his/her health. Continuous surveillance of the work area and contact with management and workers will help to recognize new hazards. This facilitates the early detection of deviations from normal health.

The occupational health nurse must be informed of proposed new machinery or altered processes or facilities for his/her input on unrecognized hazards.

7.7 Providing a treatment service

Occupational health nurses must have the clinical skills to assess any health situation and to treat or refer to a suitable outside agency and then to follow up. Effective coordination of client care requires previous liaison with emergency services, clinics, specialists and other health services.

Observation of the work methods, substances in use and factors affecting health, including the employees, family and social background, is vital for an effective treatment service.

It is imperative that the standard of treatment given by the occupational health service is maintained at a consistently high level and therefore the occupational health nurse's knowledge and skills must remain updated.

Procedures and protocol for all conditions should be drawn up and regularly updated by the occupational health nurse together with the medical officer in charge who must sign that the protocol is acceptable.

In South Africa, occupational health nurses offer a primary health service, which includes the treatment of minor ailments, supervision of chronic conditions, antenatal and postnatal maternal care, family planning and health education. This should not take up more than 20 per cent of their time, as occupational healthcare and medical surveillance is their most important responsibility.

7.7.1 Primary healthcare

Primary healthcare can be defined as: Essential healthcare that is acceptable, accessible and affordable to the community and open to participation of the individuals and healthcare workers. The same definition can be applied in industry where the occupational health nurse must provide an acceptable and accessible health service to the workforce community. In order to be acceptable, the employees must participate and their health needs addressed. The company bears the costs.

Primary healthcare components include:
- Health education
- Diagnosis and basic treatment of common diseases and injuries
- Provision of essential medicines
- Promotion of adequate nutrition
- Basic water and sanitation
- Maternal and child health
- Family planning
- Immunization
- Prevention and control of local endemic diseases.

Primary healthcare in an occupational health service includes all the above through:
- Early identification of disease in the primary health clinic or during medical surveillance
- Treatment for acute and chronic conditions such as hypertension, diabetes, epilepsy, etc. where control of the disease renders the employee fit to cope with his/her daily work
- Emergency treatment for injuries and medical emergencies
- Health education on a large variety of requested, or topical, subjects. Employees must be encouraged to accept responsibility for their own health and that of their families
- Service to vulnerable groups including ante- and post-natal services, adolescent health, chronic diseases, family planning services, etc.
- Counselling of troubled persons and rehabilitation after accidents and serious illness
- Control of the environment and provision of clean water and sanitation at work
- Correct placement of employees in jobs suited to their capacity improves self-esteem as the worker advances in a chosen field of work
- Medical surveillance for both occupational and general health
- Record-keeping of all health issues and epidemiological studies to enhance health and well-being.

Primary healthcare at work benefits both the employee and the employer through:
- Optimal physical, mental and social well-being of all individuals in the company
- Improved quality of life for all recipients
- Improved morale, productivity, job performance and job satisfaction with a resultant decrease in absenteeism, accidents and the costs involved, job dissatisfaction and malingering.

7.7.2 Approach to selected common conditions in primary healthcare

It is imperative that there are protocols for the more common or sensitive conditions in the occupational primary health clinic. Occupational health nurses require specific training and updating of knowledge to cope with the new treatments and management of conditions such as alcohol abuse, diabetes, HIV/Aids, hypertension, stress-related syndromes, sexually transmitted infections, tuberculosis, etc.

The nurse's approach should always be to:
- Provide an accessible, user-friendly service
- Have good positive communication skills
- Provide privacy for the client
- Foster mutual respect and client trust
- Obtain a full history including risk factors present
- Observe carefully and conduct a full physical examination
- Educate about the condition and to counsel in order that the employee can make choices
- Explain the effect of the treatment and that the course must be completed even though improvement occurs after two days
- Refer and arrange for treatment or to the employee-asssitance programme if necessary
- Give a follow-up date and ongoing support
- Accurately record all the facts of the consultation and intervention.

7.8 Emergency care and first aid

The occupational health nurse will have a written protocol from the company medical officer to follow in the case of each type of medical emergency. Emergency drugs and equipment are checked every day for accessibility and validity.

The occupational health nurse will train first-aid team members to assist him/her in emergencies. Emergency procedures will be practised regularly and knowledge and skills updated. Liaison with local emergency services is ongoing.

Emergencies as a result of medical conditions are less frequent if there is an efficient health service at the workplace. Pre-placement and periodic medical examinations highlight medical conditions, ensure early advice and treatment and the condition can be controlled by regular follow-up by the occupational health nurse.

A register must be kept of all known epileptics, diabetics, hypertensives, asthmatics and even those with tuberculosis and other health problems. Treatment in an emergency would be discussed with the company doctor and protocol drawn up for specific emergencies, including medication to be given in the case of cardiac arrest and anaphylactic shock. (See Chapter 9, section 9.14.17 for the management of medical emergencies including cardiac arrest and cardiopulmonary resuscitation.)

Anaphylactic shock. Anaphylactic shock is a massive allergic reaction that may be fatal within minutes and should be prevented at all costs. See also Chapter 9, section 9.14.4.

Prevention starts with good history-taking at the pre-placement medical examination and health education of the worker to emphasize the importance of reporting allergies and good record-keeping of possible signs and symptoms of previous reactions. Before administering any medication the patient should be informed as to what he/she is getting and asked if he/she is aware of any allergy to the drug, or any other substance for that matter. Skin tests before administration may prevent, but have been known to cause, a major reaction. Anaphylaxis is commonly caused by parenteral administration of a drug, serum, vaccine or venom (e.g. bee sting) to which the patient has been previously sensitized.

The first signs and symptoms include the patien's statement that he/she feels strange, perhaps with a tingling scalp or a thick tongue. He/she is apprehensive and may look flushed or have an itchy rash or paresthesia. A tight feeling in the chest, wheezing respiration, fast thready pulse, a fall in blood pressure is soon followed by laryngeal oedema, bronchospasm, unconsciousness, vascular collapse and death.

The prescribed course of drugs in the medical protocol could include an antihistamine, adrenaline, hydrocortisone and aminophyllin. These drugs are given under specific circumstances, in specific doses either intramuscularly or intravenously according to the emergency protocol and should be readily available. Also readily available in the same emergency kit are syringes, swabs and files, butterfly needles, intravenous infusions and administration sets and oxygen in a pack that can be grabbed and taken to the patient should an emergency call come through.

The patient is put into the shock position, is reassured, kept warm and given oxygen whilst being closely monitored for bronchospasm, fall in blood pressure and significant changes in the pulse rate. An open airway and an open intravenous line should be maintained while the company doctor is sent for (if he/she is on the premises or nearby), as well as an ambulance to transport the patient to the nearest casualty department. It is vitally important that the occupational health nurse clarifies the desired treatment with his/her medical officer on the first day that they work together and that he/she keeps the 'anaphylactic kit' instantly available.

7.9 Injuries on duty and occupational diseases

An injury on duty is taken to mean a personal injury sustained in an accident occurring during the performance of an employee's work. An occupational disease is like any other disease, with the distinction that it was caused solely or principally by factors peculiar to the working environment. The actual manifestation may only arise later. It is also described as a disease arising out of and contracted in the course of an employee's employment and listed in Schedule 3 of the Compensation for Occupational Injuries and Diseases Act, 1993 (No 130 of 1993). (Refer to Chapter 2.) An injury must be treated immediately, and if serious, referred to a doctor or hospital. An occupational disease is treated as soon as signs are seen or symptoms arise and also referred for the best treatment. Both must be reported to the Compensation Commissioner as described in Chapter 2, section 2.10.5. The accident or exposure must be investigated and remedial measures instituted to prevent similar accidents and incidents. Ongoing education of management and employees in the necessity of reporting all injuries and illnesses immediately, in terms of written procedures, is important. Failure to comply results in delayed treatment, unnecessary complications and excessive correspondence to the Compensation Commissioner, hospitals and private practitioners.

Occupational health practitioners require knowledge of toxicology in order to recognize early signs and symptoms of occupational disease. Toxicology is the study of the adverse effects of chemicals on living organisms and the assessment of the probability of their occurrence (Rosenstock & Cullen, 1994:116). (See Chapter 5 for more information.)

7.10 Vulnerable employees requiring special care

Employees working in risk areas and other vulnerable groups needing special insight into their health situation and support from the occupational health nurse include the following:

Employees exposed to hazards in the workplace including those in high-risk work require regular monitoring both formal and informal. The occupational health nurse will observe for possible effects of the exposure at every formal or informal opportunity and not only during the scheduled annual medical examination. The employee exposed to lead may complain of constipation – a common complaint in primary health that requires diplomatic questioning to elicit other possible lead-related effects. The employee in a 'high-powered' position may become withdrawn and the alert nurse will notice and investigate for possible burnout.

Shift workers regularly work hours outside the usual daylight hours. These employees have biological, social and cultural problems. Biologically the disturbance of circadian rhythms leads to sleep deprivation, insomnia, chronic fatigue and this may eventually lead to stress and depression. It is not at all unusual that many accidents occur during the early hours of the morning. The occupational health nurse will observe for adverse effects of shift work including gastrointestinal disorders and anxiety in the Primary Health clinic and on sick notes from general practitioners. The nurse will motivate for worker-friendly shift patterns to the human resources department and educate the workers on ways of coping with shift work and sleeping during daylight hours. (See section 5.5 in Chapter 5 for more details.)

The chronically ill employee may be fit for work but needs regular monitoring and motivation to take medication regularly. This employee must be taught about his/her condition and how to manage it through diet and lifestyle, and to accept it. Employees with a chronic disease or disablement require an adaptation of work conditions, which the occupational health nurse can arrange with management.

Women at work, particularly those with children at home, have higher levels of the stress hormone norepinephrine, during work and at home. This places them at risk of health problems and depression.

Especially in South Africa, women still assume the responsibility of child-rearing and housework after a full day at work. They often feel that they neglect their children and home – that they are not there when they are needed. The occupational health nurse will recognize this stress and counsel the individual and arrange for referral if needed. Speakers can be invited to address coping mechanisms and social workers can help if there are financial problems at home. The occupational health nurse will arrange for family planning, ante- and post-natal clinics, keep-fit classes during the lunch break, and render ongoing support.

The pregnant employee requires advice on healthcare, diet, preparation for the baby and maternity benefits. The occupational health nurse may need to arrange for a transfer of this employee to a more suitable type of job.

Being a single parent, mother or father, can be stressful and the occupational health nurse needs to be supportive and if necessary arrange counselling sessions with child guidance experts.

School leavers may need to adjust to work-life and may demonstrate attitudinal problems – too brazen or too timid. Adolescents often struggle to cope with peer pressure and are exposed to drugs, alcohol and possibly HIV and Aids. A great deal of tact and some counselling are required to help these youngsters reach their full potential and contribute to society.

Nature has a way of slowing down capabilities and the older worker may have difficulty accepting this together with pending retirement. Retrenchment to make way for younger job seekers is another fear that affects quality of life and health for the late middle-age group. The occupational health nurse will arrange sessions with appropriate agencies for counselling and advice on retirement planning and financial planning for retirement.

7.11 Education

The term education is used here to describe the different aspects of health promotion and health protection that need to be addressed in attaining the goal of a healthy workforce within the framework of quality living and work.

As we are dealing with adult education, the principle of self-directed learning is applied by involving the adult learners in setting their own goals, and then guiding them from what they know to what they need to know by giving new knowledge as they require it.

This principle and the presentation of knowledge vary according to the target group and the subject.

7.11.1 Target groups

In the occupational setting, various levels of health information are transferred to different groups:

- *Management*, who are kept informed through statistics and monthly, annual and special reports. A formal presentation may need to be made on special issues such as new legislation, or a new health programme that may impact on production. Management support is vital to the success of any programme.
- *The occupational health team*, who need to be kept informed of new legislative requirements, new occupational health information and relevant occupational health service statistics.
- *Safety committee members, line supervisors and employee representatives*, who identify health and safety needs and prepare the employees for education programmes. The occupational health nurse's task is more successful with their support.
- *Employee groups*, who are addressed in small groups so as not to disrupt production, or gender groups to address sexual or role issues, or even age groups to address issues that apply mainly to certain age groups.

The occupational health nurse presents the same health information at different levels to the above target groups so as to give them information they can accept and utilize.

7.11.2 Types of programmes
There are many different types of programmes on the market, or the occupational health nurse may devise his/her own programme to address a specific health need. Employees have a right to know about workplace health risks and should be informed about:
- What they are working with
- How it could affect their health
- What precautions they should take
- What health surveillance will be done
- How to care for personal protective equipment
- How to accept responsibility for their own health and report any change in their health.

Information about occupational hazards is a legal requirement in terms of the Occupational Health and Safety Act, 1993 (No 85 of 1993) and it is suggested that, to protect themselves and the employer, employees acknowledge receiving and understanding the information, in writing. Lifestyle programmes, identified by the employees or the occupational health nurse as a health need, and educational methods are discussed in Chapter 8.

The aim is to help all employees to learn to take responsibility for the promotion, maintenance and protection of their own and their families' health. These programmes take on a variety of forms. Group discussions are informal discussions among people with similar circumstances and are a valuable coping mechanism, as they provide information and support to those who need it. The occupational health nurse acts as the facilitator and allows the group to find solutions for their own situations.

Employees will change behaviour only when they understand what they must do and when they see the recommended action as a means to an end that they value.

7.12 Counselling and support groups
The occupational health nurse is often the first person that an employee approaches to discuss a problem. It may be that the nurse suspects a problem and encourages the employee to discuss it. All discussions should be conducted in privacy, documented later and treated as confidential.

In counselling, the nurse guides the conversation to allow the client to find his/her own solution. The nurse listens, reinforces what was said, but never interrupts or gives an opinion or possible solution. The occupational health nurse is aware of the limitations of his/her capabilities and refers the client to an appropriate agency for further assistance but remains supportive and follows up the case. (See Chapter 11 for more detail.)

7.13 Rehabilitation
An important function of the occupational health nurse is the rehabilitation of employees after serious illness or injury. Rehabilitation should begin as early as possible and the nurse liaises with the employee's doctor to establish the employee's

capabilities and mental status. The employee, the nurse and the line manager discuss the situation in order to decide on the type of work that the employee can cope with.

The occupational health nurse is the ideal person to facilitate rehabilitation, as he/she understands the employee's limitations and the job's requirements. Most persons recovering from serious illness or accidents, including drug addicts and alcoholics, need understanding and daily support, especially in the initial stages of the rehabilitation process.

7.14 Environmental monitoring

In terms of the Occupational Exposure Limits (OEL) laid down in the Hazardous Chemical Substances Regulations of the Occupational Health and Safety Act, 1993 (No 85 of 1993), identified hazards are monitored at regular intervals and when the process has changed, to control the levels of:

- Hazardous chemicals, e.g. dust, fumes, gas or vapours
- Physical hazards, e.g. atmospheric pressure, illumination, noise, radiation or temperature extremes
- Mechanical hazards, e.g. vibration
- Biological hazards, e.g. bacterial, fungal and viral.

Environmental monitoring, also known as secondary monitoring, must be done by a Department of Labour accredited occupational hygienist and the occupational health nurse must receive a copy of the report to update the exposure levels on each employee's record. More details are given in Chapter 4.

7.15 The nursing process in occupational health nursing

The nursing process is a designated series of actions undertaken to ensure the client's well-being. The general rules of assessing, communicating, planning, implementing, documenting, evaluating and researching are applicable to both the employee and the organization.

Booyens describes the nursing process as a scientific method of nursing to render personal, individualized, quality nursing. As a problem-solving technique it is an orderly systematic manner of determining the client's problems, making plans to solve them, initiating the plan or assigning others to implement it, and evaluating the extent to which the plan was effective in resolving the problems identified (1996:204).

Assessing. Occupational health nurses begin the assessment of a potential problem when they first observe their client. They will note physical or mental features, for example a limp, fatigue or anxiety, that may have a bearing on the problem at hand. Their observations, the history and a full physical examination will influence their nursing diagnosis.

Communicating. Effective communication will elicit vital information without influencing the client subjectively, for instance asking 'What symptoms are you experiencing?' rather than. 'Do you have a headache?' would give the clients perspective.

In the implementation of the nursing plan, accurate instructions can influence the outcome of the intervention, and similarly effective communication will influence the extent of success in the evaluation of the intervention.

In the occupational health service, communication takes place at all levels and nurses must use simple language to the layperson, business terms when motivating for a new programme to management and scientific terms when reporting on a medical condition to the medical officer.

Planning. Once the nursing diagnosis is arrived at, planning commences with the priorities of the problem being arranged and appropriate management decided upon.

Implementing. The intervention phase relies on the interpersonal and clinical skills of the occupational health nurse for success. This phase may be concluded once the problem is solved or it may be continuous. The complete nursing process is recorded on the employee's personal file.

Documenting. Accurate record-keeping, data collection, literature search, evaluation and report-writing are part of the nursing process and improve the occupational healthcare given. Complete and accurate documentation protects the nurse from medicolegal risks.

Evaluating. The occupational health nurse is in the ideal position to follow up cases at the workplace. Effective intervention can be reflected in the sickness absence records and statistics that the nurse monitors, and in the outcome of biological monitoring and audiometric tests. Evaluation may be the final stage of the nursing process but is often the first step of a new process.

Researching. The nursing process is complete only when research has been undertaken with a view to improving the health of all employees and the standard of care rendered by the occupational health service.

7.16 Conclusion

The occupational health nurse's clinical skills are evident in every interaction with employees in the health centre and create trust and co-operation in the occupational health programme. In pursuit of quality care occupational health nurses will use every opportunity to update and improve their skills through the attendance of clinical workshops and continuing education programmes.

The ultimate aim or goal of a successful occupational health service is to address all aspects of occupational health, but the establishment of an effective, comprehensive service takes time.

7.17 Bibliography

Acutt, J. The Policy and Procedure Manual in an Occupational Health Service. *Occupational Health SA.* 1996 2 (4), 22–23.

American Thoracic Society. 1987. *Standardisation of Spirometry Update.* American Revision of Respiratory Diseases 136:1285–1298, 1987.

Booyens, S. W. 1996. *Introduction to Health Services Management.* Cape Town: Juta.

Guild, R., Ehrlich, R. I., Johnston, J. R. & Ross, M. H. 2001. *Handbook of Occupational Health Practice in the South African Mining Industry.* Johannesburg: SIMRAC.

International Labour Organization. 1959. Recommendations Concerning Occupational Health Services in Places of Employment. Recommendation 112. Geneva: ILO.

Jarvis, C. 1993. *Physical Examination and Health Assessment.* Philadelphia: WB Saunders.

Rogers, B. 1994. *Occupational Health Nursing. Concepts and Practice.* Philadelphia: WB Saunders.

Rosenstock, L. & Cullen, M. R. 1994 *Textbook of Clinical Environmental and Occupational Medicine.* Philadelphia: WB Saunders.

Zenz, C., Dickerson, O. B. & Horvath, E. P. 1994. *Occupational Medicine.* 3rd edition. St Louis: Mosby.

8 Health promotion at work

A. J. Kotze and J. Acutt

8.1 Introduction

The concept of occupational health revolves around health promotion and maintenance to the highest degree of physical, mental and social well-being. It includes protection of the health of the workers and the prevention of deterioration of health as a result of workplace exposure, according to the World Health Organization definition of occupational health.

Hereditary, personal and environmental factors play a major role in the quality of health experienced by workers. Health education can create a more positive attitude that enables people to take an increased interest in and responsibility for their own health. Health promotion programmes, with the emphasis on disease prevention, and the promotion of positive health, can contribute to the total health of communities.

As most people spend a large part of their lives in employment, the workplace may be considered a suitable place to introduce health promotion programmes. The financial benefits of health promotion and the resulting improvement in health behaviour cannot be overemphasized.

8.2 Learning objectives

At the end of this chapter, the reader should be able to:
- Identify healthy lifestyles
- Describe the importance of health promotion
- Identify the components of a health promotion programme
- Plan and implement specific programmes for health
- Plan and implement health education programmes
- Identify the importance of primary healthcare at the workplace.

8.3 Healthy lifestyles

Human behaviour is affected by many factors. Health promotion programmes aimed at changing behaviour should address as many of these factors as possible. Motivation has always been considered an important factor in the changing of human behaviour and may be used effectively (Girdano, 1986:7). Girdano gives two essential ingredients for behaviour change:
- A reason to change (motivation)
- The knowledge to know when, where, and how to take action (1986:7).

In our multicultural society, being healthy may mean many different things to different people. To those experiencing socio-economic deprivation, health may not seem as important as food, clothing and shelter; to affluent members of society, factors contributing to an unhealthy lifestyle such as stress, overeating and the lack of exercise may cause ill health, and be a motivation to change behaviour.

Girdano (1986:9) says that in order to be healthy one must recognize and change unhealthy behaviour. At a general level this involves:
- An ability to recognize imbalance and the behaviours that promote it
- The creation of an environment that supports balance
- The ability to satisfy health-related needs with behaviour that promotes good health, rather than detracts from it by living in such a way that one's life is balanced, healthy and that there are few episodes of imbalance.

8.4 The adult learner

The adult learner is a person who acts as an adult and fulfils the role of an adult by being a responsible citizen. The adult displays the following characteristics:
- Self-concept – the adult takes control of his/her own life, making his/her own decisions
- Experience – past experience contributes to learning and new learning must be built on that knowledge
- Learning readiness is shown when the adult experiences a need to know more, especially about problems or a task in real-life situations (Muller, 2002:279).

The occupational health practitioner plans his/her health promotion programme for adult learners and respects their self-concepts and experience whilst motivating them to gain new knowledge.

8.5 Health promotion in the occupational health setting

The idea of the prevention of disease and the promotion of positive health is not a new one and in many ancient civilizations, such as the Chinese and the Greeks, health was seen as something that had to be nurtured and protected (Girdano, 1986:11).

In our own society, some form of environmental health and health education forms part of the school curriculum from a very early age. Today we realize that these programmes cannot be incidental. They must be planned efficiently and offered effectively, if we are to combat the many threats to human health.

Programmes must be continuous and cover the whole span of human development – childhood, adolescence, adulthood and old age. The workplace can be a natural and potentially effective setting for health promotion programmes, for a number of reasons:
- The workforce provides a large, readily available target group.
- People tend to make better use of programmes offered at work.
- A part of the workforce is stable and this allows for long-term intervention and evaluation.

Occupational health

- High healthcare costs and a loss in productivity may act as a motivation for industry to become involved in programmes for health promotion.
- The family of the worker also benefits from programmes offered to the worker.

Occupational health promotion relies heavily on the positive attitudes of both the worker and the employer towards promotion programmes. We could go so far as to say that the input of the employer is the major factor that will determine the success of such a programme. The employer's input is more concrete in terms of facilities, financial contribution, personnel, and all the other facets of the planning and implementation of such a programme. At present there is no legal provision to enforce such a programme, and it would therefore depend entirely upon the philosophy of the employer towards the value of such a programme.

Some firms have shown how much they value the health of their employers by instituting some form of health promotion programmes, whilst others still have to follow. Examples of elements of these programmes are:
- Health education
- Primary healthcare and medical surveillance programmes
- Recreational facilities and opportunities for social interaction
- Employee assistance programmes.

Some form of evaluation of these programmes should take place. This can be done by regular health screening for risk factors, e.g. high blood pressure, by documenting the level of participation in programmes, by evaluating absenteeism reasons and by assessing positive behavioural changes.

8.6 Components of a successful occupational health programme

Girdano (1986:21) states that 'the ideal health promotion programme is one that identifies target subpopulations with precision, intervening in those populations with selectivity based on carefully selected outcomes, modifies and tailors each intervention to maximize its individual effectiveness and delivers the programme with maximum cost-efficiency'.

The components that are essential for a health promotion programme are given below.

8.6.1 Policy
The company health policy should be characterized by the willingness of management to commit itself. Once commitment is guaranteed, active involvement of management in the programmes will act as a role model and motivate the employees to participate.

8.6.2 Planning
A well-prepared programme will be preceded by the steps of the planning process as set out below.

Establishing a philosophy
The philosophy of a health promotion programme in industry reflects that of the occupational health programme and may be to:

- Create an awareness and acceptance of responsibility for one's own health and that of one's family
- Establish positive health behaviour
- Change health-damaging behaviour to behaviour that will enhance good health
- Obtain maximum and ongoing participation in health promotion programmes.

Formulating objectives for the programme
These may include long-term and short-term objectives arising from the philosophy and are stated in measurable terms such as:
- Identifying high-risk groups within the workforce and listing them
- Establishing the interest of employees to assess the health needs that they would like to see addressed and recording these needs
- Determining the kind of programmes required to address the identified needs and implementing them
- Setting targets for employee participation in the different programmes
- Determining expected outcomes of programmes including health awareness and acceptance of responsibility of one's own health
- Compiling a data-bank for information relevant to programmes
- Determining the effectiveness of the programme through evaluation strategies.

Programme content
Objectives can be achieved by applying the methods described below.

Well-person screening. This term is used to describe the process of screening a group of employees to identify individuals who may show early signs of the condition under study, or be vulnerable to a disease. Screening can involve high costs and specialized technology, and does not end with screening, but needs to be supported by a follow-up and treatment programme. In industry the medical surveillance programme is a comprehensive screening process of well persons.

Tailoring to the participants. It has been proved that in more successful programmes, participants are able to choose the type and form of health promotion they prefer. Girdano says that this enhances individual autonomy, increases self-esteem and the likelihood of behaviour change (1986:24). Whilst aiming for maximum participation, it is important to allow for freedom of choice by employees, to obtain quality participation.

A comprehensive programme. The decision whether to plan a single focus or comprehensive programme depends on company policy, finances, resources and facilities available. A comprehensive programme that addresses all the health needs identified by the employees and those identified in screening programmes will influence the components of a programme.

A multidimensional programme offers more flexibility to the health team and more freedom of choice to the employee, while it addresses everyone's need and creates enthusiasm for the programme.

Examples of programmes that prove to be popular are:
- First aid and cardiopulmonary resuscitation
- Stress management
- Self-development
- Substance abuse prevention and rehabilitation
- Physical fitness, nutrition and weight control
- Prevention of and coping with chronic illness.

Administrative structure
The health promotion programmes cannot be offered without an administrative support system being available. Girdano says that in-house personnel, with the aid of external consultants or companies, could be contracted to offer the programme (1986:25). Programmes can be administered internally and incorporated within the existing administrative structure. Excellent health promotion videos are available commercially and from the Department of Health which the occupational health nurses could use in programmes that they have organized.

8.6.3 Educational approach
This approach needs to be decided during the planning phase. The strategies used and techniques applied should be tried and tested beforehand. Employees are most receptive to peer education, role-play and demonstrations. The provision of pamphlets and literature to take home and study at leisure has proved very effective and the occupational health nurse must be prepared for the number of questions and requests for more information following the session.

A golden 'teaching moment' occurs frequently during nursing interaction in primary healthcare and medical surveillance. The occupational health nurse must seize the opportunity to educate the client about a personal health concern.

In general, principles of good healthcare or education should be applied and regularly adapted as the programme develops and new needs arise.

8.6.4 Continuous participation
During the planning phase attention must be given to methods to motivate participants to continue taking part in programmes. Various methods can be followed, such as:
- Communication, progress reports and incentives to the participants of the programme
- Involvement of employee dependants in the programme
- Tactful encouragement of employees to be responsible for healthy behaviour
- Inclusion of methods of self-evaluation in the programme
- Use of social support systems to enhance positive behaviour
- Ensuring a safe and healthy work environment to emphasize that the efforts of the employer in health promotion are credible.

8.6.5 Evaluation
Evaluation is an integral part of the health promotion programme and general rules of

evaluation in educational settings should be applied. Evaluation should be part of the planning phase and methods of evaluation to determine the effectiveness of the programme must form part of the programme. These methods include:
- Feedback from the learners and from their representatives
- Questions or a quiz at the end of a session and at the start of the next session will indicate how much information was retained
- Questionnaires sent to all participants after a period to assess the value of the session
- Assessing results of the new information in clinic attendance, absenteeism and accident statistics.

8.7 Health education

The prevention of occupational accidents and ill health caused by harmful factors in and outside the workplace, as well as the creation of a working environment which maintains and promotes the health of workers, are essential components of a health education programme in the workplace (WHO, 1981:11).

The policy for education and training in occupational health and safety must cover all the categories of personnel involved, in order to enhance their awareness of health and safety measures.

The health education programme enhances the ability to fulfil specific tasks, and provides specialized knowledge and skills to the workers. Health and safety at work should be taught as topics inseparable from the working process itself. Safe behaviour at work, the use of protective devices, and attention to personal hygiene and general health should become an integral part of working habits (WHO, 1981:13).

8.7.1 The objectives of health education in occupational health and safety

The content of educational programmes should be organized under three broad headings for learning purposes:
1. Cognitive (knowledge) skills
2. Psychomotor (professional) skills
3. Affective (attitudes and values) skills.

Occupational health professionals and safety trainers should critically examine the learning experiences and test procedures they offer to determine whether they are appropriate to the desired level of learning.

Merely having the information does not assure it can be used. On the other hand, learning experiences and evaluation procedures directed at problem-solving will also transmit information or test its acquisition.

Attitudinal learning may have a more profound influence upon future behaviour than the informational input (WHO, 1981:20).

In terms of the Occupational Health and Safety Act, 1993 (No 85 of 1993) and the Mine Health and Safety Act, 1996 (No 29 of 1996) employees must be informed of the hazards they are exposed to and the protective measures they must undertake by

employers. To address this prescription, the following objectives of training in occupational health and safety are set:
- To train all employees to perform the functions expected of them without risks to health
- To promote a general awareness of risks associated with work
- To maintain and promote general health through occupational health programmes
- To detect physical and mental health impairment at an early stage
- To promote healthy lifestyles for all with the resultant improvement in quality of life.

8.7.2 The content of health education programmes
Content and teaching methods are determined by the behaviour to be learned.

The consumers, such as the workers' and employees' representatives, should be consulted about the health needs of the employees.

Legislation prescribes many of the occupational health programmes required for different hazardous occupations and advice may be solicited from the National Centre for Occupational Health or commercial risk management companies.

Since learning requires motivation, a realistic goal cannot be set for the content of educational programmes without incorporating the learner's desires. Individuals who are not convinced that they need to learn a particular skill will resist efforts to be taught.

Lack of motivation may be caused by:
- Difficulty in adapting to new ideas or health deterioration
- Differences in value systems and concepts of health and illness between client and health professional
- The learner's abilities and command of the situation.

Content is always determined by the learning objectives – these two should be compared – if there is content in the plan that does not relate to any objective, the content may be superfluous and should be eliminated (Redman, 1988:196).

8.7.3 Teaching methods
Each of these learning domains (cognitive, motor and affective skills) responds best to particular methods of teaching:

Facts and concepts (cognitive skills) are basic intellectual learning and are taught by means of written material; audiovisual aids representing the concepts; lectures; and discussions.

Learning of attitudes (affective skills) does not automatically follow from a knowledge of facts. Attitudes can perhaps best be taught by discussions with the client/patient; providing insight into their feelings and gaining acceptance of a new attitude by providing a model to imitate (Redman, 1988:17).

Motor skills are best learned through a demonstration of the skills, with subsequent practice, until the skill is perfected.

Group learning can save a great deal of teacher time, and provides an opportunity for people to learn from one another's experiences (Redman, 1988:17).

8.7.4 The evaluation of learning
Teaching consists of assessing what the client needs to learn, planning the lesson, and actually doing the teaching. It also includes ascertaining whether the desired behavioural change has occurred.

Redman (1988:224–229) describes various evaluation techniques:
1. *The direct observation of behaviour* can be done by making use of techniques such as video recordings; rating scales and checklists; anecdotal notes and critical incident recordings; and observing positive evidence of behavioural change.
2. *Oral questioning* is a flexible form of measurement and may be used in combination with other techniques, such as observation.
3. *Written measurement* is a method that can only be applied if the learner can read and write. It offers the opportunity to measure learning at all levels of the cognitive domain.

Evaluation is the final step in the process of teaching-learning, but the process should not stop here. It merely serves as an instrument to redirect the teaching activities (Redman, 1988:253).

Both the teacher and learner should be constantly assessing the extent to which they are progressing toward the goals set in the learning programme.

Evaluation is done during, or at the end of a lesson/learning session to determine what learning has been retained over a period of time (Redman, 1988:17).

8.7.5 Teaching plans for health education
Teaching plans can be written in many formats. The format used for a specific lesson is usually determined by the content, target group and the teaching method used.

The teaching plan is a written outline of the salient points of a specific lesson. The most important purpose is to organize the lesson by:
- Clarifying the objectives
- Selecting the methods and materials to be used
- Giving details of the content of the lesson
- Describing the activities planned for both the teacher and the learner's evaluation
- Serving as a guide for the teacher while teaching is in progress (Pohl, 1981:129).

A sample teaching plan is outlined below.

Occupational health

> **Sample teaching plan**
>
> *1 Target group/learner*
> Describe the group/learner for which the particular teaching plan is being used.
>
> *2 Main objectives of the teaching session*
> The objectives will determine the content of the lesson. Objectives should be limited in number and scope. No objectives should be included in the guide that cannot reasonably be accomplished during the lesson (Pohl, 1981:205).
>
> *3 Lesson topic/content*
> The statement of the overall topic of the lesson defines the scope of the content. It should be carefully worded to attract interest, but contain enough detail to show clearly what the content will be.
>
> *4 Methods of teaching*
> The lesson plan should show what method or combination of methods of teaching is to be used, and whether it is designed for individual or group teaching.
>
> *5 Teaching materials*
> All teaching materials for the lesson should be enumerated and the sources indicated. Teaching aids such as flannelboard, projector and posters should be included.
>
> *6 The content of the lesson*
> The subject matter should be indicated – using phrases and key words, rather than complete sentences. The written outline of the lesson content should include an introduction, body and summary of the lesson.
>
> *7 Teacher and learner activities*
> The activities planned for both the teacher and the learner should be indicated in the lesson plan, linking it with the relevant subject matter. These activities may include questions; the use of the chalkboard or overhead projector; discussions with the learners; and the answering of questions by the learners.
>
> *8 Summary of the lesson*
> Good teaching includes a summary of the main points of the lesson.
>
> *9 Evaluation*
> The teaching should indicate how the teacher will determine whether the learners have met their goals (Pohl, 1981:133).

Delivering effective health education to the client (worker) and patient remains a challenge for the occupational health team. The advantages of a well-informed workforce that values its health include benefits for the employer and the community at large.

8.8 Selected health promotion programmes

Health promotion encompasses various activities such as physical fitness, weight and stress management and smoking cessation in order to improve the quality of life. Health promotion and protection programmes should be targeted at awareness, lifestyle changes and supportive environments such as family, colleagues at the workplace, mentors in facilities such as the gym.

Some of the most important and comprehensive are being addressed in this section.

8.8.1 Primary healthcare in occupational health settings

Primary healthcare is essential healthcare based on scientifically sound and socially acceptable methods and technology made universally accessible to individuals and families in the community through their full participation and at a cost that the community and country can afford to maintain at every stage of their development in the spirit of self-reliance and self-determination (Subcommittee: Primary Health Care, 1992:2).

In the occupational health setting some of the key words take on a different meaning but the concept is essentially the same. Thus key words in this description of the services are the following:
1. *Accessibility* – this means geographically, financially and functionally accessible services
2. *Equity* – the absence of subgroup variability and discrepancy
3. *Acceptability* – a level of healthcare that is acceptable to the workforce and health worker
4. *Availability* – services must be readily available to all members of the workforce
5. *Effectiveness* – the extent to which a service does what it is defined to do
6. *Efficiency* – the end result achieved in relation to the effort expended in terms of money, resources and time.

When one considers the objectives of a primary healthcare service, it is unthinkable that an occupational healthcare service should not include such services. In terms of accessibility and availability, the health service in the workplace is most suitable to deliver such services.

Existing primary healthcare services that have now been deployed all over the country may, however, render services to the worker in or near the workplace.

If the financial implications of such services at the workplace are carefully considered and accepted by employers, primary healthcare can save many production hours and contribute toward the prevention of illness and promotion of the health of the worker.

The basic services suggested for primary healthcare are the following:
- Treatment of minor ailments, common and chronic diseases and injuries
- Provision of essential medicine
- Maternal and child healthcare services
- Immunization programmes
- Control of local endemic diseases
- Community psychiatric services
- Basic rehabilitation services.

8.8.2 The troubled employee and assistance programmes

Optimal health is a balance between physical, emotional, social, spiritual and intellectual wellness. This balance may be disturbed for any number of reasons, from changes in the workplace and loss of job security, violent crime, family conflicts, trauma and illness, substance abuse or a positive test for the human immunodeficiency virus. Whatever the cause, the effect of the person's outlook in life is severe and adversely affects his/her work performance. (See Chapter 11 on Psychological health.)

A person with this type of problem should feel free to ask the occupational health practitioner for help but is often in denial and depressed. Managers need to learn to address the performance aspect and to refer the employee to the nurse or to an employee assistance programme should one exist.

It is generally the occupational health practitioner who motivates to management for such a programme with statistics of the number of employees who would benefit. This type of programme requires management commitment and a policy and procedures in place before implementation. Human resources department officials, employee representatives, the health personnel and representatives from line management form a committee to plan the programme, the policy and the procedures to follow to ensure effectiveness. They also motivate strongly that no stigma is attached to the programme and that attendance and progress are strictly confidential.

Clinical psychologists are appointed or placed by an external company to be available for troubled employees on a consultation basis. The service is paid for by the employer and is extended to immediate family members of the employee, who are generally involved in the situation.

The benefits of this type of programme are far-reaching for the employee, his/her family and the community as a whole, as well as for the company. Increased production and decreased absenteeism and accidents improve workforce morale and loyalty to the company and are but a few of the measurable results of an effective employee assistance programme.

8.8.3 The prevention of Aids (Acquired Immunodeficiency Syndrome)

Communities should be well informed about all the aspects of this disease. The employer and the occupational health team has a specific responsibility and role to play in creating awareness of the condition and promoting positive behaviour to prevent this condition. For the person who has already contracted Aids, effective health supervision, counselling and management by health personnel with empathy and understanding are required. It is also the duty of the employer to protect other workers and personnel from high-risk behaviour, as far as this disease is concerned. An informed community can be a great asset in the prevention of Aids.

The content of the programme should be divided into two main sections:

1 Health promotion measures to create an awareness of the disease and to prevent the spreading of the condition:
- Promoting responsible relationships
- Promoting protected sexual behaviour
- Establishing Aids information groups
- Establishing screening programmes.

2 Health measures to promote the health of the Aids sufferer and the carriers of the disease:
- General health promotion programmes, e.g. nutrition and recreation

- Specific health education related to the problems experienced by the sufferer
- Safe sexual behaviour aimed at protecting partners, the family and the community
- Health maintenance and surveillance
- Health support during periods of illness
- Counselling of contacts, family and employers.

8.8.4 Promoting maternal and child welfare in the workplace

The large number of women of childbearing age in the workforce makes issues such as pregnancy and child health important. Preventive health programmes at work for women and children can eventually ensure numerous advantages to the employer in the form of a healthy workforce.

Working mothers are faced with problems, such as breastfeeding, childhood diseases, illnesses during pregnancy, and child support systems to name only a few. They can lead to a high rate of absenteeism in the workforce. If these are addressed by well-organized preventive and health-support programmes, high employee morale, work retention and good quality work are possible.

After assessing the needs of the target group the occupational health nurse decides on the content of the programme. This may include aspects of:

- Prenatal care
- Counselling and supervision of high risk groups, e.g. HIV-positive mothers, single parents and mothers with chronic diseases
- Nutrition, exercise and recreation
- Caring for an infant
- Dealing with childhood diseases effectively
- The provision and supervision of childcare facilities
- Flexitime facilities for nurturing mothers.

8.8.5 Hypertension screening programmes

According to South African statistics for 1986, the total death rate per 100 000 of the population due to hypertensive disease was 59, but the estimated number of people suffering from hypertension runs into thousands more. In America it is estimated that 15 per cent or roughly 37 million people are thought to have hypertension (Girdano, 1986:168).

Blood-pressure screening programmes can be educational and promote compliance with treatment for those who have been treated, but may also identify high-risk populations. The very many conditions of which high blood pressure is merely a symptom may be prevented, treated and controlled. Many lost workdays may be prevented with such a programme.

A successful programme for blood pressure screening should include elements such as:

- Detection of raised blood pressure
- Referral to the company physician
- Diagnosis and management of hypertension
- Follow-up clinic attendance on a regular basis
- Long-term maintenance

Occupational health

- Education about the disease and its management
- Evaluation of progress (Girdano, 1986:171).

The workplace has been identified as being a suitable site for initiating, monitoring and maintaining treatment of hypertension.

8.8.6 Physical fitness programmes

Industry is seen as an effective vehicle for the delivery of preventive healthcare. The decline in life-expectancy which is seen in modern societies today, is related to a combination of environmental health hazards and adverse lifestyle choices such as physical inactivity and cigarette smoking.

The healthcare system should move from traditional tertiary treatment to primary and secondary prevention.

Industrial fitness programmes require certain baseline data to institute such a programme. Health screening of employees, including a physical fitness test, forms the basis for this programme. Having completed a thorough physical fitness test, the next task of the occupational health team is to translate this information into an appropriate exercise prescription, compatible with company resources, societal norms and the attitudes of the individual worker.

The task of industry is now to provide some practical programme whereby the individual can respond to the advice he/she has been given. In-house programmes offer many advantages in terms of both cost and participant effectiveness. Recreational facilities may be shared by groups of companies. This may also be an acceptable alternative for the smaller industry that cannot afford extensive facilities for smaller numbers of employees.

Because of convenience and peer pressure, participation rates are 3–4 times greater for the in-house programme than for those in the community. Moreover, on-site programmes develop a corporate concern for health, so that non-participants begin to show an interest. As participation becomes more general, the entire culture of the workplace may change – a snowball effect is created. This allows the health educator to reach even the high-risk individuals.

The in-house approach is also seen as a greater opportunity for the occupational health service to develop a total lifestyle package for the promotion of the health of the worker in particular, and the community at large.

8.9 Contemporary occupational health problems in South Africa

8.9.1 The informal labour sector

South Africa is a country where social conditions of the First and Third World meet. We find a high unemployment rate, resulting in large-scale migration to the densely populated industrialized urban areas. This in turn leads to the establishment of squatter areas with the development of a large informal labour sector.

Towns and cities do not provide sufficient infrastructure to support these workers. In areas where such structures are provided by local authorities, they soon become inadequate because of the large numbers of informal workers such as street workers and vendors.

Some common health hazards/problems experienced by the worker in the informal sector:
- The absence of any formal health support system
- Physical exposure to the elements – rain, cold and heat
- Long working hours
- Heavy physical work
- Long travelling distances
- Inadequate nutrition
- Unsafe working conditions
- Inadequate water and toilet facilities
- Chronic disease and minor ailments because of poor physical condition.

Where these workers grew up as street children, additional problems such as the following are found:
- The absence of schooling or any educational opportunities
- Exposure to criminal elements and habits on the street, e.g. substance abuse
- Unavailability of formal housing.

The provision of any kind of occupational health service to these workers is certainly a challenge to the community and its structures. Accessible and affordable primary healthcare services could be the answer to provide at least some basic preventive and curative services to this group of workers.

8.9.2 Domestic workers
(Consult Chapter 2, which deals with the legislation.)
This group of workers can also be classified as informal workers. Common health and related problems experienced by these workers are the following:
- Long working hours with insufficient time off duty
- Hard physical work and high levels of work stress
- Poor housing conditions
- Long travelling distances
- Chronic disease and minor ailments
- The lack of paid maternity/sick/annual leave
- Social problems at home due to long hours absent from the family
- Non-sustenance pay.

These workers have to make use of the available formal health structures in their areas. Due to the absence of formal contracts of employment, sick leave is often granted without pay. Various structures now exist in the rural areas, which can assist the domestic worker to obtain acceptable conditions of service.

8.9.3 Agricultural workers
Agriculture is the oldest and most basic industry of all. It is also a way of life in which all family members take part – occupational aspects are difficult to separate from the

effects of living in a rural environment. Participants are often younger and older than the normal working population (Harrington, 1987:55).
(Consult Chapter 5 for Hazards in the agricultural section.)

1 Pesticide poisoning. The general adoption of intensive systems of farming has led to a number of changes in this industry – some desirable and others less so. Intensive cultivation demands the application of fertilizers, weed-killers and pesticides, which poses a great exposure hazard to the farm worker.

2 Infections, zoonoses and skin conditions. The close contact with large numbers/kinds of animals found in the industry increases the likelihood of infections in the human being. Respiratory diseases are often found in workers exposed to organic antigens such as pollen, fungal spores, grain dust and synthetic chemicals. Plant allergies can cause dermatitis.

3 Physical exposure and injuries. Hard physical labour leads to chronic muscular/skeletal conditions such as tenosynovitis. Debilitating injuries caused by accidents with heavy farming machinery are commonly found. Poor social conditions are common in the rural areas – housing, water supply and health services are often inadequate.

8.9.3.1 Providing occupational health and safety services in agriculture
Primary healthcare services are now available to these workers. The services are, however, not always accessible, due to distances from the clinics and clinic hours.

The farm labourers rely to a large extent on the goodwill of their employers to provide them with transport and financial support to obtain basic healthcare. (Consult Chapter 2 on legislation.) Some of the larger farming units in South Africa have set up their own farm health units where a nurse or health worker is employed.

International agricultural companies raising cash crops have occupational health services for their workers.

8.10 Conclusion

There are an endless variety of health promotion programmes that may be offered in the occupational setting, if the need has been expressed by employees and followed up by the occupational healthcare professionals.

Health promotion encompasses various activities such as physical fitness, weight and stress management, smoking cessation to improve the quality of life. Health promotion and protection programmes should be targeted at awareness, lifestyle changes and the provision of supportive environments.

Health promotion programmes can save the employer and the community millions of rands in healthcare costs, but in a country where occupational health is still not as readily accepted as in First World countries, a lot of work has still to be done. Primary healthcare features prominently in our present-day healthcare planning, and this is the ideal opportunity to introduce health promotion as a component of preventive healthcare programmes.

8.11 Bibliography

Cox, R. 2000. *Fitness for Work*. 3rd edition. United Kingdom: Oxford University Press.

Girdano, D. A. 1986. *Occupational Health Promotion*. New York: Macmillan Publishing Company.

Harrington, J. M. (ed) 1987. *Recent Advances in Occupational Health, No 3*. Avon: Churchill Livingstone.

Health Trends in South Africa, 1989. Department of National Health and Population Development.

Muller, M. 2002. *Nursing Dynamics*. 3rd edition. Heinemann. Johannesburg.

Pohl, M. L. 1981. *The Teaching Function of the Nursing Practitioner*. USA: WMC Brown Publishers.

Redman, B. K. 1988 *The Process of Patient Education*. St Louis: CV Mosby.

Rogers, B. 1994. *Occupational Health Nursing. Concepts and Practice*. Philadelphia: WB Saunders.

Schilling, R. S. F. 1973.*Occupational Health Practice*. London: Butterworths & Company (Publishers) Ltd.

Strategy for Primary Health Care in South Africa. Compiled by the Subcommittee: Primary Health Care. July, 1992.

The Reconstruction and Development Programme. ANC Congress 1994. Johannesburg: Umanyano Publications.

WHO. 1981. Education and Training in Occupational Health and Safety and Ergonomics. Eighth report of the Joint ILO/WHO Committee on Occupational Health.

9 Emergency care and disaster management

S. P. Hattingh

9.1 Introduction
The world is changing – technology is changing and the risks associated with it are increasingly evolving. By simply watching television or reading the newspaper, the occurrence of disasters unfolds before our eyes. On a daily basis we are confronted in the media worldwide with natural disasters such as tornadoes, and disasters of human origin such as violent workplace incidents, explosions and chemical incidents. We are also confronted with 'new' types of disasters. Today, the risks of disasters have evolved substantially to include areas far beyond the natural disasters of the past. Disasters now encompass areas such as cyberterrorism, product hampering, biological threats and ecological terrorism that were virtually unheard of a few years ago.

These disasters could have an equally devastating result as any natural disaster, however, prevention and a proactive approach to these disasters are vastly different. No matter what type of disaster occurs, it always results in substantial loss of life, money, assets, property, natural resources and productivity. The occupational health professional must adapt to the new circumstances and must be aware and prepared in order to prevent potential disasters from happening where possible, to minimize risks where prevention is not possible and to react appropriately to keep loss of life and damage to a minimum. Appropriate planning and preparedness before the disaster occurs are essentially to minimize the resulting effects. Occupational healthcare professionals work in close collaboration with an appropriately selected and trained team and should be equally trained, skilled and knowledgeable so that their reactions and decisions during a crisis are appropriate and coordinated. It is often said that few people plan to fail, but they just fail to plan. Preparedness before a disaster is the key to minimizing the potential risk and damages that may can occur in terms of human life, property and efficacy loss. Once a disaster has occurred, it is too late to plan.

This chapter gives a brief introduction to emergency care and disaster management in general and in the occupational health field. It is not at all comprehensive, as major works on this topic have been published. It is, however, one of the most important topics that needs to be explored and planned for in the occupational field.

This chapter also provides limited guidelines on the emergency care of some injuries and conditions that could be sustained during a disaster.

Emergency care and disaster management

9.2 Learning objectives

At the end of this chapter, the reader should be able to:
- Identify the risks which the occupational healthcare professional would regard as possible disaster occurrences, and plan effectively, within the multidisciplinary team, appropriate and meaningful measures to manage such disasters if they should occur
- Gather and keep appropriate information in specific workplaces in planning for disasters
- Explore causative and contributory factors which may lead to disasters in specific workplace settings
- Translate legislation and ethical issues related to disaster management
- Use effective and appropriate ways to present, practise and communicate disaster management skills and actions
- Deliver prehospital emergency care and assistance to victims.

9.3 What is a disaster?

The word dis-as-ter is defined by Blacks Law Dictionary as 'a calamitous event, especially one occurring suddenly and causing great loss of life, damage, or hardship, such as a flood, aeroplane crash, or business failure'. However, an emergency could just as easily involve only one person as it could involve the whole workforce or the whole population. A disaster may range from a minor to a major disaster, depending on the number of fatalities and injuries, the nature of the event and the cost of the destruction. If incorrectly managed, a minor event could become a moderate or even a major disaster due to increased loss of life or destruction of property. The key issue of a disaster is not the absolute number of victims but the needs of the victims and the ability of the healthcare system to meet those needs using normal operating procedures. For example, in a small rural area a head-on collision between two cars with eight injured passengers may be enough to put the disaster plan into action, whereas if the same collision had occurred in a city area, it would not have been regarded as a disaster.

Disasters are unexpected, chaotic, horrendous catastrophes in which people are initially horrified, then bewildered and confused about what to do and where to start. However, disaster management must follow normal operating procedures as much as possible. The fewer exceptions to the rules that stressed rescuers are expected to remember the better.

According to the Disaster Management Bill, 2001 (No 58 of 2001), a disaster is a progressive or sudden, widespread or localized, natural or human-caused occurrence, which causes or threatens to cause death, injury or disease, damage to property, infrastructure or the environment, or disrupt the life of a community. A disaster is further defined as of a magnitude that exceeds the ability of those affected by the disaster to cope with its effects using only their own resources.

According to the Bill, a disaster is local if it affects a single metropole, district or local municipality, and a disaster is provincial if it affects more than one metropole or district municipality in the same province or a single metropole or district municipality in the province, and if that metropolitan municipality or the district municipality, with the assistance of the local municipalities within this area, is unable to deal with it effectively.

9.4 Identifying the risk

To be prepared for a disaster is nearly impossible because there is no one basic emergency and disaster plan that fits all facilities and operations (Schneid & Collins 2000:1). It is important, however, to identify the potential risks associated with a potential disaster, and to identify the location, the process, the environment, the related structure and all other factors that lead to an initial assessment of the risks involved in the operations.

Once the potential risks have been identified and an assessment of potentially dangerous environments determined, the next step is to assess the potential outcomes of such risks and the probability of their occurrence. The probability can be determined by using formulas and other standard methodology, however, there is always a psychological factor or a subjective factor involved as will be seen in the given example of nuclear plant operations. Often risk managers and health professionals assume that, due to the strict adherence to protocol and security, there is no probability of a disaster occurring, however, many of these subjective assumptions have been proven wrong in the past. Assessment includes the human resource potential involved in such an operation, as well as the means (financial or equipment) needed to effectively manage such a devastating occurrence.

Part of the assessment and probabilities is an estimation of the potential damage to life, property, productivity, the environment, and efficacy in monetary terms. This is often called a worst-case scenario and questions such as 'what if...' are translated into monetary terms and in terms of alternative solutions. These estimations require brainstorm activity and close teamwork and all possibilities are evaluated. Only when a complete risk analysis has been conducted can the health professional team start planning the resources to eliminate or reduce all possible risks by introducing pro-active preventive plans and actions.

9.5 Natural disasters

The most sensational disasters, which are covered in the media, are the natural disasters. Devastating earthquakes, floods, hurricanes, erupting volcanoes, tornadoes and others are some of the examples of natural disasters, which occur suddenly. However, in the long term, drought, famine and epidemics can also be classified as natural disasters.

9.6 Disasters of human origin

Not all disasters have a natural cause and in this era of high speed and high technology, terrorism attacks and equipment failure are often attributed to disasters of human origin.

Disasters of human origin include war, chemical and biological terrorism and accidents, transportation accidents, food and water contamination and structural collapse.

9.7 Emerging risks

There are certain events that influence the nature and possibility of preparation, planning and response in the management of a disaster. These are given below.

Predictability of the disaster
Some disasters are predicted and can be more easily prepared for, for example advances in the field of meteorology have contributed to the prediction of hurricanes, flooding and some other natural disasters. Disasters of human origin are less predictable and these disasters often occur without prior warning. Disasters occurring in industry are not predictable and therefore need time to prepare in case they occur, for example nuclear accidents.

Frequency of disasters
Some natural disasters may occur more often in certain geographical areas, for example flooding in Mozambique, which is a tropical country with a high rainfall and large rivers, is more frequent than flooding in the Karoo, which is a desert area with a very low rainfall. People in these areas may be able to plan ahead for such an occurrence. If small accidents occur frequently in an industry, one could predict that a large-scale accident, which may take the form of a disaster, could occur in the near future.

Time of the disaster
Some disasters take a long time to develop (e.g. famine, drought or small leaks from gas pipes), and some disasters occur in a split second, for example explosions, bomb attacks and chemical spills. The time available to warn the workers and/or the population will determine the loss of life and damage. More protective measures can be taken and people can for example be evacuated. The most damage is caused by time factors such as rapid onset, no opportunity to warn the workers and/or the population, and the lengthy duration of the impact phase.

Controllability of a disaster
When there is pre-warning, certain control measures can be applied to limit or reduce the impact of the disaster. In some industries, warning signals may detect some faults or abnormal conditions within the immediate area where workers are working. The evacuation of personnel can be arranged and loss of life controlled. Applying strict safety measures, building standards, the use of certain equipment and safety and security of entry of people into the industry, may also control disasters.

Scope and intensity of a disaster
A disaster may be concentrated in one small geographical area or may involve a larger area, for example the occurrence of rare extremely contagious diseases such as Kongo fever or Marburg disease may in itself have the potential to spread rapidly to others within that area. This is a disaster situation, which must be managed with extreme care. Some disasters may be very intense and cause many injuries, whereas others may be less intense with relatively small numbers of deaths, injury and property damage. An example is the explosion, which may occur at a sewage works. There may not be loss of life, injury or there may be very little property damage, but the impact may be immense as people will be subjected to diseases and the spilling of raw sewage may cause other problems in the community.

9.8 Legislative control

In South Africa, the Disaster Management Bill, 2001 (No 58 of 2001) applies in cases of disaster and is a new approach to disaster management. Unlike previous policies contained in existing legislation that focused predominantly on relief and recovery efforts, this Bill emphasizes the importance of measures to avoid and minimize human and economic losses and establish prevention and mitigation as the core principles of a future disaster management policy. The objective of the Bill is to provide for an integrated and coordinated disaster management policy that focuses on preventing or reducing the risk of disasters, mitigating the severity of disasters, emergency preparedness, rapid and effective response to disasters and post-disaster recovery. It also makes provision for the establishment of national, provincial and municipal disaster management centres and for all matters concerning disasters.

More specifically, the Bill calls for a two-pronged approach, namely:
1. A significant strengthening capacity to track, collate, monitor and disseminate information on phenomena and activities known to trigger disastrous events, supported by institutional emergency preparedness and response capacity by both governmental and private sector role players, communities and other non-governmental agencies.
2. An increased commitment to prevention and mitigation actions that will reduce the probability and severity of disastrous events by incorporating these actions into policies, plans and projects of both government and the private sector (Disaster Management Bill, No 58 of 2001:28).

9.8.1 Key policy measures

Seven key policy measures are contained in this legislation. These include the following:
1. The urgent integration of risk reduction strategies into all development initiatives
2. The development of a strategy to reduce the vulnerability of people, especially the poor and disadvantaged communities during disasters
3. The establishment of a National Disaster Management Centre to:
   - ensure that an effective disaster management strategy is established and implemented by all spheres of government and other disaster management role players
   - coordinate disaster management in all spheres of government
   - promote and assist the implementation of disaster management measures in all sectors of society
4. The introduction of a new disaster management funding system, which ensures that risk reduction initiatives are taken, builds sufficient capacity to respond to disasters and provides for adequate post-disaster recovery
5. The introduction and implementation of new disaster management legislation, which brings about a uniform approach to disaster management, seeks to eliminate confusion by current legislation and address legislative shortcomings
6. The establishment of a framework to enable communities to be informed, alert and self-reliant and capable of supporting and cooperating with government in disaster prevention and mitigation

7 The establishment of a framework for coordinating and strengthening the current fragmented and inadequate training and community-awareness initiative.

The Bill also provides for an integrated, coordinated and common approach to disaster management by all spheres of government as a continuous and integrated multi-sectoral, multidisciplinary process of planning and implementation of measures aimed at preventing and reducing the risk of disasters, mitigating the severity or consequences of disasters, emergency preparedness and a state of readiness to deal with impeding current disasters or effects of disasters, and a rapid and effective response to disasters aimed at restoring normality in conditions caused by disasters.

9.8.2 Establishment of an Inter-governmental Committee on Disaster Management

The President must establish an Inter-governmental Committee on Disaster Management, which consists of cabinet members, MECs and representatives of organized local government. This committee reports to the Cabinet on the coordination of disaster management and makes recommendations to Cabinet regarding issues of disaster management and the establishment of a national framework for disaster management.

9.8.3 Establishment of a National Disaster Management Framework

The Bill also makes provision for the establishment of the National Disaster Management Framework, which must outline a coherent, transparent and inclusive policy on disaster management appropriate for the Republic of South Africa as a whole with a proportionate emphasis on disasters of different kinds, severity and magnitude that occur or may occur in Southern Africa. This National Disaster Management Framework cooperates with international management organizations and involves the private sector, non-governmental organizations, communities and volunteers in disaster management. It also provides incentives for disaster management, capacity-building and training and provides a framework within which organs of state may fund disaster management, including grants to contribute to post-disaster recovery and rehabilitation, as well as the payment for compensation to victims of disasters and their dependants.

9.8.4 The National Disaster Management Advisory Forum

A National Disaster Management Advisory Forum has been established which, among others, includes organized business, the Chamber of Mines, organized labour, the insurance industry, religious and welfare organizations, medical and paramedical and hospital organizations, as well as experts in disaster management. This Forum makes recommendations concerning national disasters and advises the state on matters relating to disaster management.

9.8.5 National Disaster Management Centre

A National Disaster Management Centre has been established that promotes, integrates and coordinates the system of disaster management with special emphasis on

prevention and mitigation by all role players involved in disaster management. The Centre is responsible for:
- Identifying and establishing communication links with disaster management role players
- Acting as a repository of, and conduit for, information concerning disasters and disaster management
- Gathering information on disaster management
- Setting disaster management plans and strategies
- Giving guidance to all concerned to prevent the risks of disaster and promote risk avoidance behaviour
- Monitoring and measuring performance, evaluating disaster plans, and preventing, mitigating and initiating response initiatives
- Giving advice and guidance by publishing guidelines and facilitating an electronic database
- Classifying and recording disasters and assessing the magnitude, severity or potential magnitude of an event
- Submitting annual reports to the Minister concerning, among others, particular problems that were experienced during disasters, and how they were addressed.

Should a national state of disaster be declared, the government process comes into action, which authorizes the following:
- Any available resources of the national government, which include assets such as stores, equipment, vehicles and facilities, are released
- Personnel of a national origin are released to provide emergency services (for example the SA Defence Force)
- A national disaster plan is in operation and this includes all the provisions made in the pre-impact phase of the disaster and this will be implemented in the event of a disaster
- The evacuation and provision of shelters for the disaster-stricken population or those who are threatened if such action is necessary to preserve life
- The regulation of traffic to and from the disaster area
- The regulation of the movement of persons and goods to, from or within the disaster area
- The control and occupancy of premises in the disaster area
- The provision, control or use of temporary emergency housing
- The suspension, or limiting of sale, dispensing or transportation of alcoholic beverages in the disaster area
- The maintenance or installation of temporary lines of communication to, from or within the disaster area
- The dissemination of information required for dealing with the disaster
- Emergency procurement procedures
- The facilitation of response and post-disaster recovery and rehabilitation
- Other steps that may be necessary to prevent an escalation of the disaster or to alleviate, contain and minimize the effects of the disaster
- The initiation of steps to facilitate international assistance.

The Bill clearly states that a national disaster is one that has actually occurred or that is threatening an area and that the above may be exercised only to the extent that is necessary for the purposes of assisting and protecting the public, providing relief to the public, preventing or combating disruption and dealing with the destructive and other effects of a disaster. The Bill also clearly includes regulations prescribing penalties for any contravention of the regulations.

9.8.6 Provincial and municipal disaster management

The Bill distinguishes between provincial and municipal disaster management (Chapters 4 and 5). The following Table provides the provisions in the Bill.

Table 9.1 Provisions in the Disaster Management Bill, 2001 (No 58 of 2001) of provincial and municipal disaster management

PROVINCIAL DISASTER MANAGEMENT	MUNICIPAL DISASTER MANAGEMENT
Each province must establish and implement a policy framework for disaster management in the province aimed at ensuring an integrated and common approach to disaster management in the province by all provincial organs of state, provincial, statutory functionaries, non-governmental institutions involved in disaster management in the province and local government.	Each metropolitan and each district municipality must establish and implement a policy framework for disaster management in the municipality aimed at ensuring an integrated and common approach to disaster management in its area by involving the municipality and statutory functionaries of the municipality, including in the case of a district, the local municipalities and statutory functionaries of the local municipalities in the area, the municipal entities operating in this area, all governmental institutions involved in disaster management in its area and the private sector. The district municipality must establish its disaster management policy after consultation with the local municipality in its area. The municipal disaster management policy must be consistent with all the provisions made in this Act, with the national disaster management framework and with the disaster management policy framework of the province concerned.
Each province must establish a disaster management centre for the province, which forms part of and functions within a department designated by the Premier of the province.	Each metropolitan and each district municipality must establish in its administration a disaster management centre after consultation with other local municipalities and may operate such centre in partnership with local municipalities.

Occupational health

PROVINCIAL DISASTER MANAGEMENT	MUNICIPAL DISASTER MANAGEMENT
The duties and powers include the following: ■ Must specialise in issues concerning disasters and disaster management in the province ■ Must promote an integrated coordinated approach to disaster management in the province with a special emphasis on preventing and mitigating by provincial organs of state in the province and other role players involved in disaster management in the province ■ Must act as an advisory and consultative body for the state and all other bodies stipulated ■ Must initiate and facilitate efforts to make funds available for disaster management in the province ■ May make recommendations to any relevant organ of state on draft legislation on the Act, the national disaster framework and other disaster management issues and the alignment of provincial and municipal legislation, as well as during the event of a provincial disaster may recommend that this area be declared a disaster.	The duties and powers include the following: ■ Must specialize in issues concerning disasters and disaster management in the municipalities ■ Must promote an integrated coordinated approach to disaster management in the municipal areas ■ Must act as an advisory and consultative body for the state and all other bodies stipulated ■ Must initiate and facilitate efforts to make funds available for disaster management in the province ■ May make recommendations to any relevant organ of state on draft legislation on the Act, the national disaster framework and other disaster management issues and the alignment of provincial and municipal legislation, as well as during the event of a municipal disaster may recommend that this area be declared a disaster.
A provincial disaster management centre must assist the national disaster centre to establish communication links with provincial organs of state and other disaster management and role players. They must also establish and maintain an electronic database and develop guidelines for the preparation and regular review of disaster management plans and emergency procedures. This centre may also request any relevant information free of charge in order to apply appropriate action. Any failure must be reported to the MEC of the province who is responsible for the disaster management in the province.	A municipal disaster management centre must assist the national disaster centre to establish communication links with municipal organs of state and other disaster management and role players. They must also establish and maintain an electronic database and develop guidelines for the preparation and regular review of disaster management plans and emergency procedures. This centre may also request any relevant information free of charge in order to apply appropriate action. Any failure must be reported to the municipal manager of the municipal centre for disaster management who is responsible for the disaster management in the province.

PROVINCIAL DISASTER MANAGEMENT	MUNICIPAL DISASTER MANAGEMENT
Prevention and mitigation include that the provincial disaster management centre, together with all the relevant role players as identified in this Act, assess and prevent or reduce the risk of disasters including determining the levels of risk, assessing the vulnerability of communities to potential risks, increasing the capacity of communities to deal with disasters, developing and implementing appropriate mitigating methodologies, developing plans, programmes and initiatives, and managing high-risk developments. A provincial disaster management centre must promote formal and informal initiatives that encourage risk avoidance behaviours by state, private-sector, non-governmental organizations, communities and individuals in the province.	
The provincial disaster management centre must also monitor the progress of preparation and regularly update disaster management plans and strategies and involve all relevant role players for formal and informal prevention, mitigation and response activities, and integrate these activities in the development plans. The centre must also from time to time measure performance and evaluate such progress and initiatives	
When disasters occur or threaten to occur in provinces, the centre must determine whether the event is a disaster and if so, immediately initiate efforts to assess the magnitude and severity of potential magnitude of the disaster, inform the National Centre for Disaster Management, alert disaster management role players that may be of assistance and promote and apply contingency plans and emergency procedures.	When a disastrous event occurs or is threatening to occur in the area of a municipality, the Centre must determine whether this event is a disaster and if so, must immediately initiate efforts to assess the magnitude and severity of potential magnitude of the disaster, inform the National Centre for Disaster Management and the Provincial Disaster Management Centre, alert disaster management role players that may be of assistance and promote and apply contingency plans and emergency procedures.

PROVINCIAL DISASTER MANAGEMENT	MUNICIPAL DISASTER MANAGEMENT
The Disaster Management Centre must submit annual reports to the MEC of the province about their progress, activities, disasters that occurred during the year, classification, magnitude and severity of disasters and the effects they had, and how these disasters were dealt with. The MEC submits the report to the Provincial legislature within 30 days after receipt and a copy is submitted to the National Centre for Disaster Management.	The Disaster Management Centre must submit annual reports to the municipal council about their progress, activities, disasters that occurred during the year, classification, magnitude and severity of disasters and the effects they had, how these disasters were dealt with, the problems they had and the way in which these problems were dealt with and the progress they have made. The Municipal Disaster Management Centre must submit a copy of the report to the National Centre and the Disaster Management Centre of the province concerned.
The duties and powers of provincial government are spelled out in Part 3 of the Bill and it is specifically stated that each provincial organ of state must prepare a disaster management plan that contains the principles in which the concept and principles of disaster management are applied in the functional area. The role and responsibilities of emergency response and post-disaster recovery and rehabilitation must be included in such a plan. It also makes provision for coordination with role players and the state and regular updating of the plans. A copy of each plan is submitted to the National Centre for Disaster Management. Each province must establish a disaster management plan for the province as a whole and coordinate with all other role players, regularly update this plan and provide for the anticipation of any disasters that may occur in these areas, identify communities at risk, provide any prevention and mitigating strategies, identify and address weaknesses in capacity to deal with possible disasters, facilitate maximum emergency preparedness, make provision for the allocation of responsibilities to role players during disasters, procure essential goods and services, establish communication, disseminate information and promote disaster relief and response.	Each municipality, according to Part 3 of the Bill, must prepare a disaster management plan for its area to circumstances prevailing in the area, coordinate and align the implementation of its plan with those of other role players and regularly update this plan. This plan must form an integral part of the municipal area and development plan and anticipate all types of disasters likely to occur in the municipal area and their possible effects, as well as identify all the communities at risk. The plan should contain appropriate prevention and mitigation strategies, must identify and address weaknesses in capacity to deal with possible disasters and facilitate maximum emergency preparedness. The plan should contain contingency plans and emergency procedures in the event of a disaster and for the management of a disaster by providing for the allocation of responsibilities to various role players, prompt disaster response and relief, procurement of essential goods and services, establishment of strategic communication, dissemination of information and also take any other measures appropriate to the situation.

PROVINCIAL DISASTER MANAGEMENT	MUNICIPAL DISASTER MANAGEMENT
The responsibilities during a provincial disaster, irrespective whether this is declared as a provincial state of disaster, are primarily coordination and management and are the responsibility of the provincial executive.	Irrespective of whether a local state of disaster has been declared, the metropolitan municipality or the district municipality are primarily responsible for the coordination and management of local disasters that occur in this area.
The declaration of a provincial state of disaster is made by the Premier of the province after consultation with the MEC. This may be by means of a notice in the Government Gazette, declaring a state of disaster if the following applies: ■ Existing legislation and contingency arrangements do not adequately provide for the provincial executive to deal with the disaster ■ Other special circumstances that warrant a state of disaster ■ The Premier makes regulations about the release of resources (stores, equipment, vehicles, facilities), personnel, implementation of the disaster plan, evacuation and temporary shelters, regulation of traffic, regulating movement of persons, traffic, goods, control of occupancy of premises, the provision, control and use of temporary housing, suspension or limiting of alcoholic beverages, maintaining and installation of lines of communication, dissemination of information, emergency measures.	The council of a municipality have the primary responsibility for coordinating and managing the disaster and may by notice of the Government Gazette, declare a state of disaster if the existing legislation and contingency arrangements do not adequately provide for the municipality to deal with the disaster or where any other special circumstances arise. Should a state of emergency be declared, the municipality may make by-laws which are the same as those contained in the opposite paragraph.

9.8.7 Funding of post-disaster recovery and rehabilitation

The Bill also deals with the funding of post-disaster recovery and rehabilitation subject to the Public Finance Management Act, 1999 (No 1 of 1999), which provides for funding during emergency situations. It also makes provision for national contributions to alleviate the effects of local and provincial disasters. It takes into account, however, certain aspects such as whether any preventive and mitigating measures have been taken to avoid the disaster, whether the damage caused was covered by insurance, the extent of financial assistance available to the community and the financial capacity of the victims.

9.9 The disaster management team

Disaster management according to the Disaster Management Bill, 2001 (No 58 of 2001), means a continuous and integrated multisectoral, multidisciplinary process of planning and implementation of measures aimed at the following:
- Preventing or reducing the risk of disasters
- Mitigating the severity or consequences of disasters
- Emergency preparedness
- A rapid and effective response to disasters
- Post-recovery and rehabilitation.

According to the above, disasters are multifaceted events that require expertise in many areas. It is particularly important to select the disaster management team carefully and to train the team to enable them to save the lives of others and to come prepared (where possible), and to inform team members about the protocol and procedures that need to be followed during a disaster. It is much too late to try to establish order in times of crisis when personnel have not been trained. In this regard, the Disaster Management Bill, 2001 (No 58 of 2001) states that emergency preparedness is a state of readiness which enables organs of state and other institutions involved in the disaster management, the private sector, communities and individuals to mobilize, organize and provide relief measures to deal with an impending or current disaster or the effects of a disaster. Thus, the key to effective disaster management is to be prepared.

During a disaster, a central command is established who oversees the identification of each person and group within the area of the scene. This is important because individuals will be able to know what the roles of their team members in the disaster area are and what actions can be expected from them. It is impossible for all people involved in the management of a disaster to know each other. A system of identification must be established in the pre-disaster phase and different identification systems have been developed which are easy to apply, quick and easy to fit and fasten, for example coloured hard hats, nameplates and area of specialization, different armbands with tasks printed on it, different coloured jumpsuits, overalls and vests. Police, fire, traffic and other officials associated in the daily life with various uniforms need not be identified because they will be visible unless specific ranks are allocated to them, for example an name band with 'investigation team' printed on it could be additional information. Velcro attachments are recommended and the use of coloured lettering on the front and back is advised, for example the word 'doctor' or 'nurse' is of great value in times of crisis.

When it comes to volunteers, especially where professionals are not necessarily needed or available at the impact stage of the disaster, rapid assessment should be done to determine their areas of experience, service possibilities, responsibilities and levels of command so they can fit into the team and a smooth running of the operation can be established.

9.10 Disaster planning

Lessons learnt from a myriad of disasters that have occurred in industry, have revealed that:
- A central organization is critical to the smooth management of accidents
- An overly optimistic predisposition can cause excessive allocation of safety resources to accident prevention at the expense of accident management.

Some of the world's most severe industrial incidents occurred during the North Sea Platform Bravo blowout where 12 700 tons of oil were strewn over the surface of the water, and the Three Mile Nuclear (TMI) incident where a nuclear core overheated and exploded. It appears that those in charge of both these plants were overly optimistic that accidents could not happen in these plants due to the stringent safety measures and resources for accident prevention. A lot of emphasis was placed on the pre-accident phase of the disaster management and neither of the accidents were anticipated nor prevented. Too little emphasis is placed on accident management and too much on prevention. Often people take for granted that due to the stringent measurement and training of personnel, it is impossible for accidents such as this to happen.

Often early warning signals are not recognized or are ignored due to an optimistic predisposition and perception of the impossibility of an accident to occur. In comparing these two examples, Fisher (1981:8) states that at TMI alarms and responses were designed for near-accidents, but that the responses to the alarms failed to prevent the accident and it took two to three days after the initiating event to recognize that a serious accident had indeed taken place. At the Bravo platform, the accident itself was recognized immediately, but the earlier events that combined the cause of the accident were not recognized. It would seem that accident prevention per se is as important as accident control and that emphasis must be placed on the recognition of the development of an accident.

Experts, managers and operators often refer to an accident as 'unique' – because in-depth safety measures and technology are generally much more advanced or superior to those of other industries or those applied in the past. Accidents do occur, however, and are then seen as configurations of weaknesses. Once this weakness had been accounted for and corrected, these individuals once again return to the assumption that an accident is once again impossible. It must be remembered that uniqueness is a myth.

When accidents of this nature do occur, all potentially participating individuals and organizations should have clear, pre-planned roles

It is often found that accident planning is not extensive for accidents that are considered preventable. The need here is to plan for the unexpected, to take into consideration the fact that preventable accidents can nonetheless occur. It is thus important that the roles of the government, the industry, operators of facilities, industry and government specialists, scientific experts, outside experts, high political officials, the press and representatives of groups of people who might be affected by an incident should be pre-determined.

The disaster plan specifies the roles, responsibilities and actions of all the members involved in the operational management of the disaster. These services do not only include the emergency services (hospitals, fire and ambulance services), but may involve the Defence Force, Red Cross, police and a variety of other organizations, including non-government and voluntary groups. In some disasters international links are established. This will involve close liaison with diplomatic staff of other counties and depending on the nature of the disaster, the police and healthcare authorities of those countries.

Any technology has a core of support from scientists and other specialist-trained individuals, who link their common ideology to share knowledge and interests. This highly technical information is simplified to communicate to others, including rivals and groups that may suffer from it as well as those who may benefit. For example, whereas setting a safety standard directly involves the industry or group of industries designing, manufacturing, supplying, using and servicing the technology, as well as the regulator, it also involves many other participants – unions, politicians, local governments, the community, consumers, rival technologists and research experts. These people would be influenced by the information provided to them, which is meant to promote the ideology that grows up around the technology. At the same time, these participants may generate conflict because of their differing perspectives and in some cases because of their own particular technological ideologies.

There are basically six types of groups involved in disasters. These include the following:
1. Accident response groups are agencies managing emergency situations and accidents.
2. Normal regulators are government agencies regulating the technology.
3. Inside experts are technical experts from government agencies, research institutes, companies and universities.
4. Affected groups are various social groups affected for better or for worse by the technology and the accident.
5. Outsiders are unorganized but influential individuals or factions affected by the accident such as politicians, outside experts and media representatives.
6. Other experts may also be cooperating to join the task team to manage a disaster. The relations of the individuals and groups involved in any disaster are highly complex and at times highly informal. Dealings and decisions take place under conditions of urgency, around-the-clock activity, exhaustion and frayed nerves so that the conflicts are likely.

    A successful disaster response requires coordination of many governmental agencies and services. The plan requires joint planning meetings, established lines of communication and authority, and regular agency drills.

Accident management plans can be more flexible and better designed to deal with rare contingencies if they are developed through dialectic process with all affected parties involved

There is not one single disaster plan that is appropriate and that could be universally applied to all communities or all industries. Every industry must establish their own emergency plans depending on the internal capabilities of the company, the local hospital or clinic facilities, and the available agencies that can be deployed in times of crisis. Close liaison with the identified facilities with regard to their emergency or disaster plans should be established so that an overall plan can take all possible aspects of potential disasters into consideration.

The disaster plan should be flexible and simple and each individual participant as well as each group's role and responsibilities should resemble their day-to-day activities as closely as possible. There is no time for lengthy discussions, consultations and learning new duties during a disaster. Every individual and group must know what to do and how to act during a disaster. The plan should be flexible so that it allows for a variation in the disaster and in the cause of different locations and nature. A basic structure is necessary and therefore each member of the team should know the chain of command. Participants in the disaster management plan should be willing to adapt to changes in the structure of the plan in order to meet unforeseen problems.

Assessment of the workplace
Even in the planning phase of any building before the actual design and construction work starts, the disaster plan and possibilities of emergencies, which may arise from operations, should be given priority.

9.11 Pre-planning for a disaster

Disaster drills are important in the pre-planning of a possible disaster. This drill gives the people involved the opportunity to evaluate their own shortcomings with regard to knowledge, coordination and cooperation, as well as the full impact of the plan. During a drill many problem areas, which still exist, are sorted out and identified and possible shortcomings are rectified. The use of equipment and facilities enable those practitioners at ground level to practise and to determine their adequacy during a disaster. Drill can, however, be extremely expensive and time consuming and should therefore be planned carefully and preferably be done in sessions rather than as a whole. For example, drills may be performed in appropriate areas in the industry where, for example, chemicals are used more often or in a receiving or triage area or in a medical station to which the patients will be transported. A comprehensive drill should be performed only if all the skills are mastered at the lower selected areas.

In order to conduct a well-conceived comprehensive disaster drill, certain pre-arrangements must be followed:

First there must be a formulation of a mock disaster scenario in order for all services to become involved. It should include a variety of services such as the blood bank, medicine, radiology, theatres, and procedures including evacuation, extrication, triage and transportation. There should be simulated hazards on the scene, for example cross-fire of opposing groups, gas leaks from pipes, loose-hanging electrical wires, water/liquid on the floor, mock fires, so that the teams can work together to eliminate the risks before the rescue teams can perform their duties. Simulation should also include members of the press, family members, looters taking advantage of the disaster, or people wandering around with curiosity. Realistic presentations of 'victims' who have been trained to fulfil their roles before the operations should be part of this whole scenario, for example victims with broken limbs, the deceased or those unsalvageable victims who, for example have lost both limbs, patients wandering around in a state of obvious shock, hysterical victims blinded by fire and gas or chemicals, people who cannot hear when they are spoken to due to the blast, victims with severe and minor wounds and those who are unconscious and trapped in dangerous settings.

Secondly, volunteers must be recruited and trained. Often the local schools, technikons and universities provide ideal 'victims'. They must be provided with 'vital sign' cards so that the rescuers can identify and classify them accordingly. At each particular area, 'invisible' monitors need to be placed to observe the actions and to record the problem areas. These observers are made 'invisible' by identifying them with bright orange or red jackets.

Thirdly, the disaster drill site must be chosen carefully and depending on the magnitude of the operation, for example if the victims will be evacuated by air, the site will represent the normal situation or setting where a disaster may occur, for example the shop floor with overhanging cranes. It should, however, not in any way jeopardize operations or endanger the lives or cause injury to 'victims' and 'rescuers'. The drill should be performed as realistically as possible and with seriousness. The whole disaster plan must now be placed into perspective and action must follow to perform the letters written on paper. Where the action and the written word differ, the plan must be changed. Any unforeseen circumstances should be noted, for example the breakdown of a communication line, interference caused by yet another explosion, anti-personnel mines that had not been identified, traffic problems due to peak hour traffic or changes in the conditions of the patients.

Lastly, the evaluation and recording of findings should be done. Evaluators should ask the question: What did the drill mean to the overall disaster plan, would they be performing or acting differently with the next drill, how could various problems be sorted out, did they learn anything? Recording the findings is important as these are used to update the overall disaster plan and to coordinate with other services in an organized manner.

9.12 Phases of a disaster response

Scene safety and security are essential parts of the operations. Safety is maintained by the police, defence force and traffic departments, as well as the industry safety and security personnel to prevent for example further injuries and damage, looting of property, onlookers and family of victims to be exposed to traumatic scenes and to preserve in many cases forensic evidence which could be vital in the outcomes of establishing the cause of a disaster and further investigations, particularly in industry. Scene security is also important to maintain in order to prevent speculations in the press, which could spread unnecessary panic and fear to the community. It is thus important to keep out those people who have not been identified (e.g. press, onlookers and volunteers) during the pre-disaster planning phase as authorized to provide assistance during the initial phase of the disaster. It is also the role of the safety and security personnel to provide a relatively safe working environment for rescuers during the immediate rescuing of victims, for example, experts to determine the possibilities of further bombs or explosive devices before rescue personnel enter the area where the explosion has occurred.

In high security areas where confidentiality is of the utmost importance (for example in state facilities or computer-related security systems), the police will take special precautions not to allow people in that area without the authorization of their authorities.

Examples of scene safety and security services roles include:
- Extinguishing fires to prevent chain-reaction explosions
- Inspection of buildings for further collapse
- Closing of treacherous transportation routes
- Controlling traffic
- Controlling of terrorists
- Promptly evacuating potentially dangerous sites
- Establishing and protecting transportation routes for incoming disaster management personnel and equipment
- Establishing routes for evacuees to hospitals.

The first source of information for first responders at the scene is the scene itself – the conditions, the environmental effects and the obvious first indications of the conditions of the patients. The scene can provide a great deal of information, which the patient may not be able to tell the first responders. This information must at all times be remembered as it may contribute to the effective treatment of the patient. It is important, however, for all rescue personnel and other first responders, before approaching the patient, to take a close look around them to try to establish whether it is safe to approach or not. There is no point in the rescue personnel being hurt or killed going to the assistance of a victim. The following are examples of the aspects that need to be considered:
- Possibility of fire or explosion
- Electrical wires lying around
- Hazardous cargo in the immediate vicinity
- Unstable vehicles or structural damage
- Violent or hostile crowds.

If there is any potential hazard to responders it must be eliminated before an attempt is made to reach a patient. The following slogan must at all times be kept in mind:

Dead heroes can't save lives. Injured heroes are a nuisance!

Extrication, triage and treatment are the three activities that take place concurrently in most disasters. Once the scene is declared safe and has been assessed, the central command system established and rescue teams alerted, first responders rescue teams can enter the scene to extricate, triage and treat the casualties. There are most often very rapid decisions and review of procedures, and progress made takes place within a very short time.

Extrication may range from simple removal of ambulatory patients from the scene to lengthy rescue operations where victims may be cut from wreckage, dug out of rubble, and surgical amputations being undertaken on the scene or while the victim is trapped, for example in mining operations. The first responders may be the initial persons involved in the extrication but depending on the extent of the disaster other categories of helpers may also be called in.

Triage can be described as the disaster response by sorting of patients according to the severity of their injuries, which will determine their immediate treatment and priority transport from the scene. This process saves time and lives and expedites proper treatment.

The disaster response consists of three phases: the activation phase, the implementation phase, and the recovery phase.

1 Activation phase

The first phase, the activation phase, has two components: the notification and initial response.

The first notification of a disaster usually comes from staff employed by the industry. However, disasters that indirectly affect the industry (e.g. floods, fire in the community, and disease outbreak) will usually be reported by the public. The usual route is that the public will inform the fire and emergency services or the police department, usually by a 10111 call. These departments have a system of command, which will immediately deploy/dispatch personnel to the area that is affected to determine the extent of the reported disaster and to evaluate the situation before disaster operations are activated. These are called the 'first responders' to the scene and they are trained to evaluate the situation quickly before any attempt is made to render direct medical assistance and to estimate the following:

- Specific location and accessibility to the area of the disaster
- Type of situation (e.g. fire, disease outbreak, nuclear accident) as well as the nature of the disaster (e.g. of human origin or natural)
- The number of people involved in the disaster and the extent of the damage (because this may also jeopardize the lives of rescue teams in cases where structural damage has occurred, especially in industry where for example chemicals may have serious effects on rescue teams or possible bombs or explosives may still be present)
- The effect of the disaster (e.g. the type of injuries sustained by the victims)
- Tentative cause of the disaster (note that confidentiality must at all times be maintained until the full investigation and report is officially released).

Early accurate information leads to the appropriate mobilization of disaster response personnel and materials. Once the emergency services have determined the extent of the disaster and the tentative details are available, they can use the information to follow the prescribed protocol to inform the various participating services and disaster operations will start immediately.

The second component of the activation phase is the establishment of a central command post and further assessment of the scene. The central command system for any disaster is the heart of the operations and is established immediately following the disaster. The chain of command would be established during the pre-disaster planning

Emergency care and disaster management

phase and is determined by the nature, size and number of victims involved in the disaster. For example, where there is mass casualty evacuation, the disaster central command would involve fire and rescue personnel, including specially trained nurses and doctors who will fill the positions as medical commanders. The central command post will be set up as close to the scene as safety allows. This central command post will also be established upwind and uphill due to the potentially dangerous liquids and gases, which may contaminate the area of the disaster further.

The central command works closely with the other members of the team, such as police, traffic, paramedical personnel and safety officers. The central command would have the following roles:

- Make an overall assessment of the disaster situation
- Immediately establish a communication system with key stakeholders (e.g. government health department, hospitals, management of the industry)
- Appoint a chief triage manager who will organize the treatment, manage the classification and transport of victims (could be a doctor, nurse or paramedic)
- Establish a central primary triage centre where all the victims who have been involved in the disaster would be assessed, classified, given immediate emergency care and transported in order of their classification
- Implement an identification system of staff and workers in the disaster area
- Control recruitment and deployment of rescue personnel
- Establish the need for equipment and the control thereof.

2 Implementation phase

The second phase of the disaster response is the implementation phase, which consists of three components. The first component is search and rescue, which are usually carried out by the fire and rescue personnel because of their special expertise and equipment needed in a hazardous environment. Without expertise and specialized equipment, medical and rescue personnel may also become victims.

The second component of the implementation phase involves triage, stabilization and transport of the victims. The first arriving medical providers must assess medical needs, make calls to mobilize medical resources, establish contact with central command (e.g. fire chief) and identify hazards and a safe casualty collection point. As more ambulances and helpers arrive, early treatment begins but it is limited to airway control, administration of oxygen, control of haemorrhage and back boarding. Triage has begun and the victims are now being grouped by priority within the triage or casualty area.

The third component of the implementation phase is definite management of scene hazards and victims. Victims are now transported to hospitals for care and treatment according to priorities identified by the triage officer.

3 Recovery phase

The recovery stage is the third stage of the disaster response. The first stage of the recovery phase is withdrawal from the scene after making sure that no missed victims were left behind. The second stage is the return to normal operations. Ambulances are thoroughly cleaned, stocked and checked. Standard operating procedures resume. It is also during this stage that the Red Cross and other voluntary or governmental services provide shelter and food to those victims who were not injured. Concerned family members are counselled and assisted in locating their loved ones.

The final stage of the recovery phase is debriefing. There are two types of debriefing. Firstly, debriefing about the incident operations takes place. This type of debriefing follows the disaster and is an analysis of the operation in order to improve future disaster responses. The second type of debriefing is psychological in nature and it plays an important part in the early identification and avoidance of potentially psychological difficulties among the many rescuers. Debriefing should be arranged as soon as possible after the disaster and should be followed up with sessions to identify prolonged effects and recollections of aspects during the disaster.

9.13 Triage

Triage begins with the first contact in the scene of the disaster. Triage is the process of sorting and classifying patients into categories according to priority of treatment. The aim of triage is to provide the most good for the largest number of patients. Rescuers at the scene check and correct, if possible, airway, breathing and circulation on each victim. Only rapid life-saving procedures are performed, for example ventilation is done to see if the patient does not resume spontaneous breathing. Cardiopulmonary resuscitation is not done.

Triage is again done at the triage area. Here the sorting of victims and the tagging and the identification of patients take place.

9.13.1 Sorting of victims

There is a number of triage tagging systems and there is some controversy over the value and the system. Tags, however, provide a record of critical medical interventions and prevent some redundancies in the triage survey by identifying those patients who have already been checked. It has also been found in disasters that medical personnel do not use tags because they do not use them as a daily routine. It is recommended that medical, nursing and paramedical personnel use this system of tagging as a daily activity.

The first tagging occurs when the patients are colour-coded according to their salvageability and priority of treatment starts. The following are the internationally used colour and priority classifications of patients:

- Black colour coding (also priority 4 or P4 patients) is used for victims who are not salvageable. In other words those dead or near dead – for example, who are still alive, but are so severely injured that any attempt to save them would be futile or would use up the resources (time, medical personnel and supplies) that are needed to treat the many known salvageable victims. Rescuers should, if possible, keep in mind the possibility of organ donors when coding these victims.
- Red colour coding (also priority 1 or P1 patients) is used for victims who are critically injured, but would benefit from immediate life-saving interventions.
- Yellow colour coding (also priority 2 or P2 patients) is used for patients who are seriously injuted and need medical attention soon, but not immediately.
- Green colour coding (also priority 3 or P3 patients) is used for patients who are

the so-called walking-wounded. These patients usually have minor non-life-threatening lacerations, simple fractures and sprains and require minor attention, which can be delayed for 24 to 72 hours.

All patients in every category should continuously be assessed. Triage is an ongoing, dynamic process. Victims' conditions are constantly changing and it must be remembered that a priority 3 patient may turn into a priority 1 patient in a matter of seconds. Medical personnel must not assume that those walking around do not need attention.

Which patients fall under which category will depend on the size of the disaster and the medical equipment and resources available.

9.13.2 Identification of victims

The identification of victims should be implemented through central command. The METTAG (Medical Emergency Triage Tag) System is an internationally recognized identification system used in large-scale operations to establish the condition of patients, their priority of treatment and transport and their identity. The tag is colour coded to correspond with the triage category which the patient has been assigned. The tag also contains a unique number to make identification and recording easier. In this system each victim is tagged with essential information such as the:
- Name, address and telephone number (if possible)
- Primary injuries
- Treatment, for example intravenous therapy.

The time and dosage of all medication are essential information, which must be written on the tag, for example the time, when the intravenous therapy was started, and the type of intravenous fluid. This is essential information because further treatment will depend on what and how much has been given to the patient.

In the management of victims, a record system must be established in which the essential information is written as indicated above.

Assessment, diagnosis and initiation of planned interventions are almost simultaneous activities when working with mass casualties. Several first-aid principles are followed at the scene of the disaster and this includes:
- Remove the victim from the hazard only when the risk (e.g. fire) outweighs the danger of moving the victim.
- Establish the airway, usually by elevating the jaw. Paramedics or other healthcare providers may insert an oesophageal obturator airway or suitably qualified personnel may perform endotracheal intubation.
- Initiate cardiopulmonary resuscitation as indicated.
- Control obvious haemorrhage, usually with direct pressure.
- Splint spine and extremities.
- Apply pneumatic antishock garment (PASG) (this is only done by certified personnel).
- Establish intravenous access.
- Move and transport as soon as possible.

During a disaster, victims are tagged initially at the scene and removed to the primary triage area where experienced and specifically trained medical personnel assess them and the chief triage officer reassesses tagged victims. Here they are assigned numbers, as identification is not always possible. Each patient is then assigned to predetermined areas according to their category. Here appropriately trained and experienced medical personnel will take over the treatment and care of the assigned victims. Once the patients are declared stable for transport they are removed to appropriate care facilities as arranged by central command.

Throughout this whole process, constant communication with central command is maintained to arrange for transport, backup, equipment, and to alert facilities of the category of patients who are to be transported. The most critical patients will be transported first to the nearest appropriately equipped hospital (Level 1 hospital) and the least critical will be sent last. Often the lowest category (walking-wounded) of patients are transported in large numbers by non-emergency vehicles (for example in a bus) early in the disaster management process in order to clear the scene and to facilitate the removal and care of other victims. Seriously injured persons are often transported to any nearby medical facility in order to stabilize them for transport to a level 1 facility by, for example, fixed-wing aircraft or helicopter.

Treatment at the scene of the disaster, as well as during the extrication, assessment and triage, must be simple and critical life saving.

1 Primary survey

The primary survey of the victim is designed to identify immediate life-threatening situations, treat them and to assess further treatment and immediate transport.

The first step in the primary survey of any patient is SAFETY. Once it is safe to approach the patient, the level of consciousness (LOC) of the patient can be determined by asking the patient's name, greeting the patient or speaking to the patient.

Once the level of consciousness has been determined, the rescuer can continue with the following:
- AIRWAY: if not open, open it
- BREATHING: look, listen and feel for signs of breathing
- CIRCULATION: determine if the victim has a pulse carotid/brachial and determine if there is any life-threatening bleeding.

In some cases the primary survey can be performed at a glance, for example if the patient is talking coherently then there is no problem with the primary survey. If the patient is unconscious, however, the rescuer must proceed step-by-step through the procedure of the primary survey.

2 Secondary survey

The secondary survey is usually performed in the receiving area for victims and consists of taking the history, vital signs, head-to-toe examination and evaluation of the mechanism of injury. The purpose is to get baseline data to assess whether the person's condition is deteriorating or improving and to assess for any further or other injuries, which may not have been so evident with the primary survey (for example internal bleeding or head injury).

History. The following are valuable when obtaining the history of a patient:
S = Signs and symptoms
A = Allergies
M = Medication
P = Past medical history
L = Last meal
E = Event leading to illness or injury

Vital signs are illustrated in Tables 9.2 to 9.5. These vital signs serve as baseline signs to which a patient's deterioration or improvement are measured.

Table 9.2 Taking the vital signs

VITAL SIGNS	OBSERVATION
Level of consciousness	The use of the GCS, RTS and AVPU determines the LOC of the patient
Pulse	Rate, rhythm and strength is monitored
Respiration	Monitor by look, listen and feel Normal range (adult) 12–20 breaths per minute Abnormal high > 29 breaths per minute Abnormal low < 8 breaths per minute
Skin colour	Determine colour, temperature and condition which include being: Clammy, dry, dehydrated Pink, pale, cyanosed Cold, warm, hot
Blood pressure	Hypotensive, hypertensive, normotensive
Reaction to stimuli	Painful, verbal
Pupils	Size and reaction
Capillary refill	Must be within 2 seconds
Heamoglucotest	Hypo- or hyperglycaemia
Ability to move limbs	Flexion, extension

Occupational health

Table 9.3 The Glascow Coma Scale

EYE OPENING	Spontaneous	4
	To voice	3
	To pain	2
	None	1
VERBAL RESPONSE	Orientated	5
	Confused	4
	Inappropriate words	3
	Incomprehensible words	2
	None	1
MOTOR RESPONSE	Obeys commands	6
	Localises pain	5
	Withdraws with pain	4
	Flexion with pain	3
	Extension with pain	2
	None	1
TOTAL SCORE	15	

Table 9.4 The AVPU Scale

A = ALERT	Is the patient conscious and alert?
V = VERBAL	Does the patient talk, moan to painful stimuli?
P = PAIN	Does the patient react to painful stimuli?
U = UNCONSCIOUS	Is the patient unresponsive?

Table 9.5 The Revised Trauma Score (RTS)

BLOOD PRESSURE	More than 89 mmHg (systolic)	4
	76–89 mmHg	3
	50–75 mmHg	2
	1–49 mmHg	1
	Impalpable	0
RESPIRATION	10–29/min	4
	> than 29/min	3
	6–9/min	2
	1–5/min	1
	None	0
GLASCOW COMA SCALE	13–15	4
	9–12	3
	6–8	2
	4–5	1
	3	
TOTAL RTS	12	

Head-to-toe survvey. The following table gives examples of the information that could be obtained during the head-to-toe survey. Depending on the mechanism of injury, the list will change accordingly.

Table 9.6 Head-to-toe survey

AREA OF INVESTIGATION	POSSIBLE FINDINGS
Scalp	bleeding, wounds, deformity
Ears	blood, CSF fluid draining
Eyes	blood, pupil size injury to orbit, colour of sclera
Head	deformity of face breath odours injuries to mouth loose teeth
Neck	oedema, distended neck veins, wounds, burns, deformities, trachea deviation, surgical emphysema
Chest	shape, expansion, accessory muscles use, equal air entry, abnormal sounds, trachea deviation, contusions, penetrating objects, pain, tenderness, rigidity, puncture wounds
Abdomen	pain, tenderness, penetrating objects, distension, rigidity, guarding, wounds, contusions, evisceration,
Pelvis	stability, pain, tenderness, contusion
Genitalia	Females: pain, bleeding, swelling, discharge, redness
Extremities	Males: penis, scrotum wounds – swelling, hematuria, discharge, oedema, pulses compare needle marks, bites, , wounds, deformities, loss of power, loss of sensation, medic alert tags
Back	oedema, wounds, deformities, contusions
Skin	bleeding, redness, burns, cyanosis, cold, clammy, warm, blue, mottled, smell

Depending on the availability of advanced trained medical and nursing personnel, possible delays with transport time and the total size of the disaster, as well as the logistics around the disaster area, more advanced care may be given. This may include the placement of intravenous lines, administration of life-support medicine and the application of splints, bandages, underwater drains and tubes, to name but a few.

Transport of patients takes place from the primary triage area and is coordinated with central command and the chief triage officer. In order to coordinate the activities, it is important for the central command to know of the number and type of vehicles available, as well as the level of training of the transport personnel in order to best manage their use. The red tagged victims will usually be transported first to the nearest appropriately equipped facility. Emergency personnel attending to these patients must be alerted to the fact that the condition of these patients may change very rapidly and that the triage officer must be alerted of the change of the condition of the victims.

The allocated personnel from the Department of Health must be called to the scene in order to determine the possibility of further community health risks (e.g. disease outbreak due to contamination of water, possible pollution of poisons to the area and secondary risks such as fires). These officials can arrange for shelter for the homeless (e.g. mining in remote areas), determine the need for a state of alert and involve governmental support and financial aid.

Care of the dead is an important issue to consider as forensic evidence could be of vital importance to the company, as well as to the family. Ideally the dead must not be removed from the scene until they have been seen by the medical examiner. If the presence of the body impedes the rescue of other victims, then the body must be removed. Often police or fire film crews are there to tape or film the scene and all rescuers, volunteers and medical personnel must be alerted not to disturb any evidence, which could be essential in the future. Provision must be made for the removal, identification and holding of the dead as this could cause a health risk in the community. A temporary morgue may be established at the scene and central command may allocate security-policing officials to keep relatives, bystanders and the press away from the facility.

9.14 Emergency management of certain trauma

This chapter does not intend at all to provide a course in first aid and resuscitation. It is merely a basic outline of some of the situations that could be found in times of disaster. It is advisable that all people concerned in the rescue operation should at least have a valid and updated advanced first-aid certificate (nurses, doctors and paramedics should for example have at least the Basic Trauma Life Support and if possible the Advanced Life Support which provides adequate training for those who initially treat the patient at the scene).

9.14.1 Wounds

Wounds and soft tissue injuries are always treated with respect and on the scene of the disaster, the same applies. No unnecessary movement and hasty observations must be made. A small, obviously shallow wound may in fact have large internal effects, as is the case in bullet wounds or penetrating wounds by sharp objects (missiles caused by flying objects during explosions). One must never assume that the patient's wounds are minimal at the scene. The following table provides a classification of the most important wounds and soft tissue injuries, which will be found at a scene of an incident, not necessarily only at the disaster site.

Table 9.7 Classification, description and treatment of wounds

TYPE OF WOUND	DESCRIPTION	TREATMENT AT A SCENE
Abrasion	A superficial injury to the skin, which is invariably contaminated with dirt. The mechanism of injury may be compared with sandpaper being rubbed over the skin. Only the superficial layer of the skin is usually affected. Common causes are falls, motorcycle accidents, bicycle accidents, grass burns, carpet wounds.	Clear off loose debris. Wound should be kept moist because if bandages are applied, tissue will stick to it and loosening it will cause further damage.
Laceration	Tear wound of the skin, soft tissue or internal organs due to forceful blow with a blunt object causing a wound with jagged edges. Commonly caused by cutting with instruments and unguarded machinery or any other cutting action. These wounds have rough edges.	Always treat with associated injuries, for example fractures may also occur. Assess distal pulses and function and dress with field dressing.
Incisions	Cutting usually causes these wounds, often with a knife, blade and the edges are smooth.	Assess distal pulses and apply pressure bandage if necessary or use field bandage. Important if bleeding continues, apply bandages over the soaked ones, never remove bandages except for further inspection.
Avulsions	These are tearing injuries in which the part torn becomes partially or totally separated from the limb. This kind of wound has a loose hanging flap of tissue.	Treat as for any open wound, fold flap back (gently) after cleaning. If torn off, treat as for amputation.
Puncture wounds	These are wounds caused by pointed instruments as well as low-velocity projectiles. Owing to the low energy transfer to tissues these wounds are considered to be stab wounds. The size of the wound is often misleading – more emphasis	Observe for entry and exit wounds, apply SABC (Safety, Airway, Breathing, Circulation) at all times. Clean wound, never remove an impaled object, treat for shock and prioritize transport.

TYPE OF WOUND	DESCRIPTION	TREATMENT AT A SCENE
	should be placed on the site and depth of the wound. A small entrance wound may extend very deep and result in extensive internal bleeding.	
Gunshot wounds	These are wounds caused by projectiles and are directly related to the energy transfer to the tissues. A high-velocity projectile has the capacity for greater energy transfer. The factors determining energy transfer to the tissues are velocity, instability of the projectile, shape of the projectile, consistency of the target and whether the projectile breaks with impact. These injuries cause major internal bleeding due to the shock wave they create with impact.	SABC is the first concern. Treat as for puncture wounds. Important here (and also for the puncture wounds) is to maintain and keep forensic evidence safe and not to tamper with it or to remove if not absolutely necessary.
Amputations	This injury involves the extremities and digits, which are either cut off or torn off. Jagged skin and bone are visible.	Treat as for open wounds, partially clean the limb. Place the amputated limb in a plastic bag, mark with patient's name, time of injury and date, and place bag or container on ice. Take container to the hospital with the limb. Place a firm pressure bandage on stump and prioritize transport.
Contusions	Blunt injury without penetration to the skin. This is a direct result of the rupturing of small blood vessels under the skin, causing intestinal bleeding and therefore discoloration. Major intestinal bleeding of major organs and blood vessels may not be so obvious.	Check and treat for underlying injuries and apply a cold compress if possible for swelling. Note the original size of the contusion for later comparison, as well as severe distension or swelling of the area (e.g. abdomen or chest). Observe ABCs carefully.

TYPE OF WOUND	DESCRIPTION	TREATMENT AT A SCENE
Eviscerations	These are wounds where the wall of the abdomen is opened and the bowel may be hanging out or protruding.	ABCs are important here. Leave the viscera on the surface of the abdomen. NEVER push the viscera back into the abdomen. Cover the viscera gently with soaked sterile saline or water towel to prevent dehydration. Cover patient with clean towel. ABCs are very important. Prioritize transport.

Source: Adapted from Paolini, Buchan & Dalgety, 2001:119–121

9.14.2 Burns

There is nothing more painful, debilitating and devastating than burns. Therefore, the most important aspect is prevention. Severe burns are found in patients during most disasters and the essence of treatment and management is to get the patient to a specialized unit where these injuries can get the best and immediate attention. It is important to get the following information regarding burns, namely:

- Time and date of burn
- Causative agent of the burn (e.g. fire, chemicals, radioactive materials, plastics)
- Extent of the burn (see Wallace Rule of Nines)
- Age of the victim
- Prior treatment of the burnt area
- Space or area where the burn occurred (e.g. closed space, veld fire)
- Exposure to chemicals, plastics, nuclear or radiation agents
- The level of consciousness
- Underlying medical history of the victim (e.g. diabetic).

9.14.2.1 Causes of burns

The following may cause burns:

Thermal burns, which are caused by sunburn, steam, boiling liquid, radiation and direct contact with a hot object.

Chemical burns, which are caused by chemicals such as acids, alkalis and other corrosive substances. The degree and severity of the burn depends on the nature, concentration, quantity, penetrating power and mode of action of the substance and the length of time in contact with the skin. The substance will continue to burn until it is removed from the skin or neutralized. When treating a victim with chemical burns it helps to know what kind of chemical it is and if water is the best substance to be used for flushing. Most chemicals can, however, be flushed from the skin with copious amounts of water. Should the chemical have splashed into the eyes of the victim, flush with large amounts of water. Once the burnt area has been flushed, cover with sterile dressing.

Electrical burns are not the same as thermal burns. An electrical burn is small on the surface, yet can have devastating effects on the internal organs. The extent of tissue destruction depends largely on the intensity of the current passing through the tissues. Characteristically there is an entrance burn and an exit burn. The intense heat that is produced destroys the tissues along the pathway.

Slow alternating current causes muscle spasms that 'freeze' the victim to the source. Direct current tends to 'throw' the victim away from the source. Therefore, alternating current increases the duration of contact. Injury will take place until the contact area is carbonized, then contact will break. Low voltage will travel along the pathway of least resistance, whereas high voltage will travel along the most direct pathway. Secondary injuries should therefore also be suspected due to the falling from a high place, or injury due to falling and bumping against objects while being in contact with the electrical source.

Injury from lightning may result from direct stroke, side flash (current discharged from a vertical point) and stride potential (where lightning flows from one leg through the other). Most survivors of lightning survive because they have not been hit directly. The complications of electrical burns are serious and need to be treated immediately and most often these victims perish due to severe shock reaction. Cardiopulmonary problems such as ventricular fibrillation and respiratory arrest are common. Neurological damage may occur and cutaneous wounds are seen. Vascular problems are common in the form of arterial and venous thrombosis.

Radiation burns can cause severe thermal burns. There are two forms of radiation burns, namely from light and heat (sun) and by ionising radiation which cannot be seen or heard and of which there are three types, namely alpha, beta and gamma. Exposure to alpha and beta radiation is least dangerous, but gamma radiation results from nuclear accidents and is most often fatal.

Inhalation burns are the burns caused by the inhalation of hot air, which may cause severe mucosal inflammation and tracheitis in the upper trachea. Steam inhalation causes inflammation and damage to the lower respiratory tract. Inhalation burns are suspected when the face and anterior chest are burnt, soot is seen in the nostrils and mouth, there is a history of steam burns and respiratory distress is present.

9.14.2.2 Classification of burns
Burns are classified as follows:
Superficial burns are characterized by blistering, pain and redness, and only the epidermis is involved.

Partial thickness burns are characterized by redness and blistering with slight or no pain and scarring – this means the epidermis and parts of the dermis are involved.

Full thickness burns are characterized by no pain (due to damage to nerves) and bad scarring, and the epidermis, dermis and subcutaneous tissue are involved.

Emergency care and disaster management

The extent of the burns is measured by using Wallace's Rule of Nines (see Figure 9.1).

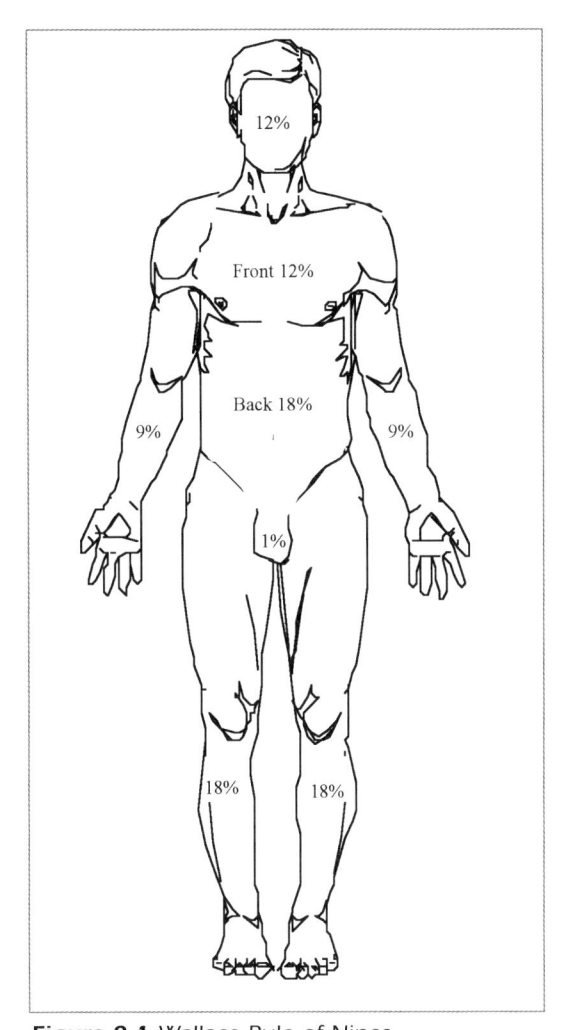

Figure 9.1 Wallace Rule of Nines

Use the palm of the victim's hand, as it is equal to approximately 1 per cent of the total body surface area, for an assessment of patches of burnt area.

The complicating factors for burns are those caused by inhalation burns involving more than 30 per cent of the total body surface area (because this now involves damage to underlying bone) and factures. Acids or electrical burns (electrical burns have a small entrance wound, e.g. the hand, and follow the shortest road/path to earth, e.g. the foot, which will have a large exit wound). People with underlying medical conditions such as diabetes and heart problems may be more seriously affected by burns.

Critical burns are those affecting the respiratory tract, the face, hands, feet and genitalia, superficial burns of greater than 75 per cent of the total body surface, partial thickness burns of greater than 30 per cent of the total surface area, and full thickness burns of greater than 10 per cent of the total body surface area.

9.14.2.3 Treatment of burn injuries

During the fire, explosion or causative source of the burning area, safety for oneself as well as the victim is important. Toxic fumes, loose-hanging electrical wires and other dangers may still be in the disaster area, which may harm the rescuers as well as the victim. Usually an officer of the fire department will declare the scene safe. Unless this is done, rescue personnel should not enter the scene.

Airway is important because burns do not occur only on the outside (skin) but the airways may be burnt as well. Ensure that the airway is opened and maintained and the victim is breathing and if available, give high percentage of humidified oxygen because of smoke inhalation.

Ensure that the victim has a pulse and monitor the pulse continuously. It is important to cut away the burnt clothing but do not attempt to pull stuck clothing out of a burn. Do not remove any impaled objects at the scene. Irrigate all burnt areas with sterile water or saline if available. Do not use tap water. Take the vital signs of the victim very often and as far as possible because this may change if the person goes into shock. A secondary survey (whole body examination) is done to determine underlying injuries and these are treated accordingly. Cover all burnt areas with burnshield as soon as possible and insert intravenous fluid if possible. It is important that these patients be transported immediately to a primary facility because of the pain a person endures.

It is important to never open any blisters due to the amount of fluid loss and because blistering prevents infections as they shield open wounds. Never apply any ointments or remedies to the burnt areas – leave for the specialists at the hospital. Cool the burnt area down for a minimum of 20 minutes if possible, but never use ice or ice water to cool the burnt areas as this may cause frostbite and further shock.

9.14.3 Bleeding

The normal average person has about 70 ml/kg blood in the body. Blood loss therefore causes a deficiency of the transport ability of the blood for organ perfusion and a decrease in the oxygen content in the blood is seen. Life-threatening blood loss in adults is approximately 1 000 ml, in children 1–4 years, 250 ml, 4–8 years 500 ml and in babies 25 ml.

Bleeding can be externally visible or subcutaneous, which is beneath the skin in the soft tissues and muscles and is usually visible as a large blue bruise or haematoma and internal bleeding. Blood is deposited into the body cavities or organs. Internal bleeding can be observed when blood is coughed up, vomited, or seen in the stool or urine, however, internal bleeding is often not visible, except when vital signs such as blood pressure reveal the precedence thereof.

There are basically three types of bleeding, namely:
1. *Arterial bleeding* is bleeding from an artery with blood spurting out – the blood is bright red and blood loss does not stop spontaneously.
2. *Venous bleeding* is more often seen because veins lie near the surface of the skin and are easier managed or controlled. The blood flow is constant and the blood is dark red.

3 *Capillary bleeding* is found with abrasions when the blood is oozing from the capillary bed and is observed by slow flow of blood loss.

Signs and symptoms of bleeding include tachycardia, tachypnoea, a narrowed pulse pressure, decreased urine output, cool clammy skin, poor capillary refill, low central venous pressure, and in later stages hypotension and altered level of consciousness. If the victim is not resuscitated and the haemorrhage progresses, with blood loss of 20 to 40 per cent, patients develop tachycardia, tachypnoea, have postural changes in blood pressure and may be confused and agitated. Late stages of unattended blood loss include hypotension and oliguria and respiration becomes quick and deeper. The skin becomes mottled. If the blood loss is more than 40 per cent, the victim also shows a marked decrease or absence of the peripheral pulses, pallor, lethargy or obtundation.

The emergency treatment of blood loss is based on two principles, namely the control of the bleeding and the maintenance of oxygen delivery. To control bleeding the immediate reaction should be to directly place a pressure bandage or the hand firmly on the wound. Dressings should not be removed at all but should be kept in position at all times. Merely place new bandages over the soaked ones. In cases of serious bleeding it should first be controlled by direct pressure before placing sterile bandages over the wound. In cases of arterial bleeding, the artery forceps may be used to locate the bleeding artery, however, this is often very difficult. Otherwise directly press the bleeding artery against the underlying tissue or against the patient's bones. It must be kept in mind, however, that blood loss cannot be controlled at the scene of a disaster or an accident and any delay in the transport of the patient is excessive.

Elevation of the affected limb above the level of the heart may be effective because the gravity helps to decease bleeding, but caution is necessary if there is a fracture, an impaled object or a spinal injury.

Pressure points are points where large arteries lie near the skin surface and directly over a bony prominence and can be used to apply indirect pressure. The following pressure points can be used to control bleeding in an emergency:

- *Facial artery*: Approximately two fingers width from the angle of the mandible over the edge of the jaw for control of bleeding from the same side of the face
- *Temporal artery*: Can be closed by pressure just anterior to the eternal auditory canal for bleeding from the scalp
- *Brachial artery*: By resting the person's upper arm in the palm of the hand and compressing the brachial artery with straightened fingers against the middle section of the humerus, bleeding of the lower part of the arm can be checked
- *Femoral artery*: Bleeding from the leg can be controlled by compressing the femoral artery with the thumb or palm of the hand against the pelvis.

Blood loss can also be controlled by the use of a blood pressure apparatus or a tourniquet, although this is not recommended for rescuers or helpers who have not been trained to do this type of procedure. It is also important that if a tourniquet is used, a trained person is available all the time to release the pressure as indicated for this procedure. Applying a tourniquet is an extreme emergency procedure and ONLY certified paramedics, trained nurses and medical doctors should use this type of measure.

Internal bleeding is the loss of blood into the body cavities and leads to hypovolaemic shock (loss of blood and fluid). Internal bleeding is suspected by the external factors, namely skull trauma, bleeding from any of the orifices of the body (e.g. anus, vagina, nose, vomiting, coughing, ears), penetrating wounds of the chest and abdomen, large bruises, blood in stool and urine and fractures of, for example, the pelvis, humerus and skull.

There is a limit to the emergency treatment that can be applied at the scene for victims suffering from internal bleeding. Emergency surgery is often the only treatment. However, the Pneumatic Anti-Shock Garment (PASG) can be applied ONLY by certified persons, but is used only under extreme circumstances. Splints can be applied to limbs where closed fractures occur (blood loss from a closed fracture of a femur is 1–1.5 litre). Victims must never receive any fluids per mouth.

The use of the MAST suit is controversial and the enthusiasm for its use has begun to wane. Only trained and experienced personnel should apply this garment in severe cases. The MAST is used with much success in pelvic fractures, however, the presence of other injuries must be eliminated. Tintinalli, Ruiz and Krome (1997:198) state that while there is no doubt that the use of the MAST will increase blood pressure, most likely through a rise in systemic vascular resistance, there is no evidence that the use of the MAST does in fact improve outcomes. In the presence of shock and chest injury, the use of the MAST may increase haemorrhage severity and mortality.

9.14.4 Shock

Although shock may have a number of different origins, it can be described as any condition resulting in inadequate tissue perfusion (decreased oxygen supply to the tissues) to body organs by the cardiovascular system. Shock is caused by three factors: failure to pump, decreased circulating volume of fluid, and significant dilatation of blood vessels.

Table 9.8 provides a description and signs and symptoms of shock.

Table 9.8 Classification and description of types of shock

TYPE OF SHOCK	DESCRIPTION
Hypovolaemic shock is a form of shock caused by the loss of fluid or blood from the body. *Signs and symptoms:* ■ Restlessness and anxiety ■ Thirst ■ Skin pale, clammy, cold, sometimes mottled ■ Tachycardia, weak, narrowed pulse ■ Tachypnoea shallow ■ Hypotension ■ Decreased urine output	Occurs usually after internal or external haemorrhage due to trauma. Can also be the result of other conditions associated with fluid volume loss without bleeding, such as burns or severe dehydration. Burns cause the loss of plasma through the skin and dehydration can occur following severe vomiting, diarrhoea, perfuse sweating, diabetic ketoacedosis and inadequate fluid intake.

TYPE OF SHOCK	DESCRIPTION
■ Poor capillary refill ■ Low central venous pressure ■ Altered mentation ■ Nausea and vomiting	
Neurogenic shock This is a form of shock caused by profound failure of the heart where the nervous system is no longer able to control the diameter of the blood vessels (as seen in spinal cord injury), and without this control, the blood vessels will dilate, thereby increasing the volume of the cardiovascular system. There is no longer enough blood to fill the entire system and the blood will pool in certain areas of the body. *Signs and symptoms:* ■ Due to decreased epinephrine secretion, the victim may not exhibit tachycardia, sweating or a pale skin, and often altered mental status and hypotension may be the only signs of neurogenic shock ■ May have diaphragmatic breathing or no breathing at all ■ Priapism in males, incontinence in female ■ 'Hands-up' or arms across the chest position ■ Flaccid paralysis ■ Loss of sensation below injury ■ Loss of bladder and bowel control	Usually due to spinal injuries or brain injuries where nerve impulses prevent impulses from the brain's regulatory system to reach the vital organs. This disruption in the sympatic nervous system prevents secretions of epinephrine, resulting in profound vasodilatation.
Cardiogenic shock This is a form of shock caused by profound failure of the heart due to cardiac arrest, dysrythmias, acute myocardial infarction, pulmonary embolism and severe acidosis. The heart is so damaged that it can no longer pump adequately, therefore tissue perfusion is not maintained. *Signs and symptoms:* ■ Systolic blood pressure < 90	In myocardial infarction, the damage to the wall of the heart may be so severe that the heart will no longer be able to contract as forcefully as it once did and cardiac output will decrease, leading to shock. These victims may suffer from severe respiratory distress due to the backup of fluid from the right side of the heart to the lungs. Chest pain may also occur.

TYPE OF SHOCK	DESCRIPTION
- Peripheral vasoconstriction - Oliguria - Pulmonary vascular congestion - Confusion and comatose - Restless and anxious	
Anaphylactic shock This is a form of shock caused by exposure to a substance to which the person is extremely allergic. Histamine is released in the body during an allergic reaction. *Signs and symptoms:* Anaphylactic shock presents a special problem because profound airway compromise can develop quickly. - Sense of uneasiness or agitation - Swelling of the soft tissues such as hands, tongue and pharynx and oedema of the eyes - Skin flushing and hives - Tachycardia, dysrhythmias - Coughing, sneezing or wheezing due to spasms - Tingling, burning and itching of the skin - Abdominal pain - Profound hypotension (late symptom) - Decreased level of consciousness and responsiveness - Sensation of lump in the throat - Nausea and vomiting - Bloating - Feeling of impending doom	This is the most severe form of allergic reaction and it never occurs the first time a person is exposed to an allergen. Once a person has been sensitized, cells patrolling the body recognize the foreign substance (antigen) and bombard the substance with histamine, which causes the severe allergic reaction. May be caused by skin contact of poisons, skin creams, perfume; injections such as penicillin; inhalation such as moulds, pollen; ingestion such as chocolate, shellfish, peanuts and medications.
Psychogenic shock This is a form of shock caused by fear, bad news and unpleasant sights and is often found during disasters. *Signs and symptoms:* - Rapid pulse - Normal or low blood pressure	A sudden reaction of the nervous system producing temporary, generalized vasodilatation resulting in syncope (fainting). Blood pools in the dilated vessels, reducing the blood supply to the brain and as a result the brain ceases to function normally and the patient faints.

TYPE OF SHOCK	DESCRIPTION
Septic shock This is a form of shock caused by an infection resulting in a massive vasodilatation of the circulatory system. *Signs and symptoms:* - Fever or hypothermia (> 38 degrees C or < 36 degrees C) - Hypotension (< 90 mmHG) - Hyperventilation - Mental confusion - Trunk of the body may be warm, but the extremities are cold due to shunting of blood from the skin of the arms and legs - Progression of septic shock is characterized by cooling off of the whole body, which is an ominous sign Other specific symptoms due to the type of infection may occur, for example in acute bacterial meningitis, patients will present with petechial rush.	Septic shock is caused by an overwhelming infection (usually bacterial) that leads to massive vasodilatation. The blood vessels dilate due to the toxins being released into the bloodstream. As in neurogenic shock, the amount of blood available for effective circulation is decreased because it is pooled up or trapped in the dilated veins. In addition, blood plasma is lost through blood vessel walls causing an additional loss in blood volume. Tissue perfusion thus results.
Metabolic shock Caused by an excessive urination, vomiting and diarrhoea. *Signs and symptoms:* - Rapid weak pulse - Hypotension - Altered level of consciousness - Cyanosis - Cold, clammy skin.	Due to the loss of body fluids there are changes in the body chemistry, including salt balance and acid base balance.
Respiratory shock Caused by severe chest injury or airway obstruction. *Signs and symptoms:* - Dyspnoea (difficult breathing) - Apnoea (no breathing) - Bradypnoea (slow breathing)	An insufficient concentration of oxygen in the blood due to the inability of the patient to breathe adequately.

The general treatment of shock is:
Follow the SABC rules, in other words ensure safety for yourself and the victim, airway (open, remove foreign objects), breathing (e.g. oxygen), circulation (e.g. stop bleeding) must at all times be maintained. Secure the cervical spine, call for backup and record all vital signs. It is important to maintain a normal body temperature and to keep the patient nil per mouth.

9.14.5 Musculoskeletal injuries
The classification of musculoskeletal injuries is described by Cardona, Hurn, Mason, Scanlon and Veis-Berry (1999) as follows:

1. Extremity fractures (open or closed fractures)
2. Traumatic amputations
3. Dislocations
4. Pelvic ring disruptions

The specific general management principles of all musculoskeletal injuries include the following:
- Early mobilization at the scene helps to preserve what function currently exists, prevents further injury, minimizes muscle spasms, decreases the risk of angulation and of overriding of bone ends so that closed fractures do not become open fractures, helps to align bone ends in a near-normal anatomical position which often restores neurovascular and lymphatic function, reduces further soft tissue damage and decreases pain.
- Immobilization techniques and devices applied in the prehospital environment should remain in place until X-rays have been taken. Proper monitoring of the device must at all times be maintained for correct placement and effectiveness.
- Massive blood loss may occur during traumatic amputations. This type of injury requires priority intervention to restore cardiovascular stability. Direct pressure dressing must be applied and immediate evacuation initiated.
- Dislocations should be immobilized in the position that they have been found because an attempt to straighten a joint will increase damage and pain.
- Pelvic fractures are extremely dangerous and are associated with early mortality due to the damage of the arteries and venous plexus of the iliac system. This network of blood vessels can easily be damaged by unstable pelvic fractures and may also include damage to the abdominal viscera, urethra and bladder, which compounds blood loss. Hypovolaemic shock usually occurs with an unstable pelvic fracture.
- The cardiovascular status of every patient who falls under these categories should be observed vigilantly and the patient frequently evaluated for shock. Vital signs must be taken every 15 minutes, general perfusion (skin colour and temperature) assessed, and capillary refill and the pulses must be monitored. Constant monitoring of vital signs is essential.
- Volume replacement should be appropriate and should start immediately.
- Pressure dressings should be applied at obvious sources of blood loss and in some cases the PASG may be considered.

- The potential for infection should at all times be considered and contamination at all costs avoided.

9.14.6 Facial injuries
Facial injuries, specifically maxillary fractures, may be classified into the following:
The Le Fort I is a transverse fracture, involving a horizontal line that separates the maxillary alveolus from the upper fracture with malocclusion and mobility of the facial skeleton. It is characterized by swelling. A Le Fort II fracture is a pyramid-shaped separation and involves the nasomaxillary segment of the zygomatic and orbital portions of the midface. It is characterized by the lengthening of the face, epistaxis, peri-orbital haematomas, malocclusion and facial mobility. The Le Fort II fracture is a complex type of fracture through the nasal bones and separates the midface from the cranium. The maxilla, one or both zygomas and the nose are all involved in this fracture. It is characterized by lengthening of the face, epistaxis, peri-orbital haematoma and movement of the face. The patient appears to have a flat face. Cerebrospinal fluid (CSF) rhinorrhoea may be seen in Le Fort II and II fractures due to the extension of the fracture through the cribriform plate.

Treatment for these fractures is the basic SABCs and vital signs monitoring. With a Le fort II, the airway may be compromised and there must be continuous observation of the patient. Transport is vital.

9.14.7 Injuries to the head, neck and spine
Injuries to the head, neck and spine can often be missed during emergencies. It is also the leading cause of death in persons up to the age of 44 years. The mortality rate due to head injuries is more than 35 per cent and functional recovery is slim. It is thus important that every victim be treated as if he/she has sustained a head, neck or spinal injury UNLESS proven otherwise (meaning by X-rays).

9.14.7.1 Head injuries
Scalp injuries
The scalp consists of five layers: the skin, coetaneous tissue, galea, areolar tissue, and the pericranium. It has a very rich blood supply and is often the source of major blood loss. Scalp lacerations are the most common head injury. These lacerations can be minor or very serious. The face and the scalp are very vascular and therefore can bleed profusely. Even small lacerations can cause significant blood loss, which can lead to hypovoleamia and shock.

Scalp lacerations are the result of direct blows to the head – they may therefore indicate a deeper, more serious injury which is often missed due to the amount of blood present or the small penetrating wound.

Treatment
- Apply SABC.
- May or may not need immobilization of the cervical spine, if uncertain, apply neck and spinal precautions.
- Control bleeding by direct pressure over the wound. Remember to replace any

flaps. If a fracture of the skull is suspected do not use excessive force when using direct pressure to control the bleeding. If the dressing becomes soaked do not remove it, cover with another dressing.
- Obtain the following because vital signs are important: eye opening, verbal response and motor response (see discussion on neurological examination).
- Do a secondary survey.
- Maintain body temperature – not too cold or too hot.
- Transport to hospital immediately as priority patient.

Skull injuries

The skull is rigid and inflexible and serves as a protection for the most vital organ in the body, namely the brain.

A fracture of the skull indicates that significant force has been applied to the head and due to the inflexible nature of the skull, increased intracranial pressure is associated with injuries to the skull. A fracture of the skull can be simple or compound. Simple linear and intact fractures of the skull do not require treatment. Severe major intracranial bleeding may occur in the skull if the larger arteries (for example meningeal artery or major dural sinus) are ruptured. Base of skull fractures can occur at any point at the base of the skull and often occur at the temporal bone.

Signs and symptoms
- Decreased level of consciousness
- Deep laceration or severe bruising
- Depression of the skull which can be open or closed
- Pain or swelling
- Deformity of the skull
- Battle sign (a late sign) usually indicates a fracture of the base of the skull (ecchymosis in the mastoid region)
- Unequal pupils
- Racoon's eye usually indicates a fracture of the base of the skull
- Sunken eyes
- Bleeding from the ears and or the nose
- CSF fluid leaking from the ears or nose (otorrhoea).

Treatment
- Maintain safety
- Immobilize the cervical spine
- Open airway, maintain suction if necessary – log roll into the lateral position
- Check breathing – oxygen – minimum of 40 per cent – may need to assist ventilation
- Control bleeding, if possible external
- Check vital signs
- Anticipate vomiting
- Be prepared for convulsions and changes in level of consciousness
- Maintain body temperature
- Arrange transport.

Brain injuries

Brain injuries account for a large number of mortalities due to the associated haemorrhage and injuries sustained to the brain centres as a whole.

Concussion is 'jarring' of the brain, possibly resulting in loss of consciousness, which is usually transient. The signs and symptoms include:
- Transient loss of consciousness
- Amnesia
- Nausea and vomiting
- Headache
- Repetitive questioning
- Dizziness
- Irritability
- Disorientation or confusion.

Cerebral contusion is the bruising of the brain. It usually results from closed blunt head trauma that injures the brain directly below the site of injury (coup), or causes the brain to rebound against the skull surface, causing injury to the opposite side of the brain to point of impact (contracoup). Bleeding and oedema occur in the area of the contusion and may occur anywhere in the brain.

Intracerebral haemorrhage is the laceration or rupture of a blood vessel inside the brain or in the meninges and causes parenchymal haemorrhage. Raised intracranial pressure is a result of this condition. Intracerebral haemorrhage is often seen only hours or days after the injury and can be extremely treacherous.

The brain is encased in a solid bony box – the skull. If there is any change to the contents of the skull there will be an increase in the pressure within the skull. Cerebral contusion and intracerebral haemorrhage increase the pressure within the skull (raised intracranial pressure).

The signs and symptoms associated with the above injuries are:
- Altered level of consciousness (ranging from confused to unconscious) or altering level of consciousness
- Lacerations or contusions of the scalp
- Deformity of the skull or scalp
- Unequal pupils
- CSF leak from the ears or nose
- Seizures
- Headache
- Nausea and vomiting
- Blood pressure rises
- Bradycardia
- Altered respiratory rate and rhythm
- Paralysis
- Combative or other abnormal behaviour
- Dizziness
- Visual complaints

- Racoon's eyes
- Battle sign
- Speech disturbances.

Treatment
- Maintain safety
- Apply suction of airway if necessary; insert oropharyngeal tube if necessary
- Arrange immediate transport to the hospital
- Administer oxygen immediately to assist with ventilation
- Check circulation (pulse) and control major bleeding
- Apply cervical collar
- Check vital signs
- Do full secondary survey
- Treat all injuries
- Package and position
- Maintain body temperature.

Impaled objects

Impaled objects MUST NOT be removed. If the object is too long it must be shortened, not removed. Stabilize the object with bulky bandages, then carefully and rigidly stabilize the object on both sides of where the cut will be made. The tool chosen should not cause the impaled object to vibrate or cause too much heat to be produced. If this cannot be done, seek advice from the emergency physician.

The neurological examination

A neurological examination is essential in establishing the severity of the head injury and the cause thereof. This examination is done rapidly and continuously while, for example, transport is in progress, in order to determine the level of deterioration or stabilization of the patient. The level of consciousness is the single most important factor to be examined. The Glasgow Coma Scale is used to do the neurological examination, which includes, as indicated in Table 9.3, eye opening, verbal response and motor response.

There are some pitfalls as described by Tintinalli et al. (1997:1146) to avoid in the assessment and management of a head-injured patient. These include:
- Inaccurate attributing decreased level of consciousness to alcohol, drugs, gases or industrial fumes. It is advisable to obtain alcohol levels and toxicological screens.
- Discharging a victim from the area during a 'lucid interval'. Rather keep a victim with a history of unconsciousness in the hospital for observation and record vitals.
- Failure to diagnose a cervical fracture or a spinal cord injury. Treat all patients with caution, until X-rays or tomogram have shown differently.
- Failure to adequately immobilize an agitated patient with a cervical fracture. When the usual restraining measures are inadequate, consider paralysing the patient.
- Failure to establish an adequate airway. All unconscious patients should be intubated and ventilated.

- Failure to recognize progressive neurological deterioration. Frequent examinations, vital signs and documentation are essential.
- Failure to rapidly and correctly manage the 'talk and deteriorate' victim. These patients are an extreme emergency.

9.14.7.2 'Talk and deteriorate syndrome'

Victims at scenes of disaster or accidents are often found wandering around and talking recognizable words and then suddenly they deteriorate and die on the scene. They have a severe brain injury, which may only show up to 48 hours after the injury. This condition occurs in 10–20 per cent of patients sustaining severe injuries to the brain. Rescuers and medical personnel often assume that victims who are talking and responding normally are not injured at all, or that the impact was not lethal at all. Once deterioration of the person's mental and physical status is observed, the reversal of the condition is too late because deterioration happens at a frightening speed. Aggressive management of these patients is necessary. All victims must be taken to hospital – irrespective of their condition – and be screened. When deterioration is observed, immediate surgical intervention is the only alternative to save the patient's life.

9.14.7.3 Neck injuries

An open neck injury can be a life-threatening situation on the scene, and secondary complications such as sepsis may occur.

Blunt trauma is one of the most commonly found neck injuries during disasters or accidents. Major problems faced with blunt trauma are usually the collapse of the larynx or trachea and swelling of their tissues, which creates a blocked airway. When a severe injury to the neck occurs a cervical spine injury must be assumed. The victims will present with symptoms such as loss of voice or hoarseness, signs of airway obstruction, external signs such as contusions to and depression of the neck, deformities of the neck and subcutaneous emphysema of the neck.

Treatment on site includes SABC principles, immobilization of the back and spine and immediate transport to hospital.

Penetrating injuries to the neck can cause profuse bleeding from a laceration of the great vessels in the neck, namely the carotid artery and the jugular vein. The symptoms include arterial bleeding, which will be profuse with bright red blood spurting from the wound, venous bleeding can be profuse with dark red to maroon-coloured blood flowing steadily from the wound. Specific management includes the management of arterial bleeding with direct pressure and/or management of venous bleeding by covering the wound with a gloved hand, then applying an occlusive dressing.

It is important with back injuries to at all times assure an open airway, immobilize the spine and back, and administer high concentration of oxygen and to transport as soon as possible.

9.14.7.4 Spinal injuries

Spinal injuries occur mainly as a result of motor vehicle accidents, penetrating injuries, diving accidents, contact sports, crush injuries, lightning strikes and polytrauma patients. Spinal injuries are devastating events, which may lead to quadriplegia if not managed correctly. The primary care of a patient with a spinal injury is of vital importance, as this will determine his/her prognosis and future outlook.

The mechanism of injury may be due to flexion, rotation, vertical compression, hyperextension, fractures, and diverse or imprecise understood mechanisms.

The symptoms of a spinal injury include the observation of the mechanisms of injury, hypotension with a systolic blood pressure of 80–100 mmHg. Despite the hypotension, the skin is warm, pink and dry and there is adequate urine output. In addition, despite the hypotension, there is a paradoxical bradycardia. Pain and tenderness over the area may occur and a feeling of numbness or weakness is experienced. The pulse is either normal or slow. The patient's breathing will depend on the level of injury and may be diaphragmatic or none. Males present with priapism and flaccid paralysis may occur. The patient often shows a 'hands up' position or crossed chest position and there may be loss of bladder and bowel control. Spinal injury may often show no signs and symptoms at all.

Treatment of this injury follows the SABC principles. It is important to maintain the airway, to suction, to apply a cervical collar, to immobilize the patient on a full spinal board, to maintain body temperature, to ensure adequate and correct package, and to position, comfort and reassure the patient.

Complications that may occur include neurogenic shock, impaired breathing – if the injury to the spine has occurred above the level of C 3 and the patient will not be able to breath. However, if the injury occurred below the level of C 3, 4 and 5 the patient may have the use of his/her diaphragm.

9.14.8 Thoracic trauma

Thoracic trauma causes 25 per cent of traumatic deaths. Thoracic trauma involves injury to the chest wall, bronchi and diaphragm. The diagnosis of thoracic trauma may be obvious, for example when the person makes no attempt to breathe or there are external signs of blunt injury where the skin of the chest is not broken.

Signs of rib fractures can also be detected by haemoptysis and there may be localized tenderness and pain during breathing efforts. Rapid shallow respiration may occur and the patient may be holding the injured side in an effort to minimize the pain. A flail chest is when more than one consecutive rib on the same side of the chest is fractured in two or more places. Therefore there is a section of the chest wall that moves independently from the rest of the chest wall (paradoxical breathing). A flail chest can also occur when the sternum 'tears' away from the cartilage.

Rib fractures are common in the elderly. A fracture of any of the four upper ribs is considered to be a severe mechanism of injury as the bony girdle of the clavicle and scapula protects them.

The symptoms for a flail chest include pain with breathing and chest pain, obvious fractures of the ribs, paradoxical breathing, dyspnoea, and signs and symptoms of shock. Tintinalli et al. (1997:1159) warn that dyspnoea and tachypnoea are non-specific and may also be caused by anxiety or pain from other injuries.

The treatment for all chest injuries includes the SABC principles and specifically giving oxygen at a minimum of 40 per cent. It is important to secure the section with a pillow over the injured side and apply an elevated arm sling.

Allow the patient to lie on the injured side, treat for shock and monitor vital signs. The patient must be transported immediately to prevent further complications and shock.

Pneumothorax occurs when there is a puncture of the pleural sac and air leaks into the pleural cavity, causing the lung to 'collapse'.

Penetrating injuries occur when there is penetration of the chest wall. In penetrating injury damage to the heart, lungs, great vessels, trachea, oesophagus and bronchi can be complicated by the accumulation of air in the pleural space. Air enters the pleural space via the hole in the chest wall as the patient tries to breathe, causing the lung on the injured side to 'collapse'. Any blood passing through the 'collapsed' lung will not be oxygenated, therefore hypoxia occurs. Characteristics of these injuries are the open sucking chest wound – as the patient inhales the air is sucked into the pleural cavity via the wound – the sound of the rushing air should alert one to this condition. The patient presents with dyspnoea, subcutaneous emphysema, and an unequal air entry on auscultation to the lungs, cyanosis, decreasing level of consciousness, tachycardia and hypotension.

A closed pneumothorax occurs when a fractured rib punctures a lung. It can also occur spontaneously. In spontaneous pneumothorax the patient has a weak area in the lung. Occasionally this area will rupture and a pneumothorax will occur. The patient presents with a sudden sharp chest pain, tachycardia, dyspnoea, decreased air entry on the side of the 'collapse' and anxiety. Non-specific causes are found. A tension pneumothorax occurs when there is a laceration of the lung and there is a significant air leak into the pleural space. This can occur if the open wound has been sealed without allowing air to escape out through the wound. A tension pneumothorax can also occur as a result of closed, blunt injury of the chest in which a fractured rib lacerates a lung. This will first cause the complete collapse of the affected lung then begin to push the mediastinum across into the opposite side of the chest, cutting off venous return. It presents as increasing inadequate ventilation, respiratory arrest, distended neck veins, deviation of the trachea to the opposite side, tachycardia, hypotension, cyanosis and decreased air entry on the side of the pneumothorax. These patients are extremely anxious and restless and there is a decreasing level of consciousness.

In both the penetrating blunt chest injuries, blood can collect in the pleural space. A haemothorax should be suspected if the patient shows signs of shock as well as signs of a pneumothorax. Haemopneumothorax is when there is air and blood in the pleural cavity. Both a haemothorax and haemopneumothorax present as a pneumothorax and are treated as such.

Pulmonary contusion is where the capillary network around the alveoli is damaged and blood leaks into the alveolus. The patient becomes hypoxic as the blood interferes with gaseous exchange. This condition usually occurs over a period of hours. The person presents with coughing of blood (frothy red in appearance), dyspnoea, and a history of injury to the chest.

A myocardial contusion is a bruising of the myocardium. When this happens the heart cannot pump effectively and is unable to maintain the blood pressure. The signs and symptoms range from an irregular pulse rate to ventricular fibrillation. The dangerous dysrhythmias are uncommon. Suspect myocardial contusions in all cases of severe blunt injuries to the chest.

A pericardial tamponade is a condition where blood and other fluid or air can collect in the pericardial sac, compressing the heart, and preventing it from filling up during the diastolic phase, therefore cardiac output is decreased. If not relieved, the heart will be compressed to such an extent that the cardiac output will drop to zero and cardiac arrest will occur. The person presents with muffled heart sounds, distended neck veins, a weak pulse, or a tachycardia out of proportion to other findings, dysrhythmia, hypotension, and narrowed pulse pressure. This condition is very hard to determine. The victim may have severe multisystem trauma and the presence of cardiac injury may be overshadowed by other, more obvious injuries. Patients with fractured sternum or first two ribs may be suspected of a pericardial tamponade.

Emergency management of all chest injuries include the basic SABCs, call for backup and immediate transport to hospital. Specific management is the maintenance of adequate ventilation, intravenous fluid, high percentage of oxygen and the management of symptomatic complications, for example open wounds must be closed, be prepared to do cardiopulmonary resuscitation, insertion of chest tubes, suction of secretions which may compromise the airway.

In open wounds to the chest, the wound is covered with an occlusive dressing. The dressing must be larger than the wound to prevent it being sucked into the wound. Tape only three sides of the dressing. The dressing will act as a flutter valve – preventing air from entering through the wound and allowing air to escape through the wound.

9.14.9 Abdominopelvic injuries

Abdominal injuries are difficult to evaluate because of the many possible injuries and their varied presentations.

There are three types of abdominopelvic injuries: blunt, penetrating, and evisceration.

Blunt trauma has three possible mechanisms of injury, namely a direct blow to the abdomen, crush of the abdomen and a deceleration injury. Blunt injuries can cause damage to one or more of the following:
- Severe bruising to the abdominal wall
- Rupture of the aorta
- Lacerations of the liver or spleen
- Rupture of the intestine
- Tears in the mesentery, injury to the blood vessels within the mesentery
- Rupture of the kidneys
- Rupture of the bladder
- Severe intra-abdominal haemorrhage
- Peritoneal irritation and inflammation
- Spinal injuries.

The patient may present with severe bruising or visible marks which give a clue to the possibility of injury to underlying organs, abdominal pain, tachycardia, hypotension, pallor, skin cold and clammy, abdomen distended rigid and if patient is conscious tender, guarding, rapid shallow breathing and difficulty with movement because of pain.

Penetrating injuries are usually visible wounds to the abdominal wall and generally the patient will have obvious wounds and external bleeding. Some penetrating injuries go no deeper than the abdominal wall. The severity of the injury can be difficult to determine. Always suspect that the object has entered the abdominal cavity and has possibly injured one or more of the underlying organs.

The patient will present with the following, namely obvious wounds or impaled objects. There may be an exit wound, however this is not conclusive. Severe pain is experienced and blood fluid loss is evident. The patient has hypotension, tachycardia, tachypnoea tenderness and guarding, the skin pale cold and clammy and the patient experiences difficulty with movement due to pain. As the condition progresses, the patient experiences a decreasing level of consciousness.

The specific management of all abdominal trauma includes log roll into lateral position, inspection of the spine, baseline vital signs and transport for surgery. If there is an impaled object – leave in position and stabilize with supportive bandage, cover wounds, and maintain body temperature.

An evisceration occurs with severe injuries to the abdominal wall, allowing the abdominal organs or fat to protrude. Any eviscerated organ should be covered with a moist sterile dressing. Do not attempt to push the organs, momentum or abdominal fat back into the abdomen. The patient must be prepared for emergency surgery.

9.14.10 Multiple trauma

Multiple trauma is usually a result of a major accident, and whether it results in several injuries to one person or injuries to several people the principles of triage remain the same.

Triage means to categorize victims according to severity of injuries in order that lives may be saved. The occupational health professional at the scene of multiple trauma would maintain an open airway, control severe haemorrhage with pressure and maintain in-line cervical spine support should the victim need to be moved. A well-trained and coordinated first-aid team, usually made up of workers, will provide invaluable support by carrying out life-saving procedures of cardiopulmonary resuscitation, haemorrhage control, wound care, the splinting of fractures and basic shock treatment.

9.14.11 Eye injuries

Another common occurrence in industry is that of foreign bodies in the eye and burns caused by acids, alkalis or hot molten metal or glass in the eye. Superficial foreign bodies may be removed by the occupational health professional (with a sterile cotton bud), but penetrating foreign bodies together with burns and any trauma of the eye should be referred directly to an ophthalmic surgeon or specific eye centre, as an extreme emergency. It is important to liaise with the specialist or unit beforehand, and for the company physician to issue clear instructions with regard to eye injuries in the event of not being available at the time of the injury.

Arc eyes, as a result of intense ultraviolet irradiation during welding, will only give symptoms of irritation as if there is gravel in the eye, followed by pain, hours after the event, and the recommended treatment by the company physician should be available in the medical centre, as protocol. The occupational health nurse has an important role to play in the prevention of eye injuries through education of the workers and the enforcement of the correct eye protection during hazardous procedures in accordance with the company policy on health and safety. The strategic placement of eye fountains and their immediate use for at least ten minutes following a chemical splash in the eye should also be taught to the workers.

Once the injury has occurred an accurate history of what the workman was using and how the accident occurred, including the direction from which the blow or foreign body entered the eye is important for the correct management of the injury by the specialist.

9.14.12 Heat exhaustion, heatstroke and hypothermia

These conditions could be emergencies in areas where extremes of temperature occur such as near furnaces, in mines or cold storage rooms and workers who work alone and do not realize what is happening when they start to feel tired.

Heat exhaustion can occur with physical exertion in a very hot, humid environment. It is the result of dehydration and electrolyte loss and presents with fatigue, headache, dizziness, thirst, muscle cramps, rapid and weak pulse, fast shallow respirations and a cool, clammy skin. Muscle in coordination, confusion, delirium and even coma could follow if the victim is not removed to a cool environment, given plenty of cool fluids to drink, if able to, and referred to hospital for intravenous fluid and electrolyte replacement. Heat exhaustion would occur more rapidly after a debilitating disease or a bout of diarrhoea and vomiting and therefore catch workers unaware after sick leave.

Heatstroke develops when the body can no longer regulate its temperature by perspiring. The first symptoms are similar to those of heat exhaustion, that is, the headache, fatigue, dizziness and thirst, but the patient soon becomes restless, the fast weak pulse becomes full and bouncing while the respiration becomes stertorous. The patient's skin becomes flushed and dry and the temperature will be over 40 °C and confusion, convulsions and unconsciousness will follow with possibly cardiovascular collapse, cardiac arrest and death if treatment is not instituted without delay. The patient should be moved to a cool environment, clothing should be removed and the patient wrapped in a wet sheet and fanned. Cardiopulmonary resuscitation may be necessary, oxygen must be administered and the vital functions monitored, whilst an intravenous infusion of Ringer's lactate is given. Medication needs to be administered according to medical protocol and the patient referred to the nearest casualty department.

Hypothermia could occur when the body temperature falls below 35 °C in an environment of below freezing point, or with prolonged exposure to low temperatures, especially with the use of alcohol and drugs, or even some medical conditions such as diabetes mellitus. The victim feels very cold and exhausted, becomes pale and shivers uncontrollably, until incoordination with slurred speech sets in. The pulse and respiration rate become very low and the patient becomes confused before lapsing into unconsciousness.

The patient must be moved to a warm area, wet clothes need to be removed and dry insulating covering applied to the whole body, except the face. Cardiopulmonary resuscitation may be necessary, after first carefully checking for a slow pulse. Vital signs must be monitored and warm sweet drinks may be given. The patient must be transferred to hospital.

9.14.13 Radiation emergencies or nuclear reactor accidents

Although uncommon, the disasters at Three Mile Island in the United States of America and Chernobyl in Russia rocked the world by the immensity of the implications.

There are three levels of radiation where the victim can be contaminated by the radioactive material ingested or inhaled, or the victim may have become irradiated as a result of exposure to gamma rays or X-rays.

Management of radioactive contamination

Radioactive material such as dust, solid particles or in a liquid form adheres to the victim's skin and clothes. The victim needs to be decontaminated in a special decontamination zone. Evaluation of the level of contamination should take place throughout the decontamination process with a suitable radiation detector. Urine and faeces samples should be saved and measured for the amount of radioactivity.

The decontamination zone

This should be a room or area away from the contamination area that should be prepared by removing all surplus furniture and other items, and placing a disposable waterproof covering on the floor. A free water supply and a large container for all contaminated water must be arranged. Protective clothing with waterproof shoe covering and respirators for the decontamination personnel, if there is a risk of airborne radioactive particles, as well as suitable containers for contaminated clothes and for urine, faeces or nasal swab samples must be arranged beforehand.

The treatment of life-threatening conditions and open wounds, which should be irrigated with copious amounts of sterile saline, take precedence over the general decontamination process; the victim is completely undressed and his/her clothing sealed in a plastic bag. Initial monitoring for the level of contamination is done and monitoring is repeated throughout the process. The nostrils, mouth and external auditory canals are swabbed with cotton wool applicators and these are sealed in glass test tubes and placed in a lead-lined container for monitoring at a later stage.

The ears, eyes and nostrils should be irrigated with a normal saline solution. The skin is then gently scrubbed with soap and water at body temperature. Vigorous scrubbing should be avoided as it stimulates the circulation and can cause breaks in the skin, which will assist absorption of radioactive elements into the body. Only if monitoring reveals persistent contamination of the skin should more abrasive scrubbing be used to remove dead skin and contaminants that adhere to the skin proteins.

Hair should be shampooed as well and if there is evidence of resistant contamination it should be cut off. (Shaving is risky as there is a chance of nicking the scalp.)

Should contamination persist, chelating agents can be used to bind the radioactive contaminant into a complex agent as it is removed from the skin. These patients are always followed up regularly and thereafter yearly for possible module formation in wounds.

Internal contamination
When radioactive material has entered the body by inhalation or ingestion, therapy must be directed at elimination and excretion of the radionuclides and decreasing the gastro-intestinal absorption. This is a medical emergency! The use of emetics, gastric lavage, purgatives and enemas and even lung lavage may be recommended by the medical officer-in-charge. Reduction of gastro-intestinal absorption will be aided by agents such as aluminium-containing antacids, alginate or barium sulphate.

Once the agent has been absorbed, blocking agents such as potassium iodide, which reduces the uptake of radio-iodide by the thyroid gland, can be used. Mobilizing agents increase the natural turnover process of some radionuclides and chelating agents bind the radioactive ion into a non-ionizing ring complex that can be excreted by the kidneys.

The time involved in carrying out the above procedures is crucial in minimizing the effects of the radiation accident and careful planning and preparation for such an event are part of the occupational health nurse's duty in an industry where radioactivity is used.

9.14.14 Exposure to toxic substances
One of the most important duties of the occupational health professional is to identify all the chemicals and gases that are brought into the workplace, how they are used and what by-products are formed during the process. In larger industries he/she will liaise with the safety officer, industrial hygienist, buyer, production manager, horticulturist or head gardener, as well as the worker him-/herself. By doing 'factory rounds' and asking workers about their work he/she will discover interesting and sometimes horrifying facts as uninformed or careless people go about making their daily tasks a little easier, albeit unsafe. Toxic substances enter the body by inhalation, skin absorption or ingestion. The most prevalent form of acute poisoning in industry is through inhalation.

Respiratory emergencies
The most common respiratory emergency that the occupational health professional has to deal with is that of occupational asthma. Careful history-taking, lung auscultation and physical examination, as well as an accurate lung function test, would preclude an asthmatic from work areas that have respiratory irritants. Allergies to natural substances such as skins, hair, fur, feathers, mites, flour, grain dust, fungi, moulds or even wheat weevils, among others, and chemicals including chromium, cobalt dust, epoxy resins, formaldehyde, gum arabic, isocyanates, nickle, organo-phosphates,

phenol, phenylene-diamine platinum salts, pyrethrin, tannic acid, toluene, tetrachloropthalic anhydride, tragacanth and vanadium, to name but a few, could result in bronchospasm.

Standard asthma treatment applies in occupational asthma and should be laid down in a medical protocol. It must be remembered that all traces of the causative agent should be removed from the patient.

Respiratory irritants

All irritants produce an inflammatory reaction of the mucous membranes of the entire respiratory tract, causing mild symptoms such as rhinorrhea and watery eyes with low-dose exposure through to oedema of the larynx and lungs followed by death in high-dose exposure or exposure to highly toxic gases.

Examples of respiratory irritants include:
- Ammonia, where the particularly pungent smell does prevent more serious accidents from happening. Used mainly in the fertilizer industry, the symptoms of exposure vary from upper respiratory tract irritation to pulmonary oedema and death. Bronchiectasis may follow as a permanent lesion after exposure.
- Bromine is a reddish brown gas used in the chemical and petroleum industries with similar symptoms and treatment as chlorine inhalation.
- Chlorine is a yellowish green gas with a sharp odour used mainly in paper, chemical and mining industries, as well as in water purification and sewage treatment plants. High-concentration exposure can cause panic due to choking, coughing, dyspnoea, chest pain and haemoptysis. Emergency treatment for shock with oxygen and bronchodilators is followed by urgent referral to hospital where patients will be admitted for observation for possible pulmonary oedema.
- Fluorine is a yellowish green gas with a pungent odour, used in the chemical, petroleum, uranium, aluminium and glass industry. High-dose exposure gives similar symptoms to that of chlorine exposure and requires similar treatment.
- Nitrogen oxides are usually colourless and odourless and are found mainly in farm silos where fodder ferments, fertilizer manufacture and in metal-cleaning processes and welding. High exposure gives similar symptoms as chlorine exposure and requires similar treatment.
- Phosgene is a toxic gas used widely in the manufacture of dyes, isocyanates, pharmaceuticals, polyurethane resins and is present in welding fumes and burning polyurethane fumes. Whilst initially causing only slight upper respiratory tract irritation, exposure is often followed by a latent period of a few hours up to three days, when pulmonary oedema arises, leading to respiratory failure if medical intervention is delayed. Admission to hospital for three days for observation is vital following exposure to phosgene gas.
- Sulphur dioxide is a colourless gas with an unpleasant, pungent odour. It is used in bleaching and paper manufacturing but is a by-product of many industrial processes, as well as fuel and oil combustion. Active high-dose exposure may prove fatal due to obstruction of airways. Treatment is oxygen, bronchodilators and even cortisone may need to be administered prior to urgent hospitalization.

Asphyxiants

Asphyxiants deprive the vital organs of the body of oxygen.

Simple asphyxiants are physiologically inert gases that displace atmospheric oxygen and thereby deprive the victim of oxygen. These gases include carbon dioxide, ethane, methane, nitrogen and smoke, which is both a chemical irritant and an asphyxiant.

Treatment can only be given once the victim has been rescued, which is a hazardous procedure. Rescuers must wear self-contained breathing apparatus. Cardiopulmonary resuscitation, oxygen and urgent hospital treatment are required.

Chemical asphyxiants are gases that disrupt cellular respiration by preventing oxygen from reaching the cells. The effect of chemical asphyxiants depends on many factors including the duration of exposure; the concentration of the gas in the area; the victim's health status and lung function; the use of personal protective equipment; the presence of other toxic gases in the area; and – most important of all – the emergency medical management. The three most common chemical asphyxiants are carbon monoxide, hydrogen cyanide and hydrogen sulphide.

Carbon monoxide is a gas that is present in any enclosed area where incomplete combustion of organic materials takes place, especially in tanks, garages and mines where ventilation may be poor. Victims will at first complain of headaches, dizziness, a tight feeling of the chest and nausea. As the carboxyhaemoglobin level rises symptoms become more severe with a shortness of breath, racing pulse rate, vomiting and eventually collapse and coma. With high carboxyhaemoglobin levels, the mucous membranes become a cherry-red colour.

Treatment of victims includes the removal of the victim from the area and oxygenating him/her and if necessary doing cardiopulmonary resuscitation. Paramedic treatment of intubation and establishing an intravenous line with a Ringer's lactate solution for drug administration may be required; monitoring for cardiac dysrhythmia and transference to hospital are required.

Hydrogen cyanide is used to make monomers for plastics and also in electroplating, fumigation and ore extraction. In a fire or an explosion, cyanide is often released and inhaled by the victims together with the smoke. It has a characteristic bitter-almond smell. Liquid hydrogen cyanide is easily absorbed through the skin.

Treatment of victims includes removing the victim from the area. Immediate use of the cyanide antidote kit, whilst simultaneously doing cardiopulmonary resuscitation and decontamination of the skin with water requires a team of first-aiders.

The cyanide antidote kit consists of Amyl nitrate capsules, and ampoule of sodium nitrate 3 per cent and an ampoule of sodium thiosulphate 25 per cent and is used in this sequence. The Amyl nitrate is crushed in gauze and held by the victim's nostrils for 30 seconds. Then the sodium nitrate is slowly administered intravenously, taking three to five minutes, followed by 50 ml sodium thriosulphate intravenously over a period of ten minutes. These injections may be repeated after two hours and must be verified in protocol from the medical officer in charge. The patient should be placed in the Trendelenburg positions and the intravenous line should be kept open. Constant cardiac monitoring is essential for early detection of dysrhythmia and atriventricular blocks.

Hydrofluoric acid is often used to remove potting, cement and lacquer from glass, ceramics and fine wires as used in the electronic industry. After exposure the skin may at first only appear wrinkled and feel strange – severe pain follows hours later as the fluorine combines with the calcium in the system to form calcium fluorine and only subsides when the fluoride ions are saturated, which may be days later. Contaminated clothing must be removed immediately and the affected area rinsed under running water for at least ten minutes to remove as much of the acid as possible, before giving the patient a jar of calcium gluconate gel to massage into the area continuously in an effort to saturate the fluoride. The application should be continued en route to hospital where the patient will be given a calcium infusion. Liaison with hospital personnel beforehand is imperative to ensure correct treatment, as permanent scarring of the affected areas and nailbeds occurs.

9.14.15 Management of hazardous material accidents and toxic exposures

Hazardous materials incidents are disastrous events that may cause mass casualties and in addition can pose serious risks to rescue and emergency personnel. Thousands of chemicals are produced and used every day. These chemicals are transported by sea, road, air and water and when a disaster occurs very few people, including emergency personnel, really are aware of the consequences and treatment of such chemicals. Millions of people use and store chemicals in their homes, garages and at their place of work, which under the right circumstances may cause a disaster of immense magnitude.

Hazardous materials can be in, for example liquid form, gases, solids, radiation, bacteria or other disease-forming agents and in many instances can spread at an alarming rate. An example is the hysteria that occurred after the American bombing of the twin towers where terrorists warned of the spread of anthrax bacteria via the post. Many postal packages and letters with suspicious white power were received by key institutions throughout the world and often these were hoaxes. However, even if one suspects a hoax, this must never be taken up lightly.

When a hazardous materials incident occurs, even on a small scale, it must be regarded as a disaster and a hazardous materials response team needs to be deployed. This team consists of experts who have undergone extensive training and practising to respond to such a disaster or potential disaster.

Rescue and emergency teams who have not been trained to manage a disaster involving hazardous materials should never be allowed to enter the scene of a disaster without the authorization of the specialist team. Contamination of people, vehicles and equipment should at all times be avoided. The wearing of protective equipment is essential and all unnecessary equipment must be removed from ambulances. Cocoon the victim in a body bag or blanket and notify the hospital. The hospital will then, where applicable, get the decontamination protocol or isolation protocol ready in order to receive and treat the patient.

The goals at the scene will be to:
- Identify the risk of the hazardous materials to life and property
- Confine the hazard to an area, workplace or container

Occupational health

- Isolate the scene from further entry
- Apply strict safety and security measures
- Evacuate people from the area
- Decontaminate those exposed
- Stabilize the injured
- Transport the injured/affected.

The management of accidents involving hazardous substances begins with good planning. The occupational health professional must know exactly which hazardous substances, whether in their original form or as a result of combination with other substances during a process, are on the premises.

Planning for accidents involving hazardous substances includes the following:
- A chart drawn up to include each substance, its trade name, its ingredients, description of colour, odour, consistency, etc., the area and the process in which it is used, the clinical signs and symptoms of exposure and the first-aid treatment.
- Education of all the workers in the area, from the manager to the floor sweeper, as well as the staff from the receiving depot and store, in the identification of hazardous substances in the area, their effects on the body and emergency procedures, including who to inform, decontamination, evacuation, first-aid procedures and personal protective equipment.
- Liaison with local emergency services to ensure good relations and correct treatment for specific toxic substances.
- Establishment of a safety and health committee, which would include the company physician, the general manager, safety officer, industrial hygienist, production manager and the occupational health professional. New procedures and substances to be used should be discussed, as well as fresh information regarding the toxic substance, its substitution or treatment of exposure. A company policy on safety and health aspects is another duty of this committee.
- Policy and procedures for the supply and the correct use and enforcement of protective equipment should be drawn up by the safety and health committee. Continual updating of information and new appliances as they become available is the duty of the occupational health professional in the absence of a safety officer.
- Establishment of decontamination zones, such as eye fountains and showers, should be provided with correct drainage so as to prevent contaminated water from entering the general drainage system and spreading the contamination. Education in the correct use of these showers for at least ten minutes while the occupational health professional is sent for is vital, rather than a quick rinse before the victim makes his/her way to the medical centre.
- Basic training in rescue and first aid for rescue and first-aid teams should be supplemented with information on specific hazards and regular practising. Team members should be issued with the correct personal protective equipment. Depending on the extent of the accident, they may need to set up a command post and secure the area.
- Follow-up is necessary. A special meeting of the safety and health committee should

be called following any spill or exposure in order to learn from the experience by ironing out any misunderstandings about procedure in an effort to reach optimal health and safety standards.
- Disaster planning and evacuation are important.

9.14.16 A disaster plan and emergency evacuation
Although the most senior official of an organization is responsible for the planning and execution of an emergency plan, he/she often liaises with other specialists and persons concerned to establish a policy in this regard.

9.14.17 Medical emergencies
Emergencies as a result of medical conditions are less frequent if there is an efficient health service at the workplace. Pre-placement and periodic medical examinations highlight medical conditions, ensure early advice and treatment, and the condition can be controlled by regular follow-up by the occupational health nurse.

A register could be kept of all known epileptics, diabetics, hypertensives, asthmatics and even those with tuberculosis and other health problems. Treatment in an emergency would be discussed with the company doctor and protocol drawn up for specific emergencies, including medication to be given in the case of cardiac arrest and anaphylactic shock. These workers are important in cases of emergency because evacuation will concern them. Pre-placement examinations are important to prevent disasters and injuries of a large scale to develop, for example a person who has epilepsy, would not be considered as a crane driver.

Cardiac arrest
Perhaps the most common cause of cardiac arrest is a myocardial infarct or coronary thrombosis. The victim or his/her co-workers usually inform the occupational healthcare professional that he/she is not feeling well, has indigestion and/or a severe chest pain. The pain could be described as a vice-like or crushing pain in the centre of the chest, possibly spreading to the left arm or throat. The victim will feel weak or dizzy, perspire profusely, be cold to touch and anxious. His/her face will become ashen-grey with the lips, tip of nose and ear lobes becoming cyanotic. It is imperative that the victim does not exert him-/herself, is reassured and placed in the semi-Fowlers position. Oxygen and medication must be administered according to medical protocol. Immediate transfer to the nearest casualty centre in a appropriately equipped ambulance with constant monitoring is required. An intravenous line should be kept open with a very slow infusion.

Should cardiac arrest occur and facilities for defibrillation not be available, the occupational healthcare professional should commence cardiopulmonary resuscitation.

Cardiopulmonary resuscitation procedure
Safety is the first concern. Look around in the area for any loose-hanging wires, sharp objects or any unsafe equipment. Detertmine the patient's level of conciousness by patting on the shoulder or arm, calling his/her name. Send for help and ask the person to return to the scene and give details of the help asked for. Take time to ascertain that

the pulse has in fact stopped by feeling carefully for the carotid pulse. If absent, place the victim on a hard surface (usually the floor) and open the airway by extending the head or lifting the jaw forward and upwards (the jaw lift is recommended if there is a possibility of a neck injury). Clear the mouth of fluid, vomitus or loose dentures.

If spontaneous respiration did not occur when the airway was opened, take a deep breath and, closing the victim's nostrils with two fingers, placing your mouth over the open mouth of the victim and sealing the lips, blow air from your lungs into the victim's mouth. The victim's chest should rise and then fall when you take your mouth away. This is an indication that the airway is open. If the air is rushing past your mouth and you cannot feel it entering the victim's airway and the chest did not rise, clear the airway again and extend the head or lift the jaw more firmly. If the airway remains blocked, try closing the mouth and blowing into the nostrils.

After two quick but full breaths, check again for a carotid pulse. If absent, measure the sternum to find the midpoint and place the heel of one hand on the centre of the lower half. Place the heel of your other hand on top of the fist, lock your fingers and lift them from the chest wall. Keeping your elbows straight and your shoulders directly over your hands, press down on your hands in order to push the breast bone 4 to 5 cm down, thereby squeezing the heart between the breast bone and to the spinal column and emptying the blood in the chambers into the circulation. Release the pressure and blood will flow into the chambers again. These compressions are kept up rhythmically for 15 counts before the airway is opened again and two full breaths are given to be followed by another 15 even compressions.

Check for a pulse again after four cycles or the first minute and thereafter after every 12 cycles.

If a first-aider comes to help, the rhythm can be changed to five compressions to one breath after initially giving two full breaths.

The procedure should be continued until the victim's heart starts beating and breathing is restored. Improvement in the patient's colour and a pulse in the carotid artery will indicate that the resuscitation is effective.

It is imperative that this procedure be practised regularly with the medical staff and first-aiders at the place of work, to perfect the rhythm which is crucial to successful resuscitation.

9.15 Communication during disasters

Perhaps the most important key to success in any disaster management system is the effective communication between the various groups. It is the key component of a meaningful and organized response. There are various routes that need to be established effectively at the scene through central command. Radio signals are not always effective, depending on the location of the disaster or the structure in which the disaster has occurred (for example at sea or in a mine). It is therefore important to plan for every possible type of disaster with regard to equipment, and to select and test various systems that can be used effectively during times of crisis.

Some of the examples of the routes that need to be established to ensure effective communication include the following:

- Communication to and from the command post to the disaster area and back from the scene
- Communication to and from police, traffic and fire departments, ensuring the safety of rescuers to move into the area and to establish continuous safety checks
- Communication to and from command post to triage and transport areas to determine the number and conditions of patients and to order more equipment, send in backup personnel, relief personnel and to sort out general problems
- Communication to and from healthcare facilities, for example hospitals, mortuary, clinics, primary care areas and other holding areas which have been identified during the planning phase – school or church halls, convention centres or any other place where victims can be treated temporarily
- Communication with and from the press is important because clear and true messages need to be communicated to the community where anxious friends and relatives await news, as well as to warn individuals about evacuating areas and advise on the possibility of secondary complications of the disaster
- According to the Act, communication channels to the authorities are mandatory and one must take into account that the departments within the government structure can assist with funds, equipment, transportation and personnel
- The management of the industry where a disaster occurred needs to be kept updated about the extent of the disaster and it is important to establish communication channels with designated spokespersons from the industry to deliver information to the press and to the rest of the management
- Continuous communication with the emergency services is necessary to update the possible risks of for example contamination or spread of a disease or possible further crises which may emerge within a matter of seconds.

Most of the communication is done by walkie-talkie systems or short-band radios. Recent techniques are that communication can be established by cellphone technology and television coverage (as seen with the Iraq war where the actual war scenes were displayed to millions of TV watchers throughout the world). Ideally, distinct radio frequencies could be designated as disaster only and used only by participants in the disaster area.

A number of problems can affect the communication during a disaster, namely:
- Overloaded radio frequencies
- Damage to infrastructure
- General equipment failure (e.g. batteries)
- Incompatible frequencies between various groups
- Noise from heavy extrication machinery.

Activation and notification of personnel is often done by a 'cascade' system, which has been proven to be highly effective. The principle here is that the people who are initially contacted call a number of key people, who in turn call a number of other predetermined people, and so this system of calling cascades. This system ensures that telephone lines from the hospital are not overloaded and that personnel within a speciality (e.g. radiology, nursing, cleaning department) are contacted by fellow colleagues.

9.16 Management of disaster victims at the hospital

All hospitals should have a detailed written disaster plan that comes into operation as soon as the report of the disaster comes through from central command. This disaster plan should include all the departments of the hospital and should be tested at least twice a year. Key personnel should keep telephone lists in their offices and at home of all the personnel working in that hospital. These lists must be updated at least monthly. It is important to deploy only half the available personnel during the disaster because they will have to be relieved by the other half after 8–12 hours. Cleaning personnel play a vital role in the smooth running of any hospital, but during the disaster their role is the key to success of the operation. The key to an effective disaster plan is that it should be as near to everyday operations as possible. When a disaster occurs, all personnel must be able to carry out their roles automatically. It is then too late to read the manual.

It is important that hospitals are adequately stocked to manage a large-scale disaster. Stretchers, extra beds and oxygen and other equipment should be brought to the receiving area immediately to get patients mobile the moment they begin to arrive at the hospital.

In large-scale disasters, all the hospitals and clinics in the area are alerted and a central control centre is established to coordinate the activities between them and the central command.

In some areas when a massive disaster occurs, community warning sirens can be sounded, alerting the public and the hospital staff to tune to radio or television for announcements.

It is crucial that patients are dispersed to various hospitals without overloading a single emergency department. Tracking patients from the scene to the various destinations is important and this requires a predetermined format of information.

At the hospital, the emergency department must be cleared of patients who are ready for discharge or those with minor complaints who can be re-routed to other facilities. Patients who are brought in from the scene of the disaster are met by a medical team who re-assess their condition and categorize the victims. The severely injured receive the first treatment and others are regularly checked for the deterioration of their condition. The dead are removed to the specially allocated area. Here clergy play a vital role in providing the needed psychological assistance to the families and in providing palliative care to the helplessly wounded or unsalvageable victims.

The hospital disaster management plan has definite designated areas to which each category of patient is allocated on arrival. The receiving and triage area is the most accessible area to receive patients from incoming vehicles and should provide enough room for secondary triage. This area should also be easily accessed for transferring victims to treatment areas. In this area the METAG is reviewed, the victims re-assessed and then transferred to predesignated treatment areas according to their coding. The area should be manned by senior medical and nursing staff, as well as administrative personnel who keep records of the patients.

9.17 Documentation

Documentation is crucial in the fields of emergency medicine and care at the scene and in the hospital. Where possible, records should include information about vital signs, Glasgow Coma Scale, incident data (e.g. type of accident, falling from a crane, involved in explosion caused by chemical), therapy received, past and previous history (e.g. diabetic Type II), time of injury, geographic location and body position. These records should be viewed very carefully by the receiving team because vital data such as the application of PASG or pain medication given may influence the well-being of the patient. Throughout the care of the victim, whether in hospital or in the wards, careful monitoring and documentation must be maintained. It often takes days or hours after the incident before the final documentation for admission and other aspects can be completed. The documentation regarding consent for operations is important and unidentified victims often have to undergo emergency operations. These aspects need to be considered and a plan worked out for which process will be followed to obtain such consent if the family is not available or the victim is not in a state to sign for the operation. Cultural aspects such as the receiving of blood should also be taken into consideration.

9.18 Post-disaster management

9.18.1 Responses of victims

Psychological factors contribute to the effect of a disaster on individuals. The nature and severity of the disaster affects the psychological distress experienced by the victims. The existence and length of a warning period and physical proximity to the actual site of the disaster influence the amount of psychological distress experienced by victims. The closer an individual is to the actual site of the disaster and the longer he/she is exposed to the immediate site of the disaster, the greater the psychological distress that he/she will experience.

The victim's perception of the disaster is the strongest influence on the type of psychological response to a disaster that the individual will experience. Individuals experience disasters in relation to how significantly they are directly affected. An individual who perceives a disaster to be less severe than it is will probably have a less severe psychological reaction than a person who perceives the situation as catastrophic. An individual's perception of a disaster may change over time as the person begins to acknowledge the full impact of the disaster. The human mind is capable of allowing perceptions to be only as disastrous as the mind can cope with at a given time.

A victim's response to a disaster will be greater if:
- There is little or no warning
- The disaster is of human origin

- The extent of damage or loss of life is great
- The victim was at close proximity to the disaster
- Support systems were not available.

The risk of an individual developing severe psychological consequences is greater if that person is emotionally close to the individuals affected, has compromised coping abilities, has experienced many losses, feels overloaded in her/his role, or has never before experienced a disaster.

Some of the more common psychological reactions to a disaster include depression, sadness, fear, anger, phobias, guilt and irritability. Feelings of guilt may arise in survivors when many victims have died. Fear of death or of another disaster occurring is a frequently seen reaction. Anger may be exhibited as general irritability or fully fledged rage and may be directed toward the cause of the disaster, displaced onto the support system, or directed inward. Anxiety may be demonstrated by hyperalertness, trembling, palpitations and tenseness. Depression is often demonstrated by frequent crying, insomnia, decreased interest in relationships, loneliness and feelings of worthlessness.

Individuals may suffer impaired intellectual functioning, have difficulty concentrating or making decisions, and experience impaired memory. Psychosomatic complaints and mental illness are also responses to disaster situations and are evidenced by loss of appetite, fatigue, intestinal upset, sleep disorders, and muscular weakness. Pre-existing medical conditions are frequently exacerbated by disaster.

If survivors do not recognize and deal effectively with these feelings, they may suffer numbness and exhaustion. Individual responses to disaster are unique, and survivors should be counselled accordingly. The psychological stress experienced as a result of a disaster may have long-terms effects, such as interpersonal or social problems. Some individuals may turn to alcohol or drugs in an attempt to relieve their stress. Others may have difficulty resuming their usual routines and relationship patterns.

9.18.2 Post-traumatic stress disorder

Post-traumatic stress disorder (PTSD) may occur in victims and in rescuers. Three criteria define the syndrome. First, the trauma must be universally recognized. Second, the individual must re-experience the trauma through flashbacks, dreams, or triggering events. Third, the individual must demonstrate psychic impairment (i.e. either numbing or decreased interest in normal events). In addition, victims of PTSD experience two or more of the following symptoms: hyperalertness or exaggerated startle response, sleep disturbance, survival guilt, decreased concentration, impaired memory, and avoidance behaviour. Reminders of the trauma increase the symptoms in victims of this syndrome. Healthcare professionals and others involved in treating clients after disasters should be aware that the symptoms of PTSD may not be evident for some time after the actual event has occurred. Health personnel need to be sensitive to the possibility of PTSD in survivors of disasters.

9.18.3 Support measures

Simple support measures may limit the devastating effects of disasters. These include:
- Keeping families together, especially children and parents

- Assigning a companion to frightened or injured victims or placing victims in groups where they can help each other
- Giving survivors tasks to do to keep them busy and reduce psychological trauma
- Providing adequate shelter, food and rest
- Establishing and maintaining a communication network to reduce rumours
- Encouraging individuals to share their feelings and to support one another
- Isolating victims who demonstrate hysterical or panic behaviour.

Some people will need more intensive support. Whenever possible, community mental health nurses will be an important asset to the healthcare team to assist in meeting the psychosocial needs of victims. A quick psychological assessment guide is a useful tool to help emergency personnel determine the psychological state of victims. Individuals at risk of suffering psychological crises after disaster may not seek help even if they need it. Therefore, it is essential that the healthcare professional assess the stress level of victims, make other rescue team members aware of this, and refer those victims who need help to appropriate professional counsellors. The healthcare professional, as a member of the disaster team, participates in rescue operations and acts as a case-finder for people suffering psychological stress, intervening to help the victim deal effectively with the stress.

9.19 Death at work

It is a devastating experience to have a death at the place of work and the occupational health nurse has specific legal and ethical responsibilities, whether the death is caused by an accident or as the result of an illness. By law most healthcare professionals may not certify death and should attempt life-saving procedures, unless it is obvious that resuscitation is impossible, as with gross mutilation. The company physician, or in his/her absence, a local practitioner may be called in this case and once death has been certified the coroner must be informed. All cases of death due to unnatural, sudden or instant causes should be reported to the coroner, the Department of Labour and the Compensation Commissioner and the scene must be left as it was found until all investigations are completed.

Accurate record-keeping of all relevant facts, including the names of witnesses is, as always, important. Ethically the healthcare professional must do all in his/her power to preserve life, but when death is certified he/she must preserve dignity in death, remembering also that to fellow workers and onlookers the body is still the person that they knew. She should carefully cover and screen the body and arrange for removal as soon as possible.

The healthcare professional will be aware of the effect of the stressful event on the fellow workers and will reassure them and arrange for them to get back to work. It is the nurse's duty to inform management of the event in a concise report. The personnel department also needs to know and it should inform any relatives who may also be employed at the same firm.

If possible, the occupational health professional and a senior member of management will inform close relatives at home. If this is not possible, the police will do it. It is at times like these that the professional status of the occupational health nurse stands him/her in good stead.

9.20 Conclusion
Disaster management has many facets. In a constant changing world of technology, economics and politics, adequate training and preparation can never be left unattended. Ignorance and lethargy cannot and should not be tolerated where disaster preparation is concerned. Significant morbidity and mortality can be prevented if adequate preparation is made before unforeseen circumstances arise.

9.21 Bibliography
Cardona, V. D., Hurn, P. H., Mason, P. J. D., Scanlon, A. M. & Veis-Berry, S. W. 1999. *Trauma Nursing from Resuscitation through Rehabilitation*. 2nd edition. Philadelphia: WB Saunders.

Fisher, A. 1981. *Lessons from Major Accidents: A Comparison of the Three Mile Island Nuclear Core Overheat and the North Sea Platform Bravo Blowout*. Luxemburg: International Institute for Applied System Analysis.

Paolini, A., Buchan, C. & Dalgety, T. 2001. Study Guide for Basic Ambulance Students. Unpublished manuscript.

Schneid, T. D. & Collins, L. 2001. *Disaster Management and Preparedness*. Boca Raton, Fla: Lewis Publishers.

Tintinalli, J., Ruiz, E. & Krome, R. 1997. *Emergency Medicine: A Comprehensive Study Guide*. 4th edition. New York: Mc Graw-Hill.

10 Epidemiology

S. P. Hattingh

10.1 Introduction

The study of epidemiology is an interesting field. Occupational health professionals have access to epidemiological data of a defined population because of the documentation they keep on, for example, workers, the environmental conditions, absenteeism, pensions, exposures and workplace conditions, accidents and investigations and many more. Industrial hygiene measurements are conducted routinely and can be used to reconstruct an appropriate grading of exposures to which workers are or were subjected. Epidemiological principles should therefore be familiar in the workplace and can be part of the daily activities of the healthcare professional. Epidemiology has its roots in Biblical times and in the writings of the Greek physician Hippocrates. The Aphorisms of Hippocrates (fifth century BC.) indicate careful observation of a large number of case studies on diseases. In ancient times, epidemiology was used to study epidemic diseases. Because of the lack of knowledge of prevention intervention in the natural history of diseases, physicians could do little more than observe and record the morbidity and mortality rate among sufferers. Up until the Renaissance, physicians rarely recorded diseases and their observations were generalized and based on impressions rather than empirical evidence. During the Reformation, people believed that disease was the result of harmful forces and spirits or punishment for transgressions, or even a trial of faith.

It was John Grant who, in 1662, made great strides for the science of epidemiology when he introduced statistics by using numerical records to interpret statistical figures of diseases. In the nineteenth century, epidemiologists developed a painstaking system of monitoring diseases, which included definitions of the causes and relationships between cases and the characteristics of the population in which these diseases occurred.

While visiting cholera sufferers in London in 1854, John Snow investigated the companies that supplied the drinking water and discovered that the people who contracted the disease got their water from the same polluted source, namely the Thames. Through this epidemiological study, he collected data about the disease and demonstrated a mode of transmission of cholera about 30 years before Koch isolated and identified the cholera vibrio (Vibrio cholerae).

In England, one-fourth of the population died of the plague in the fourteenth century and this trend continued in Europe for more than three centuries. It later spread to Japan where the Japanese scientist, Kitasato, discovered the plague bacillus after the disease had spread to Hong Kong. It was only after ten years that the web of causation of this disease was traced from rats to fleas to human beings.

Florence Nightingale (1820–1910) laid the foundations of epidemiology in nursing during the Crimean War. Forty out of 100 British soldiers were dying in the Crimea before Florence Nightingale instituted environmental and nutritional changes in the field hospitals. Through her interventions, the mortality rate dropped to two per cent. She viewed environmental conditions as the most important factors that contribute to disease and found that physical conditions, rather than psychological and social conditions, contributed to disease. She emphasized that clean air, ventilation and hygiene were of the utmost importance to combat and prevent disease.

It is during the Second World War that risks that contribute to diseases were identified, such as the risks of heart disease, lung cancer and other public health problems.

It can thus be said that the science of epidemiology has its origins in the investigations of outbreaks of infectious diseases. In contemporary medical sciences, the scope of epidemiology and its application have been greatly extended to include the full spectrum of diseases (e.g. infectious and non-infectious diseases, such as acute and chronic diseases) and conditions (e.g. suicide, alcoholism, road accidents, occupational injuries, psychological conditions and social problems such as overcrowding etc.).

The science of epidemiology today does not belong exclusively to the medical profession and it is not only the prerogative of the professional epidemiologist to find causes and solutions for problems, and to apply preventive strategies. The science of epidemiology is practised in a multiprofessional team and many individuals, not necessarily only healthcare professionals, are involved in identifying and controlling diseases.

In occupational health, epidemiology has a dual role, namely to describe the deaths, accidents and illness in the occupationally active population. It is also in search of the determinants of health, injury and disease in the occupational environment. The occupational health professional has an important role to play in the science of epidemiology because he/she has a unique privilege to serve the sick, as well as the healthy, in the work situation. If this is combined with epidemiological methods, the occupational healthcare professional may diagnose the presence of hazards before disease or undesirable conditions arise. The entire workforce is constantly under the surveillance of the occupational healthcare professional and this is vital in the prevention and control of diseases or other undesirable conditions. In the end, the findings of the healthcare professional in occupational health, which are based on facts, may contribute to promote a logical basis for managerial, political and legislative changes to benefit not only the worker, but the family and the community as a whole.

10.2 Learning objectives

At the end of this chapter, the reader should be able to:
- Plan and conduct, within the multidisciplinary team, appropriate and meaningful epidemiological studies in the occupational milieu
- Gather and keep appropriate epidemiological data in order to analyse and interpret health and health-related issues within the total work environment (physical, cultural, environmental, social, psychological and economic) context
- Explore causative and contributory factors which may influence the health and well-being of the person in the work environment
- Translate health and health-related issues into the health status of the person/persons at work
- Utilize health-related data to suggest strategies to deal with existing needs within the occupational environment
- Play a meaningful role in the transformation of healthcare delivery in the occupational health environment
- Use effective and appropriate ways to present and communicate epidemiological data to different levels of management structures.

10.3 What is public health?

The orientation of public health was initially an attempt to control epidemics, however, through the discovery of vaccines and the entry into the industrial revolution, this orientation changed to include strategies with a preventive approach and attempts to promote health. The increasing emphasis on the curative aspects of healthcare resulted in the marginalization of public health. Preventive healthcare was marginalized because the emphasis was on curative aspects rather than preventive aspects of healthcare. However, the change in disease profiles (for example, the Aids pandemic), and the costs of curative services and health policies, resulted in the public health development and intervention of preventive rather than the curative approach.

Public health is a combination of sciences with the objective of improving the health status of people. Epidemiology is one of these sciences that forms part of public health. This approach is in contrast to the medical approach, which concentrates on the diagnosis and treatment of *ill health in individuals*. The field of public health is concerned with the health needs on a larger scale, such as the community or the population of the world. To enable scientists to look at the bigger picture, the public health approach has a strong multidisciplinary tradition in which all disciplines concerned with health are involved, for example doctors, nurses, epidemiologists, environmental health officers, sociologists, psychologists, bio-statisticians, demographers, and any other profession dealing with the health and well-being of the population. These individuals and groups of scientists are equipped with a variety of skills and they are able to look at health needs from various angles and combine their efforts to ensure an effective and comprehensive approach to the health and well-being of an entire population in its many facets. A combination of skilled people and scientists are able to pool their skills, which enables them to ensure adequate planning, implementation and evaluation of the inputs and outcomes of healthcare.

10.4 Conceptualizing epidemiology

Epidemiology is a basic medical science that is concerned with the distribution and determinants of diseases in human populations. Specifically, epidemiology is concerned with the examination of the patterns of ill health in groups of people and epidemiologists try to determine why certain individuals may develop a particular disease while others do not.

Epidemiology is the study of the distribution of and changes in the patterns of diseases and conditions and its purpose is to identify variables in people and the environment that may affect the occurrence of diseases and conditions.

The science of epidemiology is also concerned with efforts to explain the aetiology of certain diseases, injuries and conditions. It identifies and describes the factors that contribute to health or illness, and provides the basis for developing and evaluating health programmes to promote health and to prevent disease.

In occupational health, the study of the epidemiology of the workforce reflects the needs of workers over time and it predicts the future human needs of this population.

Epidemiology addresses the differences in people that cause disease, the distribution of people in relation to age, sex, race, occupation and social behaviour and characteristics, as well as genetic determinants or other characteristics that are prominent in certain individuals and groups. Disease-related attributes are also identified and studied, as well as aspects such as the influence of drugs, alcohol, cigarette smoking, attitude towards life, stress, intrinsic factors such as immunological status, cholesterol levels, high blood pressure and high blood glucose, and a myriad other factors that influence the health and well-being of the population.

In essence, epidemiology deals with the following:
- The general characterization of the environment and those exposed to it
- The incidence of diseases and conditions
- The distribution, intensity and duration of diseases and health-related phenomena in groups and communities
- The determinants (causes) of diseases or health-related phenomena and the interaction between these variables
- The increase or decrease of health-related conditions and events and the changes that occur over time
- The effect of diseases and other conditions on the health and well-being of populations, communities and groups
- The application of information to control health problems
- The comparison of data with other areas (e.g. other workplaces, other countries or populations or communities).

Epidemiologists also strive to answer the following questions:
- Do certain people have special characteristics that are related to certain diseases?
- Why do some people recover more quickly than others from the same disease?
- Is one kind of treatment superior to another and if so, why?

10.4.1 The distribution of disease and health-related phenomena

Many diseases can be related to time, place and/or person. For example, malaria occurs mostly during the summer (time), in endemic areas where the mosquito thrives (place) and visitors to these areas are at risk (person).

Another example is the history of the reporting of the first Aids case in 1980 (also called a sentinel case) which is of particular interest, because of the severity of the disease and the rapid spread of the disease to others. The first Aids cases occurred between October 1980 and June 1981 (time) and were reported in Los Angeles (place). It was reported that mostly male homosexuals in their early 30s, who were previously in good health, were affected by the disease (person).

10.4.2 Determinants of the disease or health-related phenomena

The determinants of diseases or conditions refer to specific conditions or events that lead to the specific disease or condition or that contribute to the disease or condition. For example, the specific bacteria that causes tuberculosis is mycobacterium tuberculosis, but the contributory factors that lead to the development of the disease are malnutrition, a lower level of immunity (e.g. other prevailing aspects such as the frailty of the elderly and other diseases such as Aids) and socio-economic factors (unemployment, overcrowding and poverty).

With modern technology, such as rigorous surveillance and tests, many hazardous exposures at work have been reduced and as a result, many manifest occupational diseases are becoming rare.

Therefore, more sensitive indicators are needed to detect these, and again the emphasis is on prevention rather than cure, for example the rate of absenteeism for gastro-intestinal conditions was previously not looked at as an occupational risk – today more sensitive measurements are needed to determine the causative factor and to find the determinants of diseases and conditions, for example the frequency of headache, gastro-intestinal conditions and musculoskeletal pain are more sensitive indicators for diseases.

Through studying the determinants of the diseases, the factors that may cause illness can be isolated. The three broad factors traditionally described are the host (intrinsic factors), the environment (extrinsic factors) and the agent, referred to as the epidemiological triad. This triad can be used as a basis for planning interventions to restore and promote the health of workers. The epidemiological triad is depicted in Figure 10.1.

10.4.2.1 The host (intrinsic factors)

The forces within a person and the forces surrounding the person in the environment in which he/she works, plays and lives influence his/her state of health. Factors associated with the susceptibility of an individual to a specific disease include age, sex, race, genetic factors, immunological status, nutritional status, pregnancy, psychosocial factors, general health status, work experience and previous diseases. It is a fact that not all people contract the same infectious disease even though they may come into contact with someone who is suffering from a highly infectious disease. For example, a worker may have chicken-pox and live in a hostel adjacent to the place where he

Figure 10.1 Epidemiological triad

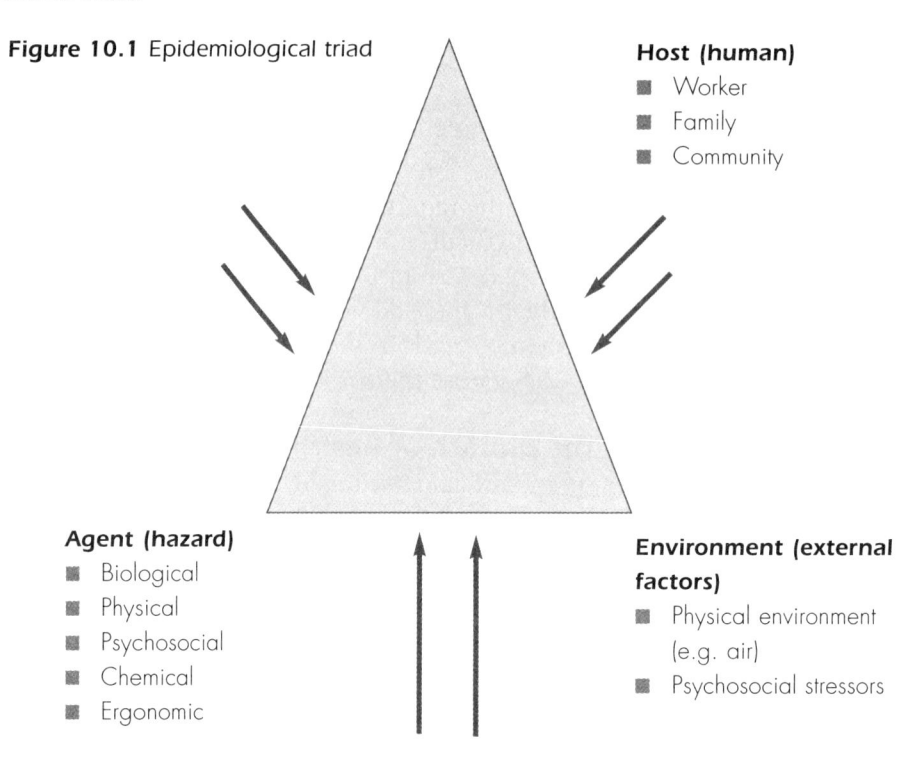

Host (human)
- Worker
- Family
- Community

Agent (hazard)
- Biological
- Physical
- Psychosocial
- Chemical
- Ergonomic

Environment (external factors)
- Physical environment (e.g. air)
- Psychosocial stressors

works. He still eats with his fellow workers, sleeps in the same dormitory and socializes with them during his illness, but not all who are in contact with him will develop the disease. A person who is HIV positive may, for example, develop the chicken-pox because of his/her lowered immunological status. This is because the human body continuously attempts to maintain homeostasis by counteracting the activities of those organisms that cause disease.

The ability of the body to defend itself against diseases may be placed in two broad areas, namely non-specific resistance and specific resistance.

Non-specific resistance
A wide variety of factors represents resistance against pathogens invading the body. These, among others, are:
- Intact skin
- Intact and healthy mucous membrane
- Phagocytosis, which is the ingestion and destruction of microbes or any foreign particle or matter by phagocyte cells
- Inflammation – when cells are damaged by microbes, physical agents or chemical agents, the injury sets off an inflammatory reaction or response and the injury is viewed as a form of stress. Inflammation is thus a defence mechanism of the body against stress due to tissue damage.
- Fever – an abnormally high body temperature caused by the infection, which inhibits the growth of some microbes and speeds up reactions that aid repair
- Antimicrobic substances are produced by the body to ward off infectious agents.

Specific resistance

Immunity, or specific resistance, involves the production of specific antibodies or specific cells against pathogens or their toxins. Immunity is developed throughout a person's life and is not inherited. Passive immunity refers to the natural immunity which a person obtains through maternal transfer of antibodies to the foetus or through breast milk. This type of immunity is temporary. Active immunity is obtained through artificial means such as immunization. It is long-lasting and may protect a person for life. A person can also obtain natural immunity by being exposed to a disease.

The components of specific resistance include:
- Antigens – any chemical substance that causes the body to produce specific antibodies and/or specific cells called T-cells, which react to the antigen
- Antibodies – a protein produced by the body in response to the presence of an antigen and which is capable of combining specifically with the antigen
- Cellular and humoral immunity is the ability of the body to defend itself against invading agents such as bacteria, toxins, viruses and foreign bodies.

Some host factors lead to the development of a disease, for example:
- The amount of the agent to which the host is exposed
- The general physical state of the individual
- The pathogenicity of the agent
- The virulence of the agent
- Host susceptibility.

There are still many unanswered questions about the interaction between the host factors and disease. There is still speculation as to why some heavy smokers do not develop lung cancer.

A number of genetic factors have been identified as contributing to either the increased or decreased susceptibility to certain diseases. Personality factors also play an important role in the susceptibility of people to disease. Psychologists, for example, believe that personality traits may contribute to cardiovascular diseases due to increased stress levels and perfectionalism. A person's lifestyle is a factor that must not be underestimated when disease susceptibility is evaluated. People in the higher ranks of society are frequently more exposed to improper diets and thus more susceptible to diseases associated with affluence.

Another example is that the population group most at risk of being involved in work-related accidents is men aged 18–25 and with less than six months experience on the job. The host factors – age, sex and work experience – are a combination that increases the risk of injuries on the job. The characteristics could be that this group is associated with greater risk-taking, lack of knowledge and experience, lack of skills, and so on. Older workers may be susceptible because of host factors such as diminished sensory abilities, the effects of chronic diseases (e.g. hypertension, diabetes) and delayed reaction time. Another group of workers extremely susceptible to some adverse exposure in the workplace is women in their child-bearing years as a result of hormonal changes, increased stress, new roles and the expectations for woman, as well as transplacental exposures. These are all host factors that may influence certain workers to respond to potential toxins.

10.4.2.2 The environment (extrinsic factors)

The environment in which a person works, plays and lives may exert an influence on his/her health, either physically or/and psychologically. Environment includes all external conditions that influence the interaction of the host and agents. It also includes the geological and atmospheric structure of the area where work is performed.

These environmental conditions include factors such as the following:
- Living conditions, e.g. overcrowded
- Unhygienic conditions
- Environmental conditions, such as pollutants, extreme temperatures
- Occupation, employment conditions
- Climatic and seasonal changes
- Geographic location
- Lifestyle of the individual (e.g. dangerous hobbies)
- Shiftwork
- Inflexible management styles
- Stressors (physical, psychological, social and environmental).

Environmental factors thus include all the conditions of living and there is a significant association between determinants in the environment and disease. Diseases, however, arise from within a ecological system and therefore cannot be attributed to one factor alone. Host and environment each play an important role in producing a disease. By recognizing this important interrelationship, the occupational health professional may discover clues for preventive actions.

Unhygienic conditions create opportunities for toxins to threaten the health and safety of the worker. Social aspects in the environment, such as economical and political factors, affect the health of not only the worker, but also of the family and the community as a whole.

10.4.2.3 The agent

Agents that can be found in the workplace include biological, chemical, ergonomic, physical and psychosocial aspects of worklife. Agents are those factors associated with illness and injury. It should be kept in mind that the route of entry of an agent may affect the signs and symptoms associated with an agent, for example if a chemical agent enters the body through intact skin or through inhalation, the effect may be different or prolonged.

The principles of epidemiology are based on the complex interaction between the three variables that influence the interventions to prevent injury and illness, to restore health and well-being, and to promote health and well-being. To understand these variables and to design effective healthcare strategies for dealing with these variables, healthcare practitioners working in the occupational health setting need to look at how each element influences the others.

Biological agents
Biological agents are those living organisms capable of causing human disease, for example viruses, bacteria and other pathogenic organisms. Biological agents include substances of vegetable and animal origin, and micro-organisms and the products of their metabolism. These pathogens can be transmitted from worker to worker, from client to worker, or from worker to client. Airborne pathogens are of specific importance in the workplace as many of these pathogens can be spread to a large population in a short time. Other important pathogens are those spread by the blood and excretions of humans and animals, for example human exposure to the blood of other humans in the case of medical personnel by needle sticks (HIV, haemorrhagic diseases and hepatitis) and animals, for example rabies. Transmission of tuberculosis is an extremely important aspect to be considered in workplace settings. Many workers who are employed as maintenance, cleaning and security workers may, for example, be exposed to soiled filters in air conditioners, soiled equipment while doing repairs, soiled linen or contaminated dressings or specimens.

Workers may be exposed to the following biological agents:
- Vegetation and vegetable dusts
- Substances of animal origin
- Combination of substances of vegetable and animal origin
- Micro-organisms and their products of metabolism
- Insects (e.g. ticks, mites, mosquitoes, ants, fleas).

Chemical agents
Stanhope and Lancaster (2000:949) mention that less than 0.1 per cent of the 2 million known chemicals produced have been tested for their effects on humans.

Chemical agents used in the workplace are linked to a variety of effects when workers are exposed to an amount that exceeds the dose for the capacity of the body to deal with. These long-term effects include:
- Carcinogenic agents
- Mutagenic agents
- Atherogenic agents
- Schlerogenic agents
- Gonadotropic agents
- Embryotropic agents.

Nerve poisons cause spasmodic and neuroparalytic effects, narcotics affect the parenchymatous organs and some substances have a purely narcotic action. Some chemical agents produce blood changes when the dose is exceeded or if there is a cumulative effect. Many agents are bone-marrow depressants, some substances react with haemoglobin and others cause haemolysis. Irritants and corrosive substances cause eye, upper respiratory, skin and mucous membrane damage.

Chemical compounds used to inject or feed animals that serve as food sources for the general population, or used for spraying on crops are important compounds that may cause chronic and deadly diseases. Industrial wastes, either accidental or deliberate, may contribute to the pollution of water and soil and cause increased tissue damage in the population.

In many workplaces, significant exposure to a daily low-level dose of chemicals may be below the exposure levels, but cumulatively their action over years may be severe to the health of the worker.

Chemical agents often combine with other agents, and this combination has adverse effects on workers exposed to these substances. The effect on a worker depends on the level of exposure, for example the toxic effect of brief exposure to a high concentration is frequently different from prolonged exposure to a low concentration.

Epidemiological studies of chemical agents have identified the following chemicals as being toxic to the human body. These compounds are carefully monitored to identify the toxicity of chemicals to the human body, and agents such as lead, mercury, cadmium, nickel and zinc are all compounds which are carefully monitored. Since data for predicting human responses to many of the chemicals found in the workplace is inadequate, workers should be assessed for all potential exposures and take precautionary measures when handling these agents. High-risk and sensitive or vulnerable workers should be carefully screened and monitored for optimal health protection.

Epidemiological studies, therefore, are concerned with the raw materials and intermediates of the manufacturing process, their physical and chemical properties and their possible transformation in the surrounding medium. These studies also examine the environmental effect that these substances would have if they were spilled into the environment, and the effect this would have on workers and the population.

It is therefore essential that all healthcare practitioners should have a good understanding and knowledge of the basic principles of toxicology, which include the sources, routes of exposure, dose-response relationship, and the acute and chronic effects of chemical agents in a specific workplace.

Ergonomic agents

Ergonomic agents are those factors that are related to the work process. The intensity of an activity and the workload involved in certain types of work are ergonomic factors that determine the health of workers. These agents may cause illness or/and injury, for example, postural strain may result from performing certain tasks, such as lifting heavy objects; or working with vibrating equipment, such as jackhammers. Carpel tunnel syndrome, musculoskeletal injuries, back injuries, tendonitis and tendosynovitis are all examples of mechanical injuries related to the work a person performs. Injuries sustained from these ergonomic agents are often referred to as cumulative trauma and may lead to disability claims later in a worker's life. These injuries should be carefully recorded and the most important strategy to prevent them is by means of re-engineering and re-designing machines and processes.

Recent risk factors that have arisen in industries are monotony, lack of physical activity and mental overload. These agents cause nervous tension and functional strain, which may influence the physiological and neuroendocrine regulation of a worker.

Physical agents

Physical agents are those that produce injuries and adverse health effects through the transfer of physical energy. Examples of these agents are extreme temperatures, vibration, noise, radiation, lighting and extreme humidity. All these factors make up the microclimate in which a worker performs his/her daily tasks.

Epidemiological research, close scrutiny of workers and physical examinations are necessary to limit exposure to these agents and to prevent rather than cure. Workers should be taught safe working habits and encouraged to wear protective clothing. Monitoring exposures is important and the results should be directly related to the workers who are at risk. This class of agent is considered to be the most easily controlled.

Psychosocial agents

Psychosocial agents are those conditions that threaten the psychological and social well-being of the worker. Important factors are work-related stress and burnout, which are associated with professions such as police officers, nurses and paramedics. However, people working in other non-medical occupations are also susceptible, for example workers who are subjected to armed hold-ups, non-fatal violence at work, and people who perform dangerous jobs such as deep-sea diving. Shiftwork is one of the major contributors to the disturbances in homeostasis and has the potential to lead to a variety of psychological and physical problems, such as exhaustion, depression, anxiety, gastro-intestinal disturbances, sleeping disorders, eating disorders and aggression.

Workers react selectively to their environment in an attempt to maintain homeostasis. When this relationship fails and the harmonious relationship is broken, stress occurs. The stress, burnout and often post-traumatic stress associated with work are often severe and may affect interpersonal relations at work, home and socially and may lead to an increase in absenteeism and sick leave. Epidemiological studies are important to identify and eliminate the hazards of work-related stress. Table 10.1 summarizes the types of occupational hazards and associated health effects that can be identified through the interaction by the host, the agent and the environment.

Table 10.1 Examples of occupational hazards and associated effects

CATEGORY	EXPOSURE	EFFECT
Biological	Blood or body fluids	Bacterial, fungi, viruses
Chemical	Solvents	Liver disease, dermatitis, headache, central nervous system dysfunction
	Lead	Central nervous dysfunction
	Asbestos	Dermatitis, asbestosis
	Acids	Burns
	Glycol ethers	Reproductive effects

CATEGORY	EXPOSURE	EFFECT
	Mercury	Ataxia
	Arsenic	Peripheral neuropathy
	Pesticides	Poisoning, 'farmer's lung'
	Chlorine, alkalis, isocyanates	Ocular damage
	Propylene, glycol, mercury	Auditory nerve toxicity
	Chlorine gas, hydrogen cyanide gas	Respiratory system damage, hypoxia and asphyxia, cardiovascular collapse, systemic poisoning
	Hydrocarbon solvents	Cardiovascular toxicity, cardiac arrhythmia
Ergonomic	Static or non-neutral postures	Musculoskeletal disorders
	Repetitive or forceful exertions	Back injuries
	Lighting	Headache and eye strain
	Shiftwork	Sleep disorders
	Electrical	Electrocution
	Slips and falls	Musculoskeletal injuries
Physical	Noise	Hearing loss
	Vibration	Raynaud's disease
	Radiation	Reproductive effects and cancer
	Heat	Heat exhaustion and heat stroke
Psychosocial	Stress	Homeostasis affected, which results in drug and alcohol abuse, anxiety, depression, aggression, poor interpersonal relations

10.4.3 Health-related conditions and events

As in the past, epidemiology is concerned with communicable diseases, but now includes chronic diseases, such as hypertension, cancer, occupational diseases, rheumatic diseases, nutritional disorders and disabilities, as well as other health-related conditions such as suicide, divorce, criminal acts, rape and drug abuse. Health is thus viewed from a holistic perspective and in the field of epidemiology, physical, psychological, social, cultural, environmental and economical issues are taken into account on an equal basis.

10.4.4 Populations
It is important to realize that epidemiology essentially focuses on conditions and events in human populations, however there are many diseases that occur in animals which effect the human populations, for example anthrax, some worm infestations and rabies. It is important to realize that, although epidemiology is essentially concerned with conditions and events in human polulations, many diseases that affect humans are related to animals, for example anthrax, worm infestations and rabies. For this reason epidemiologists are also involved in the science of epizoology.

10.5 The application of epidemiology
Epidemiological methods can be applied for various purposes, including disease surveillance, searching for the measurements of morbidity and mortality, incidence and prevalence rates, searching for causes, diagnostic testing and determining the natural history of disease.

Risk assessment plays a key role in every occupational setting. This involves the assessment of or likelihood that an individual may contract a disease or condition in the workplace. Prevalence means the number of cases of the disease already present in the workforce or individual. Incidence means how fast new occurrences of the disease arise.

10.5.1 Risk
Risk or cumulative incidence is the likelihood that an individual will contract a disease and is a measure of the occurrence of new cases in the population. Applied to occupational health, risk can be seen as the observation of a particular population, for example miners working in a gold mine for a specific period of time, for example during January 2003 to January 2004 (the risk period). All members of the group are free of the disease at the start of the investigation. Risk or cumulative incidence is calculated as:

$$R = \frac{\text{New cases}}{\text{Persons at risk}} = \frac{A}{N}$$

R = Estimated risk
A = Newly affected cases
N = Number of unaffected persons in the population under study

> **CASE STUDY**
>
> On 1 January, 10 new miners were employed in a specific mine. Their ages were between 25 and 30 years. During their physical examinations, all were found to be in good health and fit. All were placed in the same working area and worked on the same shift for the next three months. All were subjected to the same moist conditions. After three months, two of the miners reported itching of their feet and redness and swelling between the toes. They were given medication, but

three weeks later the condition deteriorated and they reported off sick. During the same two weeks another miner reported at the clinic with the same condition. An investigation of the seven others revealed that two others were also showing mild symptoms of the same condition. The five others were not affected.

The risk of the disease therefore is estimated by:

$$R = \frac{A}{N} = \frac{5}{10} = 50\% \text{ affected during the first three months of employment}$$

Risk factors are characteristics or habits that are consistently more common in those people who suffer from a disease than those people not exposed to these risk factors. Some people are thus more susceptible or vulnerable to a specific disease or condition, for example people who smoke are more susceptible to cardiovascular diseases, people who experience adverse stress are more vulnerable to infections such as cold and flu, people exposed to severe traumatic experiences are more likely to develop post-traumatic stress disorders and poor people who live in overcrowded areas with limited access to proper nutrition are more vulnerable to contract tuberculosis. When applied to occupational health, one can from the example given in the case study above say that employees who work underground in moist conditions and who have poor hygienic habits are most susceptible to infections of their feet.

10.5.2 Disease surveillance

In occupational health the question is often asked: 'How often does a disease/condition occur?' In other words, healthcare workers and management and other people often ask about the frequency of a certain condition or disease prevailing in a specific workplace. To answer this question, the occupational healthcare worker must know the number of persons (workers) who acquired the disease or the number of cases reported of such diseases or conditions over a specific time and the size of the unaffected population. To be able to do this, the occupational health professional must have information of the current development and of a specific condition.

Workers with a specific condition can be identified through mechanisms such as physical, psychological or other investigations and/or laboratory tests. Generally, surveillance data in occupational health relates to general characteristics such as gender, race, age, place of work, type of work, and so on. Through surveillance data, high-risk groups can be identified and specific measures applied to prevent further occurrences of the condition. The identification of high-risk groups leads to more in-depth investigations into personal characteristics, environmental characteristics and behaviour.

10.5.3 Morbidity and mortality

Morbidity (the effect of illness) is particularly useful when a disease or condition does not have a high mortality rate, for example rheumatoid arthritis, hearing/visual impairment and mumps. There are many facets to mortality and not a single agreed measurement. Morbidity rates are often used to clarify the reasons for mortality. In the workplace, morbidity rates are of the utmost importance because these rates may indicate preventive treatment and measures to be taken. They are also an indication of the success of preventive strategies.

Morbidity is classified in three major groups, namely impairment, disability and handicap.
Impairment is organ-based and describes failure or loss of an organ to function, for example renal or cardiac. *Disability* is when a person is unable to function effectively, for example wash him-/herself, walk, see or hear. *Handicap* is socially based and means there is a deficiency in the social functioning of the person and that a person cannot fulfil his/her role, for example if the person is unable to function as a parent.

Statistics of mortality rates (death rates) and morbidity rates (illness rates) are collected routinely in every occupational setting. These rates are used as indicators of the frequency of death and disease as they occur in time, place and persons. The concept of morbidity also includes measures related to specific symptoms of diseases and conditions, days off from work and the number of clinic visits of workers. These statistics contribute to the overall determination of trends of diseases and conditions, not only in the workplace but also compared with other industries and the country as a whole.

Mortality rates contribute in providing invaluable data on the trends in the health of the population. How valuable this data is for the occupational setting, depends on the completeness of records, the accuracy of the diagnosis, the monitoring of the workers and the records of autopsies to confirm the diagnosis.

The death rate (crude mortality rate) is calculated as follows:

$$\text{Crude mortality rate} = \frac{\text{Number of deaths in a specific period in a specific year} / 100}{\text{Average total population during that period}}$$

The crude mortality rate does not take into account the age, sex, occupation, socio-economic class and other factors, however, specific mortality rates are used when specific groups in the community are studied, for example age, sex, occupation and race. The specific mortality rate is calculated as follows:

$$\text{Specific mortality rate} = \frac{\text{Number of deaths in the occupation for a specific period in a specific year} / 100}{\text{Average number of people in that specific occupation/ period}}$$

10.5.4 Prevalence

Prevalence refers to the number of existing cases in a specific population. It is calculated as follows:

Occupational health

$$P = \frac{C}{N}$$

P = Prevalence
C = Existing cases
N = Number of persons under observation

CASE STUDY
During 2002 the floods in Mozambique caused havoc and 780 workers were deployed to repair damages to roads and bridges. A mobile medical facility was established to diagnose and treat minor injuries and diseases. During the first three weeks, 143 workers reported diarrhoea and cholera was cultured from the specimens of stool. The prevalence of cholera can thus be determined as:

$$P = \frac{143}{780} = 0.18 = 18\% \text{ of the workers were affected by cholera for a specific period of time}$$

Prevalence is thus calculated as the number of people in a population (e.g. road workers) who have the disease either at a particular time or over a stated period of time. Prevalence rates are often used in decisions to intervene medically. It is also used to plan health services. High rates can suggest that the nature of the work (population) and the environment are generating new cases.

The prevalence rate is all the existing, as well as all the new cases of a condition. The prevalence rate is influenced by the number of people who became infected and the number of people who die or do not recover from the disease or condition. Prevalence rates are important in determining measures of chronic illness in the workforce and are affected by the factors that influence the duration of the disease. Thus, prevalence rates have relevance to the planning of services, personnel and for evaluating treatments that prolong life.

10.5.5 Incidence rate

This rate measures the rapidity with which a newly diagnosed disease develops over a period. To estimate the incidence rate, the total population is observed, and the number of new cases of a disease in the population and the net times or person times are needed.

$$IR = \frac{A}{PT}$$

IR = Incidence rate
A = Number of new cases of the disease in a specific population
PT = Patient time (the net time in which the disease developed)

CASE STUDY

During 1990 a mining industry reported that they had 200 workers employed at a specific mine.

During routine X-rays and screening in June that year, 25 workers were found to be affected by tuberculosis. The remaining 175 workers were free of any lung disease. During the first two years, one other case was reported, seven years later another case and two years later another.

Thus, the total number of new cases of the disease reported were: 3

Person time (in years) = 2 + 7 + 2 = 11 (years)

$$IR = \frac{3}{11} = 0.27 \text{ cases/person-year} = 27\%$$

Incidence rates are often difficult to determine because the population studies may change over a specific period of time, for example a year. Therefore, the incidence rate should take into account the variable time periods individuals are disease-free and the risk of developing the disease.

In occupational health, incidence rates refer to the rate at which a specific condition develops in the workplace. It is the number of new cases of a disease, injury or any other condition that occurs within a specific time. These rates are used to study the patterns of both acute and chronic illnesses that may occur in the workplace. These rates are of the utmost importance in the workplace because they reflect a direct measure of the magnitude of new conditions in the workforce and provide an assessment of the risk associated with a specific condition.

10.5.6 Searching for causes

Epidemiologists often rely on interviews, records and laboratory examinations as sources of information to determine the risk factors associated with a specific condition.

10.5.7 Diagnostic testing

The purpose of diagnostic testing is to obtain specific objective and undisputed evidence of the presence or absence of a specific condition. This evidence can be obtained to detect diseases at the earliest stage among asymptomatic persons. It is referred to as screening. Diagnostic testing can also be used to confirm a diagnosis among persons with existing symptoms.

10.5.8 Determining the natural history

The natural history of a disease refers to the natural development of a disease when this development is not interrupted by prevention and treatment. The disease is allowed to develop and take its natural course. It is often not necessary to treat some diseases because a person may fully recover (e.g. the common cold), however, some diseases may result in complications, leading to disabilities or even death if there is no intervention (e.g. tuberculosis). Another possibility is that an untreated disease could become chronic, impairing the normal functioning and also having an impact on that person's family, social and economic life (e.g. diabetes and some forms of psychiatric illness).

HIV cannot be cured – this means that the disease will follow its natural course until the death of the person. Tuberculosis, on the other hand, can be prevented and treated and, if detected early by screening, the health professional may realize that this disease can be spread to people who share the same geographical area, workplace facilities, water sources, and so on and that these people may share the same disease pattern. Making sense of such phenomenon, identifying the commonalities and in doing so identifying the causes of the phenomenon, is exactly what epidemiologists do.

10.6 Types of epidemiological investigations

Epidemiology uses observational rather than experimental approaches to research design. There are basically two major types of epidemiological studies, namely observational studies and experimental studies.

10.6.1 Observational studies

With observational studies, the researcher observes, but does not intervene, in other words, it allows nature to take its course. There are two major observational types of studies, namely descriptive and analytic studies.

10.6.1.1 Descriptive studies

The leading causes of death in developing countries are infectious diseases, such as tuberculosis, measles and HIV/Aids; and chronic and non-infectious diseases, such as poisoning, malignancies and cardiovascular diseases. To develop strategies for the prevention and control of these conditions, it is important that the specific priorities must be determined and specified. The use of descriptive studies is of importance here. These studies describe the amount and distribution of disease within a population. This approach relies primarily on the use of existing data and answers the following questions:

Who is affected?
The most important variables are age, sex, marital status, education, occupation, income, cultural and religious group, family size, nutritional status and immune status. In occupational health, the clinic attendance and non-attendance might be answered with this question.

Where is the disease distributed (place)?
The place where people live and work may partly determine which health and disease problems they suffer from and what use they make of the available health services, for example town, village or isolated dwelling, high or low altitudes, proximity to rivers, forests, wild animals or sources of toxic substances and the distance they are from a dispensary, healthcare centre or hospital (Vaughn & Morrow, 1998:11).

When is the disease present (time)?
The time factor is important to determine when health problems are the most severe or when the incidence of new cases is greatest. To show this, cases, episodes or events can be grouped according to new cases per day, week, month or year.

What is the overall effect of the disease?
The effect of the disease can be determined as acute or chronic or leading to death. Descriptive studies are important in occupational health because they are based on routinely available data or on data obtained in special surveys and these studies are often the first step in an epidemiological investigation. They are of great importance in occupational health because without them, it would be impossible to set up effective programmes for health protection for the working population. Descriptive studies make no attempt to analyse the links between exposure and effect, and are therefore often criticized. Caution should therefore be exercised in drawing conclusions from such studies. They are usually based on death statistics and may examine patterns of death by age, sex, occupation, ethnicity and religious affiliation during specific time periods or in various countries. Descriptive statistics also describe the frequency of occurrence of health phenomena, for example morbidity, sickness and absenteeism in the general population. By comparing these results with the data collected among different populations and in different periods leading up to a disease, changes with time can be identified in order to provide a basis for organizational action, planning and evaluation of healthcare and the formulation of hypotheses on cause-effect relationships.

10.6.1.2 Analytic studies
Epidemiological studies are mostly analytic in nature. An analytic study goes further than a descriptive study by analysing relationships between health status variables. Analytic cross-sectional studies in occupational health provide information on interesting questions relatively quickly and with an acceptable level of expenditure. There are four types of analytical studies, namely correlation (ecological) studies, prevalence (cross-sectional) studies, case-control (case-reference) studies, and cohort (follow-up) studies.

Correlation studies (ecological studies)
In correlation studies, groups of people are studied, rather than individuals. In this type of study the relationship of various factors pertaining to a disease or condition are investigated and correlations are made between various countries. Although this type of study is usually simple to conduct, the interpretation of findings may be problematic because it is almost impossible to compare populations from different countries, and because there may be many variables, such as the socio-economic status, culture, religion, en so on.

Prevalence studies (cross-sectional studies)
This type of study measures the prevalence of certain diseases or symptoms with regard to work-related factors. These studies are often easy and more economical to conduct

and are useful for investigating given characteristics of individuals such as age, sex, ethniticity and blood group, and can measure the true differences in morbidity between people. In sudden outbreaks of diseases where measurements of several exposures must be investigated, these studies are most often the most convenient first step of the investigation.

Data obtained in the case of prevalence studies is mainly from medical examinations or from individual questionnaires or screening procedures. These studies are often concerned with the etiology of work-related diseases rather than with pathogenesis. For example, cross-sectional studies may be used to determine which exposures to chemical of physical factors and which physical or neuropsychic loads give rise to health disturbances and also which occupations, in which activities, and under which additional conditions such disturbances occur. These studies are often used as a baseline for cohort studies and are most often used to test the acute and subacute effects of, for example, a new chemical or other potential noxious factor in the occupational environment.

Case-control studies (case-reference studies)
Case-control studies are aimed at looking at the causes of diseases and are used with much success in the study of rare diseases. These studies include people with the disease and a suitable control group of people who do not have the disease. The occurrence of the possible cause is compared between cases and controls. These studies are retrospective in nature because they look backward from the disease to identify the cause. A case-control study starts with the selection of cases which should represent all the cases from a specific population. The most difficult task is to select controls in order to sample exposure prevalence in the population that generated the cases. Case control studies are often an effective and convenient alternative to other designs in epidemiology; however, the validity is often difficult to control and to evaluate.

Beaglehole, Bonita and Kjellstrom (1998:37) mention that 'an important aspect of case-control studies is the determination of the start and duration of exposure for cases and controls'. It is thus important that those affected by the disease be questioned about their experience of the disease. It is important to record detailed and accurate information, such as employment records, specifically in industry where exposure is sometime determined by biochemical measurements (for example for lead and cadmium).

Cohort studies (follow-up studies)
Cohort studies begin with a group of people (a cohort) who are free of a disease or who have a low exposure to a specific agent. This group may also be classified into subgroups according to exposure to a potential cause of disease or outcome. This group is then followed up to see if new cases of a disease are developed with and without exposure.

Cohorts may be established in two ways, namely prospectively (at the present time) or retrospectively (historically). The value of a prospective study is that it can be planned in detail by the investigator so that the risk factors can be identified. Most commonly though, cohorts are established retrospectively.

Cohort studies provide the best information about the causation of disease and are the most direct measure of the risk of developing a disease. Many investigations are of a long-term nature and need accurate collection over long periods.

Beaglehole et al. (1998:39) refer to the following incident:

> One example is the catastrophic poisoning of residents around a pesticide factory in Bhopal, India in 1984. An intermediate chemical factory in the production process, methyl isocyanate, leaked from a tank and the fumes drifted into surrounding residential areas, killing more than 2 000 people and poisoning 200 000 others.

The writers also state that the acute effects of this incident were easily studied with a cross-sectional design, but the chronic effects of the poisoning and those effects that developed long after this incident are still being studied using a cohort design.
Certain important aspects need to be considered when finding a cohort, among others:

- Sample size must be determined before the search for the cohort begins and the number of workers must be sufficiently large to permit detection of the hypothesized health outcome.
- The time in which the cohort takes place must be sufficient to allow the development of diseases.
- The levels of exposure must be adequate to allow for a definite disease, e.g. asbestosis.
- Exposures other than the one of interest complicate the interpretation of the study. It is desirable to find a cohort exposed only to the agent of interest.
- Historical exposure data should be available in order to permit interpretation of the study findings in relation to the level of past exposure.
- Records and definite identification must be available to establish who was exposed (Karvonen & Mikheev, 1986).

Cohorts follow some major steps, as described below.

Formulation of a hypothesis
Cohort studies test a well-formulated hypothesis. For example, miners who had worked for a certain asbestos mining company for the last 30 to 40 years developed asbestosis. These findings were the basis for the hypothesis that asbestos miners were at greater risk than the general public to develop certain chronic diseases, especially asbestosis.

Study design and cohort definition
Once the hypothesis was formulated, an investigation was lodged in the form of a historical cohort morbidity and mortality study. After claims had been received of asbestosis, the documentation of the miners was scrutinized. Investigators studied the proof supplied to them by the mining company and the former workers and their next-of-kin, autopsy reports were studied and the data contained critical information necessary to identify cohort members and trace them through time. This information

contained the dates on which the miners were employed by the company, the type of work each worker performed, in which mines the miner had worked, and the related exposure to the product mined. The medical history was also scrutinized and, being a notifiable disease, records of treatment of these miners did exist. Prior industrial hygiene records were also identified and used to estimate the exposures.

Follow-up
An attempt to determine the vital status (alive or dead and cause of the death), of at least 95 per cent of the cohort is desirable. In the above-mentioned study, the vital status for all cohort members for a specific period was determined. The last date represents the closing date or cut-off or study-end date for the study. The investigation and data analysis were stopped at a specific date, even though the study had the potential to continue. The time lag allowed for completion of the study and preparation for the court case that was to follow.

Analysis
The observed morbidity and mortality experience of the cohort was compared with the expected outcome. The mortality and morbidity of the cohort were calculated by taking into account the age, employment and disease/treatment history, the calendar time and the exposure to the substance.

10.6.2 Experimental studies
Intervention or experimentation involves attempting to change a variable in one or more groups of people. In occupational health this could mean, for example, testing a new hand-cleaner on a specific group of mechanics to determine the effectiveness for hygiene. The effects of an intervention are measured by comparing the outcome in the experimental group with the control group. Ethical considerations are of paramount importance in this type of study and no workers should be subjected to any harm or denied treatment as a result of participation in such an experiment. The treatment must be ethical, legal and scientifically acceptable in the light of current knowledge.

Experimental studies are carried out in three ways, namely:
1　Randomized controlled trials (clinical trials)
2　Field trials
3　Community trials (community intervention studies).

10.6.2.1 Randomized controlled (clinical) trials
Randomized controlled trials or clinical trials are epidemiological experiments that are applied to study new preventive or therapeutic regimens. Participants are randomly selected by choosing them to be equivalent, and then allocated to the experimental group, while another group is allocated to the control group. The intervention may be a test for a new drug, new ear protection devices, different make of breathing apparatus and a new treatment regime for people who are sick. The results are assessed by comparing the outcome in the two groups.

Because of the ethical concerns of this type of study, strict protocols are maintained

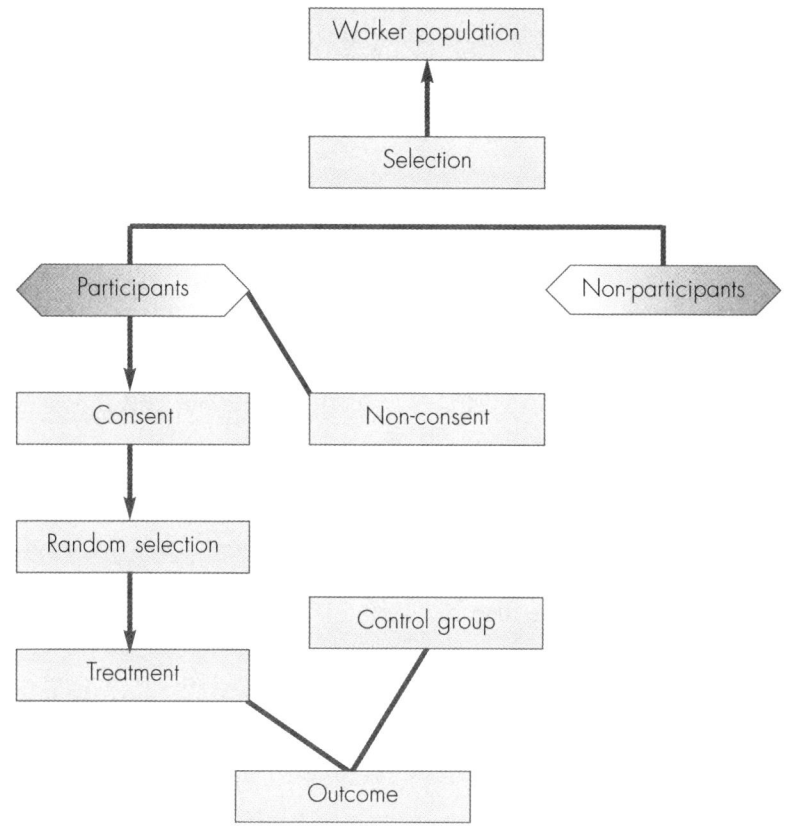

Figure 10.2 Design of a randomized (clinical) trial

throughout the study and rigorous measures must be taken not to cause harm to the person or the company.

10.6.2.2 Field trials
Field trials involve people who are disease-free but presumed to be at risk. These trials are undertaken to evaluate interventions aimed at reducing exposure without necessarily measuring the occurrence of health effects. Data collection takes place among the general population, since the subjects are disease-free and the purpose is to prevent the occurrences of diseases at a low frequency. Field trials are huge and costly undertakings, for example the Salk vaccine for the prevention of poliomyelitis which involved more than one million children. In occupational health, field trials may be used to determine the effectiveness of a variety of protective methods used by workers who are exposed to pesticides. This method may also be used to determine the levels of lead found in workers in the petrol-chemical industries by eliminating lead from petrol. Some of these field trials can also be carried out on a smaller scale and at a lower cost in industry.

10.6.2.3 Community trials
This type of trial concentrates on communities rather than on individuals. Community trials are appropriate for diseases and conditions that have their origins in social

conditions, which in turn can most easily be influenced by intervention directed to a group as well as in individuals. The prevention of HIV infection is a good example of such interventions.

10.7 Sources of data

Epidemiological studies may be conducted by:
- Data collected for routine purposes, for example routine physical examinations that are of immense value in descriptive epidemiology and may be useful in case-control or prospective cohort studies.
- Special recorded data on exposure at the workplace, of the worker and in the environment. This data is collected in cross-sectional surveys and prospective cohort or experimental studies.

Three main sources of data may be used, namely:
- Official statistics, which are kept by official corporate bodies and include the variety of morbidity and mortality statistics, for example pension, funeral, mortuary, register for notifiable diseases, sickness absence, medical aid records, accidents and occupational diseases and hospital records
- Records of employment and other data in workplaces include, for example, the area, places of work, type of work done, the dates of employment, reasons for leaving employment and other specific information regarding the specific employment at a given time.
- Records kept by occupational health services are details of routine medical examinations, tests (e.g. hearing tests, blood results), consultations, environmental monitoring (e.g. dust, lead), treatments at work (e.g. back injuries, psychological treatment), results of occupational-oriented inspections and enquiries, sickness and absences, results of special medical examinations and clinical examinations (e.g. blood tests, X-rays) on high-risk groups, audit records of morbidity of cases which needed specific medical attention (e.g. injuries on duty) and records and data on acute and chronic occupational poisonings.

10.8 The uses of epidemiology in occupational health

The workforce can be regarded as a community within a community. This workforce community has its own unique environment in which it functions and therefore also has its own specific health problems. Not all the health problems found in this working community are caused by the occupational exposures and conditions that workers are exposed to, but most of the health problems are related to natural ageing, diseases of lifestyle (e.g. drugs, alcohol abuse or obesity) or the 'general' morbidity patterns of the larger community. However, these 'general' problems do have an influence on the day-to-day functioning of the individual, since every disease can interfere with the working capacity of the worker and may influence or interfere with his/her ability to cope with occupational exposures, conditions and stressors. For this reason, the complete profile of the working community should be taken into account when assessing the total picture of the worker.

To achieve a complete picture of the workforce, the general state of each employee must be established by conducting a survey. Through this survey, the following aspects may be identified:

- The incidence or prevalence of important diseases specifically related to the workplace, for example asbestosis, may be detected.
- Minor illnesses may be cured or correctable measures taken in order to prevent deterioration of the condition (e.g. seemingly insignificant skin rashes may be treated before dermatitis occurs and more severe and expensive treatment is required).
- The early stages of chronic diseases may be identified, often without the person being aware of a simmering illness, for example diabetes or hypertension.
- Persons who are at risk of developing specific diseases such as obesity may have a high cholesterol level and consequently develop coronary heart disease – preventive and corrective measures may therefore be taken to address such diseases.
- Some people are restricted to do certain jobs, for example people with epilepsy may not become a crane operator, or colour blindness may be identified, which would restrict the person to performing only certain tasks.
- People with unfavourable health behaviour, for example heavy smokers or physically inactive people, may be identified and their suitability to perform certain jobs questioned.
- Health information about the importance of certain aspects may be provided, such as wearing ear protection and other safety attire, personal hygiene and smoking.
- Beliefs, customs and health behaviour in the workplace may be taken into account, for example traditional medicine treatment.
- Risk identification may be the first clue pointing to unrecognized health hazards, for example a sudden increase of dermatoses in a group may indicate wrong handling of a new chemical.
- Follow-up of changes in the occurrence of illness among employees may lead to observed changes in health patterns, to the identification of new health problems or to examining known health hazards and their changes after corrective measures, new treatment or any other measures have been applied.

The data collected from surveys is often used to identify people who have been exposed to specific conditions in order to:

- Identify the location of the exposure or hazard
- Quantify the hazards, for example to measure it in the air or in blood or stool
- Provide a basis for the prevention of diseases/disabilities associated with the hazard
- Assess the need for follow-up and regular health surveillance
- Monitor the trend of the hazard
- Provide data on the effect of the hazard on a specific community
- Monitor the progression of the disease/condition.

Surveys are the most useful way of collecting additional information that is not available from routine health information or surveillance systems. Because resources are limited (e.g. staff, time and money), the purpose and objectives of a survey must be clear from the start and management and health professions must agree that it is desirable and necessary.

Equally important is the selection of the screening methods to be used in the survey. These methods must be applicable, sensitive, objective and specifically related to the conditions as applied to a specific working community. If these basic aspects are not taken into consideration, false positive findings may lead to unnecessary further examinations which are often costly, may pose a risk and cause unnecessary anxiety. Five main stages are involved in an epidemiological investigation. These include:
1. Clarification of the need for the survey and stating the objectives
2. Determination of the sample and methods to be used in the survey
3. Organization and implementation of the survey
4. Analysis, interpretation and presentation of the findings
5. Use of the findings in health planning, prevention and control of diseases.

Healthcare professionals use epidemiological data in various ways. Epidemiological research serves as an aid to decision-making, planning, implementation and evaluation. Scientific epidemiologic research serves the following functions:
- It extends human knowledge.
- It serves as an aid to making practical decisions.
- It limits mistakes made in the past.
- It confirms or rejects previous findings.
- It compares population groups.
- It gives exact, quantified information.

Decision-making
Management use epidemiologic data to base their decisions on. These decisions must often be made in situations where alternatives are supported by results obtained from the data that healthcare professionals produce. It must, however, be kept in mind that epidemiological results alone do not serve as a basis for decision-making in practice, but that case histories, histories of accidents, engineering progress, financial aspects, cost-effectiveness and other considerations are part of the overall picture of decision-making.

Planning
Records kept by healthcare professionals provide a basis for annual reports which are presented to management. According to these records, the trends and tendencies of diseases and the overall health/disease profile of the workforce can be estimated. For example, production loss may occur during winter months when flu and colds are common. By estimating the production loss, management may plan an immunization campaign during the autumn to protect workers (and sometimes their families too) against the adverse effects of flu. Comparative studies may indicate whether or not this campaign was successful.

Planning of healthcare facilities and emergency services are also based on records, for example more advanced equipment such as audiometry equipment would be considered where data could be provided for such a need.

Data provided is also a valuable tool for the identification of training and education that is required, and may give an indication of recklessness, burn-out among workers and the attitude of workers.

Implementation
The implementation of various measures to identify disease patterns among the workforce is part of the total health surveillance programme in the workplace. Mass screening is aimed at identifying and diagnosing medical conditions that are related or may not be related to the job. Screening enables healthcare professionals to detect the initial stages of diseases and this early case finding may improve prognoses and serve as an important source of savings (in monetary terms and human resources) for the industry because it prevents absenteeism, sick leave pay-outs, promotes productivity in the healthy worker and limits disability claims. Examples of the implementation of early screening are X-rays and tuberculin tests for lung diseases (cancer and tuberculosis). Another important recent development is the voluntary HIV/Aids testing available to workers. This provides an opportunity for healthcare professionals to better understand the affected worker's opportunistic infections and to treat and counsel the worker more appropriately. These tests, however, still raise serious ethical concerns which need to be addressed.

Evaluation
The evaluation of numerous studies and recordings leads to the conclusion that prolonged exposure to, for example, different substances and conditions, even at low concentrations, may cause a variety of adverse effects on the human body. Evaluation allows for the determination of the degree of deviation from the general health of the workforce.

Evaluation of the workers' health records enables healthcare professionals to rank the workers according to the degree of risk incurred. Namely:

Group 1: No risk category, which indicates that workers are in a state of homeostasis.
Group 2: Potential risk categories, which indicate that the workers are in a steady state of equilibrium, that some risk may be attached to their health and well-being.
Group 3: These are the workers who are definitely at risk and are in an unsteady level of equilibrium with the environment.
Group 4: These are the workers who have been exposed and need follow-up and their equilibrium has been distorted.

10.9 Planning an epidemiological study
Planning an epidemiological study has definite steps according to a sequence of events.

The planning of an epidemiological study follows the following steps:
1. Identify the problem for investigation.
2. Determine the priority of the problem.

3. Formulate a hypothesis.
4. Formulate objectives.
5. Select a sample/population.
6. Determine research methods.
7. Conduct the survey.
8. Collect the data.
9. Analyse and interpret data.
10. Write report.
11. Present findings.
12. Take action: apply findings or recommend and implement changes.
13. Evaluate the outcome.

10.10 Ethical considerations in epidemiological research

In the light of the highly confidential nature of the information obtained in epidemiological research and the possible legal consequences of any breach of confidentiality, the healthcare professional is bound to maintain a high professional standard regarding all issues of confidentiality. Consideration is therefore given to the ethical considerations as described by the international declaration concerning ethics, set out in the Declaration of Helsinki as well as the Belmont Report. The World Health Organization (WHO) proposed international guidelines for biomedical research involving human subjects and these were framed with special reference to developing countries and problems of informed consent from certain disadvantaged subjects such as children, the mentally ill and prisoners.

The practice of epidemiology in occupational health settings requires workers and the community to adhere to the basic principles of biomedical ethics and carries special obligations to individuals and the community, not only those participating in this study, but also those whose health may be protected or improved by application of the results. People who have been exposed to a health hazard should realize that epidemiological studies carried out on them may not improve their personal situation but may help to protect thousands of others.

10.11 Conclusion

This chapter provided a brief introduction to the science of epidemiology as applied to the occupational healthcare environment in the understanding of health, disease and conditions related to the workplace. It described in broad terms the major and basic formulas and methods used in epidemiological investigations. The chapter attempts to make the professional healthcare provider aware that a wealth of information is collected every day and that by understanding the multiple factors of diseases, preventive measures can be taken to eliminate many of the occupational diseases known to them. However, this must be based on sound epidemiological research and factual information.

10.12 Bibliography

Beaglehole, R., Bonita, R. & Kjellstrom, T. 1998. *Basic Epidemiology*. Geneva: World Health Organization.

Karvonen, M. & Mikheev, M. I. (eds.) 1986. *Epidemiology of Occupational Health*. Geneva: World Health Organization.

Nies, M. A. & McEwen, M. 2001. *Community Health Nursing*. Philadelphia: WB Saunders.

Stanhope, M. & Lancaster, J. 2000. *Community and Public Health Nursing*. 5th edition. St Louis: Mosby.

Vaughn, J. P. & Morrow, R. H. 1998. *Manual of Epidemiology for District Health Management*. Geneva: World Health Organization.

11 Psychological health and adjustment in the work context

Z. C. Bergh

11.1 Introduction

As a health worker, in general and in your work, you must have observed many examples of people or employees with psychological and related problems. Think of drug and alcohol dependency, Aids, anxious employees, or employees responding with excessive suspicion, aggression or dependency, suicide, industrial injuries, people always complaining of illness while medical experts can find no cause or cure for such ailments, or employees who are always over-worked compared with those who mostly fail to perform. You may even have considered a whole work group or organization as 'unhealthy' because of dysfunctional relationships, negative and disloyal work behaviours or poor working conditions.

Psychological health is a multidimensional concept incorporating physical and mental (psychological) health, since more often than not both body and mind are involved in the illness–health relationship. This holistic emphasis is also reflected in the recognition that various factors – cultural, social, psychological, biological, environmental, economical, political and work – must be considered in assessing and managing people's health status. The *effects of illness and maladjustment* also spread further than the individual or immediate place of incidence because of the interactive nature of human behaviour in different systems. There can be a *circular relationship* between a psychological problem, a social problem, a work problem and their symptoms. Thus the policy on such a problem and the responsibility for it could become an individual, organizational, economic and even a political problem, an example being the ongoing controversy about Aids/HIV-infected people. Considering such multiple influences and consequences also emphasizes the importance of team approaches or various disciplines in healthcare of which psychological and occupational health nursing interventions should be important components.

Physical illness and related healthcare issues fall in the field of occupational health in which the medical disciplines, like occupational health nursing, are involved in the promotion and management of occupational health and safety. The field of occupational health entails an interdisciplinary study of all occupational health issues, which relate to the delivery of effective health services in work organizations and their environments, to ensure healthy and safe workplaces and effective work performance, but with special emphasis on physical illness of any type and the services related to it.

In this regard, psychological problems are recognized as one aspect of occupational healthcare.

Psychological or *mental health* as a comprehensive concept refers to certain behaviours and conditions in individuals, which in the context of their environment or situation and related norms, characterize their psychic or psychological well-being. Psychological adjustment or maladjustment can include behaviours such as the degree of life and job satisfaction, emotional stability, kinds of interpersonal relationships, social behaviour, actualization of potential and skills, stress experiences, as well as the presence or absence of psychopathology or psychological or psychiatric disorders, even physical handicaps and the influence of conditions such as Aids and unemployment. The degree of psychological adjustment also refers to people's coping behaviours, for example how they act in their environment, solve problems and handle life demands and work stress.

Because work is central and meaningful in most people's lives, personal success and psychological adjustment are often linked to job or career success. The study of work *adjustment or occupational mental health* is about the adjustment or maladjustment of employees in the context of work organizations. Therefore, an individual's occupational health cannot be separated from the individual's personal adjustment, nor from the organization's health, nor from the environment in which both the individual and the organization exist and function. Thus, it is also necessary to understand the interaction between employees and the organization because the degree of adjustment or maladjustment is not caused only by the situation or the individual's traits, but may instead be the result of the type of congruence or fit between the individual and his/her work situation. In this regard note, for example, Davis and Lofquist's theory (1984) of work adjustment, which in essence states that the level of job satisfaction and adjustment is determined by the congruence of work environment features and employee needs. An understanding of work, working, and both the individual and the organization and their interaction, will not only aid our assessment or diagnosis of causes and symptoms, but also help us to manage and promote occupational health, for instance, counselling the problem employee or intervening with aspects of organizational and even environmental functioning. In our modern times surely psychological work adjustment should be of equal importance to aspects such as the quantity and quality of products and services, the physical health of the worker and the hygiene of the workplace. The interaction between employee, workplace and environment and the complex nature of occupational health also indicate that occupational healthcare requires varied knowledge and multiple skills, for example, with regard to primary, occupational, clinical, community, social and psychological healthcare. Health psychology, for example, entails a new approach to thinking about and practising health matters in a multidimensional and interdisciplinary way. As such, health psychology brings together various disciplines, such as psychology, the medical sciences, and other social and behavioural disciplines in the understanding, assessment, treatment, management and promotion of health at individual and community levels.

Health, especially mental health, remains one of the world's greatest and most expensive problems. In this regard, however, Mickleberg also views occupational mental health as a neglected service in the industrial world (1986:426–434). Statistics on the incidence, prevalence and costs of health and mental health are often inaccurate and merely the tip of the proverbial iceberg. In most cases they underestimate the cumulative negative effects of physical and mental dysfunctions on the individual, families, workplaces, organizations and the community. It is estimated that up to 30 per cent of the world's population suffers from at least one type of psychological disorder such as anxiety and depression. If less serious stress and emotional problems are also considered, this figure may even be higher than 50 per cent (cited in Louw & Edwards, 1998; Lowman, 1993). A well-known fact is that only about 25 per cent of reported cases with psychological problems receive treatment. In this regard also, it is estimated that, depending on the condition, up to 60 per cent of patients who consult medical doctors on physical or organic complaints are actually experiencing psychological problems, especially anxiety, depression, stress reactions and psycho-physiological conditions.

In the work context it is generally accepted that stress-related disease is one of the highest by-products of business success. In this regard, cardiac diseases, which are normally associated with stress and psychosomatic conditions, are responsible for more than half of all the deaths and lost working days, and amount to a cost of hundreds of millions per annum. It is estimated that for every death resulting from an industrial accident, 50 people die because of cardiac disease. While it may be easy to assess the direct costs of physical and mental health problems, the indirect costs in terms of people's psychological pain and loss can never be calculated.

11.2 Learning objectives

At the end of this chapter, the reader should be able to:
- Describe the study field and related concepts of occupational health
- Identify, with examples, the roles and tasks of the occupational health worker
- Explain the interaction between employees, work organizations and environments
- Relate the importance of work in personal and work health and adjustment
- Give a description of psychopathology, mental health and psychological optimality
- Explain occupational health and work dysfunctions
- Cite criteria for psychological work adjustment
- Identify and illustrate, by examples, causes for personal and work adjustment problems
- Explain methods to assess and diagnose the status of occupational health in employees and organizations
- List certain psychological disorders
- Explain psychological work dysfunctions related to employees
- Describe work-related problems related to organizations' environments
- Discuss personal or self-management strategies to promote work adjustment
- Explain organizational and therapeutic approaches to improve work adjustment.

11.3 The role of the occupational health worker

The literature on psychological work adjustment stresses the interactive roles of management, the employee and other parties in health promotion. These roles include the treatment of occupational health problems, but also facilitating activities to manage and improve occupational health for all employees and in the organization as a whole (Cooper & Payne, 1994; Ross & Altmaier, 1994; Carroll, 1997; Dejoy & Wilson, 1995; Lowman, 1993; Bowerman & Collin, 1999). Health promotion and workplace counselling should not be merely 'lip service', but should form an integral part of effective human resources management and a service of caring and assisting employees to cope better, and adapt to the continuous changes in the workplace (Carroll, 1997). In our view, and according to D'Alonzo and Belinson (in Noland, 1973), and also more recently, Harrison (1984) and Carroll (1997), the role of the occupational health worker and psychologists can include the following functions:

- Executing, if necessary, needs analyses to determine the status of existing resources and occupational health problems
- Assessing, treating and referring troubled employees, in both serious and less serious cases
- Assessing the capacity of employees after rehabilitation or treatment for re-utilization in their work
- Executing emergency measures in crises or for employees in need, for example, debriefing and treatment during traumatic events
- Counselling and supporting troubled employees to empower themselves with health-related knowledge and effective health-promoting coping mechanisms
- Monitoring, controlling and influencing the factors in the workplace and environment that cause or support emotional maladjustment and other health problems
- Giving ongoing training to medical and human resources and health experts to manage workers with emotional problems, acting correctly towards rehabilitated workers, and implementing health programmes for employees
- Consulting with medical and other parties about troubled employees
- Consulting with and advising management on matters such as occupational health hazards, health policy, rehabilitation, health-promotion strategies and facilities
- Aligning health promotion activities and programmes with existing policies, ethical, legislative and social-sensitive issues
- Planning and designing strategies and methods for assisting individuals and groups with emotional or behaviour problems, also with regard to social and cultural differences that are present in a diverse work force
- Promoting organizational change in culture and attitudes towards health promotion
- Mediating between employers, employees and external sources with regard to health issues
- Advising involved parties on the selection, placement and rehabilitation of emotionally troubled employees or workers who receive(d) treatment
- Managing or supervising specific cases or processes in conjunction with colleagues and other interested parties, which may include non-work involvement such as house visits and community service
- Knowing the scope of own knowledge, competencies and experience by referring, if necessary, to other health experts in order to best serve the needs of employees, the organization and the community

- Keeping accurate records, for example, the number of cases, types of problems (epidemiology), causes of problems, interventions and recurrences
- Being able to manage health promotion initiatives, for example, employee assistance programmes, or components of it
- Evaluating the effectiveness of health promotion strategies, programmes and methods.

These tasks and roles involve very specific professional knowledge and skills, as well as many cognitive, interpersonal and other personal attributes and competencies. These tasks and roles may also be described as diagnostic, preventive and remedial in nature, and as having a research function. These health-promoting actions should be directed at the well-adjusted employee, but more must be done in diagnosing and managing the problem employee in, and outside the workplace. The health-promotion actions, programmes and interventions offered must be directed at achieving certain health objectives and needs, for example, to give information, motivate, influence and change behaviour, attitudes and values at individual, group, organizational and community or environmental levels.

11.4 Systemic understanding of occupational adjustment

It is a necessary task and role of the health worker to understand employees in the *context of the work organization and its related environment*, how all these attributes may influence and interact with employees and work groups, and how the work environment can be managed to promote optimal occupational health.

In psychology, many approaches and theories can be used to explain and understand psychological adjustment and maladjustment. The most important of these ideas can be summarized in the following statements or assumptions about the nature of human behaviour and psychological adjustment and health:

- People's genetic and biological endowment and attributes
- Unconscious factors and traumatic past experiences
- Learning of behaviour patterns and the influence of cultural and other physical and social environmental factors
- People's unique experiences and efforts to find meaning in life and work
- People's knowledge and thinking about themselves, ideas and the world
- The type of psychological attributes or traits people obtained from their genetic make-up and during their development.

However, a systems-interactional model, as shown in Figure 11.1, can accommodate all or most other explanations on human and organizational behaviour, but can explain all interactions and not only certain elements. It provides a valuable tool to understanding the employee-organizational interaction and also to remind us to interpret and act upon occupational health problems in context, that is, what the meaning and functions are of such problems for employees and organizations (Cummings, 1980). This systems model will help you to understand and integrate occupational health as a field of study, but also the various aspects in this chapter, for example, the causes and influences, processes and dynamics that direct employee and organizational behaviours, and the consequences for the employee, organization and their surrounding environments.

Organizations and individuals or groups form and cooperate to achieve objectives and satisfy needs which would be difficult or impossible to accomplish on their own. The type and quality of *interaction* between the employee and organization will contribute to the organizational and individual objectives and success, namely efficiency, effectiveness, and employee and organizational health.

A main premise is that individuals as self-systems in all their modes of behaviour (e.g. biological, intellectual, social and psychological) can be best understood by first examining their functioning in the context of the organization and the wider and hierarchical systems that surround them (Littlewood, 1990).

11.4.1 Operational explanation of a systems model

Individual employees as *self-systems* bring unique qualities and characteristics to the work organization, for example, developmental experiences, personality and health status, which in turn will determine their behaviour and relationships in the organization. The *organization* also has characteristic inputs, for example, its culture, certain structures, rules, policies and business plans, which will determine the type of contact and behaviour towards and control over employees. Through this reciprocal and continuous *interaction process*, by way of specific behaviours and processes, communication, rules and transactions, the individual and the organization define a certain type of relationship or contract and associated attitudes and a certain type of psychological climate. In this regard organizational culture is a powerful influence on employee and organizational behaviour and also on their health (Ahia, 1991; Prince & Tcheng-Laroche, 1987; Varma, 1986; Lewis-Fernandez & Kleinman, 1994; Carroll, 1997). This will motivate or discourage employees and lead to certain outputs (*attitudes, behaviour, feelings, etc.*) by the individual and the organization, which in turn finally will result in certain *consequences* for the individual, the organization and for the surrounding environments. The consequences reveal the extent to which individual and organizational objectives, needs and expectations have been satisfied and whether the interaction is healthy or dysfunctional. The interaction between individuals and between individual and organization is constantly monitored by means of *feedback*, for example, by means of social interaction, performance management, evaluation or audits of processes and business results and customer feedback, which also determines the extent to which the individual and organization accepts or rejects the interaction, outputs and consequences. The conclusions from the feedback processes will in turn serve as an input for employees, the organization and environments to continue, improve or terminate their working relationships. It is important to remember that there are certain *dominant influential factors* in both the individual and the organization, and from the environment. In the individual it may be his/her previous experiences, family, religious values and training, for the organization these coalitions may be in its management style, certain departments or certain customers and business objectives. These dominant coalitions can determine the extent to which individuals and organizations are selective in their interactions, observations and acceptance of each

Occupational health

other, so as to gain the maximum benefit from events and situations. In all these processes employees and organizations may be influenced by their associated *environments*, for example, family, societal roles, customers, unions and governmental demands. If boundaries and expectations between employees, organizations and certain environmental influences (e.g. customers, family and government) are not clearly defined, conflicts with resultant problems may arise. An example is the emotional strain in families and couples due to the overload in and between work and family roles.

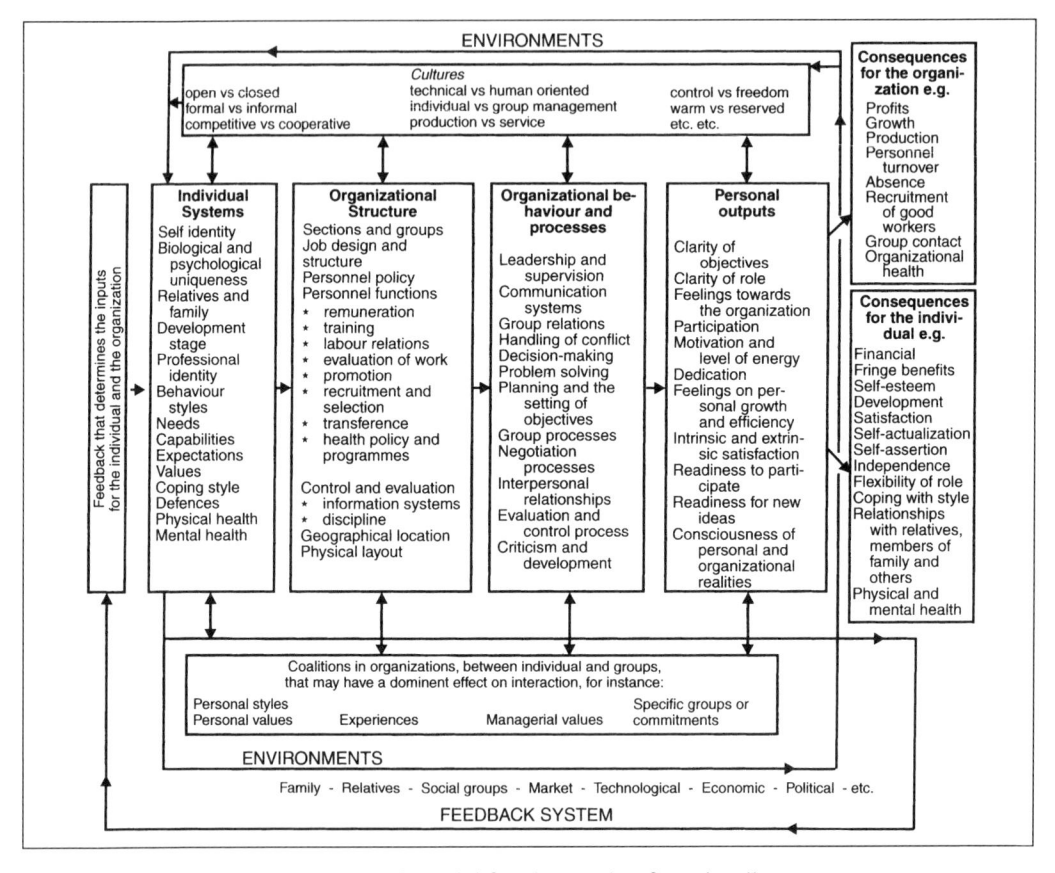

Figure 11.1 A systems-interactional model for the study of work adjustment

In summary, you should realize the importance of assessing individual problematic behaviour in the context of the influencing environments. It is, for instance, necessary to assess individuals as total entities, realizing that dysfunctional behaviour may often be a function of not only their behaviour, but rather their interactions and the rules and boundaries that control their actions. Furthermore, it is often of no avail and often counter-productive to treat the individual only when he/she is merely a symptom-bearer of a broader problem. In contrast, a health promotion intervention aimed at changing bad working conditions may alleviate many stress reactions and change employee attitudes and feelings of dissatisfaction. Similarly, change in only one person or department in an organization may cause frustration for another employee or work group. It is important to realize that the health worker also forms part of the diagnostic or treatment systems. This means that, based on our own frame of reference, we will always influence others, either positively or negatively. The healing or helping factors in interventions like counselling and therapy are really embedded in the characteristics of the relationship between the helper and the client or those we assist. People with problems learn other or more acceptable behaviour because they see and experience examples of such behaviour within the helping relationship.

11.5 Work and human behaviour

Work is generally defined as a *purposeful and meaningful activity*, which people execute in order to meet and fulfil various physical and psychosocial needs. Work, like family life, religion and sex, is a central and essential part of life and people's health. Work, perhaps more than any other life interest, defines a person's self-image and personal identity. The importance of work is mostly defined in terms of psychological, social, ethic-moral, religious, economical and even political *values and meanings*, thus the serious impact of unemployment on people and their dependants. Theories and research on work values point to the fact that positive work values and strong work ethics contribute towards work motivation, involvement, commitment and good work adjustment (Furnham, 1984:1990). With regard to the so-called Protestant Work Ethic (which stresses prosperity and promotes work as good and noble and as humankind's duty and life's mission to develop potential, while laziness and idleness are condemned), Georgi and March (1990) found cultural differences with regard to the work ethic – it being strongest in Protestant communities (Denmark, Britain), whereas there is a lot of variation in and between Catholic and 'mixed' cultures (Spain, France, Italy, Germany).

Most people work for one of the following reasons, these also being those factors most severely impacted on during work loss or prolonged unemployment. It is also true that if health workers understand the dynamics of work and working in people's lives, these influences can be used as healing factors when counselling a troubled employee:

- Work contributes to finances whereby people can provide for basic physical needs, such as housing, security, clothing, food and healthcare.
- To work is to exercise, obtain and develop a variety of knowledge and cognitive and social skills.
- Social and friendship needs are met in the workplace because people work in groups or interact with other people.
- Work provides for intellectual stimulation and physical activity as people are faced with challenging tasks and problem-solving situations.
- Entering and practising work is to express adulthood and fulfil a productive role in society.
- As a source of self-esteem, the individual obtains a sense of worth and responsibility to provide for his/her loved ones (e.g. family).
- Work, as a source of personal identity, allocates a certain role and place (status) to individuals within society and the family.

- Some people may work for the sheer pleasure of working or even for the achievements that work can generate.
- Work is a source of time management for many people, thereby fighting boredom and filling the long hours of living.
- Work represents a progression or continuation for families in terms of jobs/work, wealth and status in that each family tries to ensure a better quality of life for the next generation.
- Work provides a sense of creativity and mastery in the sense that people use their knowledge and skills to exercise personal control over things and the environment.
- Work is a religious and moral obligation for many as in some societies the virtues of work are taught, maintained and rewarded, for example according to the so-called Protestant Work Ethic (PWE) or Work Ethic in which work is seen as good whereas laziness and idleness are viewed as wrong.

Work in some form or another is here to stay and will always have a strong influence on the individual and the community. Camus (in Levitan & Johnson, 1982:63) expresses this unavoidable interaction between people and work as follows: 'Without work all life goes rotten. But when work is soulless, life stifles and dies'. O'Toole (in Healy, 1982:115) says: 'Effective performance of challenging, socially meaningful work enhances self-esteem and overall mental health, while labouring in an unchallenging, undesirable job, reduces self-esteem and correlates with many physical and mental disorders'. Citations like these support the view that bad work and no work cause melancholy, whereas meaningful work can be a cure for many miseries. In this respect research shows the positive long-term effects of work on personal adjustment, general life satisfaction, career satisfaction and family life (Cooper & Payne, 1994; Morris, 1989; Ross & Altmaier, 1994; Eckenrode & Gore, 1990; Long & Kahn, 1993; Zedeck, 1992).

Employees, working and careers, workplaces, organizations, the surrounding environments and the interaction between these variables, have characteristics that affect occupational health in general and mental health in particular. It is interesting to note that although unemployment must be detrimental in most cases, for some people such a state of non-work may be better for their health compared to working in a 'bad' employment situation. From a broad spectrum of literature on work and human behaviour (e.g. Warr, 1987; Argyle, 1992; Leatz & Stolar, 1993; Lowman, 1993; Morris, 1989; Cooper & Payne, 1994) the majority of *complaints about work* revolve around the following factors: constant and unfair supervision, control and constraint to work; lack of diversity and variety in work; lack of autonomy and decision-making; boring and meaningless work; repetitive work; isolation in the work; lack of participation and decision-making in the work; too much technological change (automation, computers) which may lead to alienation, de-skilling, boredom and unemployment.

Things that people *most wish to experience in their work*, not necessarily in order of preference, are the following: interesting work and significant work; having an impact on others; sufficient information, help and equipment to do the work; adequate authority to plan and execute work tasks (autonomy); adequate compensation;

opportunities to develop specific skills and use a variety of skills; work and physical security; task identity, to be able to see the results in and of the work (feedback); opportunity for interpersonal/social contact and recognition of personal value and position.

Contrary to the positive effects of work, however, work also *contributes negatively* to psychological maladjustment through unfavourable working circumstances, which may overwhelm people, thereby creating stress and illness; by demeaning a person, thereby undermining a sense of self-worth; through meaningless work activities, thus preventing problem-solving abilities, a sense of mastery and coping skills to fully develop; by demanding obedience to authority and some times amorality, people's own sense of authority, identity and honesty is undermined; by exhausting a person to such an extent that he/she finds him-/herself with little energy to pursue psychological rewards after work; by demanding that a person do meaningless tasks, thus giving rise to feelings of cynicism and alienation; by encouraging excessive competitiveness and hostility towards others and by failing to provide adequate material rewards, thus creating chronic financial strain for the individual.

Although work in general, poor working conditions, meaningless work and unemployment, influence physical and mental health negatively, most people (50–85 per cent) are satisfied or fairly satisfied and only 10 per cent definitely dislike their work (Argyle, 1989). The degree of work satisfaction and adjustment, however, is influenced by many factors, which also vary for individuals. The task of the human resource and health worker is to create and sustain jobs and job environments which will not only provide for basic needs but facilitate optimal growth and health. This must be achieved in ever-changing work environments, changing perceptions, attitudes and values about work; changing interfaces in work forces (e.g. between cultural and race groups, male and female etc.); changing management styles and organizational structures; increased use of technology; increased numbers of unemployed and retired workers; more leisure-oriented work; shorter working lives (earlier retirement); more home-based and part-time workers; increasing intellectual requirements and demands on individuals to be entrepreneurs themselves, for instance in South Africa, to create more jobs, to be self-employed even in the informal job market. It seems necessary for the individual to realize and develop a mental set that will foster psychological adjustment and coping in an environment with the possibility of fewer formal paid job opportunities. 'Joblessness' need not mean to be workless and worthless! It also seems a fact that stress, which can be a positive factor and is an integral part of personal and industrial success, might increase even more in work context, thereby putting stricter demands on coping resources of all employees and organizations.

11.6 Describing mental health

Unlike physical diseases where norms or criteria for health are generally clear, psychology does not always have generally accepted criteria or theories and models to explain and diagnose adjustment (health, normality), maladjustment (disorders, abnormality) and excellent adjustment or psychological optimality.

For psychological disorders or psychopathology, however, the well-known classification of the American Psychiatric Association, the Diagnostic and Statistical Manual of Mental Disorders (DSM), enjoys acceptance by most (Carson, Butcher & Mineka, 1996; Nevid, Rathus & Greene, 2003). Occupational mental health or psychological work dysfunctions, on the other hand, still do not have an accepted classification system, though classifications exist, for example those by Miner (1966), McClean (1970), Kornhauser (1965), Neff (1977, 1985), Baker et al. (1969), Morris (1989), Campbell and Cellini (1981), Lowman (1993) and Sperry (1996).

A problem in explaining occupational work dysfunction is that psychological disorders described in the DSM-classification seldom manifest as a complete clinical condition in the workplace, but rather as certain symptoms that impair work performance. Many work adjustment problems may result from emotional problems, stress-related and occupational diseases, Aids, certain behaviour and attitudinal problems, as well as specific work-related problems like absenteeism, unemployment, minority group problems, and dysfunctional work conditions.

Figure 11.2 represents mental health as a term for the nature and quality of adjustment (normality), maladjustment (abnormality) and optimality.

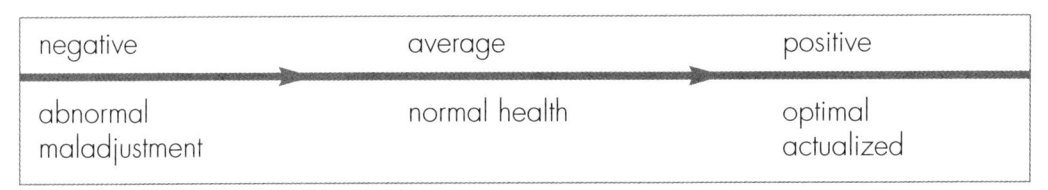

negative	average	positive
abnormal maladjustment	normal health	optimal actualized

Figure 11.2 Maladjustment to optimality

11.6.1 Psychological disorder/psychopathology

The American Psychiatric Association (APA) (1994) defines *mental disorders* (also referred to as psychological or psychiatric disorders or psychopathology), as:

> ... a clinically significant behavioural or psychological syndrome or pattern that occurs in an individual and that is associated with present distress (a painful symptom) or disability (impairment in one or more areas of functioning) or with a significantly increased risk of suffering death, pain, disability, or an important loss of freedom. In addition, this syndrome or pattern must not be merely an expected and culturally sanctioned response to a particular event, for example, the death of a loved one. Whatever its original cause, it must currently be considered a manifestation of a behavioural, psychological, or biological dysfunction in the individual. Neither deviant behaviour (e.g. political, religious, or sexual) nor conflicts that are primarily between the individual and society are mental disorders unless the deviance or conflict is a symptom of a dysfunction in the individual, as described above (American Psychiatric Association, 1994: xxi–xxii).

The persistence and intensity of patients' physical, subjective and psychological pain and discomfort necessitates psychiatric or psychological or other treatment or admission in an institution.

Authors who are more concerned with people's *social context*, communication and interpersonal relationships believe that congruent and honest communication between people is the basis of mental health. They describe behaviour and symptoms of maladjustment as tactical communication or behaviour styles to obtain benefits or to create meaning for themselves, often though in a manipulative manner, while pretending not to do it (Erikson (in Haley, 1967; Van Kessel, 1974; Kiesler and Anchin, 1982; Sullivan, 1953; Haley, 1963; Szasz,1966; Kanfer, in Swart and Wiehahn, 1979). Thus, the ills of the individual are not really separable from the ills of the social context they create and inhabit, and one can't really isolate the individual from his/her cultural context and label him/her as sick or well. In this regard too, authors like Carson (1969), Minuchin (1974), Byng-Hall (1980) and Andolfi (1979), stress the fact that the individual is the *symptom-bearer* of his/her greater systems, for example, children or spouses having emotional problems as a result of marital conflicts.

11.6.2 Psychological well-being

Good or *positive mental health* in people exist if they, in physical, intellectual and emotional respects, can develop and are compatible with other individuals. They show no or few of signs of mental disorder, and are reasonably free from undue pain, discomfort, disability and emotional conflicts, they have a satisfactory capacity for work, and are sufficiently adapted to life's demands, also with regard to others and the community. Allport (1961) and Rogers (1961) believe that healthy, adult or fully functioning people act rationally, openly and free, are congruent in themselves and with their environment, responsible and in control of what happens to them, and self-motivated for growth and development to achieve their potential or to self-actualization.

11.6.3 Psychological optimality

Although the concept and condition of *psychological optimality* are not defined clearly in literature, growth and health psychology has moved the emphasis away from negative, pathological or abnormal behaviour towards a positive view of *healthiness* and emphasizes the human motivation to grow and to actualize potential. Concepts like individualizing, superiority, productivity, self-realization, emotional integration, adulthood, self-actualization, the fully functioning person, self-transcendence, winners' behaviour, high-level health and wholeness, stand for what is positive and excellent in human functioning (Cilliers, 1984).The so-called coping theories also stress certain intrinsic personality dispositions and support from external sources and successful coping behaviour by which some people show more resistance to internal and external influences.

Psychological optimality, shown in personality or behaviour repertoires, represents integrated behaviour patterns, cognition and emotions, which enable individuals to have personal control, experience balance and behave effectively in their environments. Kobasa (1979), for instance, uses the concept of hardiness, Antonovsky (1987) the sense of coherence, Rotter (1966) refers to locus of control, and Meichenbaum (1977) to learned resourcefulness, Bandura (1977) refers to self-efficacy, whilst potency (Ben-Sira, 1985) and stamina used by both Thomas (1981) and Colerick (1985) also refer to the enduring qualities of people against stress and difficult circumstances (in Strümpfer, 1995).

The emphasis on healthiness or wellness and the above-mentioned concepts are perhaps best expressed by Antonovsky's concept of 'solutogenesis' (1984, 1987) and related concepts of fortigenesis and psychofortology (Strümpher, 1995; Coetzee & Cilliers, 2001). Salutogenesis indicates people's ability to manage stress and stay well, that is, to modify conditions that create stress, to modify the meaning of stress factors, and to use effective methods of coping with stress experiences.

From all these descriptions it is clear that psychological health is more than the mere absence of symptoms or even adjustment. It is a transcending well-being, wholeness or totality in the human psyche, an ability to succeed in and adjust in various areas like work, love, play, religion, interpersonal relations, and to solve problems, which enables people to adjust and function excellently in different environments, and to develop and realize their potential. If we utilize these concepts of health, health promotion activities should focus on improving troubled employees' sense of personal control, self-efficacy and effective coping.

11.6.4 Describing occupational mental health

As an applied field, for example, of clinical and abnormal psychology and of behavioural medicine, occupational mental health is about the adjustment or maladjustment of individuals and groups in a work and organizational context. This field of study is also referred to as industrial or occupational clinical psychology, industrial mental health, psychopathology of work, occupational health, ineffective work behaviour, work stress, industrial stress injuries and work dysfunctions.

In his view of the psychopathology of work, Neff (1977:1985) regards the *work personality* as 'a semi-autonomous area of the general personality'. He believes that work psychopathology implies some area of deficiency or defect in the development of the work personality. Since work-maladjusted persons have not learned a productive role through their development and experiences, they lack certain work competencies and display certain styles or responses that do not satisfy the requirements of the work situation.

Lowman (1993) defines *work dysfunctions* as psychological conditions in which significant impairment in the capacity to work is caused by either attributes in the individual or by the interaction between the individual and the working environment. This approach includes psychiatric disorders or psychopathology, but also work dysfunctions related to employee attitudes, perceptions, feelings and behaviour, that determine an individual's overall level of personal effectiveness, success, happiness and excellence of functioning as a person.

In the literature on occupational mental health, one or more of the following issues are included in defining occupational health:

- Work performance impairment as a result of physical disease, injury and disability
- The problem employee with a psychopathological or psychiatric disorder
- The troubled employee whose work performance is impaired by dysfunctional perceptions, attitudes, feelings and behaviour
- Causes or stressors in the work environment, organization, management and external environment will also contribute to stress reactions and other work dysfunctions or can be problems in themselves

- Management, employees and expert health workers all have a role and responsibility in occupational health promotion
- Occupational mental health as an interdisciplinary field of study and research.

Thus, a comprehensive definition of occupational mental health is needed, of which the following is the author's own example:

> Occupational mental health is the scientific study of the causes, symptoms and characteristics of individuals and groups, organization and management, the work situation and the external environments that lead to and support various forms of occupational maladjustment, and the study of the treatment, management and utilization of problem or rehabilitated workers.

11.6.5 Criteria to assess occupational mental health

Criteria for mental health refer to *standards or characteristics* to explain or assess human behaviour and mental health in general or to diagnose specific psychological disorders, for example, according to the DSM classification system, when manifested symptoms, assessment data and behaviours of troubled employees are compared with diagnostic indicators, illness history, previous functioning in work, family and cultural contexts, and the diagnostic knowledge of experts.

We refer only to general criteria for occupational health, some of which are implied in a few of the above-mentioned descriptions. Criteria for psychological disorders, however, can also be applicable in work context to assess work performance impairment caused by psychological disorders or their symptoms, and because employees use all their capacities in their work.

In a cross-cultural study in four countries (Greece, USA, Germany and France) Minsel, Becker and Korchin (1991) found agreement that positive mental health is best explained by a positive attitude towards others, optimism, good problem-solving skills, autonomy and responsibility.

In analysing psychological optimality, Cilliers (1988) describes the following intrapersonal, interpersonal and work performance characteristics:

- *Intrinsic or intrapersonal characteristics* are related to healthy physical, cognitive, emotional and conative (motivational) functioning
- *Physical characteristics.* Optimally functioning individuals are physically active, healthy and fit. This provides them with enough energy and stamina to cope effectively with stress. They are realistically aware of their somatic or physical functioning and able to accept their condition without preconditions or objection.
- *Cognitive characteristics.* People use their cognitive abilities optimally. They experience their world objectively and rationally; they are also disciplined in their thinking and reasoning, are lenient, and make well-thought-through, optimistic cognitive assessments and judgements which help them to have insight into the meaning of life.
- *Emotional characteristics.* Optimal-functioning persons are open, aware and sensitive to their emotions, feelings and needs, which they can accommodate and verbalize.

They also take responsibility for their emotions, which leads to emotional independence, and a rich emotional life.

These behaviours lead to self-insight and knowledge, which help them to form a realistic self-image with self-valuing, self-respect and self-acceptance. These qualities decrease anxiety and lead to eustress – a pleasant, exhilarating and facilitating form of stress. These people experience fullness of life – while they continue to explore and grow – rather than a situation of stability.

From their own self-acceptance, such people show optimistic and unconditional acceptance and respect towards others; a preference for qualitative, deeper and richer *interpersonal* relationships. This type of relationship is characterized by responsible, spontaneous, natural and open, genuine behaviour, they understand their own feelings, but are also considerate towards others and in a relationship of love for others.

This type of behaviour in people, for example, managers, also encourages and facilitates similar behaviour on the part of subordinates and colleagues. These characteristics are represented in the so-called person-oriented psychotherapy by four essential conditions for effective interaction, that is: respect, empathy (insightful emotional understanding), honesty and concreteness.

Psychologically optimal persons are totally *involved in their work*. All the intrapersonal and interpersonal characteristics mentioned above are therefore preconditions for optimal work performance. More specifically, optimal work performance requires purposefulness, productivity, responsibility, motivation, lenience, initiative, concentration, creativity and optimal time management. People who perform their work best are focused on the here and now, yet are aware of the past without being a victim of their history while also being future directed. Such people are cooperative, which shows that they are able to transcend opposites and to experience their role in the organization realistically.

Optimally functioning people's style is based on humanitarian values, and is therefore democratic. They plan and organize proactively by prioritizing their activities and by delegating appropriate tasks. By doing this they create a safe and permissive climate in which subordinates and colleagues are permitted to develop their own potential and to be more responsible for their own behaviour and the working environment. In this way the subordinate's working behaviour becomes more productive, directed at the organization's working objectives, without denying their own needs. This indicates an authentic working relation in which optimally functioning people increase their own and other people's awareness and acceptance in such a way that their subordinates are enabled to do the same. In this way choices that are characterized by negative feelings and repressed energy are transformed into positive growth situations, resulting in higher productivity and a better quality of life.

Robinson and Howard-Hamilton (1994) propose an *Afrocentric paradigm* to understand and manage mental health. Based on the Nguzo SABA principles, an African value system, it includes the following seven principles, which are also reminiscent of Ubuntu principles:

1 Unity (*umoja*), which refers to solidarity and harmony between persons and groups
2 Self-determination (*kujichagalia*), which emphasizes internal influences and self-knowledge rather than external influences
3 Collective responsibility (*ujima*), which denotes connectedness with other people in terms of things like family, meaningful work, a common destiny, etc. Progress means to struggle also in order to achieve objectives
4 Cooperative economics (*ujaama*), which means that people must share in wealth, thus excluding individual favouritism
5 Purpose (*nia*), which entails an individual goal-directedness but strongly connected to other people's objectives, even if it means delaying gratification
6 Creativity (*kuumba*), which stresses the ability to use intelligence, imagination and ingenuity to improve existing things and the quality of life
7 Faith (*imani*), which denotes empowerment by past, present and future events; it means to live now but also to leave something of value behind.

Kasl divides the characteristics of psychological health in the work situation into four categories:
1 Functional effectiveness or role behaviour, which refers to employees' inability to perform their daily tasks and social activities – including factors such as hospitalization, absence, and a change of work
2 General welfare, which relates to emotional conditions (depression, etc.), symptoms such as stress and trembling, and measurements for self-esteem and contentedness (self-evaluation, job satisfaction, contentedness with life and need satisfaction)
3 Mastery and efficiency, which include features such as development, self-actualization, efficient performance, the exploitation of abilities and the achievement of predetermined objectives
4 Psychiatric symptoms as in disturbed reality testing, disorientation, etc. which may impair work performance in total (in O'Toole (ed.), 1974).

It must be obvious that not all these criteria are behaviour specific, and that the diagnostician has to convert the general characteristics into observable and appropriate behaviour for every person, for example, according to known psychiatric diagnostic indicators (e.g. the DSM-system or indicators for occupational and medical or organic diseases).

11.7 Aetiology or causal factors in mental health problems
11.7.1 The nature of causation
In the above-mentioned discussion on work, some positive and negative factors that influence human behaviour and adjustment have been mentioned. Also, from the preceding definitions and criteria, you will know that the cause and effect (problem) relationship is not always clearly distinguishable. Although a single factor or stressor can have a dominant influence, mental health can best be understood by considering

the sudden or persistent interaction between a complex number of factors. The same factors or stressors that facilitate healthiness and adjustment may also, under certain circumstances, be responsible for illness and maladjustment. In this connection the systems and interactional theories stress that one should not try to explain behaviour too simplistically from a linear model or from your own frame of reference only. It is necessary to note that the individual is a whole system consisting of a number of subsystems (such as body, mind, intelligence, emotions and motivation), which are influenced by and function within many other systems and sub-systems, for instance political government, nation, culture, work group, religion, family relations and marriage. The interactive and circular influence of factors on people and their behaviour and their circumstances or context should always be taken into consideration. For instance, a man's alcohol problem could have a specific functional meaning if he obtains secondary gains (e.g. sympathy) through it or if the family or work group functions according to it. To the outsider, however, who does not consider all the implications, it is sometimes easy to say, on a linear basis, that the man has a drinking problem because he is weak, unsuccessful and so forth. A faulty consequence of such over-simplification could be the planning and implementation of less effective methods for the prevention, cure and promotion of health.

Causal or etiological factors may be considered in terms of the following causal attributes:
- Necessary causal factors that must occur for a disorder to be diagnosed
- Sufficient causes which may indicate illness (if present) that will lead to certain disorders
- Contributory causes, if present, are factors that will increase the possibility of disorders occurring.

This approach also coincides, for instance, with the so-called *diathesis-stress model* (Nevid et al., 2003) which proposes that certain people may have *predispositions* to certain forms of maladjustment or illness if certain biological, psychosocial or other causes are present. In contrast, however, you are reminded about the salutogenetic model which proposes health protective or resiliency factors in people even in detrimental circumstances.

11.7.2 Classification of etiological factors
In conjunction with the theories of personality and personality development and approaches to abnormal psychology, the aetiology of maladjustment can be subdivided into a few main groups (Carson, Butcher & Mineka, 1996; Nevid et al., 2003):
- *Biological causes*, which have an organic or biological basis. The concern here is with the influence of the nervous system, heredity, hormones and neurohormones, physical neurochemistry, nutrition, infections, intoxication, brain injuries and tumours, and degenerative changes in the human body (e.g. due to age).
- *Psychosocial influences*, which are caused by individual factors such as motivation, especially unconscious motivation, conflicts and frustration and emotions in, say, marriage, work, friendships, family and so forth. Various approaches are dominant

here but in general all emphasize the influence of unconscious factors, emotional and social factors as a result of development, learning, culture and social interactions.
- *Sociocultural influences*, which emanate from culture, family dynamics and work, and the immediate environment, for instance, socio-economic factors, urbanization, religion, ethnic groupings, marital state, educational and social status, and numerous other influences.

If you prefer to work from a stress model, stress may arise from any one or a combination of the above-mentioned factors. Stress is sometimes viewed as a generic determinant for many psychological symptoms and adjustment problems.

This classification also applies when work-related *causal or influencing factors* are considered. There are, however, also more specific classifications such as those by Miner and Brewer in Dunnette (1990), Neff (1985), Warr (1987), Lowman (1993), Cooper and Payne (1994), Ross and Altmaier (1994).

An important task of the occupational health worker is to prevent and manage negative causing factors and assist employees in preventing such factors or to adapt optimally to the presence of certain working conditions or other influencing factors. The following aetiological factors are discussed only briefly and include aspects that relate to psychological occupational health problems.

11.7.2.1 Stress, conflict and frustration

The *stress model* explains psychological adjustment and maladjustment as a function of the individual's ability to display effective (or ineffective) *adaptive or coping behaviour* when internal and/or external *stressors* lead to physical and/or psychological *stress*. Stress is a condition that develops when the demands made of individuals exceed their physical and psychological adaptive (coping) abilities.

In the first instance, stress can act as a *stimulus* or *stressor*. Internal factors (e.g. needs, physical functions) and external influences (e.g. pressure at work, finances, death in the family, or natural disasters) create a state of tension in the individual. Frustration and conflict are two important sources of stress. Holmes and Rahe (in Carson et al., 1988) compiled a list of stressors that make serious or less serious demands on an individual's adaptive ability (see Table 11.1). Stressors that continually affect individuals reduce their effective adaptation and resistance, and this in turn may have grave consequences.

Secondly, stress refers to a *specific response* by the individual, for instance a physical reaction such as pulling away a hand when experiencing pain or withdrawal during unsafe situations, and physical illness. The effects of stress may be slight (e.g. physical exhaustion or fright), moderate (e.g. a physical disease or pain, or feelings of anxiety), or serious (e.g. cardiac diseases, stomach ulcers, anxiety, fear and psychotic conditions, and even death). Added to this, reactions to stress may be purely physical, purely psychological, or psycho-physical, the latter in cases like a cardiac disease and conversion disorder (impairment of physical function without any organic cause) which is a physical reaction to psychological stress.

Thirdly, following on the explanation of stress response, stress can also refer to the individual's *coping behaviour*. Coping behaviour in response to stress may be either very direct, for example, physical flight, withdrawal, attack, or compromise – or more indirect, like psychological defence mechanisms and techniques such as physical recreation and exercise, diets, and psychological therapy. These adaptive behaviours are always aimed at achieving a state of physical and psychological homeostasis (balance). Salutogenetic protective factors such as hardiness and potency may also be regarded as coping resources, as are external resources, such as social support from family and colleagues.

The effects of stressors, and the individual's response to them, will be *moderated* by the following factors which determine the *intensity* of stress:
- The importance, duration and number of demands
- The proximity of the stressor, for instance the death of a close member of the family, or the day before an examination
- The individual's perception of the stressor, an aspect which might be the most important component of stress reactions, that is, stress is experience if we perceive stressors as threatening
- People's stress thresholds or ability to tolerate frustration, and their resilience and adaptive abilities
- A person's external resources of support, for instance family, relatives, religion and work.

Holmes, Rahe and other colleagues (in Carson et al. (1996, Nevid et al., 2003) have developed the Social Readjustment Rating Scale (SRRS), an objective method for measuring the cumulative stress to which an individual has been exposed over a period of time. This scale measures acute life stress in terms of 'life-change units' (LCU) involving certain events.

For persons who had been exposed in recent months to stressful events that added up to an LCU score of 300 or above, these investigators found the risk of developing a major illness within the next two years to be very high, approximately 80 per cent.

A promising and perhaps more valid way of measuring stress is the assessment of daily stress experiences and coping in various contexts by using so-called daily hassle and uplift-scales (De Longis et al., 1982), aimed at diagnosing and preventing continuous, irritating or chronic stressors, for example in student life, at home, while working, driving, buying, and so forth.

Hans Selye's General Adaptation Syndrome (GAS) model helps to explain previous approaches and how people react physically and psychologically to stress. It describes how the human body and psyche reacts by means of immune systems like the nervous system and endocrine functions when it experiences stress from internal or external influences (in Carson et al., 1996).

In the *alarm-and-mobilization phase* the individual prepares to counteract stress and its effects. The functions of the central and autonomous nervous system are especially important in this phase.

The second phase, *resistance*, is also characterized by alarm and mobilization, but the rate of adaptive reactions increases since the endocrine system comes into operation. For instance, the cortex may facilitate the secretion of adrenaline, or hormones may be released into the blood to stimulate blood circulation. At this stage the individual actually experiences the alleviation of stress at the psychological level through effective defensive or genuine problem-solving behaviour. On the other hand, the individual's adaptive behaviour may be less successful; there may be more serious physical and psychological problems and his/her adaptive behaviour makes no progress, because they cling to unsuccessful methods of coping and solving problems.

In the third phase of *exhaustion and disintegration* the sustained stress exceeds the individual's capacity for physical and psychological adaptation. Serious physical and psychological symptoms or conditions may follow, for instance metabolic changes, physical diseases, and psychosomatic conditions, such as cardiac or stomach diseases and paralysis. At the psychological level there may be symptoms that indicate the serious decompensation caused by stress and emotional strain. These symptoms include extreme anxiety, phobia, breaking with reality, delusions and hallucinations, thought and speech disorders – in other words, symptoms associated with psychoses – and may lead to death.

Table 11.1 The social adjustment scale of Holmes and Rahe

Events	Scale of impact	Events	Scale of impact
Death of spouse	100	Change in responsibilities at work	29
Divorce	73	Son or daughter leaving home	29
Marital separation	65	Trouble with in-laws	29
Jail term	63	Outstanding personal achievement	28
Death of close family member	63	Wife begins or stops work	26
Personal injury or illness	53	Begin or end school	26
Marriage	50	Change in living conditions	25
Fired at work	47	Revision of personal habits	24
Marital reconciliation	45	Trouble with boss	23
Retirement	45	Change in work hours or conditions	20
Change in health of family member	44	Change in residence	20
Pregnancy	40	Change in schools	20
Sex difficulties	39	Change in recreation	19
Gain of new family member	39	Change in church activities	19
Business readjustment	39	Change in social activities	18
Change in financial state	38	Small mortgage or loan	17
Death of close friend	37	Change in sleeping habits	16
Change to different line of work	36	Change in number of family get-togethers	15
Change in number of arguments with spouse	35	Change in eating habits	15
		Vacation	13
High mortgage	31	Christmas	12
Foreclosure of mortgage or loan	30	Minor violations of the law	11

Selye's model really explains how people try to *conserve coping powers* and create balance by using various strategies, as does Hobfoll's conservation of resources model (1988, 1989). These approaches, as well as developmental, biopsychological, sociobiological and evolutionary approaches, are largely responsible for the fact that human behaviour and mental health are now regarded as a process and a function of the interdependence between body, psyche and social environment. People do not *have* bodies and spirit; they *are* both, and are in constant interaction with a variety of environmental influences (Corballis & Lea, 2000).

Stressors can also be grouped together under what is known as frustration and conflict.

Frustration arises when people are prevented in some way or another from attaining their objectives. The type of reaction or frustration can also be determined by the importance of the objectives, the intensity of the needs for them, the period of frustration, and so forth. What is more important, however, is people's *tolerance for frustration*. Tolerance for frustration is, apart from biological determination, largely a function of people's acquired behaviour, how they have learnt to have their needs satisfied.

Conflict is a condition that arises when people want to satisfy several needs at the same time. People's problems arise from the fact that they then experience choice anxiety, especially if they have strong negative and positive feelings about an objective (approach–avoidance conflict), and have to choose between equally attractive objectives (double-approach conflict) or have to choose between equally unattractive objectives (double-avoidance conflict).

11.7.2.2 Factors unique to the individual

These influences include people's *idiosyncratic or unique characteristics* that result from their biological equipment, and development and learning experiences they bring with them when entering a job. These features characterize their behaviour, actions, and methods of solving problems in their environment. Both Furnham (1995) and Cooper & Payne (1994) report extensively on how individual differences influence employee work performance and psychological adjustment in many areas. The following factors are important:

- People's intellectual abilities and skills – or the lack of them
- People's genetic biological and physical equipment – and possible deficiencies – which may affect their skills in the physical work environment and determine their ways of coping and stress management
- Typical styles of behaviour and methods of communication and interaction learned in the family and other contexts, which govern a person's behaviour towards others and his/her methods of dealing with and solving problems from the environment
- Special needs, attitudes, values, and interests that direct work behaviour
- People's motivation – unconscious needs that, though unsatisfied because of repression, still activate and direct behaviour, or, on the other hand, their lack of motivation for work and achievement
- People's occupational concepts, in other words, acquired attitudes to, and values about work and their occupation

- People's self-image or ego identity, which includes everything they know, learn and feel about themselves through learning and experience – problems will develop if a person's self-image concepts are not confirmed in the work situation
- People's perception of their role in the work organization, their understanding of their tasks at work, and their job satisfaction
- Possible psychiatric problems, such as neurotic, psychotic and organic conditions, personality disorders, alcoholism, and drug addiction, which have an adverse effect on work adjustment
- Work-related problems, for instance absenteeism, or accident proneness, which may affect work adjustment
- Physical disease influences from a person's family and other groups, which may affect his/her work behaviour
- Aspects such as sex, race and other group links, which may affect work behaviour
- Job alienation, which may be the result of the isolation that often occurs in a large organization and may affect a worker's psychological adjustment to the work.

Some of these factors are discussed in some detail below.

11.7.2.2.1 Mental health as a function of human development and change
Differences and similarities in and of personalities, as well as in adjustment and maladjustment among individuals, are strongly impacted on by the quality of continuous physical and psychological development. Human development progresses though several stages in which crucial and even critical development tasks must be established. People are exposed to various influences, which make human development one of the main determinants of healthy functioning and adjustment (Hook, Watts & Cockcroft, 2002). Heredity, positive or traumatic environmental influences, experiences and learning in the formation of the self-image are fundamental determinants of development and characteristic behaviour patterns. Neff (1977) also explains the 'work personality' as a process of differentiation and development out of which a productive role grows. Thus, possible work dysfunctions may be caused by the successful or unsuccessful development of a work personality. Healthy career development and effective work coping skills are coupled to the knowledge, skills and other qualities the individual has acquired in the development process. Many career developmental theories maintain that career development is a lifelong process of self-image development during which people pass through a number of crucial phases and where the acquisition of certain skills and career concepts is essential for the choice of a career, good work performance and successful work and career adjustment (Mortimer and Borman, 1988; Schreuder & Theron, 2001).

When intervention techniques are applied to the individual, to groups or to components of the organization, the developmental stages and crucial events of employees and organizations must be taken into account. Interventions should also address better coping skills with changes in people's personal lives, careers and in their environments.

11.7.2.2.2 Personality, health and illness

One should guard against labelling people, or seeking the cause in the personality of the individual for each problem. However, personality, as an important individual differences factor, has a strong influence on health, but is also influenced by physical and psychic adjustment problems. The critical role of personality in psychological maladjustment is recognized in the fact that a separate category exists for personality disorders in the DSM-classification system. It is also a well-known fact that personality clashes are an important determinant in work conflicts. Personality is also coupled to the development of productive roles and specific career choices, and to health and illness, in the latter instance a concept like the disease-prone personality is a case in point (Friedman & Booth-Kewley, 1987; Friedman 1990).

Certain genetic and psychological traits in a person may lead to illness and adjustment problems, because they may, genetically and as a result of lifestyle, predispose a person to the occurrence of certain illnesses. Psycho-physiological or psychosomatic disturbances are examples of this interaction between personality, biology and adjustment. Coronary/cardiovascular diseases, cancer and asthma are some of the best-known conditions in which personality is recognized to have an increasingly greater causal role.

The personality that is prone to heart attacks, the so-called A type, originated after a long history of research into the relation between emotional reactions and coronary/cardiovascular diseases. Further research, with Friedman and Rosen (1975) in the forefront, confirmed that the personality that is prone to heart attacks is characterized by specific emotional, psychological and social behaviour patterns that also find expression in a certain orientation towards time and job involvement (Eysenck, 1991). The Type A personality is defined as a person with a great need for achievement, who tries to do increasingly more things in less time, and who even pursues goals by means of aggressive behaviour, often at the expense of recreation and good relations. A great deal of research supports the relationship between Type A behaviour and coronary/cardiovascular diseases, but there are still conflicting findings, some maintain that type A behaviours are not always destructive and may have health resiliency factors.

In the *disease-prone personality type* an effort is made to find the underlying factors in the personality that cause particular pathological conditions, in this regard asthma, headaches, stomach ulcers, cardiac diseases and arthritis in particular were studied. Though the validity of the disease-prone personality repertoires and types still lacks construct validity, research shows that emotions, especially depression, as well as anger and hostility, are linked to many diseases. There are also sufficient research findings on the connection between personality traits such as anxiety, self-image evaluation, neuroticism, aggression, guilt-proneness and psychological health status. Karen Homey speaks of the neurotic tendencies that indicate an orientation towards, away from or against people; Jung refers to introversion and extroversion, which together with certain attitudes will influence behaviour in many spheres. Adler stresses four life orientations, namely dominance, dependence, avoidance and social utility, which characterize the type of social interest of the person as well as his/her interpersonal relationships. Fromm refers to a productive orientation with undesirable behaviour styles, such as symbiosis, narcissism, compulsiveness, aggression, conformity and rigid defence. In occupational psychology literature, Roe and particularly Holland distinguish various occupational orientations among people, which are based on congruent (and often incongruent) fitting between six personality types and accompanying types of occupational environment (Bergh & Theron, 2003; Schreuder & Theron, 2001).

Coping theories refer, among others, to specific types of emotional, cognitive and direct *modes of adaptive behaviour*, or particular integrated personality dispositions, that enable people to remain healthy and to adjust and cope more effectively with stress and its consequences. In this regard mention was made of the concepts of salutogenesis and fortigenesis and related concepts (e.g. hardiness, optimism, self-efficacy), which are integrated personality dispositions or repertoires and 'opposites' for pathogenesis, and refer to resiliency factors or sources for health, how people stay well even in the presence of intense or continuous stress.

A *personality repertoire* refers to a pattern of behaviour, cognition and emotions through which people act towards themselves, others and their environments (Friedman and DiMatteo, 1989). In many health promotion interventions, efforts are made to improve troubled employees' sense of personal control and self-efficacy through which more effective coping skills can be learned. Below are brief descriptions of some of these integrated personality or behaviour repertoires.

- Locus of control, as initially defined by Rotter (1966), refers to the degree of control or mastery which people feel they have over events (e.g. stress factors) and how they think and act (problem-solving and decision-making) in problem situations. Internal locus refers to coping with life by means of internal sources, while external locus of control means that a person is predominantly under the influence of external factors.
- Personal hardiness (Kobasa) refers to the behaviour patterns that indicate a feeling of control and influence over and involvement in events, and change is considered to be a challenge. In much of the research in this field (in Friedman & DiMatteo, 1989), hardiness is represented as a moderating factor in the relationship between stress and illness.
- Positive thoughts (Scheier & Carver, in Friedman & DiMatteo, 1989) refer to optimism and the general expectation that events will be positive.
- Sense of coherence (Antonovsky, 1987) refers to a person's convictions that events are understandable, controllable and meaningful. This construct is the core of Antonovsky's salutogenesis theory, which explains how people endeavour to remain healthy. Kalimo and Vuori (1990) find high levels of sense of coherence to be related to high levels of job satisfaction and competency.
- Acquired or learned resourcefulness (Meichenbaum, 1977; Rosenbaum & Ben-Ari, 1985) refers to people who, once they have acquired certain skills for coping with stress, such as self-evaluation of negative thoughts, feelings and behaviour, problem-solving, control of emotions and other methods of self-control, believe positively that they can handle stress.

11.7.2.3 Factors in the work situation

Many factors in workplaces determine the psychological climate in an organization. Employee perceptions of these factors will determine employees' attitudes and feelings about their work, which will be the basis for job and career satisfaction or dissatisfaction and possibly more serious work dysfunctions.

11.7.2.3.1 Task demands

Like people, various jobs and work environments make different demands on employees, for example, with regard to tasks, hygiene factors and working hours. In Table 11.2, research by Cooper on the stressfulness of various job types, like that of nursing, is summarized (in Auerbach & Gramling, 1998).

Table 11.2 Stress levels in different jobs

Extremely stressful	Very stressful	Above average stressful
pilots, policemen, prison warders, journalism, acting, advertising, mining jobs, building construction, dentistry	firemen, ambulance workers, broadcasting, musician, film production, personnel workers, social workers, teaching, medical doctor, nursing	publishing, professional sport, management, marketing and export, public relations, sales and retailing, secretary, printing, psychologist, business endeavours, public transport, stockbroker, barrister

Job incumbents in the same job under similar or different circumstances, or in different jobs in similar circumstances may experience work stress differently, because of individual differences, like certain predispositions (e.g. sensitivity for light, noises, substances, reaction levels) gender, age, work experience, personality traits associated with for instance, anxiety, locus of control and stress reactions.

Work demands also relate to employees' perceptions of their roles in the organization and in relations with other employees and management. Employees may experience uncertainty because of role conflicts due to various work and non-work roles. Role conflicts may also result from role ambiguity (unclear task descriptions), role overload or underload (too much or too little involvement), and low levels of autonomy, participation and decision-making and responsibility. Role stressors, caused by perceptions and role execution may lead to intense feelings of dissatisfaction, frustration and, even more serious, conditions of burnout and psycho-physiological illnesses (Auerbach & Gramling, 1998).

Role stress may also lead to work alienation, which refers to the worker's feelings of being alienated in the work, experiencing feelings of aimlessness, hopelessness and work that has lost its positive meaning, because employees no longer feel part of the work processes and end results.

11.7.2.3.2 Organizational and management processes

Employee perceptions, attitudes and feelings will be about structural aspects and processes which should direct, motivate and control employees.

Organizations, as sociotechnical systems, achieve their objectives by many formal and informal structures to coordinate, utilize and control the behaviours, competencies and energy of employees. These structures refer to management, leadership, communication, administrative processes, reward and development systems, health policies and facilities, disciplinary and communication systems. The type of relationship or contract between the employer or organization and employees, either congenial or conflictual, will determine employee and organizational health. A crucial element in mental health for employees is probably the extent to which an individual's needs for care, independence, interpersonal relationships and achievement have been satisfied. High morale and cohesion in the workplace are powerful positive health factors. Employees must also feel and experience that they belong and have a fair chance of achieving and being equally rewarded if compared with colleagues and other groups.

Organizations are also developing systems and these organizational cycles of development are related to individual development and adjustment. Constant changes and transformation, like in South Africa and in organizations, for example, with regard to sociopolitical issues, affirmative action, work design, interpersonal and intergroup relations, management, decision-making, objectives and production standards, increased unemployment and job losses are important stressors for employees and employers. This illustrates that individual, organizational and environmental problems cannot be separated. In many instances, employers and employees suddenly have to fulfil new roles and meet new demands that may represent primary sources of tension.

11.7.2.3.3 Employee relations

Relationships, characterized by positive regard, trust and consideration, with co-workers, management and clients are linked to good mental health. Social support at work from colleagues and supervisors is related to job satisfaction and a good resiliency resource against work stress and ill-health. *Social support* includes emotional, instrumental (physical support in the workplace), informational and appraisal or feedback support, the latter especially with regard to the level of work performance (Bennett & Murphy, 1996). Relationship stress with, for instance, symptoms of burnout, are highest among the ranks of people-oriented professionals such as psychologists, nurses, hospice workers, teachers and medical doctors. One symptom of burnout in the helping professions is emotional bluntness, which may result in low levels of caring towards clients and colleagues. More formal relationships, for example, between employee groups and employees, employers and unions, should promote working circumstances and occupational health, but are often the source of conflict and hardships for employees, for example, during strike actions, slow-downs and retrenchment of workers.

11.7.2.3.4 Physical factors in work and in the work situation

Work stress is often equated with particular *physical working conditions* and circumstances in the workplace. Dysfunctional working conditions are viewed as a separate type of work dysfunction (Lowman, 1993). In this regard, a discipline like ergonomics will apply, as it is concerned with work design that optimizes the interaction between employees, their work equipment and the physical place of work. Concepts such as industrial hygiene, occupational safety and occupational diseases are closely linked to the impact of the physical work environment and in particular to the physical and physiological well-being of workers. Some related issues include pollution by toxic substances, working hours, work pace, repetition of work, shift work, noise, lighting, temperature, automatization, work load and mass production. The impact of the physical working conditions is illustrated by the so-called sick-building syndrome, which conveys the idea that poorly designed and equipped workplaces can contribute to physical and mental illness. The latter is recognized in employee attitudes and feelings (e.g. irritability, anger and frustration) about their workplaces, which may result in job dissatisfaction and decreased motivation. With regard to work equipment, Statham and Bravo (1990) also indicate the health implications of new technology.

The following are some physical factors that could be taken into consideration when assessing the suitability of workplaces with regard to the influence on occupational health.
- Sustained concentration and physical exhaustion
- A work rate that is too fast or too slow
- Physical dangers in the workplace
- Extreme temperatures
- Toxic conditions and radiation
- Poor ventilation
- Badly designed work stations and equipment.

The health worker should also be fully conversant with governmental legislation for health and safety (e.g. the Health and Safety Act of 1993) in general and for specific situations.

11.7.2.4 External influential factors

A systems model also indicates the interaction and influence between employees, the workplace and their surrounding environments. Real and perceived non-work stressors, such as sociopolitical changes, economic recessions, wars and other traumatic events, as well work and family conflicts, can have direct and indirect consequences for employees and organizational health. For many employees, real and important non-work stressors are work and family conflicts, because each area may have spill-over effects on the other, for example, aggressive behaviour of a male employee towards a supervisor at work because of his unsolved negative feelings towards a dominant father figure. Or a mother neglecting her family at home, because she feels drained as a result of overload in her work and at home. In the modern world, the rapid *changes and discontinuity* that occur in the world of work, communications media and in the socio-economic, political and technological spheres make life uncertain and unpredictable, and may be too much for some people. The organization is also affected through its environmental systems, for instance the type of technological, marketing, labour, product and service demands it constantly has to face.

11.7.2.5 Stressors related to occupational health nursing

Although the above-mentioned factors are applicable in occupational health nursing as well, specific aspects will influence the health worker's occupational health more than in other professions.

The nurse's task of caring, interacting with patients, clients and the public, and managing and facilitating their pain and anxieties, is demanding and creates stress. Though many factors may influence the experience of stress, for example, culture, age, work experience and specific situations, the following are some of the stressors for nurses in training and for qualified nurses that are reported in nursing literature (Bailey & Clarke, 1989; Harrison, 1984; Niven & Robinson, 1994; Clark, 1999; Derstine & Hargrove, 2001).

- Adapting to the culture and social climates in different institutions and wards
- General lack of control, decision-making and problem-solving caused by too much supervision, of which the latter in turn is often required by medical and healthcare responsibilities and expectations
- Interpersonal problems at work
- Involvement in, knowledge about and fears for own mortality, during experiences of death and dying
- The diverse demands, work-overload, lack of interpersonal communication and lack of control experienced by nurses working in intensive healthcare units (ICU)
- Specific task demands in the nursing occupations, for example, patient admission, patient care (e.g. cases of surgery, coronary heart disease, chronic problems, change in body image, cancer and bereavement)
- Work and organizational problems, such as under- and over-promotion, opportunities for further development, role clarity, job security, lack of work equipment, and problems of communication and consultation with management.

11.8 Assessment of occupational mental health

11.8.1 Various methods

Diagnosing mental disorders (e.g. by DSM-classification) is mostly done by considering all information on a person's behaviour with regard to biological/neurological, social and psychological aspects. The person's health history and personal experiences, as well as diagnostic signs used by an experienced diagnostician, are taken into consideration. Factors such as the intensity and duration of symptoms are also considered before coming to a conclusion on a person's mental health status.

It is not in the scope of this chapter, nor is it the task of the health worker (except if a qualified psychologist) to do in-depth psycho-diagnostic assessments of troubled employees. However, the occupational health worker should be able to assess the troubled employee's ability to work using available expertise, techniques and criteria for general and occupational adjustment.

In the management of occupational health a sound *evaluation programme* should form part of the personnel and organizational functions. Besides the fact that evaluation can be useful, the aim should be to constantly monitor causative factors of work dysfunctions and of employee behaviour and attitudes. This will result in timely identification of problems and their causes and functions so that preventive or corrective measures can be planned and implemented.

Lowman's (1993) classification of work dysfunctions makes provision for a distinction to be made between psychopathology, that is, classified psychological disorders, and specific work-related problems. In addition, it is necessary to determine the mutual relationship between psychopathology and work dysfunctions.

The type of psychopathology or work dysfunction will determine what course of action is to be taken. Lowman proposes, among others, the following types of question to be asked in order to determine the type of work adjustment, either psychopathology or work dysfunction:

- What is the duration of the unhappiness at work?
- What are factors in the work situation that could trigger the maladjustment?
- What are the symptoms, reactions and behaviour?
- What were the circumstances when the reactions occurred?
- Did the employee choose his/her own career or not (possible career dissatisfaction?)
- What are the types of symptoms/psychopathology/work dysfunction according to all the evidence?

In the assessment of employee and organizational health, the following methods should be used:

- Psychological tests, questionnaires and checklists to be used by qualified health professionals to assess psychological adjustment, ways of coping, stress management, and so forth
- Recognized medical diagnostic techniques to assess the incidence of occupational and other diseases
- Psychiatric and other diagnostic interviews and observation of behaviour to evaluate behavioural signs and symptoms
- Self-assessment, in which employees can be taught to observe and note their own biological and psychological responses
- Analysis of individual work performance compared with expected norms, for example job descriptions and objectives
- Production and cost analysis with regard to employee and organizational inputs and outputs
- Analysis of occupational health status in the form of absences, accidents, personnel turnover, numbers of reported medical and psychological cases, admissions to clinics, recurrences, and so forth
- Organizational diagnostic assessment, for example, survey techniques to measure employee attitudes and perceptions with a view of assessing the dynamics of organizational culture, climate and job satisfaction.

11.8.2 Diagnostic and Statistical Manual (DSM) for classifying psychological disorders

While the DSM classification system is the most used and acceptable system to classify psychological disorders, its main assessment properties are discussed. Assessments

Psychological health and adjustment in the work context

made according to the DSM are based on all available information on a psychologically troubled person.

DSM is a multi-axial classification system of psychological disorders and is based on all aspects of a person's behaviour, that is, biological, cognitive, psychological and social dimensions and also work, because all these other dimensions are involved in work. In addition, DSM also adheres fairly well to the criteria for an effective classification system, that is, it attends to the causes of maladjustment, uses language familiar to many professionals and researchers, provides information of the context (e.g. duration) of disorders, describes the characteristics, symptoms and illness processes, as well as implications for treatment and prevention. DSM is used by clinical assessors to order their assessment data in order to make a diagnosis and to plan and apply treatment and health-promotion activities. According to a diagnostic decision based on DSM a person's condition can be described as acute (duration of less than six months and possibly of high intensity), chronic (long-standing, possibly permanent and mostly with low intensity of symptoms). Descriptive terms such as *mild, moderate* and *severe* are used to indicate the levels of seriousness or severity of symptoms or a condition. The concepts *episodic* and *recurrent* are used to describe unstable or unpredictable symptoms or disorders, because these may come and go across time and situations.

DSM uses the five axes given in Table 11.3 below to classify psychological disorders according to all available information on a person's condition:

Table 11.3 *DSM-axis for diagnostic classification of psychological disorders*

Axis	Contents
I	Most possible disorders, except personality disorders, which may apply to an individual are reported here and the principal diagnosis is listed first.
II	Personality disorders and mental retardation are considered here, because these may be long-standing and already started in childhood. If a definite diagnosis for a personality disorder cannot be made, this axis is also used to consider certain maladaptive personality attributes and defence mechanisms that do not meet the full criteria for a personality disorder. Childhood development orders, however, are coded under axis I.
III	Any medical condition and medical illness history that seems relevant to a person are listed here, for instance, depression due to chronic pain or a history of heart attacks.
Iv	Psychosocial causing factors/stressors are considered here, e.g. checking possible causes in the family, economic factors, and legal aspects, also if the disorder created some of the adjustment problems for the person.
V	A global assessment of functioning (GAF) of a person with regard to psychological social and psychological behaviours is executed on a 100 point rating scale. The more information available, the easier it will be to make a global assessment and to differentiate between people, even if they have the same symptoms.

The *first three axes* deal with a person's clinical condition and a person may be diagnosed with more than one syndrome on any of the three axes until a definite diagnostic decision is made. *Axes IV* and *V* deal with the broader context and other aspects of the person's condition. Axes IV and V need not necessarily be included in a diagnosis, for instance, they should not to be misused in cases of assessment for insurance claims and obtaining insurance policies. The *global assessment scale for axis V* ranges from a point of 100 through to 0 and intermediate points can be used, for instance 100 and 91 represent high and lower dimensions on the same behaviour description, as do 60 and 51, and 1 and 10. A point of 100 indicates superior functioning, with no problems, a point of 50 indicates serious symptoms, for instance, frequent stealing behaviours, suicidal tendencies, severe obsessive behaviours, *or* serious impairment with regard to school, social and occupational functioning and 10 through to 1, indicates persistent violence and danger of severely hurting others and self, *or* a persistence to take care of personal hygiene, *or* serious suicidal acts and expectations of death. A zero (0) point is rewarded if no or inadequate information is available.

11.8.3 Programme and process evaluation

In a broader context the occupational health nurse should also have knowledge and be involved in process and *programme evaluation*. This means that the health promotion initiatives, programmes and specific activities in organizations should be evaluated on an ongoing basis. This should be valuable in determining current and future resources, the effectiveness and success of health promotion, and the possible implementation and changes to programmes or specific activities. The following issues and questions could be valuable in a cost and viability assessment:

- The current budget with regard to employee and organizational health
- The current status of personnel resources and future needs
- The current status with regard to health-promotion facilities
- Current and new reported cases with occupational diseases and work dysfunctions
- The perceived and actual direct and indirect cost factors
- The direct perceived and actual direct and indirect costs
- An answer to whether planned interventions and changes could be achieved
- An answer to whether impaired work behaviour could be corrected without other major life disruptions, and if not, whether other interventions would be achievable
- The number of remissions in treated cases
- The cost of treatment for remissions
- Whether there is or was a commitment from management and employees to change and, if so, how long-lasting this would likely be
- Whether the employees and organization have a history of unsuccessful change and what caused such short-lived changes.

11.9 Psychological work dysfunctions

In this section we deal mainly with general adaptive reactions and specific work-related problems or work dysfunctions. Psychological disorders are not covered fully, but only some aspects deemed relevant in the field of occupational or work dysfunctions. Remember that the study of occupational mental health can be viewed as an applied field of clinical and abnormal psychology, and the health worker should have a good knowledge of psychiatric disorders, as described in many standard text books (e.g. Nevid et al., 2003; APA, 1994, 2000), because of its implications for work dysfunctions.

Before we discuss the specific conditions and situations, it is necessary to refer to Lowman's (1993:43–44) classification of psychological work-related dysfunctions in Table 11.4.

Lowman relates psychopathology, according to the DSM-classifications, to work maladjustment, but also distinguishes certain manifestations as pure work-related dysfunctions in which psychopathology need not have a role. He defines a work dysfunction as any psychological condition as a result of personal attributes in employees, or the interaction between the employee and the work environment, which might impair the ability to work and work performance. Lowman (1993) emphasizes that health workers need to assess correctly and to first determine the relationship between psychopathology and work functioning, or equally importantly, to assess the influence of work dysfunctions on psychopathology. Such assessment is important for planning and executing treatment interventions. It is, for instance, unproductive to use career counselling or performance feedback for employees with severe emotional problems, for example, depression, schizophrenia, paranoia, personality disorders and severe anxiety, unless these problems are first addressed.

The following discussion is not a discussion according to Lowman (1993) but rather an integrative approach, firstly of psychological and work dysfunctions in the individual, including a listing of psychiatric disorders and adaptive reactions, followed by work dysfunctions with regard to organizational functioning.

11.9.1 Psychological work dysfunctions in employees

The following discussions are about psychological disorders, adaptive reactions and work dysfunctions which may occur in employees as a result of their own attributes or in interaction with the work environment.

11.9.1.1 Psychiatric or psychological disorders

Though psychological or *psychiatric disorders* are not discussed, a detailed list of disorders according to the APA's DSM-classification (APA, 2000; Nevid et al., 2003) is included here. These disorders may cause the impairment of work performance or be related to work dysfunctions.

- Stress, psychological factors, and health (adjustment reactions and psychological factors and physical disorders), in which dysfunctional responses are caused by temporary and other stressors, and psychological problems
- Anxiety disorders, characterized by fear, panic and anxiety
- Dissociative and somatoform disorders, which refer to disruption of identification, memory and consciousness and complaints of unexplainable physical symptoms

Table 11.4 Classification of psychological work-related dysfunctions

I DETERMINING THE RELATION BETWEEN PSYCHOPATHOLOGY AND WORK DYSFUNCTIONS
  A Affecting work performance
  B Not affecting work performance
  C Affected by work performance
  D Not affected by work performance

II DISTURBANCES IN THE CAPACITY OF WORK
  A Patterns of undercommitment
    1 Underachievement
    2 Temporary production impediments
    3 Procrastination
    4 Occupational misfit
    5 Organizational misfit
    6 Fear of success
    7 Fear of failure

  B Patterns of overcommitment
    1 Obsessive-compulsive addiction to work role (workaholism)
    2 Type A behavioural pattern
    3 Job and occupational burnout

  C Work-related anxiety and depression
    1 Anxiety
      (a) Performance anxiety
      (b) Generalized anxiety
    2 Work-related depression

  D Personality dysfunctions and work
    1 Problems with authority
    2 Personality disorders and work

  E Life-role conflicts
    1 Work-family conflicts

  F Transient, situational stress
    1 Reactions to changes in the work role (e.g. new job) whose impact on the work role is time limited

  G Other psychologically relevant work difficulties
    1 Perceptual inaccuracies

III DYSFUNCTIONAL WORKING CONDITIONS
  A Defective job design (role overload, ambiguity, etc.)
  B Defective supervision
  C Dysfunctional interpersonal relationships

- Mood disorders and suicide, characterized by serious inflated manic and depressive feelings and destructive behaviours
- Personality disorders, in which learnt deviant behaviours, like aggression, suspicion, disinterest, avoidance, dependence and manipulation occur
- Schizophrenia and other psychotic disorders, characterized by serious distortion in about all spheres of human functioning, that is, thought, speech, perception and emotions
- Substance abuse and dependence is the result of abuse of and dependence on alcohol, drugs and other substances
- Eating disorders, obesity and sleep disorders are characterized by excessiveness, either too little or too much
- Gender-identity disorder, paraphilias and sexual disorders, which include dysfunction in some form of gender identification and sexual functioning
- Cognitive disorders and disorders of aging include psychoses and impairments as a result of organic brain damage due to genetics, substances, injuries and age
- Abnormal behaviour in childhood and adolescence
- Violence and abuse refers mostly to aggression and aggressive and sexual abuse of other people and children
- Other disorders, for example:
    - impulse control disorders not classified elsewhere (e.g. explosive behaviour, kleptomania, pyromania, pathological gambling)
    - adjustment disorders (e.g. related to anxiety, depressed mood, conduct, mixed emotions and conduct, mixed anxiety and depression)
    - disorders that may also get clinical attention (e.g. psychological factors affecting medical condition, other medication-induced disorders, relational problems, problems related to abuse and neglect).

11.9.1.2 Adjustment or adaptive reactions

All people use adaptive reactions to cope with life's demands, which are quite acceptable if such behaviour is not dysfunctional. Stress, frustration, conflict and other factors that put physical and psychological strain on all or many people, and require some form of adaptive reaction or *defence mechanism* to maintain or acquire *homeostasis, balance* or *equilibrium*. Though it is possible to single out some acceptable adjustment reactions, it is impossible to describe all the kinds of adjustment, or defence mechanisms. In fact, there are as many kinds of adaptive reactions as there are people, situations in which they behave, and ways in which people have learnt to adapt. In a sense, all our behaviours in our daily lives are based on adaptive reactions. However, it is also possible to indicate certain adaptive or defence reactions in all forms of psychiatric disorders and in work dysfunctions. The best known of these are probably the so-called personality disorders where clearly defined defence mechanisms can be identified. In some cases also, without necessarily belonging to a type of disorder, certain behaviours or a certain type of behaviour (e.g. aggression, suspicion, cleanliness) in people may be so disturbing and defensive, that it can be viewed as maladaptive.

The many forms of everyday adaptive reactions and the fact that everyone manifests adaptive reactions, often make it very difficult to distinguish clearly between adaptive reactions or defences and maladaptive reactions or defenses. The difference is probably mostly in the frequency, duration and intensity of certain reactions. In this regard, for example, ordinary eating habits are essential for life and survival, yet excessive or inadequate eating habits constitute a behavioural disorder with serious biological and psychological implications. It is also accepted that all people may occasionally be disoriented with regard to time and place, or that we sometimes mistrust people's intentions, yet when disorientation of time and place and suspicion become repetitive and intensive to a level where the daily and expected forms of behaviour are disrupted, a certain form of psychological disorder may be possible.

Types of adaptive and defence mechanisms are identified and classified in different ways.

Adjustment and defence

First, a distinction is sometimes made between adaptive or adjustment reactions and defence mechanisms. *Adaptive reactions* refer to everyday forms of behaviour which individuals (children and adults) use to handle problems and crises so as to satisfy possible physical and psychological needs and to alleviate anxiety or stress. These adaptive reactions, or ways of coping, whether positive or negative, can be classified as either problem- or emotion-focused, and people will solve adaptive demands by applying certain behaviours, emotions or ways of thinking. Examples are the following:

- Touch, for instance a child seeking the protection of the mother's arms
- Music, which has a calming effect on many people
- Eating and drinking when experiencing emotional problems
- Crying and scolding (negative emotions)
- Talking things out and praying
- Work or more work, e.g. by analysis, and taking on two jobs
- Games, recreation, travelling and vacation
- Physical acting out of feelings
- Shopping and buying habits
- Physical habits, such as grooming one's hair and nails
- Withdrawal or isolating oneself from people or problems, e.g. avoidance, daydreaming, denial
- Purposive relaxation techniques, such as progressive relaxation of the body and meditation
- Cognitive adaptive reactions, such as reassessment of problems and imaging of problems.

Many of these types of behaviour can also form the basis of more serious behavioural disorders. In contrast too, many of these adjustment reactions also are the basis of techniques and programmes for handling stress, for instance in therapy and vocational guidance.

Defence mechanisms, also referred to as *ego-defence mechanisms* (Bergh & Theron, 2003) are more comprehensive patterns of behaviour, usually unplanned (automatic) and unconscious, which the individual uses to relieve or avoid emotional conflicts and resultant anxiety and stress. This view of defence mechanisms as intra-psychic, unconscious patterns of behaviour to protect the ego or self against threatening impulses (primary impulses like sexual and aggressive needs) is primarily the Freudian or psychoanalytic view. Conscious defences may signify manipulation indicating that the individual purposively behaves differently or tries to mislead others in order to attain certain objectives. In our discussion of specific types of defence mechanisms the intra-psychic defence mechanisms are emphasized.

Direct as opposed to indirect defence mechanisms
The distinction between adaptive reactions is directly related to the distinction between adjustment and defence.

With *direct defence reactions*, the individual mostly behaves in a conscious and overtly perceptible way to adapt to conflict, frustration, anxiety and stress. Examples of direct behaviour are aggression and withdrawal from a situation. In the case of *aggression* it can be associated with physical attacks, overt rage and violence. Otherwise aggression may occur in a more inhibited way so that rage, for instance, is not as demonstrable. In the latter instance, aggression is therefore internalized and can manifest in somewhat displaced forms, such as verbal sarcasm, refusal to work, strikes and hunger strikes. Although *withdrawal* is mostly reasonably directly observable, in exceptional cases behaviour is found that indicates total inactivity or apathy and depression. In such cases people regard their chances of adapting or coping as being so hopeless that they actually stop trying. Examples were observed during wars where soldiers under severe war stress simply stopped fighting and waited to be taken prisoner. The post-war stress reactions (or so-called post-traumatic stress reaction) could contain an element of inactivity after severely traumatic experiences or protracted experience of stress.

Another form of direct defence reaction, but which manifests in a displaced form, is the so-called *symptom-directed* way of behaviour. Examples are the use of liquor and drugs, as well as more acceptable narcotics such as sedatives, prescribed medicine and (excessive) cigarette smoking.

Indirect defence mechanisms refer to the previously mentioned intra-psychic, unconscious adaptive reactions. Some of the best known are discussed in more detail below.

Repression implies that individuals seek to exclude threatening, undesirable and painful impulses, ideas and memories (experiences) from their consciousness. This reaction can also be described as a form of psychological loss of memory (amnesia) where the person uses selective forgetting or, in other words, selective remembering. Repression can be viewed as the main defence mechanism which is basic to many of the other defence mechanisms. Repression is sometimes regarded as a 'successful' adaptive mechanism because it can provide immediate relief from traumatic events or even for longer periods until the memory of certain ideas or events is safer again, for instance after therapy or as an adult. The disadvantage is that repression does not really solve the problem (for instance guilt feelings), since repressed contents can manifest in disguised or indirect ways, for instance, in dreams, fantasies and slips of the tongue (e.g. addressing your partner by another name). It is also said that in extreme cases, 'repressed' persons behave so defensively and rigidly that they cannot live and experience spontaneously.

Examples of repression can be the apparent amnesia of soldiers after other soldiers next to them were decapitated or the total repression of sexual needs because of traumatic sexual experiences, for instance in sexual assaults such as rape and incest. In anxiety-based forms of behaviour (previously known as neurosis) the individual may, for instance, forget his/her date of birth and address or be apparently unable to remember acquaintances. In the work situation, repression could manifest in the form of forgetting to perform tasks and forgetting appointments with a supervisor.

It is necessary to distinguish between repression and *suppression*. Whereas the first is an unconscious process, suppression is a conscious, rational attempt to keep unpleasant ideas and experiences from the conscious mind. For example, a family could decide deliberately not to speak about a lost member of the family or someone could consciously bear in mind that he/she finds a task unpleasant.

Denial is related to repression and is based on a total denial of the existence of certain facts or events. In children denial is regarded as a reasonably acceptable defence mechanism because the child's repertoire of problem-solving mechanisms is still limited, for example, a boy who denies that his father has left home or a child who denies that she was a baby or is angry. Conversely it is said that in adults a pattern of denial behaviour is based on limited adjustment and problem-solving behaviour, for example the alcoholic or glutton who denies his/her problem. More extreme cases occur in people who deny that they are seriously ill, for instance someone suffering from terminal cancer, or parents who deny that their child is seriously ill or even dead. Protracted denial of reality, for instance, people who deny that they were abused as children and therefore deny their negative feelings towards their parents, can eventually lead to a schizophrenic reaction. In a work context denial can manifest when someone denies that he/she was not promoted, has become unemployed and so forth.

As a very common and simple form of defence, denial has the value of relieving the stress of severe trauma. In general, however, a protracted pattern of denial can have only detrimental effects on an individual.

In *projection*, people ascribe their undesirable characteristics, impulses, behaviour, or errors to other people or even inanimate objects. Projection is reasonably common in children in that they use all sorts of stories about other children and things to overcome or reduce their fears. In adults, projection is less successful and actually indicates people's inability to handle their own mistakes, feelings of inferiority, and so forth effectively. Examples of projection are seen when people who experience strong aggressive impulses ascribe them to others; the mother with guilt feelings about her early sexual experiences who accuses her young daughter of permissiveness; workers or students who produce poor work and ascribe their failure to their supervisors' prejudices against them; sportsmen who loose blame their failure on poor equipment, playing surfaces, and so forth. In extreme pathological conditions, projection is a characteristic of the paranoid personality and schizophrenic and paranoid psychosis. Such people have strongly entrenched ideas that others threaten or persecute them.

Reaction formation involves defence reactions where the person manifests behaviour or attitudes that are the direct opposite of the undesirable impulses. Examples of this are mothers who overprotect their children while they actually harbour feelings of hatred; the apparently self-sacrificing love of a husband for his invalid wife, while he might wish she were dead; people who over-zealously preserve moral values but who are actually using this to defend their own sexual needs; the boastful Don Juan who is actually secretly afraid of female sexuality; and students who fail and then maintain that they actually do not care whether they pass or not.

Regression refers to a return to earlier or less responsible patterns of behaviour which are inappropriate to the present situation. Regression is common in children, for instance the child who begins wetting the bed again (to gain attention) when a baby arrives in the family. In severe forms, this is a continual regression to a narcissistic self-love which could inhibit the young child from growing emotionally and socially. Regression is also observed in prisoners who could become so dependent that they can't think, act or plan for themselves. In everyday life, forms of behaviour, for example outbursts of rage in the work situation or an inability to complete work, could indicate inappropriate regressive forms of behaviour.

Fixation is related to regression and implies that with regard to certain behaviours the person's psychological development has progressed only to a certain stage. So mother fixation refers to the fact that a young man could find it difficult to put another woman in his mother's place.

Identification involves the internalization or adoption of the characteristics of another person or even group. Many authors, like Freud, regard the process of identification as an integral part of personality development, particularly the development of cultural values (super-ego) and the development of sexual identity. According to Freud it is through identification with the father that the boy overcomes his Oedipus complex and concomitant feelings of aggression and fear of the father and male figures (Bergh & Theron, 2003). Another extreme case of identification with the strongest person or body was observed in concentration camps where some prisoners tried hard to assume the appearance and behaviour of their oppressors or aggressors. Identification occurs throughout life – in children particularly with hero figures, pop stars, sports stars, and so forth, and in adults often with leaders and organizations. Although identification has positive aspects, it can also have negative consequences. Aggression and crime could be the outcome of faulty learning through identification. When identification figures are unsuccessful or die, the effects are sometimes detrimental: it is well known that with the death of figures such as Martin Luther King, John F. Kennedy, Elvis Presley and John Lennon some people experienced serious emotional disturbances and even committed suicide; and when soccer teams lose, match violence often erupts between opposing supporters.

Displacement occurs when people direct or channel intense negative feelings or attitudes away from themselves to other people or objects. Some of the best-known examples are the displacement of aggressive feelings, for instance, the aggression of a high-school pupil towards his/her father is directed at the teacher or school in rebellious behaviour; the worker's aggression towards his/her supervisor is taken out on the family at home; and the childless couple displace their needs by working very hard for child-care organizations. Although displacement is an effective form of release for tension and prevents more extreme behaviour, the basic problem often remains.

According to Freud, displacement is a characteristic way of converting unacceptable id impulses (sexual and aggressive drives) into more socially acceptable behaviour. In these ways also, as in identification and sublimation, cultural values are acquired and people can live in greater harmony.

Sublimation is closely related to displacement and is sometimes regarded as a special form of displacement. Sublimation is used to apply the energy of unacceptable sexual and aggressive instincts in such a way as to lead to more acceptable and exemplary behaviour. So it is said in some cases that jobs of minister or surgeon could be chosen to sublimate aggression, a sexually frustrated person could become a physiotherapist, a baby might suck his thumb or another object instead of the mother's breast and the school girl could fall in love with her teacher out of admiration for her father. Another good example is the premise that Leonardo da Vinci's preference for painting women (such as the well-known Mona Lisa) arose from an intense longing and need for his mother.

Rationalization is when a person finds socially acceptable reasons for his/her behaviour or events, while the real reasons are repressed. People who rationalize mislead themselves (and sometimes others as well) by justifying their behaviour or the course of events. Rationalization is, however, not necessarily lying behaviour but an attempt to adapt and to alleviate or avoid disappointment or stress. Rationalization is one of the most common forms of defence, also in everyday life. For instance, unsuccessful students could contend after the examination that the paper was in any case unfair or that they did not really study or want to pass. Employees who are not promoted maintain that they are actually glad to remain in their old post, or that they would actually lose too much by changing jobs. Aesop's fable 'the fox and the grapes' illustrates how the fox, when he could not get the delicious bunches of grapes, concealed his disappointment by accepting that the grapes were sour – hence the saying 'sour grapes'. Other proverbial rationalizations are expressed in sayings such as 'every dark cloud has a silver lining' or 'tomorrow is another day'.

Negative or very unreasonable rationalizations are illustrated by some political leaders' war crimes, for instance, which they claimed were done for love of the fatherland, or the family murderer who kills his wife and children and claims that he wanted to save them from the suffering of a difficult life on earth.

Intellectualization, also regarded as a form of isolation, occurs when people isolate threatening emotional experiences or behaviour or events from themselves by speaking about such events in an excessively intellectual or rational way. In ordinary life intellectualization often occurs among people in careers where they have to work with human pain and suffering. For instance a medical doctor, nurse and even the commander of soldiers will give intellectual reasons for events. An individual is regarded as an object of study who can be used to save other lives.

When intellectualization becomes so intense that people mislead themselves and lose contact with their feelings and therefore have limited emotional experiences, this form of defence becomes maladjustment. For instance, a young man could have severe sexual fears. He tries to appear to be 'adjusted' in this respect by philosophizing and speaking rationally about sex, marriage and so forth, also in his contacts with women. Another form of isolation is referred to as *emotional insulation*. In this case the person will begin to behave passively, apathetically and despairingly during or after traumatic events such as unemployment, imprisonment, war or death. Someone like this is, however, merely hiding behind a protective 'wall of emotionless' behaviour in an attempt to avoid further shocks. Although such behaviour can relieve acute traumas, protracted emotional withdrawal will amount to an isolated and rigid way of experiencing life.

Compensation amounts to protecting the self-image by overachieving in some or other inadequate or inferior area of behaviour. Direct compensation occurs when an unattractive woman uses too much make-up or follows a mannequin course or when a slightly built man takes up a course in body building. In history, people such as the American president, Theodore Roosevelt, and the Greek orator and statesman, Demosthenes, are cited as examples where compensation for weaknesses led to great achievements. In the world of sport, also in South Africa, there are many examples of people who have achieved a great deal irrespective of a physical handicap or other drawbacks.

Indirect compensation is reflected in a different type of behaviour than is indicated by an apparent deficiency. For instance, someone who is poor at sport could perform well academically or politically and a slightly built, short person (such as Napoleon) could behave in a very domineering manner, or a young man from a poor family could do well academically or financially to compensate for his family's shortcomings. Even Freud and the musician, Haydn, it is said, were outstanding in their fields because they in fact had few opportunities.

Fantasy consists of the fulfilment of unsatisfied needs, wishes and desires through imagination, wishful thinking and also daydreaming. In this way the individual creates images of people, things or events in order to try to satisfy needs or as a way of finding a temporary escape from frustration, conflict and tension. Fantasy is mostly not negative and is found particularly among children but often also among adults. In this connection you can note how often adults participate in children's games or television programmes and enjoy fairy tales that are actually intended for children. Fantasy is also regarded as an element of creativity. When fantasy becomes pathological, it actually means that the individual cannot handle reality and therefore lives in a naive or childlike way in a fairytale world of flights of the imagination. Many psychopathological conditions, such as schizophrenia and psychopathy, contain elements of fantasy in the disordered patterns of behaviour.

As indicated, these defence mechanisms are ways of coping and sometimes of handling conflicts and tensions. However, defence mechanisms entail maladjustment when they become the only or a dominant way in which people can handle reality, their problems, conflicts and tensions. In such cases people rob themselves of energy, spontaneity and creativity with the result that they cannot experience events, themselves and interactions with others fully. Such persons continue to mislead themselves and their problems are never really solved.

11.9.1.3 Negative work motivation, attitudes and perceptions

Though these are employee perceptions about various aspects in their workplaces and not psychological dysfunctions per se, they distort behaviour and are fundamental in many work dysfunctions. According to Lowman (1993) these negative behaviours underlie the employee's capacity and willingness to work. In this regard work motivation, work attitudes and perceptions can be part of what Lowman in his classification refers to as dysfunctions of under- and overcommitment and perceptual inaccuracies. The nature of work motivation, work attitudes and related perceptions can be influenced by many factors, for example how work values and productive roles were socialized and reinforced, career development and the acquisition of the necessary career choice knowledge and skills, the extent to which the individual's needs have been satisfied and the characteristics of jobs and workplaces.

Job satisfaction, as a specific aspect of work motivation and indicated by attitudes and perceptions about work and workplaces, can be a function of the need for achievement, recognition, responsibility, interpersonal relationships and of the physical aspects of the job, for example job specialization. Other *causative factors* include organization and management processes, supervision, salary and working conditions.

Job dissatisfaction is associated with physical illness, stress reactions like cardiac diseases, frustration, hostility, accidents, absence, change of work, anxiety and fear of failure, lower standards of performance and practices that have little connection with the tasks of the job in question.

The individual's job satisfaction and work attitudes, for example loyalty, can also be a function of the *work group's cohesion and morale*. People may find the type of psychological climate in the group which confirms their self-esteem and contributes to behaviour which will promote their own objectives and those of the group. Individual complaints and symptomatic behaviour may be merely the manifestation of the fact that the work group is experiencing stress.

11.9.1.4 Stress reactions, psychological factors and health

We have referred to stress as an important aetiological factor in physical and psychological decompensation. With regard to Lowman's classification for work-related dysfunctions (Table 11.4), the dysfunctions of under- and overcommitment and transient situational stress can partly be related to adjustment disorders, psychological stress reactions and psycho-physiological diseases, as well as less serious work-related anxiety and depression. Following is a brief description of more extreme examples of stress reactions.

In the so-called *adjustment disorders*, stress reactions are the result of adverse life events. Reactions such as depression, anxiety, behavioural disorders, emotional outbursts, loss of work capacity, and withdrawal, can follow acute or severely traumatic stress or chronic (protracted) stress. Examples of life events that can lead to adjustment disorders are unemployment, divorce or separation, enforced relocations, and loss or bereavement, such as the death of a loved one. Although these types of stress reactions are associated with intense emotions and often progressive reaction phases (such as shock, rage, denial, withdrawal, depression and acceptance), recovery is usually complete as soon as the stressor has faded or the individual has learnt to adapt. These types of stress reactions are also referred to as transient or situational stressors, and the impact is temporary until the cause of the stress has been alleviated (Carson et al., 1996; Lowman, 1993).

Workaholism and burnout

Workaholism and psychological burnout are conditions of overcommitment to and in work, and result in various type of stress reactions. Reasons and causes of overcommitment are many, like anxieties as a result of low self-esteem, strong abilities and creative powers, too high aspirations, obsessive-compulsive personality, efforts to compensate for failures or childhood trauma, avoidance of intimate relationships or other social and non-work roles (Sperry, 1996; Lowman, 1993).

Workaholism, or the obsessive-compulsive addiction to work roles indicates employees who have an irrepressible need for work. They are always or continuously working, without necessarily achieving. A distinction is often made between workaholism and work addiction in the sense that the work addict enjoys his/her work, while the workaholic is totally unable to manage his/her work time-effectively. The workaholic's work load never decreases. Gherman (1981) also describes workaholism as a stress reaction under pressure of time and as a defence mechanism, which is employed in an attempt to associate self-induced work overload with success, while it is in fact a withdrawal reaction, for example, from unpleasant domestic problems or an inability to relax.

To assess whether you are, or a person you know is a workaholic, tick 'yes' or 'no' to the following statements.

- Intense, energetic, competitive and self-driven to make more money, to gain more knowledge or just to compete.
  ❐ yes ❐ no
- Seriously doubts own abilities, hard work can be an attempt to compensate for inabilities, often in spite of an apparent attitude of self-confidence and arrogance.
  ❐ yes ❐ no

- Prefers work to relaxation, hates being away from work, finds weekends and holidays depressing and fears the day of retirement.
  ❏ yes ❏ no
- Will use any place and opportunity to work.
  ❏ yes ❏ no
- Uses time efficiently or 'safe' time, for instance, sleeps no more than six hours, often combines meals with work, does not wait for elevators, uses note books and computers to organize work and time.
  ❏ yes ❏ no
- Draws no clear distinction between work and recreation activities.
  ❏ yes ❏ no
- In hobbies or activities such as jogging, does it with the same intensity as work.
  ❏ yes ❏ no

According to Machlowitz (1978), a 'yes' answer on most items may mean that you, or the other person you know, may be a workaholic or addicted to work and working.

Psychological burnout is a stress-related concept, associated with many illnesses and possible outcomes of doing things in excess, and is a multidimensional concept with similarities to a few other psychological states, like (job) dissatisfaction, fatigue, depression and (work) stress. Seriously burnout fatigue in employees will manifest in job and occupational burnout.

Burnout, initially defined by Freudenberger (1974) and confirmed by later research, refers to physical, mental, emotional and psychological overload, and patterns of overcommitment that influence the work behaviour and physical and mental health of workers. This can be true in many jobs, but is particularly true in people-oriented career groups, such as medical practi-tioners, nurses, psychologists and attorneys (Evans & Fisher, 1993). In these occupations employees are very busy helping and facilitating other people and their problems, but leave little time for their own 'debriefing' from shared stress experiences of clients or while working with clients. A problem in burnout is employees' denial that they are experiencing symptoms of burnout.

Maslach's definition (in Muldary, 1983:11) of burnout shows that a combination of symptoms, behaviour and attitudes can be involved. 'The loss of concern for the people with whom one is working includes physical exhaustion and is characterized by an emotional exhaustion in which the professional no longer has any positive feelings, sympathy, or respect for clients or patients.' Most definitions of burnout contain elements of physical, psychological and social exhaustion or burnout, which influence physical health and psychological adjustment.

We contend that burnout refers to a bio-psycho-social state of fatigue in which a person's energy for most purposeful activities is depleted. In general, burnout is accepted to refer to three progressive psychological states, which is depersonalization, which leads to a lower sense of accomplishment, followed by emotional exhaustion. Each of these psychological dimensions may relate more or less to one or a combination of people's stress and experiences in and the demands of various life roles, for instance, work, family life and personal achievements.

Table 11.5 (adapted from Muldary, 1983:6) illustrates the wide range of physical, psychological and behaviour problems that can be associated with burnout. The consequences for work performance of these symptoms are self-evident and predominantly negative.

Post-traumatic stress disorder reactions (PTSD)
PSTD occur during, immediately or some time after an intense, traumatically acute or chronic stressor. These reactions are more intense than the adjustment reactions and are difficult to diagnose since the condition has diverse symptoms and recovery is more difficult. A distinction is made in post-traumatic stress reactions between *acute* (begins during or within six months of the stressor), *chronic* (lasts longer than six months) and *delayed reaction* (begins at least six months after the stressor).

Table 11.5 Various symptoms and consequences of burnout

Physical	Psychological	Behavioural
Fatigue	**Feelings of:**	Dehumanization of clients
Sleep disturbances:	Anger	Victimization of clients
Difficulty in sleeping and getting up	Boredom	Critical, blaming
	Frustration	Defensiveness
Stomach ailments	Depression, anxiety	Impersonal
Migraine headaches	Apathy	Poor communication
Frequent colds, flu	Guilt	Derogatory perceptions
Lingering colds	Suspiciousness	Physical distancing
Backaches	Helplessness	Withdrawal, isolation
Nausea	Pessimism	Postponing behaviours
Muscle tension	Irritability	Sticking to rigid rules
Shortness of breath	Resentment	Clock watching
Frequent injuries	Hopelessness	Absenteeism
Weight problems		Making mistakes
Weakness	**Attitudes**	Unnecessary risks
Change of eating habits	Cynicism	Substance use
	Indifference	Marital and family conflict
	Self-doubt	Conflict with co-workers
	Loss of empathy	Workaholism and obsessiveness
	Poor concentration	Humour as a buffer from emotions
	Discouraged	
	Moodiness	Decreased job efficiency
	Low self-esteem	Suicide
		Over-commitment/ undercommitment

In general, post-traumatic stress reactions are characterized by repeated experience of anxiety about the stressor, a lack of responsiveness to the environment (apathy) and a variety of symptoms such as fright reactions, irritation, fatigue, insomnia, intolerance (for instance for noise), nightmares, loss of concentration, memory impairment, depression, heightened aggression and withdrawal. Examples of experiences that can or have evoked post-traumatic stress reactions are catastrophes (such as collisions, floods, earthquakes, fires, explosions) assault and rape. Wars such as the First and Second World Wars with resultant events such as the atomic bombs on Hiroshima and Nagasaki, the mass deaths of Jews in the Nazi concentration camps, as well as wars such as those in Vietnam and the situation in Israel and Iraq, and the Twin Tower bombings in the USA, drew renewed attention to the intense influence of traumatic stressors. Concepts such as 'shell shock', 'operational fatigue', 'war neuroses', 'combat exhaustion', and more recently 'burnout' are used to refer to post-traumatic stress reaction. Although a great deal of research is still required about post-traumatic stress reactions with regard to diagnosis and treatment, particularly delayed reactions in Vietnam veterans and survivors of concentration camps illustrate the protracted and possible irreversible effects of acute and chronic stress. Treatment requires intense medical, psychiatric and psychological intervention and the emphasis currently is on early identification and treatment of potential post-traumatic reactions.

Psychological factors and physical illness

These conditions, previously also called psychosomatic disorders, refer to the manifestation of physical symptoms as a result of psychological stress and negative emotions. There is sufficient evidence to prove that negative stress and emotions, for example anger, aggression, hostility and worry, are harmful to physical health, while positive emotions and attitudes, like optimism, create an increased ability to counteract physical illnesses (Nevid et al., 2003). In this regard you are also familiar with Selye's stress response syndrome (general adaptation syndrome) where he indicates how the nervous and hormonal systems, among others, affect the body during stress. Moreover, he maintains that certain lifestyles such as those filled with stress, rich diets, smoking and drinking and little exercise, are additional contributory factors to psycho-physiological diseases. Although a multitude of psycho-physiological symptoms are reported, particularly stomach ulcers, anorexia nervosa, migraine and tension headaches, hypertension and coronary heart diseases are classic examples.

Stomach ulcers are caused by excessive secretion of acids and digestive juices that damage the stomach or intestinal linings. Although diets and other organic conditions can cause stomach ulcers, they are ascribed particularly to emotions such as worry, rage and anxiety. These physical symptoms are, in turn, followed by further emotional reactions.

Coronary diseases are probably the most frequently related to negative stress conditions. In this connection the A-type person is described as having the kind of personality which entails a high risk of coronary disease because of a stressful lifestyle and over-involvement with work, achievement and time. Coronary diseases are in most cases preceded by prolonged emotional strain.

Other stress-related illness can be chest pains, headaches, hypertension, dysfunctional eating, gastro-intestinal problems, menstrual irregularities, muscle tensions, panic attacks, hyperventilation, sexual difficulties, etc.

Work dysfunctions of overcommitment may also manifest in *obsessive-compulsive thinking* and *behaviour* of employees who have anxiety-based behaviour or who may manifest symptoms of the obsessive-compulsive personality disorder. Their work may be characterized by an overemphasis on orderliness, neatness, structure, repetition and other forms of excessiveness, which are encouraged in some jobs and tasks and may therefore maintain and disguise the problem.

In summary, sustained stress affects the individual's work behaviour at various levels, namely his/her physical, physiological, emotional, motivational and cognitive functions. In the case of serious decompensation, this may lead to psychiatric disorders, as job stress is associated with emotional disorders such as anxiety, fear, depression, aggression and anger, poor interpersonal relationships, and gives rise to absenteeism, high staff turnover, accidents and underachievement.

11.9.1.5 Anxiety-based disorders and depression

Anxiety-based disorders are characterized by anxiety panic and fear, as well as other emotions, such as depression, which individuals often handle by adaptive behaviour and defence mechanisms (Carson et al., 1996). According to Lowman's classification (Table 11.4) the work dysfunctions in undercommitment and work-related anxiety, manifested by generalized feelings of anxiety and work-performance anxiety, and work-related depression will be applicable here. Persons with different types of phobic disorder will find it difficult to work in certain work environments and tasks, for example, in narrow and high places, among other people, with animals, in hospitals, in nature, and so forth. The individual's emotional behaviour may lead to an unrealistic evaluation of the demands of reality, which can result in evasive and fearful rather than in positive and achieving adaptive behaviour. With some employees, work performance may be marked by so-called fear of failure (FOF) and fear of success (FOS), and helplessness which all denote being afraid to achieve. This type of work commitment can be explained in terms of an over-emphasis by parents and other agents of work ethics, which render people afraid of being rejected if they fail or if they cannot cope with success and its demands, e.g. being promoted. Obviously, generalized anxiety and fear can have an adverse effect on the general adjustment and work behaviour of an individual.

It must be emphasized that *depression*, as part of mood disorders, is a separate clinical condition from anxiety-based disorders. It is, however, obvious that many of the milder depressive and manic symptoms will influence work behaviour. In many research projects so-called emotional strain is often measured as anxiety and depression.

It may be a faulty assumption to assume that excessive emotional reactions will always immobilize the individual completely or impair work effectiveness totally, as a certain level of anxious energy (like stress) may enhance performance, as in some compulsive work behaviours where accuracy and neatness are enhanced. Also, in certain cases, anxiety-stricken employees may work more to defend against anxiety and to satisfy certain needs, for instance the need for authority, to achieve, to be accepted and to please others. This may represent an overinvolvement in that work can actually reinforce and support particular styles of behaviour. Thus, this type of work involvement may possibly also explain the sometimes almost self-destructive and anxious work behaviour of the so-called workaholic, work addicts and type A behaviour patterns that may lead to psychological burnout.

On the other hand, intense anxiety, such as phobias, obsessive-compulsive behaviour, panic disorders and even generalized anxiety and depression, will incapacitate the employee, for example, when fear, panic attacks, depression and obsessive thoughts and compulsive actions dominate a person's work behaviour. This could lead to poor motivation, negative attitudes and perceptions, job dissatisfaction, poor self-esteem, helplessness, dependence, disturbed interpersonal skills, withdrawal behaviours (e.g. absenteeism), procrastination and production impediments, work disinterest, passiveness, very poor performance or underachievement and even an inability to start a task at all. Anxiety tends to incapacitate people's beliefs of self-efficacy and resourcefulness about themselves and in their own cognitive ability. Psycho-physiological reactions may be observed in illness complaints, risky work behaviour which may cause accidents, inaccurate cognitive judgement, visual perception problems, inaccuracy, slow rate of work and psychomotor activities, and have an effect on functions such as respiration, heartbeat and muscular tension (Warr, 1987; Lowman, 1993; Eckenrode & Gore, 1990; Carson et al., 1996).).

11.9.1.6 Personality disorders and work performance

As indicated in a previous section, personality, because of its directive influence, has a strong impact on many dimensions of human behaviour and health. Personality disorders involve dysfunctions that can be described as characteristic *deviant acquired, persistent and repetitive behaviour*. The individual behaves and defines his/her relationships and communicates in ways which may be negative and destructive and inconvenient towards others and eventually themselves. These type of symptomatic behaviour are frequently the only behaviour the person is familiar with; they may seem to be unaware of such behaviour (ego-syntonic), pretend that they cannot help it or deny that they have acted in a certain way. This is in contrast to anxiety disorders, which are ego-dystonic, because such persons usually perceive anxiety as unpleasant, not part of the real self and are anxious to be helped. The main personality disorders are characterized in behaviours like aggressiveness, dependence, impulsiveness, depressiveness, antisocial behaviours, dishonesty, manipulation, avoidance and suspiciousness (Nevid et al., 2003). Examples of personality-related work dysfunctions can manifest in so-called anti-social behaviours and intentions. Such employees behave in destructive ways towards employers and colleagues, for example, by way of arson, blackmail, workplace aggression, harassment, sabotage, espionage, fraud, revenge, extortion, violations of regulations, lawsuits, litigation and unfair claims.

Most people with personality disorders are also characterized by being unpredictable and having poor interpersonal relationships. The antisocial personality type and criminal show a total disregard for other people's feelings and belongings. As in the case of anxiety-based disorders, people with symptoms of personality disorders may sometimes be very effective in their jobs, however, they will often run into difficulties as a result of personality clashes with other employees. Behaviour and attitudinal problems in the work situation frequently coincide with personality disorders, and, together with anxiety-based disorders, depression, psychosomatic conditions and alcoholism, may constitute the chief problem in the industry (Roberson, 1986; Leary (in Carson, 1969), Neff (1985), Steinmetz (1969) and Lowman (1993).

The classification of vocational maladjustment made by Neff (1977, 1985) can be regarded as a description of *personality styles or responses in the work situation*. This relates to Neff's view that mental health in the work situation is a function of the work personality, which is characterized by a productive role. Thus, people differ in this respect; some cannot be productive since they have not learned to be efficient in their environment. The development of the dysfunctional work personality is largely a lack of work-related motivation, work competencies and occupational self-image. Neff's types of occupational maladjustment coincide in ways with the classification of personality disorders and in some instances also with Lowman's categories of personality dysfunctions, undercommitment and perceptual inaccuracies (Table 11.4).

People with poor motivation and a negative role conception of work and of their roles as employees

People's personality structure in this category does not contain acquired cultural norms with regard to work, because of their education and background. For them the community, and hence work, poses a threat to their ego; they are against or negative towards the community and work, and they have little or no sense of responsibility. They do not satisfy the basic requirements of the work situation and are ignorant of the meaning of productive role fulfilment. They generally display symptoms such as absence, ignorance of rules, arriving late, poor production and passive or indifferent attitudes to work. They do not associate work with need satisfaction and their motivation is based on impulsive action such as aggression, theft and dishonesty (immediate need satisfaction). They show little initiative, are inclined to justify their mistakes and defend themselves by often nursing grudges. Accidents, revolt against authority and even alcoholism and drug addiction are safety valves for their impulsive motivation and inadequacy. The most severe manifestation of these symptoms is found in the antisocial or sociopathic personality disorders. Their inadequacy in their work is merely an extension of such behaviour in other spheres, for instance in marriage.

There is relatively little to be done for these people, since their type of work behaviour is fundamentally an attitude towards life. In practice, therapists sometimes use group behaviour therapeutic techniques to achieve the long-term objective of changing their attitudes and deviant behaviours.

People who respond to work mainly with fear and anxiety

In this type of person we find that cultural norms with regard to work have probably been too strongly impressed upon them, with the result that there is tremendous motivation for achievement. However, the motivation is handicapped by vague or even more serious feelings of anxiety and fear, tenseness, touchiness, discomfort, distress and fear of interpersonal relationships. They doubt their own capabilities, with the result that they are unable to fulfil a productive role. The irony in this type of work dysfunction is that although such people have the intention of being very committed and even overcommitted, the performance usually comes over as underachievement.

Other symptoms include varying standards of achievement, poor interpersonal relationships, withdrawal symptoms, depression, absence, self-imposed absence ('sick leave'), little enterprise, an accident record, psychosomatic complaints and a compulsive possessedness with the successful performance of a task, which sometimes succeeds but usually fails. Fears about losing a job and even paranoid traits can be characteristic. People in this category have probably experienced failure in several other spheres, for instance the disappointment of parents and poor achievement at school. This type might coincide with patterns of undercommitment and underachievement, as well as behaviour described as people having a fear of failure and fear of success and procrastination (Lowman, 1993).

Causes are sought in a too strict upbringing, too high expectations by parents, repeated failures, too high aspirations in comparison with abilities, and so on. In other words, work stress is an extension of the individual's personal anxieties. Criticism in the work situation exacerbates the condition, competition is a threat and even group work (cooperation) creates anxiety. Although symptoms of this nature can be manifested generally, they are typical of life-stress conditions, anxiety disorders, psychosomatic disorders and depression, while the obsessive-compulsive personality disorder can also fall in this category. In these cases occupational maladjustment is a function of the degree of anxiety that is experienced. Corrective procedures based on positive motivation will probably be the best, for instance supportive supervision in workshops where a person will learn to trust his/her capabilities.

People whose chief responses in the work situation are openly hostile and aggressive
Because of possibly negative cultural influences, personal shortcomings and limited abilities, people with these types of responses regard work and its requirements as restrictive and as a punishment. The slightest stress and provocation cause aggression where such people are prepared to defend themselves and to attack others. These types of employees are moody, abrasive, frequently cross, negative, inclined to argue and to do things to annoy others, and they are sarcastic and insulting. Accidents may occur because of their impulsiveness. In other words, their energy is used in a constant struggle against their co-workers and against management and authority. Their problem is to keep their jobs and they frequently change jobs by resigning from their present job or because of dismissal. The main reason for their dismissal is their poor interpersonal relations. Comparative psychopathological symptoms or conditions may be looked for in the characteristics of paranoid schizophrenia, paranoid personality, explosive personality and passive-aggressive personality.

People who respond mainly with dependence and immaturity to job requirements
This type of person is uncertain about his/her own capabilities and retains a childlike need for the help and support of others – an analogy with the child–parent

relationship. They are constantly trying to please authority figures, they only work effectively under supervision, and they display little initiative and independence. Because of their search for security and support, these workers are a burden to their fellow-workers and to supervisors, mainly because it is difficult to create a supportive atmosphere in a task-oriented work situation. Certain personality disorders can fall into this category, for instance dependent, histrionic, narcissistic schizoid symptoms, hysteria and inadequacy. This type of personality can benefit from rehabilitation workshops where independent behaviour is reinforced.

Occupational maladjustment can also be a characteristic of the socially naive person

Cultural norms about work have not been impressed upon this type of person, since they have never perceived work and work requirements probably because of too little exposure to work or because of insufficient ability. Their responses are based on ignorance rather than on resistance, aggression, etc. These workers accept working conditions as they are, they experience little stress and show little initiative. Socially naive people are unpredictable in their feelings for others, they fail to realize the effect of their behaviour and they are generally ignorant of how to act socially. The avoiding personality type may fall into this category and they are marked for their inadequacy in interpersonal relationships. They need well-defined and structured work environments (Lowman, 1993). Overprotected children, for instance, if they had been overprotected because of a physical handicap, may have this type of response. In rehabilitative work situations such a person must be exposed to the work and to work-related requirements.

According to Neff and Kultuv the above-mentioned types are fairly reliable and relatively independent. However, much research is still needed. Neff describes two additional types, namely the *reserved* (apathetic) type and the *self-deprecatory* type. The former type of response is characterized by a lack of vitality, by indifference towards everything, emotional unresponsiveness, non-involvement and nonchalance. Self-deprecatory types are critical towards themselves, distrust themselves, their own capabilities and qualities, and like to talk about their weaknesses (Neff, 1985).

Steinmetz's (1969) *criteria for underachievement* are very similar to Neff's classification. He describes the following additional characteristics of poor achievers: persons who do not wish to discuss their ineffective work behaviour because of their natural reserve or their somatic inadequacy; the formation of cliques in the work situation which leads to 'group defence mechanisms', which in turn give rise to poor achievement. 'Group resistance' includes resistance to small social groups, reactive individualism as a response to the informal group (e.g. keeping information from the group), mutual fault-finding and self-imposed absence. Steinmetz also describes the following types:

- The blind spot syndrome, which appears in an individual who is ignorant of his/her limitations
- 'A lack of just one more skill type', which applies to the type of worker who attributes poor achievement to the fact that he/she lacks the capabilities for the job

- The 'OK on routine, weak on troubleshooting type', who easily performs simple tasks but who cannot cope with unusual tasks
- The 'tenacious individual syndrome' is characteristic of the hard-boiled type of person who always thinks he/she is right.

Steinmetz (1969) also describes other forms of unsatisfactory work achievement in the following behaviour types: resistance to change; moodiness; disorganization of work and work methods; the inability to communicate effectively; the person who rarely takes the initiative; intolerance; the individual who invariably wishes to appear blameless; the emotionally sensitive worker; unimaginativeness; and the worker who is always defensive.

In many sources on the relationship between personality disorders and work stress reference is made to the so-called A and B personality types. These two personality types represent two different ways in which people react in the work situation, perform tasks and cope with stress. Type A is associated with the following behaviour patterns, as well as with a high-risk factor for coronary heart diseases and other stress-related problems (Lowman, 1993; Nevid et al., 2003).

- *Intense aspirational behaviour* and conscientiousness – this style of behaviour is characterized by traits of high ambition, strict performance criteria, willingness to work hard, suppression of tension, working long hours, displaying very responsible behaviour and linking production to self-esteem, competing even during recreation.
- An irrepressible *tendency towards urgency*, characterized by virtually impossible time limits for the completion of tasks, impatience, restlessness, a feeling and sensation of constantly working under pressure, doing everything quickly, for instance eating, walking and talking fast, quick emotional reactions, attempting to do several things at once and even attempting to project occurrences.
- Interpersonal relationships display *a lack of caring for other people*. Characteristics of this style of behaviour include hostility, sometimes aggression and anger, egotism, difficulty in following someone else and accepting his/her point of view and often displaying frustrated reactions towards others with less insight, should they receive negative feedback on their interactions.

The Type A personality therefore continually wants to be in control. Sometimes, however, in the midst of unrealistic aspirations, they simply do not command the physical, emotional, cognitive and social adjustment mechanisms, with a resultant loss of control which may lead, among others, to total helplessness and stress reactions in the form of coronary heart diseases in particular. However, the behaviour problems of the Type A person should never be likened to those of the neurotic. Sir Peter Medawar (Nobel Prize winner) describes the Type A person as follows: 'Type A's are without doubt the great doers of the world. Even if Type A's lead shorter lives they live more life while they are living it' (in Friedman & Rosens, 1975:iv).

The Type B personality represents behaviour on the opposite behaviour continuum to that of the Type A. Behaviour is characterized by greater work satisfaction, shorter work hours, satisfaction with less compensation, a more relaxed attitude, less competitiveness, more patience, hard work, but without an intense drive and constraint and they do not set such critical time limits. Type B's like to relax and maintain sound interpersonal relationships.

11.9.1.7 Substance abuse and dependence

Narcotics problems are caused by alcohol or drug abuse and by physical and psychological dependence on these substances. Addictive problems may take the form of behaviour problems because of the use of alcohol or drugs; the problems can also be the *after-effect*s of the excessive use of some form of addictive drug. Examples of these are the chronic stage of alcoholism where the individual is unable to function effectively at the personal, social and work levels; psychotic-induced conditions because of alcoholism and drug abuse; physical diseases; intellectual deterioration and even death.

Industry in general acknowledges narcotics problems, especially *alcohol problems*, as a 'disease', which entail high costs with regard to work loss and intensive internal and external programmes to treat workers with alcohol problems and to re-employ rehabilitated persons. On the other hand, the existence of narcotics problems in the work situation is often denied with no policies and treatment procedures in this regard; insensitive interpersonal and managerial styles which contribute little to the recovery or re-utilization of this type of problem worker. Contemporary general and work context attitudes and policies with regard to smoking, alcohol and drug abuse are, however, encouraging.

The main personal problem of alcoholics and of drug addicts are in their *denial* that they are having difficulties. This is probably a reaction to the condemnation by the community of these types of problems. Denial of problems can have serious consequences in the work situation, for instance, in terms of interpersonal relationships, inaccurate work, unimaginativeness, absence, poor quality work, accidents, vocational immobility (e.g. the fact that the person makes no progress or refuses to undergo training), and feelings of uncertainty, dependence, and aggression – all of which make heavy demands on other workers; there are also financial and material losses (Miner & Brewer, in Dunnette, 1990; Leatz & Stolar, 1993; Cooper & Payne, 1994). The same inefficient behaviours and interaction will occur outside the work situation too, for instance in family and marital problems, financial problems, clashes with the law and traffic offences which, in turn, affect work behaviour and general health.

Different types of drugs have different effects. In the work context drug and alcohol abuse and dependence have more or less similar negative effects. Figure 11.3 illustrates the progressive reactions and work behaviour during the different stages of alcohol addiction.

The chart in Figure 11.3 depicts the working life of an employee in his/her chosen field of endeavour after the point of addiction. This chart was compiled from 230 case studies.

The job efficiency percentage rating decreases in direct proportion to the number of years of addiction if a company does not have treatment programmes, for example an Employee Assistance Programme.

Occupational health

Detecting work-performance deterioration is extremely difficult during the first seven years of addiction. Any referrals in this area would be mostly self-referrals.

The area of greatest cover-up is in the seventh to eleventh year of addiction. This is where early *identification* by means of proper documentation and a control programme is most effective because the greatest number of employed alcoholics fall into this category.

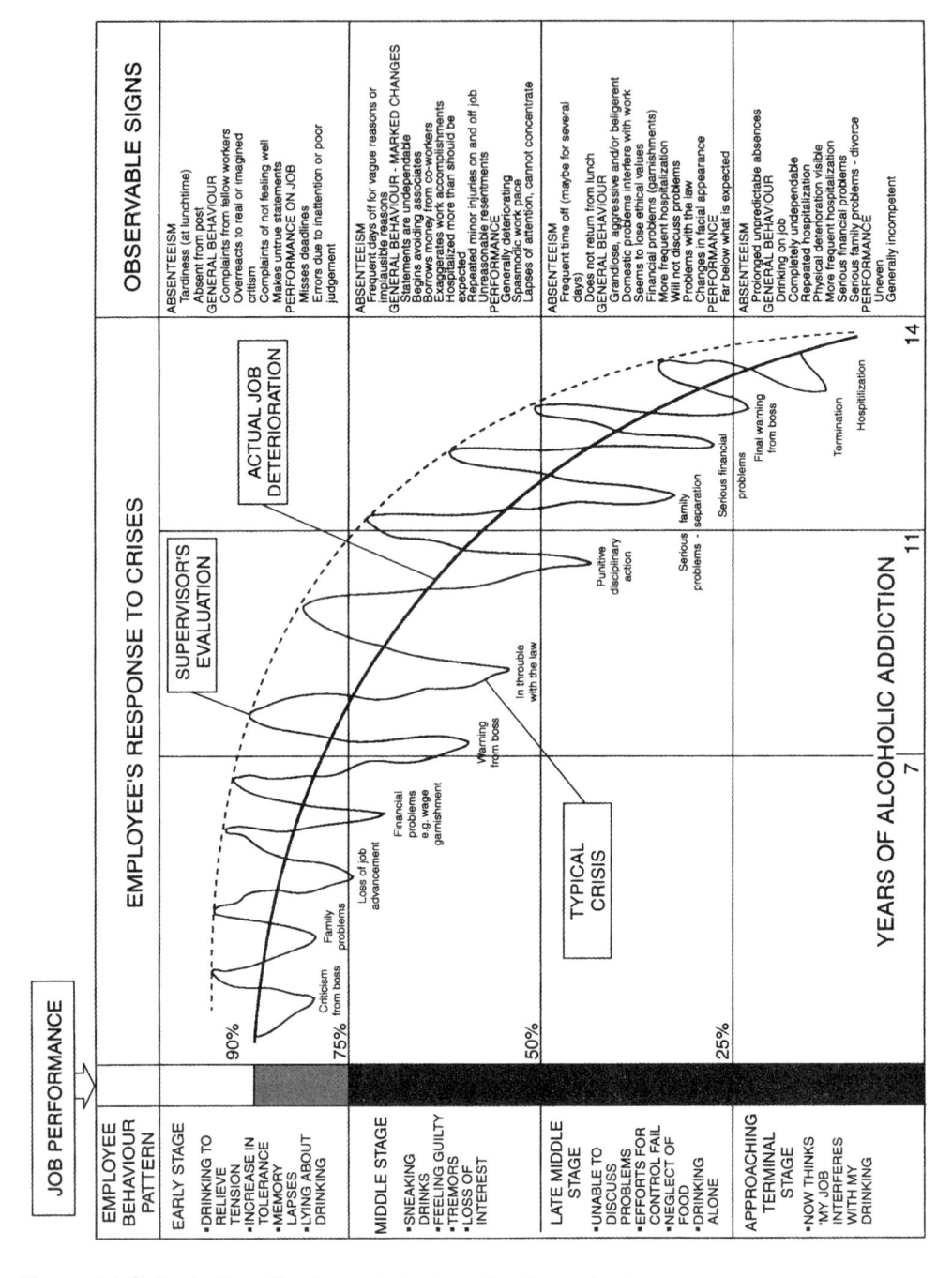

Figure 11.3 Alcoholism: Employee behavioural pattern chart

As the disease progresses beyond the eleventh year, alcoholics are no longer able to conceal their illness and find that work is interfering with their drinking. This also is the area where the employee shows up in the medical department with clinically detectable symptoms, and where many valuable employees are dismissed or resign to take up work that is less demanding.

On the right side of the chart you will note the general deterioration pattern that takes place which is *observable*, such as absenteeism, excessive sick leave, general work performance, attitude and general behaviour.

11.9.1.8 Cognitive and ageing-related disorders

In these conditions, previously referred to as organic psychosis, the emphasis is on *biological aetiology*, particularly on the *brain functioning*. Brain dysfunction could be a result of injury or the abuse of a substance. Treatment is usually based on a medical model, although behaviour problems and occupational rehabilitation can belong to psychological and related disciplines. Cognitive syndromes are characterized by brain damage, which affects intellectual capabilities and the associated functions of speech, concentration, memory, movement, and so forth, either completely or partially. Examples are delirium (mental confusion), dementia (mental deterioration), and amnesia (decline in memory). Dementia due to general medical conditions are Pick's disease, Parkinson's disease, Huntington's disease, HIV disease, head trauma and neurosyphilis. Mental retardation is characterized by underdeveloped intellectual functioning. In both instances there are emotional and physical problems apart from the intellectual impediment.

Because of the nature of these conditions, serious problems can make the individual totally unsuitable for work in the ordinary labour market. Special positions have to be created for these people, or they can work in sheltered working places during and after rehabilitation. The place of work must often be designed to suit the worker's related physical handicaps.

The *age psychoses*, where there may be serious or less serious brain dysfunctioning because of physical and psychic processes of change, constitute a special problem area. The problems of older or retired persons are of particular importance for the industry. Work problems in this case are due partly to cultural norms, namely that 'old people' are dependent and no longer able to play a productive role, and partly to the individual's subjective feelings about retirement, age and uselessness. However, research, for example by Miner and Brewer (in Dunnette, 1990) has proved that older workers, although slower from a motor point of view, are still able to work accurately. They may, however, experience problems with memory processes, with the physical demands of the job and with complex abstract intellectual tasks. Perceptual and motor retardation may also be a safety factor, and poor physical health may be a problem. Examples of specific problems as a result of aging are anxiety disorders, depression, sleep disorders, as well as Alzheimer's disease. On the other hand, the writers point out that the older worker can offer wisdom, better integrated knowledge, greater responsibility, positive work attitudes and management skills.

11.9.1.9 The impact of other psychological disorders
Other psychological disorders or their symptoms may also manifest in work dysfunctions, for example dissociative and somatoform disorders, schizophrenia and other psychotic disorders, sexual disorders and specific development *disorders of childhood and adolescence*, the latter because early development problems may influence later career behaviours. In the dissociative disorders, symptoms relating to the loss of identity, memory and even consciousness will have a serious impairment on many aspects of occupational and job performance, and may also be related to other psychiatric disorders, for example, personality and anxiety disorders. The disorientation which *schizophrenic disorders and other types of psychoses* cause in about all spheres of human functioning, will seriously disrupt career and job performance in about all areas. These symptoms include distortions and peculiarities in thinking, speech, attention, vision, perception, emotions and even movement in some cases. Gender identity and sexual dysfunctions and disorders are important with regard to people's gender (male or female) and sexual identification which may relate to perceptions about work roles, power and relationships at work. These aspects may be important in work dysfunctions relating to sexual harassment and other sexual offenses, for example exhibitionism, violence, abuse and rape. *Sexual harassment* in the workplace is rather commonplace and plagued by prejudice and misunderstanding and quite often the subject of litigation. Sexual harassment refers to any observable or implicit behaviour and actions that suggest unwelcome or hostile sexual advances and actions between employees, usually to obtain certain advantages (Fitzgerald, 1993).

11.9.1.10 The physically disabled and related problems
We contend that emotional or psychological troubled employees are also 'handicapped', as indicated in the larger part of this chapter, however, this section is about the occupational psychological adjustment of the physically ill and the physically handicapped employee.

Real and 'invented' physical ailments
Physical illness or complaints of physical ailments, real, imagined or faked, might still be the most prevalent of all occupational diseases, and also a symptom or contributing factor in many psychological disorders or complaints of related symptoms.

Typical occupational physical diseases are not easily distinguishable from non-occupational diseases, for example, non-specific symptoms like head and body pains, nausea, insomnia, fatigue and anorexia may manifest in many types of diseases with a wide variety of causes. Most psychological disorders also have physical symptoms or in some conditions such people may develop physical illnesses more easily. *Occupational diseases* are those that can be related to causal factors in the workplace, for instance, injuries and accidents due to unsafe work methods, unhealthy and unsafe workplaces and unsafe equipment, pollution and poisoning through toxic, high-risk substances and chemicals, as well as extreme temperatures and poor ventilation. Some of the well-known occupational illnesses and injuries are lung diseases and cancer, musculoskeletal injuries, amputations, fractures, trauma, eye loss, cardiovascular diseases, reproductive disorders, noise-induced hearing loss, dermatological diseases, as well as certain psychological conditions like anxiety, stress, depression and substance abuse.

Psychologists are involved in the psychological or emotional pain, caused by real or imagined physical diseases and symptoms. In previous sections the relationship between physical and psychological health is emphasized in almost all the psychological disorders, especially the physical symptoms of anxiety, stress and psycho-physiological disorders. These physical symptoms, like fatigue, diarrhoea, ulcers, insomnia, upset stomach, nausea, various types of body and head pains, allergies, anorexia nervosa, asthma, diabetes, enuresis and cardiovascular-related diseases, may even last longer than physical illnesses not related to emotional problems, with associated decreases in work performance and increased medical expenses. In the DSM-diagnostic criteria for many of the psychological disorders, the possibility of medical illness, which may contribute to the psychological symptoms, is emphasized (APA, 1994, 2000). These are predominantly real diseases in which physical and psychological symptoms are not 'invented', such troubled employees do not consciously control their symptoms by faking or malingering. These physical and related psychological symptoms, and vice versa, interact and can markedly impair work behaviours and other life roles. In some conditions, for example, in conversion disorder (loss or impairment of physical function without apparent organic cause), troubled employees may also consciously or unconsciously fake or control physical symptoms to avoid problems or to gain advantages.

Paradoxically to real psycho-physical symptoms, it seems as if some people consciously or unconsciously prefer illness or assumed illness to being healthy. In some psychological disorders, *factitious symptoms* (feigned physical and psychological symptoms to assume a sick role), *faking of symptoms and malingering* (the intentional production of false or grossly exaggerated physical or psychological symptoms for an exterior motive, for example, to avoid responsibilities or to obtain other advantages), are also considered before final diagnoses are made. In factitious, faked and malingering of illness symptoms, the employee's motivation is manipulative and either externally motivated (e.g. to obtain medical benefits, have more leisure time, avoid an unpleasant supervisor) or internally, that is, to assume a *sick role* and thus obtaining secondary gains, such as attention, avoiding work or other responsibilities, for fear of failure or to mask a lack of competencies. In all these cases, the mind is consciously and possibly unconsciously conditioned to take control and to convert a psychological problem into physical symptoms, through which such employees can avoid internal and external problems, or gain something from the external world, which would not otherwise be obtainable. Due to the manipulative nature of feigned illness symptoms and the fact of obtaining personal gains without really being sick, such behaviours are not easily changed, as verified by paradoxical responses to treatment. Malingerers will assert to be even more ill, despite intensive or the best treatment and no clear signs of real illness, which will delay any prognosis.

Whatever the cause and nature of physical illness in the work context, physical impairment mostly also has other disabling effects, like cognitive, emotional and social impairments, which will impact on effective work behaviours. Added to ineffective work performance, are the loss in work hours, absenteeism and high direct and indirect costs for medical and related treatment.

The physically disabled

Physical handicaps, that may be caused by genetic and related metabolic factors, organic brain damage, accidents, toxic and nutritional influences, and which include disabled limbs, blindness, deafness and paralysis, are health problems that may severely impede an individual's general and work adjustment. These problems in the work experience are partly due to the disability symptoms, but also the attitudes of the disabled person, employers and the community at large, which translate in certain 'traditional' attitudes towards the 'dissimilarity' of handicapped people compared with able people. The many prejudices and stereotyped views about handicapped people often result in a type of special treatment or job reservation in the labour market, even if legislation prohibits any discrimination. Even competent disabled people do not always have a free choice of vocation, jobs and tasks. This is contrary to present and past examples of handicapped individuals, blind, deaf and crippled, who have been very successful as people and as professional people. Ferreira (1999) finds that the frustrations of disabled employees are related to many aspects in training at school and post-school level, job opportunities, discriminatory people, management practices in work situations, and unfair attitudes and perceptions about disabled employees. Ferreira also discusses various unfounded stereotypes about the work ability of disabled employees, for example, high personnel turnover, less productivity, high safety risk, expense of employing disabled people, being demanding and an embarrassment for the organization. In Ferreira's (1999) research on the subjective work experiences of disabled employees, task and role characteristics, organizational climate and their general attitudes about work were found to have the strongest influence on the disabled employee's work experiences. Negative perceptions of these organizational factors may have a negative influence on the disabled person's feelings about the organization, commitment and stress experiences.

While unrealistic expectations and demands should not be made on competent handicapped workers, who often are exemplary in their positive attitude to work and excellent performance, they should also not be treated differently, except that the work design must also fit their impairments. Similarly to physically able employees, the physically handicapped employees' problems should be evaluated in context, their capabilities and skills should be considered and they should be utilized optimally, taking into account the requirements of the job, work design and practical considerations such as their health and safety.

Because of the close relationship between the physical and emotional aspects of a person's functioning, even temporary physical handicaps may have an intense emotional effect on employees. Generally speaking, the work adjustment of physically handicapped people is good, often better than that of emotionally handicapped people, even if it is motivated by the knowledge of restricted job opportunities. Absences and accidents do not necessarily occur more often than among other workers, and personnel turnover among physically disabled employees is often lower than for other groups. Obviously the type of physical disablement will also contribute to the level of work and work performance and related emotional problems.

HIV/Aids: A general and work problem

The *acquired immunodeficiency syndrome* (Aids) is a fatal contagious pandemic disease that can be transmitted by unsafe sexual intercourse practices, rape, blood transfusions, and injections. Even if much controversy about HIV/Aids exists, its potential devastating influence on human health and other life roles are widely recognized in all parts of the world. In Africa and South Africa, especially, HIV/Aids is assuming drastic proportions, and figures for infection on a daily basis are already higher than those for deaths resulting from violence, tuberculosis, road accidents, cardiac diseases and smoking put together. It is estimated that more than 12 per cent of the world's population resides in Africa, but that more than 60 per cent of all HIV/Aids sufferers are also in Africa, while it is spreading at an alarmingly fast rate.

Aids has a profound affect on every individual, family, group, work organization and nation. Because it is not only a medical or health problem, but also influences behaviour patterns, values and attitudes, it has become a community, country and global health problem. Aids has also become an economic problem, since its consequences (e.g. due to medical care and death) are, and will become astronomical in respect of decreased human resources, productivity, unemployment and medical care. Aids has probably also become an educational problem, because in all spheres people's behaviour patterns, knowledge, thinking and attitudes will have to be influenced in respect of prevention of Aids. It is also a socio-economic problem, because improvements in living standards can prevent the spreading of the HIV/Aids virus. Aids has also become a legal and moral issue, with regard to, say, liability for spreading the virus, the rights of Aids sufferers, and legal protection. Aids has also become a work problem. As in their personal lives, in the workplace too, there is still a stigma attached to HIV/Aids sufferers, despite legislation which prohibits any form of discrimination. Employed HIV/Aids sufferers do create a 'problem' for the organization management and co-workers, because of the real needs of such employees, but also perceptions and misperceptions about the disease. The incidence of HIV/Aids in the workplace affects the formulation of policies regarding employment and work benefits, as well as interaction with other employees.

Health workers and psychologists in particular, have a special role in general and in the workplace with regard to prevention and the following tasks, among others:

- Aids prevention education, for example, information, training and education of prospective employees and present employees with regard to the implications of HIV/Aids and other sexually transmitted diseases
- Formulation of rights, policy and procedures with regard to the handling of Aids sufferers in the workplace. Current legislation prohibits any discriminatory practices against HIV/Aids sufferers, and requires them to be treated like any person with any other life-threatening disease
- Training of management and other employees in respect of work accommodation, that is, the handling of and behaviour towards Aids sufferers, their work design and provision of health-care services
- Therapeutic and counselling services for Aids sufferers, because they, and often their relatives, often have to bear a stigma and social isolation and are in need of empathic support as badly as they need medical care. HIV/Aids sufferers

experience similar feelings (e.g. grief, anxiety, fear, depression, guilt) as other people with a serious physical illness, and in some cases may experience similar grief processes as terminal patients, for example, cancer sufferers (Jason & Glenwick, 2002).

The management of HIV/Aids in South Africa remains a controversial issue, especially with regard to treatment aspects and the governmental perceptions, role and contributions in treatment. However, the Code of Good Practice on HIV/Aids provides guidelines and also serves to prohibit any measures of discrimination and unfair workplace practices against HIV/Aids sufferers. The HIV/Aids Code of Good Practice with regard to employment, concerns policies and actions related to recruitment, continued employment, termination, promotion and development, illness, benefits, grievances and disciplinary procedures, education and prevention of sexually transmitted diseases, testing, management of colleagues and clients, confidentiality, dispute resolutions and healthcare. In summary, all these measures require employers to treat HIV/Aids sufferers the same as any other employee and actions must only relate to the person's ability to do the tasks or whether illness prevents a person to work efficiently.

11.9.1.11 Career development and work performance problems

As a further elaboration and because it primarily integrates problems during career transitions and in the workplace, the taxonomy of career and organizational performance work dysfunctions by Campbell and Cellini (1981) serves as a valuable reference. Many career performance problems may be coupled to career immaturity, caused by emotional problems and personal uncertainty, a lack of career-related knowledge and values, and a lack of adequate career choice skills, which may cause career choice uncertainty, other career decision problems and stagnation in career progress. The following discussion involves a number of specific career development psychological problems which can manifest because of work-related factors or even because of psychological or emotional dysfunction.

Table 11.6 Campbell and Cellini's taxonomy of work dysfunctions: Problem categories and sub-categories

---

I PROBLEMS IN CAREER DECISION-MAKING
  A Getting started
   1 Lack of awareness of the need for a decision
   2 Lack of knowledge of the decision-making process
   3 Awareness of the need to make a decision but avoidance of assuming personal responsibility for decision-making
  B Information gathering
   1 Inadequate, contradictory, and/or insufficient information
   2 Information overload (i.e. excessive information that confuses the decision-maker)
   3 Lack of knowledge as to how to gather information (i.e. where to obtain, organize, and evaluate information)

---

4 Unwillingness to accept the validity of the information because it does not agree with the person's self-concept

C Generating, evaluating, and selecting alternatives
   1 Difficulty deciding owing to multiple career options (i.e. too many equally attractive career choices)
   2 Failure to generate sufficient career options because of personal limitations such as health, resources, ability, or education
   3 Inability to decide because of the thwarting effects of anxiety such as fear of failure in attempting to fulfil the choice, fear of social disapproval, and/or fear of commitment to a course of action
   4 Unrealistic choice (i.e. aspiring to goals either too low or too high based on criteria such as aptitudes, interests, values, resources, and personal circumstances)
   5 Interfering personal constraints that impede a choice (e.g. interpersonal influences and conflicts, situation circumstances, resources, health)
   6 Inability to evaluate alternatives because of lack of knowledge of the evaluation criteria (e.g. criteria could include values, interests, aptitudes, skills, resources, health, age, and personal circumstances)

D Formulating plans to implement decisions
   1 Lack of knowledge of the necessary steps to formulate a plan
   2 Inability to use a future time perspective in planning
   3 Unwillingness and/or inability to acquire the necessary information to formulate a plan

II PROBLEMS IN IMPLEMENTING CAREER PLANS
A Characteristics of the individual
   1 Failure to undertake the steps necessary to implement plan
   2 Failure or inability to successfully complete the steps necessary for goal attainment
   3 Adverse conditions of or changes in family situation

III PROBLEMS IN ORGANIZATIONAL OR INSTITUTIONAL PERFORMANCE
A Deficiencies in skills, abilities, or knowledge
   1 Insufficient skills, abilities, and/or knowledge on position entry (i.e. underqualified to perform satisfactorily)
   2 Deterioration of skills, abilities, and/or knowledge over time in the position because of temporary assignment to another position, leave, and/or lack of continual practice of the skill
   3 Failure to modify or update skills, abilities, and/or knowledge to stay abreast of job changes (i.e. job obsolescence following new technology, tools, and knowledge)

B Personal factors
   1 Personality characteristics discrepant with the job (e.g. values, interests, work habits)
   2 Debilitating physical and/or emotional disorders
   3 Adverse off-the-job personal circumstances and/or stressors (e.g. family pressure, financial problems, personal conflicts)
   4 Occurrence of interpersonal conflicts on the job specific to performance requirements (e.g. getting along with supervisor, co-workers, customers, clients)

> C Conditions of the organization/institutional environment
> 1. Ambiguous or inappropriate job requirements (e.g. lack of clarity of assignments, work overload, conflicting assignments)
> 2. Deficiencies in the operational structure of the organization/institution
> 3. Inadequate support facilities, supplies, or resources (e.g. insufficient lighting, ventilation, tools, support personnel, materials)
> 4. Insufficient reward system (e.g. compensation, fringe benefits, status recognition, opportunities for advancement)
>
> **IV PROBLEMS IN ORGANIZATIONAL OR INSTITUTIONAL ADAPTATION**
> A Initial entry
> 1. Lack of knowledge of organizational rules and procedures
> 2. Failure to accept or adhere to organizational rules and procedures
> 3. Inability to assimilate large quantities of new information (e.g. information overload)
> 4. Discomfort in a new geographic location
> 5. Discrepancies between individuals' expectations and the realities of the institutional/organizational environment
>
> B Changes over time
> 1. Changes over the life span in one's attitudes, values, lifestyle, career plans, or commitment to the organization that lead to incongruence between the individual and the environment (e.g. physical and administrative structure, policies, procedures)
>
> C Interpersonal relationships
> 1. Interpersonal conflicts arising from differences of opinion, style, values, mannerisms, etc.
> 2. Occurrence of verbal or physical abuse or sexual harassment
>
> Source: Campbell & Cellini, 1981:179–180, adapted by Lowman, 1993:61–64.

11.9.1.12 Spill-over effects from work and non-work conflicts

The close relationship or *interaction between work and many non-work roles* (e.g. family, education, religion, leisure, and other societal roles) may bring conflict and frustration in both areas, which will result in stress reactions and even more serious consequences like physical illness, work loss, divorce and family tragedies. The work and family interaction is of special importance, and in this regard special issues relate to the problems of single parents, role conflicts between working married couples or dual career couples (e.g. Greenhaus & Parasuraman, 1989; Eckenrode & Gore, 1990; Long & Kahn, 1993). In a sense, a disruptive work or family environment can be viewed as problem area in itself. An explanation for some of the work and non-work conflicts is that the traditional roles are changing, sometimes even reversed, as the labour market changes, women increasingly enter work at all levels, often both parents (dual career couples) or more members of households are working, and more children are alone at home and young adults are dependent on parents for financial support for longer periods during studies or while they search for jobs. The accumulation of more or multiple family and work roles in the life of families or between working couples, can provide more opportunities, life and work satisfaction, but also more stress, conflicts and emotional problems. Most of these work and non-work conflicts result from factors such as conflicting responsibilities and roles at work and at home, conflicts at home with regard to household and family care tasks, time constraints and conflicts, financial matters and possibly also conflicting work interests and even competition and jealousy about types of work and income. Greenhaus & Beutel (1985) summarize the various type of work–family conflict as belonging to one or more of the following three types:

1 Time-based conflict results from too little time for either work or non-work roles, because of the time taken by either one of these roles.
2 Strain-based conflict follows when physical and emotional symptoms experienced in one area have negative consequences in the other area.
3 Behaviour-based conflict arises when behaviours expected in one area are incompatible with behaviour expectancies in the other area.

Many research results (Cooper & Payne, 1994; Eckenrode & Gore, 1990; Loscocco & Rochelle, 1991) show that non-work roles may have positive and negative influences on work satisfaction. It seems as if married working couples often experience higher levels of work satisfaction than single working parents. Such research outcomes are obviously determined by the types of relationships at home and work, as well as work satisfaction experienced. It is probably true that work impacts more on the family than the family does on work. Work overload, for instance, may contribute even more to the parents' (especially mothers') perception and even guilt feelings of having to fulfil various life roles, while work stress of men and women may spill over at home in reactions such as frustration, anger, sexual disinterest, illness complaints, excessive alcohol intake, violence and abuse. In general, work-role stressors (role conflict, role ambiguity and role overload) have been reported to impact on mental health in symptoms such as tension, irritability, anxiety and fatigue. Greenhaus and Parasuraman (1989) concluded that the influence of stress between family and work among dual or two-career couples will to a large extent be determined by task characteristics in the work, work schedules and the importance of the work for each person (Thompson & Bunderson, 2001).

11.9.1.13 Executive pathology

It is possible that *executives, managers and supervisors* of our present-day large industrial organizations experience more stressors than many other employees or their subordinates. We define executives as all levels of supervision and management in organizations, because all these levels of executives are more or less involved in leadership, planning, decision-making, organizing, controlling and administrative tasks and responsibilities. Management, through their executive functions in people management, is arguably a very strong contributing factor in the occupational adjustment of their subordinates. However, individual differences and the level of managerial work will influence their psychological adjustment. In this regard Sperry (1996) observes that female executives in some respects manage differently from their male counterparts. Male management styles are characterized by a strong personal identification with their work and managerial roles, are strongly business and achievement oriented, work at a fast pace, face conflicting demands and few breaks, experience many time pressures, do not like unscheduled interruptions, are very busy with their daily activities and business planning, they prefer face-to-face contact to communicate about business matters, and do not make much time for personal matters or self-reflection. Female managers, on the other hand, view their work and managerial position as only a part of their multifaceted roles, prefer to work at a steady pace, but with breaks, do not mind unscheduled interruptions, use face-to-face and other methods of business communication, like to do long-term planning, and make time for personal matters during their work time. According to Sperry (1996), it is possible that given the changing work environment, the future manager will have to be more multifaceted, creative and nurture new ideas, services and products. It seems that female management styles with the characteristics of flow and leniency, interaction, access orientation, networking, nurturance, creativity and involvement, might be needed more in the future business organization.

Intense stress effects are attributed to the executives' positions, their roles, responsibilities and the expectations linked to all these aspects. Since managers are leaders, decision-makers, innovators, coordinators, administrators, conflict-solvers and risk-takers, many stressors may affect their occupational health. Job overload, a non-supportive work environment, competition for executive positions, power struggles in organizations (politics), and unethical and illegal practices are some of the critical crises which executives face. Blotnick (1985) in turn, relates causes of executive adjustment problems to the various life and career stages as follows:

- In their 20s, managers are faced with the problems of making a good corporate impression and behaving correctly.
- Managers in their 30s are expected to mature in their managerial competencies and to be good team members.
- In their 40s, executives are required to become indispensable by keeping abreast of knowledge and other demands and not be become redundant.
- During their 50s executives must guard against stagnation, but must develop into good mentors for younger executives.
- In their 60s, executives must be busy developing and training their successors or selecting a right successor.

Moreover, many managers' work behaviours are expected to be exemplary and achievement-oriented (e.g. compare type A behaviours). The issues of career plateaus and related boredom and frustration, limited opportunities for further progress, increasing health problems, dwindling competency levels, as well as oncoming retirement and isolation, may further create stress for many older executives. All these roles, expectations, behaviours and factors are indications of the possible incidence of high levels of stress and stress-related diseases, like cardiac illness and psychological burnout.

Except for the generic sources of stress, managers in contemporary industrial settings and changing work environments also experience other types of demands, such as merging and acquisitions of companies, retrenchment and downsizing of work forces, uncertainty of managerial jobs due to structural changes in organizations, economic declines, affirmative action and personnel policies, which may limit career development scope for certain groups and put greater demands on managers to achieve better results, sometimes with even more restrictions on resources and more pressure from employees and unions on managers to negotiate better working conditions, financial income and other benefits. In current re-engineering or restructuring practices in many organizations, the middle management levels are drastically decreased, which not only weakens organizational management, but puts even more pressure on the higher executive levels.

Sperry (1996) distinguishes between the distressed and the impaired executive.

Distressed executives are still functioning well in their various life roles, but may experience temporary distress and occupational dysfunction, due to work stressors like work overload and strict time constraints. Distressed executive symptoms, which may correlate with symptoms of burnout and adjustment disorders (according to the DSM) can manifest in marital problems, poor work relationships, suppressed emotional reactions at work and home, aggression and hostility, problems with authority, and anxieties about dependency, success or failure. Severe stress, much compulsory socializing (possibly excessive drinking), long hours, work compulsiveness, and heavy work loads in the distressed executive may also be associated with illness complaints and insomnia.

The term *impaired executives* refers to executives whose functioning, in their various life roles, especially their fit in their occupational roles and the work environment, are substantially impaired due to physical and/or psychological illness. Impairment of executives can be the result of many illnesses or psychological adjustment problems, of which substance abuse and related disorders, stress-related disorders, anxiety, depression, schizophrenia and personality disorders and marital problems are the most prevalent. Severe work dissatisfaction and underemployment can also lead to executive impairment. These types of impairments will cause the executive to lose some contact with reality, behave incoherently, inappropriately, strangely and unpredictably. Their work behaviours can further be characterized by indecisiveness, forgetfulness, being apathetic and confused, demonstrating poor judgement and business sense, and also overreacting or showing aggression on insignificant stimuli. The impaired executive cannot handle the challenges of business life, has poor coping mechanisms and recuperation will take time.

In the current competitive business world, managers/executives may often be the symptom-bearers for possible other problems inside and often outside the organizational system. Managers spend much energy, as representatives of employers and negotiators between employees and employers, which may leave them devoid of sufficient resources to cope with their own personal stress. Thus, executives find themselves in the position where the climate for the incidence of emotional, stress, physical and even psychiatric problems, is optimal. However, they are also in a position where acknowledgement of health-related problems may be seen as a weakness. In some organizations executive illness and adjustment problems may even be 'rewarded' by peers and authorities, for example, to deny the existence of problems, allow or put up with mistakes for long periods of time. Such reinforcement behaviours will only increase problems and delay treatment and recovery. Although many managers, because of their expected good qualities and coping resources, may function well initially, they may be inclined to overtax these mechanisms. Thus, any warnings of possible psychological impairment are often very late. It seems as if in many cases the saying 'cowboys don't cry', may be applied with regard to executive health. On the other hand, in many organizations, executives have even better health promotion services than other employees.

Prevention, curative and health promotion strategies may overlap in methods like health education and training, effective stress, time and goal or objectives management, best use of leisure time, social support systems, like family and friends, use of fitness facilities, regular health status assessments, appropriate group and individual psychotherapy and medication, as well as executive coaching and consultation with regard to their managerial and career issues and frustrations. Preventive treatment strategies can include effective selection, promotion, career development and training functions to ensure optimal fit, performance and expectations of employees in executive positions. According to Sperry (1996), executive treatment in organizations include three overlapping areas: psychotherapy, consultation and coaching. These aspects do not indicate only the possible problem areas, but also the skills repertoire that the health professional or psychologist in organizations should have. Executive psychotherapy mostly involves personal problems, like overcommitment, interpersonal conflicts, conflicts between career development and non-work issues (e.g. family matters), loss, marriage and family problems, specific personality disorders and other behavioural problems. Executive coaching involves teaching, training and directing executives with regard to their various roles, especially their people management and interpersonal skills – the latter are essential to handle individual employees and to be effective in team work. Corporate or executive consultation with an individual or executive team includes the knowledge and skills to listen, question, advise on and facilitate managerial decisions and actions, with regard to the various organizational sub-systems, policies, strategies, structures and functions.

11.9.2 Organizational and environmental work-related dysfunctions

The causes of the following work dysfunctions may be related more to work, organization and the environment, but may still have psychological components relating to individual employees and their psychological health problems. When defining organizational health various approaches can be followed, for example, according to the organization's business objectives, that is, whether it is profitable and productive, and if not, the organization and its employees may be diagnosed as ineffective. Another approach is to concentrate on the dynamic human and related processes, that is, the status of the employees' health and how employee capacities are developed and optimized in an organization. In research by Levering (1988), and Jacques and Clement (1991), the following factors were identified for successful organizations:
- Mutual trust and confidence
- Pride in jobs being done

Psychological health and adjustment in the work context

- Enjoyment in working with other people
- Dignity and respect for employees
- Fairness, justice and recognition of employees' personal and work achievements
- Expectations of mutual integrity, initiative, cooperation and reliability
- A climate of openness without fears of authority.

Work dysfunctions, which may be viewed as collective or organizational health problems, can be classified, according to, for example, Lowman (1993) and Sperry (1996) as described below.

11.9.2.1 Dysfunctional group dynamics in organizations
- Problematic organizational culture
- Impaired work group or team functioning
- Authority-follower problems
- Culturally estranged and minority employees.

11.9.2.2 Dysfunctional internal organizational environment
- Incompatibilities in organizational mission and strategies
- Dysfunction in organizational structures and functions
- Organizational and work design problems
- Unhealthy and unsafe or dysfunctional working conditions
- Personnel turnover and absenteeism
- Inability in organizational transformation and restructuring.

11.9.2.3 Macro-organizational/external environmental problems
- Unemployment
- Problems as a result of change and transformation.

With regard to organizational problems, five interdependent areas in organizational functioning important for diagnosis and assessment are: power and authority, morale and cohesion, norms and standards, goals and objectives, and roles and communication.

Similarly, Sperry (1996) refers to the six interdependent sub-systems in organizations from which all problems may also arise, and which must be considered in organizational diagnosis. These are the sub-systems of strategy, culture, structure, employees, leaders and the surrounding environment. Though change in one area will or may influence change in the other areas, it is crucial for the health practitioner to identify the most troubled area in order to focus interventions on that area. Only a few comments about some of these issues are given below.

Another approach is to explain organizational health within the context of the corporate paradigm, for example, culture, values, climate and management philosophy (Cox, 1991; Sperry, 1996; Robbins et al., 2001). *Dysfunctional organizational culture* can be a disruptive influence in an organization and for all employees. Corporate culture is the pattern of basic assumptions, shared beliefs, experiences, values, customs, rules, rituals, secrets and conscious and unconscious behaviours, that a given group like an organization has invented, discovered or developed in learning to cope with its problems of external adaptation and internal integration and control, and that have worked well enough to be considered valid, and therefore, to be taught to new members as the correct way to perceive, think and feel in relation to those problems. In a sense, corporate culture represents an organization's collective personality and temperament.

The assumption here is that all functional and structural processes in the organization according to which employees function have their foundation in basic organizational values. Thus an organization's 'personality' and employee behaviour patterns are formed and maintained as in the selection and promotion of certain types of personalities (organizational men and women). Phenomena such as 'group think' and 'dominant coalitions' that can influence decision-making in organizations can also be explained in these terms. Thus, if any unhealthy influences exist in the organizational culture, for example, in poor managerial style and behaviours, favouritism, dishonest business practices and ethics, this may work through to all employees and subordinates and their actions with colleagues and customers.

Ketz de Vries and Miller's theory (1984), for example, on *neurotic styles and 'organizational pathology'* relates to the influence of corporate values. A similarity exists between organizational pathology and individual pathology as defined in clinical psychology/psychiatry and as explained by psychoanalytical and psychiatric literature. Top and company managers may have specific fantasies and neurotic tendencies that can lead to organizational disorientation. Because top management, especially in centralized organizations, directly determines and influences organizational culture and climate, structure and processes, these negative tendencies will have negative effects, although positive influences can also result from such orientations. Specific types of managers will, for example, be appointed and this could lead to an undesirable kind of uniformity and conformity. It stands to reason that individual employee behaviour can also be detrimentally influenced. These authors identify five 'neurotic styles' that manifest themselves in five organization types:

The *paranoic organization* is based on the fantasy of mistrust of others and manifests a neurotic style of suspicion about the accompanying risk of reality disturbance and defensive attitudes. In an organization this style manifests in careful analysis and strict control, cautious decision-making, centralized control and reactive rather than proactive actions. In business activities, such as marketing, diversification rather than specialization is emphasized. Weaknesses in this style are lack of a consistent strategy, no outstanding skills and uncertain action towards employees.

The *compulsive organization* is based on the fantasy of dependence, mastery and control which can result in the neurotic style of perfectionism. A risk factor is excessive internalization and indecision. Organizations with this style function according to definitive routines, processes and structures, with a great deal of emphasis on thoroughness, completeness and conformity. Formal control, standardization and hierarchical structures are the order of the day. Management is centralized and excessive emphasis on planning leads to fixation and delay in growth and decision-making, which may ultimately be fairly compulsive. Positive characteristics are sound control and skilled action and clearly defined business goals. Negative characteristics are rigidity, over-structuring and inhibition of responsibility and decision-making.

The *histrionic organization* is influenced by a fantasy to attract attention and impress, with a resultant neurotic style of 'narcissism' – dramatic expressiveness and attention seeking with feverish activity and over-reaction. In this type of centralized organization, corporate culture and strategy are based on boldness, risky action and diversification. The result is uncontrolled proactivity with mobility in business transactions. Positive characteristics are potential for growth and creativity, whereas negative characteristics are inconsistent, risky and uncontrolled action.

The *depressive organization* is influenced by a fantasy of hopelessness with a concomitant neurotic style of feelings of guilt, uselessness and ineffectiveness. A risk factor is pessimism which inhibits actions and decision-making. Activities and structures in this type of organization, which is usually established bureaucratically, are extremely conservative and autocratic, and are characterized by poor leadership, passivity, lack of self-confidence and aimlessness in planning and decision-making. Trivialities are emphasized – there is an internal locus of control and the goals of strategy and planning are narrow and limited. Positive characteristics are effectiveness of internal processes and clearly outlined strategies, while negative characteristics are stagnation, limited growth, passivity among employees and poor competitive ability.

The *schizoid organization* is based on the fantasy of failure and withdrawal, with a concomitant neurotic style of alienation, uninvolvement and lack of interest in people. Risk factors are isolation, which results in other people's dependence needs not being satisfied. This in turn leads to aggression. This type of organization is characterized mainly by absenteeism and uninvolvement on the part of leaders, with consequent internal conflict between levels of leadership and management. Transactions and structures are characterized by manipulation and changing coalitions to achieve goals. Individual rather than group goals are pursued. Because there is a strong locus of control this can also result in passivity, lack of control and contact with the outside world, as well as impulsive decision-making which often contains hidden motives. Although this type of organization can facilitate participation by all employees, negative characteristics are an inconsistent strategy, hidden motives that have to do with internal politics, lack of leadership and a climate of suspicion and mistrust.

A systematic study of organizations will provide a useful framework for understanding and classifying organizational health and pathology.

In conclusion, Herman (1963) (see also Krantz, 1985) refers to the following symptoms in organizations that are in conflict: an increase in withdrawal behaviour (dissatisfaction, low production, absence and personnel turnover), an increase in and an intensification of conflict situations, fewer communication channels, an increase in authority structures, so that only a few people take part in decision-making, greater stress for authority figures as the authority becomes more centralized, authority figures evade responsibilities as the stress increases, a decline in standards because of the stress effects on authority figures, the further reduction of communication channels increasing conflict between management and other units in the organization, more people withdraw from tasks and activities because of the increasing conflict, fewer communication channels for the collection and distribution of information as the conflict and problems increase, the further increase of conflicts and withdrawal behaviour as organizational standards become even lower, and the reduction of specific communication which will lead to further withdrawal and less available information.

Personnel turnover, absenteeism, industrial accidents, unemployment and problems of change may be indicators of poor adjustment and dysfunctions in employees, but possibly more so of ineffective organizational functioning, poor working conditions and influences from the surrounding environments.

Personnel turnover and absenteeism may relate to general *job dissatisfaction* with regard to workplace and organizational variables, for example, the quality and nature of working conditions, remuneration, security communication, equity and fairness. Obviously, employee dysfunctions, like anxiety, depression, personality disorders, alcohol and drug addiction, physical diseases and age can contribute to absenteeism and personnel turnover.

Personnel turnover is an *expensive* industrial phenomenon and though mostly negative may also have advantages if managed efficiently. *Functional personnel turnover* comes into question when the organization summarily allows the individual with a negative evaluation to leave. *Dysfunctional personnel turnover* comes into question when the organization allows an individual to leave without trying to stop him/her, although it would like to retain his/her services. When analysing personnel turnover, aspects like voluntary, non-voluntary, unavoidable and controllable turnover and desertion, have to be taken into account.

Absence from work, a form of withdrawal behaviour, can be a main indication of organizational stress, and it involves great costs, especially with regard to the loss of productivity. *Ilness*, especially respiratory problems, stomach disorders, gynaecological problems (menstruation, menopause, spontaneous abortions), and stress conditions such as headaches, insomnia, fatigue, heart problems and endocrinal disorders are responsible for most absences. Other factors that contribute to absence include dissatisfaction with organizational and work factors, for instance insufficient training and supervision, disturbed work relationships, poor work group cohesion and morale, and the physical job design. Follman (1978) refers to the psychological determinants of absence by describing the following characteristics of persons with an extensive record of absences: uncertainty, stress, self-pity, anxiety, the incidence of compulsive tendencies and phobia, paranoid and schizophrenic qualities, conversion hysteria, neurosis, alcoholism, broken marriages, behaviour that indicates defence, suspicion, unhappiness, the inability to make friends easily, dissatisfaction, hostility and resistance to change.

From the literature it also becomes clear that personnel turnover and absence are complex problems and are often closely related. More accurate assessment procedures are necessary, and there should be a clearer distinction between types of personnel turnover and also different forms of absenteeism in order to plan a more effective course of action.

Industrial accidents refer to occurrences in the workplace and work behaviour that may give rise to unsafe working conditions, injuries, death, and loss to workers, their colleagues and the work organization. Errors and accidents still represent one of the biggest cost factors of occupational stress (Ross & Altmaier, 1994). Research has revealed a strong connection between situational factors and worker behaviour which leads to either the occurrence of or can contribute towards the prevention of industrial accidents.

Accident proneness is a theory that states that particular human characteristics will lead to accidents, no matter how safe the working conditions are. However, such an assumption may be invalid, especially in the light of factors such as high-risk tasks, the effects of factors such as employee personality, fatigue, noise, poor ventilation, alcohol abuse, drug addiction, poorly designed work equipment and work stations, and ignoring safety regulations. Training of workers, with regard to health and safety, particularly in respect of perception and motor skills, no longer keeps track of the technology of modern work environments.

The occurrence of industrial accidents is also coupled to personal factors like age (e.g. high accident rates between the ages of 17 to 28 and in people aged 60 years plus). It is also possible that around the age of 30 many employees may experience temporary maladjustment problems due to possible career and life changes, for example, the so-called mid-career crisis, may be accompanied by emotional instability, risky behaviour, and so forth. Some authors like Hirschfield and Behan (1963) argued that accidents may be motivated behaviour, for instance self-destructive needs and an attempt to withdraw from the work situation. The combination of specific personality traits and situations which repeatedly lead to accidents, could rather be described as accident repetitive behaviour, according to McCormick and Ilgen (1981). Other personality traits which may be associated with industrial accidents are expressed by Miner and Brewer (in Dunnette, 1990) and Miner (1966) as follows: physical handicaps and inefficient task skills; inadequate training; feelings of hate, aggression, etc. towards management; depressive and self-destructive tendencies; negative work attitudes; characteristics such as impulsiveness, tenseness, immaturity, social irresponsibility and lack of intimate interpersonal relationships.

A so-called theory of *biorhythms* explains industrial accidents on the basis of the interaction between the individual's physical, emotional and cognitive functions. When one of these aspects reaches a low, such as poor cognitive judgement or emotional tension, accidents can occur. This theory could not be confirmed.

In respect of the management of and actions regarding industrial accidents, the astronomical costs incurred through bad accident reporting and inadequate criteria are often pointed out. Better selection procedures, more systematic training and improved work design are recommended as possible areas of improvement as regards accident prevention.

Unemployment refers to people who want to work but who can't find a job or are denied a job. Unemployment, which can start with job loss due to involuntary withdrawal from work as a result of layoffs, downsizing of companies and personnel and firing, is a state of worklessness, exclusion and non-involvement; being a non-member of the working society. Even retirement, which is not unemployment but compulsory non-employment, can have severe consequences, such as intense boredom, a loss of interest in life and income, and physical and emotional deterioration and even premature death (O'Meara, 1977). In this regard work loss and continuing unemployment can be seen as a state of bereavement, a personal loss, even an ongoing 'terminal' condition as Greenwood (in Smith 1987:7) illustrated: 'Nothing to do with time; nothing to spend; nothing to do tomorrow nor the day after; nothing to wear; can't get married; a living corpse; a unit of the special army of three million lost men.' In our times it can be said that unemployment is a 'social illness' because social-economic and political conditions in countries (societies) create such workless status for millions of individuals, families and societies with serious impacts on their quality of life, health and mental well-being.

Research on job loss and continuing unemployment established that, in general, unemployment significantly impairs mental health (Warr, 1987; Feather & O'Brien, 1986; Hayes & Nutman, 1981; Leana & Feldman, 1988; Smith, 1987). Clearly, such effects can differ between individuals, families or societies in terms of factors such as work values involved, duration of the unemployment, support structures and other factors. We would best understand the consequences of unemployment if we carefully consider the various positive meanings and functions of work (employment) in people's lives, because unemployment mostly impacts negatively on these same values. The consequences of unemployment must be assessed with regard to employees' subjective experiences, the physical and mental health problems and social pathology that impact on individuals, families and society at large.

In terms of *physical health*, the general agreement is that unemployed people have poorer physical health than employed persons, because of possible excessive substance use and abuse, changes in blood pressure, more visits to the doctor, more medication, more illness complaints and staying sick in bed, increase in smoking which may relate to cancer, whilst increases in suicide and para-suicide (self-injuries) have also been reported (Warr, 1987).

Mental health problems are related to increased mental hospital admissions, increased figures for homicide, crime, suicide, imprisonment, alcoholism and death. Specific symptoms related to unemployment are a decrease in general mental well-being, decreased feelings of happiness, pleasure and life satisfaction, also increased feelings of anxiety, being strained (stressed), depression, incompetency, not being in control, being bored and demotivated.

Both mental and physical well-being will be influenced by the duration and transitional progression of unemployment, especially due to dwindling financial resources, loss of social and other support sources and increasing hopelessness if job-seeking efforts are repeatedly unsuccessful (Hayes & Nutman, 1981; Warr, 1987).

The *social pathology* is relevant because families and societies may lose many of their benefits in a state of unemployment. Unemployment results in loss of income; affects the family and family members' position and status in society negatively; decreases the development of knowledge and other cognitive skills; increases the development of negative working attitudes and negative perceptions towards non-working parents and adults; increases the spillover effects between work and family interaction such as negative behaviour, and emotions at home; in total – as a result of loss of resources, the family and society's general quality of life, health and mental health will decrease. Many specific family problems have been reported such as increased family strain, relationship and marriage problems, higher levels of anxiety and depression, increased divorce rates, child neglect and abuse, as well as increased family violence (Warr, 1987).

As health workers we have much to do in managing unemployment and its consequences. Our primary task may be in physical health caring and mental counselling. We may, however, also have a task in redesigning existing jobs and creating more jobs. Another task can be to change people's values and perceptions about being unemployed, they must realize that being jobless does not mean to be workless and worthless, thus facilitating entrepreneurship, self-help and work/job creation! This will also facilitate the views that unemployment can be an opportunity; have a positive side. We must teach people to make 'bad unemployment' into 'good unemployment' in the same way as we must change 'bad employment' into 'good, meaningful employment'.

It is also possible and often true, that re-employment does not necessarily reset the psychological equation but may leave a legacy of perceived worthlessness, stigma, cautiousness, self-doubt, weariness, anxiety and depression.

Continuous change and transformation in the nature of work, working, organizations and the world at large, is a consistent stress factor in the lives of people in general and employees. For many people these changes may mean continuous efforts to adapt and feelings of insecurity of uncertain expectations and not knowing what will happen next. Modern employees must continually adapt to new technologies and changes and develop their intellectual and other knowledge, skills and other attributes to be relevant in labour markets. Employees cannot necessarily depend on a long career in one company because career prospects now demand multiskilling and the ability to be effective and competitive in the types of organizations, jobs and tasks which in specific places and time are required to provide in the increasing demands for services and products.

A necessary task of health workers is to facilitate improved self-help and entrepreneurial skills in employees and to be more self-efficient and execute personal control, not only to create opportunities and jobs, but also to be more efficient in the organizations and jobs they are in.

11.10 Managing and promoting occupational adjustment

Work adjustment problems are too often only coupled to stress management or health and safety only. Although such programmes are important, it should not be the only strategies and can be an oversimplification of occupational health management and promotion.

Occupational health management and promotion refers to the total process of preventing problems, the treatment of troubled employees and correction of dysfunctional work conditions, the utilization or re-utilization of the employee suffering from the effects of stress or some form of diagnosed occupational illness or psychological disorder or related symptoms. In a more specific context, it can refer to the management of the problem employee only, in which case we are more concerned with curative or corrective intervention. Another level of health promotion to consider is whether interventions should be on the individual, group or organizational level. Added to this it is crucial to decide what to instill, influence or change, for example, does the programme aim at giving information, changing behaviour and attitudes, motivating employees or must the culture in a group or organization be influenced or changed? *Behaviour change* is used as a blanket term to refer to any technique or approach (intervention) for the influencing (rehabilitation or treatment) of people exhibiting symptomatic behaviour so that the behaviour of the individual or the group will change and their functioning become more effective. *Manpower utilization* is a process associated with behaviour change and development and can either be part of the usual human resources or organizational functions or be specific methods in health promotion programmes, like in an Employee Assistance Programme (EAP).

There are various *approaches or levels* to occupational health promotion, for example, preventative, diagnostic and remedial (curative, corrective) approaches. Some authors differentiate between primary, secondary and tertiary functions in the remedial approach. Others differentiate between preventive, therapeutic, self-development and disciplinary measures in the management of the problem employee. Some sources, in turn, distinguish between personal, organizational and external procedures for the management of work stress (Cooper and Payne, 1994; Ross and Altmaier, 1994; Santer, Murphy and Hurrell, 1990) in their systems model for the management of work stress. It is also important to emphasize that the individual, the organization and the community all play a role at the different levels of occupational mental health management.

11.10.1 Personal or self-management strategies

In previous sections we referred to the importance of improving employee coping skills in order to be more in control and self-efficient. According to the so-called coping theories people make use of different intrinsic and extrinsic preventive and healing coping resources to handle stress and cope with life's demands. These resources include personality dispositions (e.g. optimism), as well as cognitive, emotional, and direct and indirect coping behaviours. In many views the individual's strategies for managing general wellness really boils down to a healthy lifestyle, good health attitudes, behaviours and habits. Interventions will therefore emphasize the effects of personal counselling, diet, physical fitness and sleep, and other healthy habits.

We have pointed out that if we believe people to be capable of development, they are also *capable of helping themselves if they have self-knowledge*, for example, about their bodies and their type of psychological responses in situations. People should be given responsibility, and experience for themselves that change is possible or that it is taking place in themselves or in their environments, for example, at home or work. Personal coping mechanisms are people's skills in handling responses or behaviour from other people, or to cope with events and change in their surrounding environments. These adjustment mechanisms can include the following:

- People need to have an understanding of aetiological factors (stressors) in themselves, the organization and the external environment.
- People need to know themselves and their physical and psychological responses to stressors. This could mean that they should know and experience the pros and cons of stress. In other words, they need to understand the stress process, e.g.

according to Hans Selye's general adaptation syndrome, so that they will be able to monitor their physical and psycho-physical responses.
- People can take steps to identify their strong and weak points, for instance, by means of medical examinations, psychological evaluation, therapeutic procedures and self-analysis.
- On the basis of such evaluation processes, people can plan their daily objectives and activities, for instance their tempo of doing things, social activities, people whom they wish to associate with, and financial affairs, in other words, they need to determine and of prioritize their needs.

Personal strategies to manage psychological stressors or their effects
These could include the following:
- People could work toward the acquisition or improvement of *interpersonal skills* in order to make interaction with other people more effective. This can include the clear expression of feelings, frank and open communication, self-assertive action, sensitivity (warmth, empathy and congruence) towards other people's behaviour, decision-making and the handling of conflict. They can reinforce these social skills by being aware of their conduct and by participating in counselling and development groups.
- People can easily teach themselves *physical and psychological adjustment techniques*, which include relaxation techniques, physical exercises, controlled breathing, positive thinking, meditation, self-hypnosis and various therapeutic techniques.
- *Biological feedback processes* include steps to determine how the body responds to stress or how it has already responded. It can take the form of an ordinary medical examination, or techniques such as training in biological feedback by means of feedback thermometers, the electromyograph, the electroencephalograph, the psycho-galvanometer, etc.
- People should learn to *avoid and control stressors or environments* that they know will cause stress.
- *Counselling or therapeutic techniques* can be valuable. By learning the principles of therapeutic approaches, for example being conscious of their own and other people's transactions and interactions, self-assertion, responsibility, relaxation techniques, psychological desensitization, and listening and response skills, people will be able to apply self-help, especially by responding to the reactions or problems of others. Self-help programmes or techniques can be directed towards assessing own health status, career development, stress management, etc. Other techniques that can produce positive results for the personal management of stress include diets, a change of environment (e.g. changing one's job), training, a change in work methods, better sleeping habits, holidays, and even increased stress, such as more work or exercise. The purpose of personal or self-management programmes should be the optimal functioning of the individual in order to actualize his/her potential and overcome obstacles in life more effectively.

11.10.2 Behaviour change in the work situation: Organizational strategies

As indicated earlier, occupational mental health includes a management policy or philosophy about the responsibility for occupational adjustment and health promotion. Thus the emphasis should be on steps that will make the interaction or resemblance between individual and organization with regard to their needs and objectives, and the fit between employees and their work optimal or as congruent as possible. Miner and Brewer (in Dunnette, 1990) refer to this as a *control model*, which they base on the setting of criteria for measuring (identifying) occupational maladjustment so as to permit corrective interventions in the worker's conduct. The four steps of a programme for the *reduction of ineffective work behaviour*, are as follows:
- The selection of people for employment in whom the risk of failure is low
- The determination of work standards so that poor achievement will not occur easily
- The identification of causative factors and the immediate implementation of corrective procedures
- The dismissal of poor achievers as soon as they have been identified.

Many authors regard the management of occupational maladjustment (underachievement) as a planning function which forms part of the management policy. The concept and practice of *management by objectives* are used for the identification of underachievers. This implies that the worker's objectives have to be included in the organizational policy and objectives, and that management plays an important role in the achievement and evaluation of these objectives. These steps are as follows:
- Define the organizational requirements and objectives
- Make the worker's responsibilities with regard to the organizational objectives clear
- Make sure there is consensus between employer and employee about the latter's objectives in relation to the global organizational objectives. This means that employees are certain about what they should do to perform satisfactorily, and that management has a definite structure for evaluating employee achievements
- Encourage management to support employees in their endeavours to satisfy the predetermined criteria for achievement
- Compare employees' achievements with their objectives
- Ensure that management discusses employees' achievements with them (apply a process of performance management).

This approach, with regard to managing underachievement by objectives, has the advantage that management is actively involved and that employees fulfil a *self-therapeutic role*, as it were. In other words, it is an approach by which conflicts between organization and employees can be reduced, since not only the organization's production objectives, but also the individual's needs are recognized.

Planning, policy and management with regard to occupational mental health are increasingly regarded as an integral part of modern management in the organization as a sociotechnical system. In this regard you could try to establish in your work situations the extent to which this assumption is true, and also try to determine what the extent of your involvement as a health worker should be.

Effective management of mental health and positive work adjustment, high achievement and organizational success are functions of effective organizational functioning. Health professionals should therefore understand occupational health problems with regard to the total organization and not treat only specific problems in isolation. This also means that occupational maladjustment will be minimized if individual employees are optimally utilized and developed by means of the normal personnel and management functions, which will ensure the best fit between employees and their tasks and work environments. In other words, many of the usual personnel and organizational functions are nothing less than preventive and even corrective methods that are used to combat occupational maladjustment. These personnel and organizational processes, structures, policies and programmes should also continually be monitored and revised in order to create a better climate for work adjustment. Many modern workplaces, human resource practices and management styles may still be 'dehumanizing' and as such create much stress for employees.

11.10.2.1 Organizational and work structures and processes

We can make the following classification of organizational strategies that involve individual and organizational functioning, which can be preventive, remedial and rehabilitative, and which apply to the management of mental health in the work, the biological and the psychosocial context.

Evaluation and employment procedures

These procedures are used to place *the right person in the right post* by means of person and job descriptions. An effective employment policy provides for task and worker specifications, determines minimum cut-off points and considers the applicant's early work history so as to predict or identify the potential for successful work behaviour or for problems. Further requirements include familiarity with the diagnostic symptoms of psychological disorders and work dysfunctions, and a sound training in diagnostic measuring instruments. Through ineffective selection a certain type of person may be placed in a position, for example, being under- or over-promoted, in which the demands can precipitate underlying psychopathology or ill-health. Effective employment procedures must include a policy on such matters as placement, promotion, transfer and job rotation. It is essential for organizations to have identification programmes by which stress and other mental health problems can be identified at an early stage. Such a programme should also include organizational diagnostic (OD) techniques, according to which the physical and social job design can be adapted if necessary. The complete and accurate 'diagnosis' of problems and existing resources is essential for the planning of effective and appropriate interventions. However, *evaluation processes must be executed with care, since it can also cause anxiety, frustration and aggression* because employees are weighed against success or efficiency criteria.

Training and development

Training and development programmes can have a major preventive function. In organizational development functions, the possibilities for *job expansion and enrichment* must be optimized so as to offer the worker sufficient opportunities. Individual competencies, traits and capabilities can be important factors in maladjustment, if such shortcomings impair work performance. The worker who is incapable of fulfilling the task requirements may use defensive behaviours or inappropriate work behaviours, such as anxiety, aggression and withdrawal. A sound management policy makes provision for definite training requirements at different levels to furnish employees with the necessary knowledge and skills required in their work environments. If needed, special training and development facilities must be created for underachievers or other vocationally maladjusted workers. In some organizations there are specific programmes for certain problem areas, for instance for physically and culturally deprived persons and for alcoholics. Organizations may also cooperate with external bodies in this regard, for instance, institutions for the treatment of alcoholics and sheltered work environments for emotionally and physically handicapped persons. A major problem when such rehabilitated persons are re-employed is that they have acquired their experience in a simulated situation, with the result that their chances of adjusting to the realistic work environment may be difficult. Their progress should therefore be assessed.

The matter of *career development* is an important aspect of training and development (Schreuder & Theron, 2001). The role of the manager in personnel counselling and career development is extremely important. In this regard, aspects such as various career opportunities and decisions, preparing for promotion, and retirement are some of the issues that can be addressed. An important emphasis also is the ability of employees to self-manage their own occupational progress, thereby being able to be more responsible and to adapt to change and stress more effectively.

Training in health and aspects of mental health

The training of all employees at all levels in health and aspects of occupational health is probably the most important element of any health promotion programme. Such an educational programme must contain information about general health and safety aspects, causes, symptoms and effects and the nature of psychological health in general, particular conditions such as alcoholism, drug addiction, HIV/Aids and other occupational diseases. It must also be aimed at the attitudes of management, the worker and other people involved, for instance, worker unions. Training in interpersonal and communication skills and self-assertive behaviour and the handling of conflict and stress management can be very valuable for all employees and especially for management in personal adjustment behaviour and in the handling of problems. If a better understanding of, and more sensitivity towards, occupational and mental health problems can be created, these factors will perform a therapeutic role.

In this regard the use of group techniques such as focus groups, training groups, and sensitivity training can be used for improving the mutual understanding in relationships. This type of training has the advantage that management, for instance, supervisors, will be better equipped to handle problem cases, which implies that the stressors in the social environment of employees can be reduced more rapidly.

Change in the physical and social work environment
Change in the worker's physical and social work environment can contribute to greater *congruence between individuals and their work*. Physical and social working conditions can easily lead to dissatisfaction. Hackman and Oldham (in Argyle, 1992) proposed that five job characteristics in particular, that is, skill variety, identity with a task, task significance, autonomy and feedback, will motivate employee performance. Unless management makes changes, the individual will respond with stress reactions, possible illnesses, absences, work errors, accidents, resignations and negative attitudes.

As far as possible, the *physical work environment must be ergonomically designed* to suit the capabilities of employees, whether the physically able or the physically handicapped worker. To further prevent physical and psychological fatigue, matters such as lighting, noise, pollution, safety, work methods, rest periods, shift work and flexitime – apart from the best fit between employee and machine – must be carefully considered.

Changes in the *social design of the work* can include matters such as supervisor–subordinate interaction, the consideration of the workers' preferences in physical job design, opportunities for decision-making and participation, job expansion and enrichment, and recognition of and awards for achievements and services rendered.

Health and mental facilities
In many work organizations, medical-related health workers play an important role. Their services vary from medical examinations for selection, medical guidance and treatment for physical ailments to chemotherapy for stress conditions. Some organizations have internal health facilities, such as clinics, rehabilitation centres, workshops for sheltered labour and placement services. Organizations frequently follow a team approach in which medical, psychological, psychiatric, nursing, social and other services are offered, often in the form of integrated health promotion initiatives, such as Employee Assistance Programmes (Dickman, Challenger, et al., 1988; Cooper & Payne, 1994; Plaggemars, 2000). Apart from medical, therapeutic and counselling services, services such as health education, legal and others may also be offered. In many instances organizations may offer services in conjunction with other organizations or external health services and make use of the services and products provided by private organizations and persons. Private services are often used in cases of severe illness and psychopathology where the patients are referred to or placed for rehabilitation. The systemic nature of work behaviour influencing non-work situations also frequently makes it imperative to involve the worker's other systems in the rehabilitation programmes, for instance family, spouse or relatives.

Labour relations for healthcare management
Industrial and organization psychology and related theories emphasize the interaction between employer and employee in terms of roles, expectations, abilities, objectives and needs in the process of achieving personal and business objectives. If legislation provides for employee rights, modern organizational theory still does not provide for an employer–employee interaction based on mutual rights. This results in the employer, but

more so the individual employee, often being at a disadvantage, for example, in cases of work loss, poor production and bargaining sessions. For their protection and own well-being, employees therefore often join unions and thereby ensure that their rights and relationships are determined and managed in a fair and orderly way.

Labour relations, currently also referred to as *employee or employment relations*, are aimed at labour peace by maintaining cooperative relationships between employer, employees, unions and government. Such beneficial relationships or interaction, which also include physical and psychological well-being, are maintained by certain rules, regulations and disciplinary and grievance procedures, for example during resolution of conflict or differences. Handling of grievances or conflict between employees, unions and employers is managed by a negotiation process known as collective bargaining. Though labour relations is a separate field of study and cannot be dealt with in full here, it is sufficient to say that labour relations and their management by the different parties have important implications for the quality of work life and the employee's general well-being.

Employees have certain needs, and are contracted to work in a certain capacity and under certain circumstances. Employees have the right to physical, social and psychological working conditions that will enhance an optimal quality of work life.

Such expectations might be:
- Fair and humane treatment
- Adequate compensation
- Reasonable leave benefits
- Safe physical working conditions
- Challenging and interesting work
- Freedom of speech and participation
- Opportunities for growth and development
- Access to management.

Coupled to such needs, it is also recognized internationally that employees have certain rights, for instance the right to work, to be trained, to enjoy protection, freedom of association, to negotiate and the right to strike. By the same token, the employer also enjoys certain rights which must be respected by the employee or union. These may be:
- Determining policy and procedures
- Determining pay structures
- Setting work standards
- Setting organizational objectives
- Managing the organization
- Providing and changing facilities.

The management of labour relations and the part played by unions have particular implications for organizational management, for instance, on employment practices, supervising, training, assessment of workers, communication structures, remuneration policies, promotion and disciplinary procedures. The quality of labour relations and related actions in an organization has definite influences on productivity, motivation, work satisfaction, personnel turnover, absenteeism, feelings of loyalty, security, etc. The costs of physical damages, loss of work hours, injuries and even deaths can be calculated, but the costs and hardships of psychological pain (fear, anxiety, depression, etc.) can never be assessed, sometimes having continuous and long-lasting effects.

It is essential for healthcare workers and management to be able to identify and handle conflict, thus utilizing it constructively and avoiding the destructive powers of conflict, which, for instance, may increase problems such as unemployment, stress reactions, loss of income and jobs, etc. It is a fact that the cornerstones of creativity and productivity lie in the constructive use of conflict and differences. The symptoms of destructive conflict, according to Robbins (1989; Robbins, Odendaal & Roodt, 2001) can be as follows:

- Counter-productive acts such as strikes and stay-aways
- Verbal and physical aggression
- Continuous grievances
- Poor communication
- High absenteeism
- Many industrial accidents and even sabotage
- Poor motivation and work attitudes
- High personnel turnover
- Low productivity
- More trespassing and disciplinary cases
- Mutual strife and rigid attitudes.

A further input from management could be the establishment of proper grievance and disciplinary procedures and policies, thereby ensuring that all parties at least know how to act technically and correctly in such cases.

11.10.3 Therapeutic or counselling approaches

In relevant sources various approaches to psychotherapy or counselling are discussed (Nevid et al., 2003; Ivey, Ivey, & Simick-Morgan, 1997). Thus, the interventions of helpers can be based on different assumptions and on different evaluation techniques. The fact that a therapist supports a specific approach or technique in all circumstances, may render him/her to be a *rigid* helper and the therapy to be a closed system, because it may not encourage cure and growth for all types of problems. It is impossible to use the same approach or technique for all the clients or symptoms. In this respect various authors propose cultural sensitivity in treatment and diagnosis as variables, for example race, class and ethnicity often influence these processes (Gobodo, 1990). One has to realize that every person's problems or symptoms manifest themselves in a unique manner and that such problems and symptoms may have particular functions in the context of the person's conduct, for instance in the family, towards a marriage partner, the supervisor or in the work group. The aim of helping, like therapeutic or counselling techniques, should be to plan appropriate and purposeful intervention and to implement it consistently, always in terms of the client's (individual's, work group's) behaviour, its context and its meaning. In a more specific sense we can ask the question: What type of intervention at what time (crucial point for a change) and place and by which 'helper' will be the most effective for a particular client?

Irrespective of the helper's premiss, effective helping (e.g. therapy) in practice is always based, to a greater or lesser extent, on the following principles:

- It is a process of events through the medium of the interpersonal relationship that can be defined between therapist and client.
- The relationship between helper and client(s) can be regarded as a helping or therapeutic system with all the special systemic qualities. The nature of the processes in this system can determine the client's development and the helper's effectiveness.
- The helper–client relationship should create a psychological climate in which the helper acts in such a way that the client will experience and recognize his/her self-esteem, that they will be able to speak about the things that are important to them, and that they will experience the possibility and reality of change.
- The essential conditions for an optimal psychological climate can be described as follows:
  - acceptance of and respect for the client as a person without prejudices and external frames of reference
  - positive esteem for the client's positive health and mental health – in other words, for the fact that the client has potential that can be developed and which he can personally help to develop
  - empathetic understanding for the client's verbal and non-verbal behaviour and the ability to communicate the empathy and understanding to the client, also with regard to what is happening in the helping situation
  - honesty and congruence, which implies that helpers can be spontaneous, genuine and transparent (open) about themselves and in their relationships with clients, without the facade of defences or a 'therapeutic' role, so that the client will also be able to act congruently
  - concreteness, which is the helper's skill in transmitting the messages clearly, specifically and unambiguously so that the client will understand exactly what the helper's actions mean
  - a facilitating by the helper/therapist of the helping process intentionally and purposefully, so that the behaviour will develop in the direction of the helping – and, hence the client's – objectives
- Skilled use by the helper/therapist of interpersonal and other skills purposefully and strategically to achieve the objectives of the helping intervention.
- All the above-mentioned points presuppose that the helper has certain interpersonal and communication skills. They include accommodation or the creation of rapport, skills to initiate a relationship and to obtain credit from the client, listening, verbal and non-verbal responsive skills, skills to structure the helping process, confrontation and diagnostic skills, and skills to terminate interventions when necessary. Note that these skills are not propagated for clinical psychologists only. Many lay counsellors are trained according to the same assumptions or curative factors, and these skills are also necessary for effective personnel counselling and communication.

With all this information in mind, the author compiled the following definition of a helping process, like therapy:

> Therapy is the process (system) of purposeful reciprocal communication in the interpersonal relationship between two or more persons. Therapy or counselling takes place through verbal and non-verbal interactions during which the helper collects, exchanges and evaluates certain information under certain essential conditions by means of purposeful and planned interpersonal strategies and techniques in order to facilitate optimal behaviour and attitude changes in the client.

Counselling and therapeutic facilities should be available to any employee, and are particularly essential in cases of psychopathology and adjustment problems, and also in matters such as career progress and development, performance assessment counselling, exit interviews, group conflicts and financial counselling.

Still, helping processes, like individual and group therapeutic work, rarely take place in the work situation, where clinical, counselling or therapeutic psychologists or other qualified experts have been appointed. In most cases individuals are referred to outside organizations, or psychologists are appointed internally on a session basis. Important reasons for this lack of services in side organizations are the few well-paid job opportunities for well-qualified counsellors and therapists, scarcity of well-qualified therapists and counsellors and a lack of knowledge and insight by employers and management about the human resources development value of therapy or counselling; and the fact that management frequently fails to regard the worker's health as part of their responsibility and to include it in personnel policy. These facts therefore make it more important for occupational health workers, like nurses, to be well trained in the basic helping processes and skills of counselling and therapy. This is also important for the initial helping of troubled employees, before serious cases are referred to institutions and other experts. Health workers must be aware of multi-cultural and client-centred approaches, because the troubled employee must be treated in context and also have the opportunity of participating in the helping process, to assume responsibility, to explore feelings, to set objectives, and to evaluate alternatives – thus actualizing their potential.

Health workers must also be trained in using *group techniques* in practice. Not only therapeutic groups are used in the industry, but also T-groups – especially for training purposes – which have strong underlying therapeutic power factors. The group leader must have the same skills as those applying to individual therapy or counselling. The effectiveness of group work lies in the group dynamic processes, in other words, in the 'helping' or 'curative' factors facilitated by group activities and interactions. Yalom (1975) describes the *power factors* as follows: the perception of similarity between group members (universality); group members care for one another (altruism); group members find it easy to speak of feelings or experiences (catharsis); group members identify the group leader and other group members in 'family roles' (the group as the second family, etc.); in the group the members easily become aware of their personal feelings and of verbal and non-verbal behaviour; group members are involved with one another (group cohesion); group members learn from one another and from the leaders (modelling); group members believe that the group process will work (trust); and group members help and support one another (support).

Because of the complexity of groups (e.g. work groups, families and relatives), group skills, such as accommodation, activation, intervention, diagnosis and evaluation, are difficult to acquire and require intensive training. Most writers acknowledge the positive effect of group workers, but they also warn against the emotional damage that may be caused by unscientific, unplanned and uncontrolled group influences.

In some instances the conversational techniques of psychological counselling and therapy or the chemotherapy of the biological approach may be too narrow for some people. Furthermore, the rehabilitation of the problem worker often takes place away from the work situation where there is no task-oriented or work-related reality testing. In this regard *rehabilitation workshops* are oriented towards placing the individual in the work situation or in simulated work situations (including sheltered work situations) where they can experience practically what the return or the adjustment to the real situation will mean. The maladjusted or rehabilitated worker has to experience the demands of *productive role fulfilment* both physically and psychologically. The requirements of the real situation should be duplicated in the simulated situation as far as it is possible to do so. The role of the supervisor varies from task leader to 'therapist', and conditions in the workshop could be varied to achieve certain effects. The workshop also provides the opportunity for supportive group and individual conversational interventions. In practice, the workshop technique is frequently used for the rehabilitation of physically and emotionally handicapped people.

11.10.4 Crisis intervention

A crisis can be defined as a situation or event that has reached a critical phase, a turning point for better or worse, and which can have damaging consequences for individuals, groups and organizations if allowed to continue.

From a business or service-oriented point of view a crisis is any situation that runs the risk of:
- Escalating in intensity
- Coming under close media or government (authority) scrutiny, interfering with the normal operations of business or services, and damaging the image a company enjoyed
- Damaging or interfering with the company's basic objectives, e.g. income, training, etc.

From a behavioural perspective, a crisis may be a state of disorganization in which clients face frustration of important life goals or profound disruption of their life cycles and methods of coping with stressors. The term crisis usually refers to the client's feelings of fear, shock and distress about the disruption, not the disruption itself.

The healthcare worker, the client and all parties involved in dealing with a crisis call for crisis intervention techniques that are flexible and rapid and will offer alternatives and new goals to the stressed person in such a way that he/she can be functional again as soon as possible.

The skills for crisis intervention call for coping skills that have to be learned like any effective intervention method. Although it is more complex, crisis intervention or management comes down to:
- Identifying the crisis and its causes quickly
- Isolating the crisis and its manifestations quickly
- Managing the crisis quickly.

Referring to Brammer (1985:19) in more detail, these coping skills for crisis intervention entail the following:
- Perceptual skills (seeing problematic situations clearly, as challenging or dangerous, and as solvable)
- Cognitive change skills (restructuring thoughts and altering self-defeating thinking)
- Support networking skills (assessing, strengthening, and diversifying external sources of support)
- Stress management and wellness skills (reducing tensions through environmental and self-management)
- Problem-solving skills (increasing problem-solving competence through applying models to diverse problems)
- Description and expression of feelings (accurate apprehension and articulation of anger, fear, guilt, love, depression and joy).

In a way, crisis intervention or management really involves the management of decision-making. A lot will depend on how accurately and swiftly decisions are made and applied.

Only some hints or aspects concerning crisis intervention will be discussed further. The *causes* of a crisis may be complex but may generally relate to the following, which will also indicate the type of crisis dealt with: *severe loss* (bereavement, divorce, unemployment, disaster, imprisonment), *internal distress* (hopelessness, despair, fatigue, drug-taking, suicidal attempts, depression), *life transitions* (job change, pregnancy, relocation, new family member, job choice, family conflict, illness). In this regard, Holmes and Rahe's social adjustment events apply (eg. see Table 11.1).

To identify a crisis it is also necessary to recognize the phase of crisis development. Generally, a crisis may progress through the following stages, which are similar to Selye's GAS model (see 11.7.2.1):
- During the *pro-dromal crisis stage* the initial tension is experienced and may be accompanied by warning signs and habitual adaptive responses.
- The *acute crisis stage* is marked by increased tension and lack of success in coping and efforts to reduce tension. Frustration is increased by feelings of inefficiency and distress.
- The *chronic crisis stage* is marked by events that are beyond turning point in cases, tension increases and some release may only be experienced because emergency

internal and external resources are mobilized. Certain damage may have been caused, such as behaviour dysfunctions and loss of emotional control.
- The *crisis resolution stage* is when healing starts under the influence of self-management skills or the influence of external interventions.

In more detail and in terms of behaviour, typical reactions in crisis situations may be as follows:
- Shock and disorganization
- Expression of anguish and/or relief
- Experience of denial and minimization of the loss
- Sadness and lowered self-esteem
- Taking hold of a new way of life and letting go of the past
- Final acceptance of change and planning for the future
- Reflections on learning from the transition experience.

Although simplified, the following clues for crisis intervention or management skills might be useful. Suffice to say that in-depth training in certain of these aspects is necessary. In very general terms crisis intervention might be helpful by following the steps below:
- Liberal use of emotional support through close contact, reassurance and listening to feelings
- Changing of the client's environment, such as ensuring a safe place and understanding people
- Starting to change or influence the client's perceptions about his/her crisis situation.

Specific crisis intervention techniques can be varied and may involve some of the health management methods discussed previously. As was said, the process of crisis intervention entails firstly the accurate appraisal of the situation and/or the person involved and the options that are available; secondly by a decision on the type of help and available resources; and thirdly by concrete and purposeful acts of help, followed by resolution of the crisis in which the person and/or situation once again experiences some balance and calm.

The following strategies are mentioned only briefly:
- Multiple impact support strategy involves a combined effort of several disciplines to ease distress – for example in a family crisis the family as a whole will be treated in an intensive two-day round-the-clock programme, preferably away from the familiar environment.
- Individual or group counselling or therapeutic interventions must be based on building and maintaining hope and attempts to foster renewal and growth. These objectives will only be achieved if the helper is trained in using acknowledged therapeutic skills as described previously.
- Creating or renewing a client's support systems involves identifying people, places and things that may be physically and emotionally helpful to the person.

- Referral skills involve the helper being informed about community and other resources in times of crisis.

In conclusion, it is necessary to observe that crises cause stress and without some stress life will be sterile. Uncontrolled stress, such as in acute and chronic crisis stages, however, may be damaging. On the positive side, stress and crises may have productive and creative outcomes. A prerequisite for these positive outcomes will, however, be determined by our ability to manage our decisions when intervening in crisis and conflict situations.

11.10.5 Community mental health and research

Although there is a universal desire for intellectual, economic and political security, most people fail to achieve these. There should probably be more emphasis on the close relationships between human emotional security and mental health as prerequisites for the other qualities. This requires a shift in emphasis from the individual as 'sick', to the individual as the symptom-bearer of his/her environments. In this light the emphasis on family and marriage therapy and on therapies such as group work, rehabilitation programmes, and diagnostic and development strategies in the organization are hopeful signs. Training and educational programmes that disseminate information about health and mental health all over the world by means of various media, and the involvement of the community in the accommodation and employment of physically and emotionally handicapped people underline a concept that is gradually gaining acceptance. In the work organization this requires the continued influencing of management and managerial practices, so that people and their behaviour become the focal point, rather than an over-emphasis on 'hard criteria', namely technology, production, economy, etc. In this regard, health workers with community-based training and experience, like community health nurses and social workers, will be a valuable asset for organizations and troubled employees.

The best strategy for the effective management and promotion of occupational health will be based on research into the issues mentioned in this chapter, that is: aetiology, specific mental health and other occupational health problems, better assessment evaluation methods, the relationship between work behaviour and occupational health problems, and the success of preventive and corrective actions. There is still a need for systematic evaluative research on the effectiveness of managing stress and other occupational health problems.

11.11 Conclusion

There are some indications of an improved awareness of health in general and of employee or occupational wellness. Some of these are the interest in health psychology, an emphasis on and support for healthier lifestyles, improved legislation and policies with regard to health-related matters, an awareness of health issues with regard to our environments, training of health workers to be more available and of value to more people and communities, as well as suggestions for innovative strategies for health and mental health promotion across the lifespan and in various contexts (Stroebe & Stroebe, 1995; Jason & Glenwick, 2002).

Psychological disorder and the concomitant occupational dysfunctions create a human resources problem, which health workers and organizational management have to deal with. We refer to a few of these implications.

The potential of an organization's human resources lies in the quality of the human potential within the organization, and especially in the environment. The quality of the 'organizational life', which includes its effectiveness, efficiency and health, is also a function of the feedback between the organization and the systems surrounding it. In this context occupational and mental health or maladjustment can become part of the organization and its functioning, irrespective of whom management wishes to hold responsible for it or of its policy on health. In its policy and functions, management must consistently tackle the prevention, diagnosis, treatment and promotion of occupational maladjustment. In this way the risk of and financial investment in, say, research, health promotion programmes and in its management will become a profitable rather than an unprofitable venture.

Every organization has its own problems with regard to the interaction that takes place inside it and with its surrounding systems. Because of its heterogeneity or diversity and rapid development, South Africa now has to face new challenges in general, and in relation to global economic competition which puts more demands on employee relationships and adjustment. The work scenario is characterized by ongoing change and even discontinuity. In this regard, work forces are more diverse and the new labour legislation requires ongoing change and transformation in many work-related policies and practices. A projection of the future employee–work interaction seems complex. Organizations become bigger, more differentiated, technologically more refined, perhaps more impersonal for the worker. As jobs become scarcer and more demanding and intellectual demands are higher, workers are becoming more sophisticated and sensitive, and they want to know and participate more and take more decisions. They want to become more deeply involved and want to communicate more. In the midst of these more intense stressors, effective employees will want to satisfy their social and achievement needs. It is the task of occupational health experts and management to use their professional knowledge and skills to create an optimal working environment to prevent the alienation of the worker from his/her place of work, and to facilitate improved employee health, adjustment and coping skills.

11.12 Bibliography

Ahia, C. E. 1991. Cultural Contextualization of Diagnostic Signs, Symptoms and Symbols in International Mental Health: A Focus on DSM-III-R. *Journal of College Student Psychotherapy*, 6(l):37–51.

Allport, G. W. 1961. *Pattern and Growth in Personality*. New York: Holt, Rinehart and Winston.

American Pscyhiatric Association. 1994. Diagnostic and Statistical Manual of Mental Disorders (DSM-IV) 4th edition. Washington DC.

American Pscyhiatric Association. 2000. Diagnostic and Statistical Manual of Mental Disorders (DSM-IV-TR) 4th edition, Text revision. Washington DC.

Andolfi, M. 1979. *Family Therapy: An Interactional Approach*. New York: Plenum Press.

Ankrah, E. M. 1991. AIDS and the Social Side of Health. *Social Science and Medicine*, 32(9):967–980.

Antonovsky, A. 1984. A Call for a New Question – Salutogenesis – and a Proposed Answer – the Sense of Coherence. *Journal of Preventive Psychiatry*, 2:1–13.

Antonovsky, A. 1987. *Unravelling the Mystery of Health: How People Manage Stress and Stay Well*. San Francisco: Jossey-Bass.

Argyle, M. C. 1989. *The Social Psychology of Work*. Harmondsworth: Penguin.

Argyle, M. C. 1992. *The Social Psychology of Everyday Life*. London: Routledge.

Ashforth, B. S. & Lee, R. T. 1990. Defensive Behaviour in Organizations: A Preliminary Model. *Human Relations*, 43:621–648.

Auerbach, S. M. & Gramling, S. E. 1998. *Stress Management: Psychological Foundations*. Upper Saddle River, NJ: Prentice Hall.

Baker, F., McEwan, P. J. M. et al. 1969. Industrial Organizations and Health, Vol 1. *Selected Readings*. London: Tavistock.

Bailey, R. & Clarke, M. (1989). *Stress and Coping in Nursing*. London: Chapman and Hall.

Bennett, P. & Murphy, S. 1996. *Psychology and Health Promotion*. Buckingham: Open University Press.

Bergh, Z. C. & Theron, A. L. 2003. *Psychology in the Work Context*. Cape Town: Oxford University Press.

Blotnick, S. 1985. *The Corporate Steeple Chase: Predictable Crisis in a Business Career*. New York: Penguin Books.

Bowerman, J. & Collin, G. 1999. The Coaching Network: A Programme for Individual and Organizational Development. *Journal of Workplace Learning: Employee Assistance Counselling Today*, 1918:291–297.

Brammer, L. M. 1985.*The Helping Relationship: Process and Skills*. New Jersey: Prentice-Hall.

Byng-Hall, J. 1980. Symptom Bearer as Marital Regulator: Clinical Implications. *Family Process*, 19(4):355–365.

Campbell, C. A. 1991. Prostitution, AIDS and Preventive Health Behaviour. *Social Science and Medicine*, 32(12):1367–1378.

Campbell, R. E. & Cillini, J. V. 1981. A Diagnostic Taxonomy of Adult Career Problems. *Journal of Vocational Behaviour*, 19:175–190.

Carroll, M. 1997. *Workplace Counseling: A Systematic Approach to Employee Care*. London: Sage.

Carone, P. A. & Kiefer, S. M. (eds.) 1978. *Misfits in Industry*. New York: S. P. Medical and Scientific Books.

Carson, R. C. 1969. *Interaction Concepts of Personality*. Chicago: Aldine.

Carson, R. C., Butcher, J. N. & Mineka, S. C. 1996. *Abnormal Psychology and Modem Life*. New York: Harper Collins College Publishers.

Carson, R. C., Butcher, J. N. & Coleman, J. C. 1988. *Abnormal Psychology and Modem Life*. 8th edition. Glenview, Illinois: Foresman & Co.

Cilliers, F. v. N. 1984. 'n Ontwikkelingsprogram in Sensitiewe Relasievorming as Bestuursdimensie. Thesis, D.Phil. Potchefstroom: PU vir CHO.

Cilliers, F. v. N. 1988. Die Konsep Sielkundige Optimaliteit in Bestuur. *IPB-Joemaal*, 7(5):15–18.

Clark, M. J. 1999. *Community Health Nursing Handbook*. Stamford, Connecticut: Appleton & Lange.

Clegg, C. W. & Wall, T. D. 1981. A Note on Some New Scales for Measuring Aspects of Psychological Well-being at Work. *Journal of Occupational Psychology*, 54:211–225.

Coetzee S. & Cilliers, F. 2001. Psychofortology: Explaining Coping Behaviours in Organizations. *The Idustrial-Oganizational Psychologist*, 38(4):62–68.

Cook, J. D., Hepworth, S. J., Wall, T. D. & Warr, P. B. 1981. *The Experience of Work: A Compendium and Review of 249 Measures and their Use*. London: Academic Press.

Cooper, C. L. & Payne, R. (eds.) 1994.*Causes, Coping and Consequences of Stress at Work*. Chichester: Wiley & Sons.

Corballis, M. C. & Lea, S. E. G. 2000. Comparative-Evolutionary Psychology, in K. Pawlik & M. R. Rosenzweig (eds.) *International Handbook of Psychology*. London: Sage Publications.

Cox, T. 1991. Organizational Culture, Stress and Stress Management. *Work and Stress*, 5(1):1–4.

Cull, J. G. & Hardy, R. E. 1973.*Adjustment to Work*. Springfield: G. C. Thomas Publishers.

Cummings, T. G. (ed.) 1980. *Systems Theory for Organization Development*. Chichester: Wiley.

Davis, R. V. & Lofquist, L. H. 1984. *A Psychological Theory of Work Adjustment. An Individual Differences Model and its Application*. Minneapolis: University of Minnesota Press.

Dejoy, D. M. & Wilson, M. G. 1995. *Critical Issues in Worksite Health Promotion*. Boston: Allyn & Bacon.

Delongis, A., Coyne, J. C., Dakof, C., Follman, S. & Lazarus, R. S. 1982. Relationship of Daily Hassles, Uplifts, and Major Life Events to Health Status. *Health Psychology*, 1:119–136.

Derstine, J. B. & Hargrove, S. D. 2001. *Comprehensive Rehabilitation Nursing*. Philadelphia: WB Saunders.

Dickman, F., Challenger, B. R., Emener, W. G. & Hutchison, J. R. 1988. *Employee Assistance Programs: A Basic Text*. Springfield: Charles C. Thomas.

Dunnette, M. D. 1990. *Handbook of Industrial and Organizational Psychology*. Chicago: Rand McNally.

Eckenrode, J. & Gore, S. (eds.) 1990. *Stress Between Work and Family*. New York: Plenum Press.

Evans, B. K. & Fischer, D. G. C. 1993. The Nature of Burnout: A Study of the Three-factor Model of Burnout in Human Service and Non-human Service Samples. *Journal of Occupational and Organizational Psychology*, 66(1), 29–38.

Eysenck, H. J. 1991. Personality as a Risk Factor in Coronary Health Disease. *European Journal of Personality*, 5(2):81–92.

Feather, N. T. & O'Brien, G. S. 1986. A Longitudinal Study of the Effects of Employment and Unemployment on School Leavers. *Journal of Occupational Psychology*, 59:121–144.

Ferreira, A. 1999. Probleme en Subjektiewe Ervaringe van die Gestremde Persoon in die Ope Arbeidsmark. Ongepubliseerde verhandeling. Pretoria: University of South Africa.

Fitzgerald, L. F., & Shullman, S. L.1993. Sexual Harassment: A Research Analysis and Agenda for the 1990s *Journal of Vocational Behaviour*, 42:5–27.

Folkman, S. 1984. Personal Control and Stress and Coping Processes: A Theoretical Analysis. *Journal of Personality and Social Psychology*, 46(4):839–852.

Follman, J. F. 1978. Helping the Troubled Employee. New York: AMACOM.

Freudenberger, H. J. 1974. Staff Burnout. *Journal of Social Issues*, 30:159–165.

Friedman, H. S. 1990. *Personality and Disease*. New York: Wiley.

Friedman, H. S. & Booth-Kewley, S. 1987. The Disease-Prone Personality: A Meta-Analytic View of the Construct. *American Psychologist*, 42(6):539-555.

Friedman, H. S. & Di Matteo, M. R. 1989. *Health Psychology*. Englewood Cliffs, NY: Prentice-Hall.

Friedman, M. & Rosen, R. H. 1975. *Type A Behaviour and Your Heart*. London: Wildworld House.

Furnham, A. 1984. The Protestant Work Ethic: A Review of the Psychological Literature. *European Journal of Social Psychology* 14:87–109.

Furnham, A. 1990. *The Protestant Work Ethic: New Psychology of Work-Related Beliefs and Behaviour.* London: Routledge.

Furnham, A. 1995. *Personality at Work: The role of Individual Differences in the Workplace* London: Routledge.

Georgi, L. & March, C. 1990. The Protestant Work Ethic as a Cultural Phenomenon. *European Journal of Social Psychology*, 20:499–519.

Gherman, E. M. 1981. Stress and the Bottom Line. New York: AMACON.

Gobodo, P. 1990. Notions about Culture in Understanding Black Psychopathology: Are we Trying to Raise the Dead? *South African Journal of Psychology*, 20(2):93–98.

Greenhaus, J. H. & Beutel, N. J. 1985. Sources of Conflict Between Work and Family Roles. *Academy of Management Review*, 10:76–88.

Greenhaus, J. H. & Parasuraman, S. 1989. Sources of Work–Family Conflict among Two-Career Couples. *Journal of Vocational Behaviour*, 34:133–153.

Griffiths, R. D. P. 1977. The Prediction of Psychiatric Patients' Work Adjustment in the Communit *British Journal of Clinical Psychology*, 16:165–173.

Grossman, H. Y. 1991. *The Experience and Meaning of Work in Women's Lives* Hillsdale: N. J. & Erlbaum.

Haley, J. 1963. *Strategies of Psychotherapy.* New York: Grune & Stratton.

Harris, C. 1984. (ed). *Occupational Health Nursing Practice*. Bristol: Wright.

Harrison, B. M. 1984. *Essentials of Occupational Health Nursing*. Oxford: Blackwell Scientific Publications.

Hayes, J. & Nutman, P. 1981.*Understanding the Unemployed: The Psychological Effects of Unemployment*. London: Tavistock.
Healy, C. C. 1982. *Career Development. Counselling through the Life Stages*. Boston: Allyn & Bacon.
Herman, C. F. 1963. Some Consequences of Crisis which Limit the Viability of Organizations. *Administrative Science Quarterly*, 8:61–82.
Hirschfield, A. H. & Behan, R. C. 1963. The Accident Process: Ethological Considerations of Industrial Injuries. *The Journal of the American Association*, 186:193–199.
Hobfoll, S. E. 1988. *The Ecology of Stress*. New York: Hemisphere Publishing Co.
Hobfoll, S. E. 1989. Conservation of Resources: A New Attempt at Conceptualizing Stress. *American Psychologist*, 44(3):513–524.
Holland, J. L. 1973. *Making Vocational Choices: A Theory of Careers*. Englewood Cliffs: Prentice-Hall.
Hooks, D., Watts, J., & Cockcroft, K. (eds.). 2002. *Development Psychology*. Landsdowne: UCT Press.
Hurrell, J. J., Murphy, R. L. R., Sauter, S. L. & Cooper, C. L. 1988. *Occupational Stress: Issues and Developments in Research*. New York: Taylor & Francis.
Hurrell, J. J., McLaney, M. A. & Murphy, L. R. 1990. The Middle Years: Career Stage Differences. *Prevention in Human Sciences*, 8(l):179–203.
Ivey, A. E., Ivey, M. B. & Simick-Morgan, L. 1997. 4th edition. *Counseling and Psychotherapy: A Multicultural Perspective*. Boston: Allyn & Bacon.
Jacques, E. & Clement, S. 1991. *Executive Leadership: A Practical Guide to Managing Complexity*. Cambridge: Blackwell Business.
Jason, L. A. & Glenwick, D. S. (eds.) 2002. *Innovative Strategies for Promoting Health and Mental Health Across the Life Span*. New York: Springer Publishing Company.
Kalimo, R. & Vuori, J. 1990. Work and Sense of Coherence Resources for Competence and Life Satisfaction. *Behavioural Medicine*, Summer 1990:77–89.
Kenrick, M. & Luker, K. A. 1995. *Clinical Nursing Practice in the Community*. Berlin: Blackwell Science.
Kets de Vries, M. F. R. & Miller, D. 1984. Neurotic style and organizational pathology. *Strategic Management Journal*, 5(35):35–55.
Kiesler, D. J. & Anchin, J. C. 1982. *Handbook of Interpersonal Therapy*. New York: Pergamon.
Kobasa, S. C. 1979. Stressful Life Events, Personality, and Health: An Inquiry into Hardiness. *Journal of Personality and Social Psychology*, 37(l):1–11.
Kornhauser, A. 1965. *Mental Health of the Industrial Worker*. New York: Wiley.
Krantz, J. 1985. Group Process under Conditions of Organizational Decline. *Journal of Applied Behavioural Science*, 21(l):1–17.
Leana, C. R. & Feldman, D. C. 1988. Individual Responses to Job Loss: Perceptions, Reactions, and Coping Behaviour. *Journal of Management*, 14(3):375–389.
Leatz, C. A. & Stolar, M. W. 1993. *Career Success: Personal Stress: How to Stay Healthy in a High-stress Environment*. New York: McGraw-Hill.
Levering, R., Moskowitz, M. & Katz, M. 1988. *The 100 Best Companies to Work for in America*. New York: American Library.

Levitan, S. A. & Johnson, C. M. 1982. *Second Thoughts on Work*. Michigan: Upjohn Institute for Unemployment Research.

Lewis-Fernandez, R. & Kleinman, A. 1994. Culture, Personality and Psychopathology. *Journal of Abnormal Psychology*, 103(l):67–71.

Lindegger, G. & Wood, G. 1995. The AIDS Crisis: Review of Psychological Issues and Implications, with Special Reference to the South African Situation. *South African Journal of Psychology*, 25(l):1–11.

Littlewood, R. 1990. From Categories to Contexts: A Decade of the 'New Cross-Cultural Psychiatry'. *British Journal of Psychiatry*, 156:308–327.

Long, A. (ed.) 1999. *Interaction for Practice in Community Nursing*. Houndsmills: Macmillan.

Long, B. C. & Kahn, S. E. (eds.) 1993. *Women, Work and Coping: A Multi-disciplinary Approach to Workplace Stress*. Montreal: McGill-Queens University Press.

Loscocco, K. A. & Rochelle, A. R. 1991. Influences on the Quality of Work and Non-work Life: Two Decades in Review. *Journal of Vocational Behaviour*, 39:182–225.

Louw, D. A. & Edwards, D. J. A. (red.) 1998. *Sielkunde: 'n Inleiding vir Studente in Suid-Afrika*. Johannesburg: Heinemann.

Lowman, R. L. 1993. *Counseling and Psychotherapy of Work Dysfunctions*. Washington: American Psychological Association.

Machlowitz, N. H. 1978. *Determining the Effects of Workaholism*. Ann Arbor: Yale University.

Massel, H. K. & Liberman, R. P. 1990. Evaluating the Capacity to Work of the Mentally Ill. *Psychiatry*, 53:31–43.

McClean, A. 1970. *Mental Health and Work Organizations*. Chicago: Rand McNally.

McCormick, E. J. & Ilgen, D. R. 1981. *Industrial Psychology*. London: George Allen.

Meichenbaum, D. 1977. *Cognitive Behaviour Modification. An Integrative Approach*. New York: Plenum.

Mickleberg, W. E. 1986. Occupational Mental Health: A Neglected Service. *British Journal of Psychiatry*, 48:426–434.

Miner, J. B. 1966. *Introduction to Industrial Clinical Psychology*. New York: McGraw-Hill.

Miner, J. B. & Brewer, J. E. 1990. The Management of Ineffective Performance. In M. D. Dunette (ed.) *Handbook of Industrial and Organizational Psychology*. Chicago: Rand McNally.

Minsel, B., Becker, P. & Korchin, S. J. 1991. A Cross-Cultural View of Positive Mental Health: Two Ortogonal Main Factors Replicable in Four Countries. *Journal of Cross-cultural Psychology*, 22(2):157–181.

Minuchin, S. 1974. *Families and Family Therapy*. Cambridge, Massachusetts: Harvard University Press.

Morris, L. E. 1989. *Industrial Stress Injuries*. Los Gatos: Bourne & Allerton.

Mortimer, J. T. & Borman, K. M. 1988. *Work Experience and Psychological Development Through the Life Span*. Colorado: Westview Press Inc.

Muldary, T. W. 1983. *Burnout and Health Professionals: Manifestations and Management*. Norwalk: Appleton-Century-Crofts.

Neff, W. S. 1977, 1985. *Work and Human Behaviour*. Chicago: Aldine.

Nevid, J. S., Rathus, S. A. & Greene, B. 1997, 2003. *Abnormal Psychology in a Changing World*. Upper Saddle River, New Jersey: Prentice-Hall.

Niven, N. & Robinson, J. 1994. *The Psychology of Nursing Care*. Houndsmills: Macmillan.

Noland, R. L. 1973. *Industrial Mental Health and Employee Counselling*. New York: Behaviour Publications.

O'Meara, J. R. 1977. Retirement. *Across the Board*, January:4–9.

O'Toole, J. 1974. *Work and the Quality of Life*. Cambridge: M.I.T. Press.

Plaggemars, D. 2000. EAPs and Critical Stress Debriefing: A Look Ahead. *Employee Assistance Quarterly*, 15(4):77–95.

Prince, R. & Tcheng-Laroche, F. 1987. Culture-Bound Syndromes and International Disease Classification. *Culture, Medicine and Psychiatry*, 11:18–23.

Robbins, S. P. 1989. *Organizational Behaviour – Concepts, Controversies and Applications*. New Jersey: Prentice-Hall.

Robbins, S. P., Odendaal, A. & Roodt, G. 2001. *Organisational Behaviour: Global and Southern African Perspectives*. Cape Town: Pearson Education.

Roberson, C. 1986. *Preventing Employee Misconduct: A Self-Defence Manual for Business* Massachusetts: Lexicon Books.

Robinson, T. R. & Howard-Hamilton, M. 1994. An Afrocentric Paradigm: Foundation for a Healthy Self-image and Healthy Interpersonal Relationships. *Journal of Mental Health Counselling*, 16(3):327–339.

Rogers, L. R. 1961. *On Becoming a Person: A Therapist View of Psychotherapy*. Boston: Houghton Mifflin.

Rosenbaum, M. & Ben-Ari, K. 1985. Learned Helplessness and Learned Resourcefulness: Effects of Noncontingent Success and Failure on Individuals differing in Self-Control Skills. *Journal of Personality and Social Psychology*, 48(l):198–215.

Ross, R. R. & Altmaier, E. M. 1994. *Intervention in Occupational Stress: A Handbook of Counselling for Stress at Work*. London: Sage Publications.

Rotter, J. B. 1966. Generalized Expectancies for Internal versus External Control of Reinforcement. *Psychological Monographs*, 80(l), Whole No. 609.

Santer, S. L., Murphy, L. R. & Hurrell, J. J. 1990. Prevention of Work-Related Psychological Disorders. *American Psychologist*, 45:1146–1158.

Schreuder, A. M. G. & Theron, A. L. 1997. 2001. *Careers: An Organizational Persperctive*. Kenwyn: Juta

Schuler, R. 1982. An Integrative Transactional Process Model of Stress in Organizations. *Journal of Occupational Behaviour*, 3:5–19.

Shareef, R. 1991. Ecovision: A Leadership Theory for Innovative Organizations. *Organizational Dynamics*, 199:50–162.

Shirom, A. 1982. What is organizational stress? A facet analytic conceptualization. *Journal of Occupational Behaviour* 3:21–37.

Smith, R. C. 1987. *Unemployment and Health: A Disaster and a Challenge*. Oxford: Oxford University Press.

Sperry, L. 1996. *Corporate Therapy and Consulting*. New York: Brunner/Mazel.

Statham, A. & Bravo, E. 1990. The Introduction of New Technology: Health Implications for Workers. *Women and Health*, 16(2):105–129.

Steffy, B. D., Jones, J. W. & Noe, A. W. 1990. The Impact of Health Habits and Life Style on the Stressor–Strain Relationship: An Evaluation of Three Industries. *Journal of Occupational Psychology*, 63:217–229.

Steinmetz, L. L. 1969. *Human Relations: People and Work*. New York: Harper & Row.

Stroebe W. & Stroebe, M. S. 1995. *Social Psychology and Health*. Buckingham: Open University Press.

Strümpfer, D. J. W. 1995. The Origins of Health and Strength: From 'Salutogenesis' to 'Fortigenesis'. *South African Journal of Psychology*, 25(2):81–89.

Strümpfer, D. J. W. 1990. Salutogenesis: A new paradigm. *South African Journal of Psychology*, 120(4):265–276.

Sullivan, H. S. 1953. *The Interpersonal Theory of Psychiatry*. New York: Norton.

Super, D. E. 1980. A life span, life space approach to career development. *Journal of Vocational Behaviour*, 16:282–298.

Super, D. E. & Bohn, M. J. 1970. *Occupational Psychology*. Monteray: Brooks-Cole.

Swart, N. & Wiehahn, G. 1979. *Interpersonal Manoeuvres and Behaviour Change*. Pretoria: H & R Academia.

Thompson, J. A. & Bunderson, J. S. 2001. Work–Non-Work Conflict and Phenomenology of Time. *Work and Occupations*, 28(1):17–39.

Van Kessel, W. & Van der Linden, P. 1974. Een Interactioneel Model voor Gestoord Gedrag en voor Psychotherapie. Unpublished lectures. Instituut voor Clinische en Industriële Psychologie: Utrecht.

Varma, V. K. 1986. Cultural Psycho-Dynamics in Health and Illness. *Indian Journal of Psychiatry*, 28(l):13–34.

Warr, P. B., Cook, J. & Wall, T. D. 1979. Scales for the Measurement of Some Work Attitudes and Aspects of Psychological Well-being. *Journal of Occupational Psychology*, 52:129–148.

Warr, P. 1987. *Work, Unemployment and Mental Health*. Oxford: Clarendon Press.

Wolfgang, A. P. 1988. Job Stress in the Health Professions: A Study of Physicians, Nurses and Pharmacists. *Behavioural Medicine*, Spring 1988:43–47.

Yalom, I. D. 1975. *The Theory and Practice of Group Psychotherapy*. New York: Basic Books.

Zedeck, S. 1992. *Work, Families and Organizations*. San Francisco: Jossey-Bass.

12 Environmental health

S. P. Hattingh

12.1 Introduction

The responsibility of industry does not end at the factory wall. It extends to all human activity. Human environment is dependent on environmental health and stability. All elements in the human environment contribute to a complex cycle of total health – physical, psychological and socially. If one of these elements surrounding human beings are removed, the total health of the human being is affected.

All people have the right to a standard of living adequate for the health and well-being of themselves and their families, including food, clothing, housing, healthcare, and the necessary social services. Human beings are in constant interaction with all the aspects of their environment, be they natural (e.g. water, air, soil, plants), manufactured (materials, machines, tools) or animal in origin.

12.2 Learning objectives

At the end of this chapter, the reader should be able to:
- Define, discuss and analyse environmental health
- Establish the place of environmental health within the broader framework of healthcare
- Identify the critical factors for a healthy human race in the future
- Indicate environmental factors that may enhance/affect sustainable living
- Discuss the developments in health and environment within the South African perspective
- Define, discuss and analyse the concept of primary healthcare
- Describe the position of primary healthcare in environmental healthcare
- Identify the basic principles of primary healthcare
- Indicate how the declaration of Alma-Ata contributed to health and environmental care
- Discuss the importance of preventive rather than curative care
- Describe the impact of development in a country.

12.3 Conceptualizing health and environment

12.3.1 Definition of health

To the general public, the term health is a very subjective and personal experience and health to most people refers to the way they experience and perceive their immediate environment. The World Health Organization (WHO) defines health as 'a state of complete physical, mental and social well-being and not merely the absence of disease or infirmity' (WHO, 1986).

The concept of disease, disability and death tends to be much easier for health professionals to address than the concept of health. As a result, health sciences have largely been *disease sciences*, since they focus on treating illness rather than enhancing health.

The definition of health acknowledges the broader dimensions of health. It states that health is... 'physical, mental and social well-being, and not merely the absence of disease and infirmity'. This implies that health is seen as a product of a person's positive interaction with the total environment and that all environmental factors need to be taken into account.

To be able to attain optimal health, the multidisciplinary approach must be followed. In occupational health, the multidisciplinary team will consist of professionals and scientists from very different backgrounds, but all with the same objective, namely maintaining health, preventing disease and controlling those factors that may affect the health and well-being of the working and living environment. For example, air pollution in any industry is indirectly closely monitored by healthcare professionals (e.g. nurses, doctors) by performing lung function tests and examining workers for potential signs of illness related to air pollution. More directly, safety officers, hygienists, microbiologists, engineers and other scientists monitor the air around workers to determine the amount of pollution to which the worker and the community is exposed. Human interaction with the environment is thus multifocused and multidimensional, and one discipline alone cannot attain the goal of optimal health for workers and the community on its own. Industry is also closely linked to the community. It is a mistake to think that pollution, for example, extends only as far as the boundaries of the factory and that this is also the margin where responsibility of the industry ends. In fact, the responsibility extends far beyond the individual industry.

12.3.2 Definition of environment

A population does not exist in a vacuum, but is part of a living, vibrant environment in which it plays various roles. The environment manifests itself at the natural, political, social, economical, cultural and psychological level.

Last (1995) defines the environment as 'All that which is external to the individual human host. It can be divided into physical, biological, social, cultural, etc., any or all of which can influence health status in populations'. This definition is based on the notion that an individual's health is basically determined by two factors; the genetic make-up of the individual and his/her environment.

Internal environment

The internal environment is determined by a person's genetic make-up which he/she inherits from the parents. Every person's genetic make-up is different. Some people have more resilience and resistance towards psychological and physical detrimental factors than other people. Some theories suggest that the genes have a time clock that leads to self-destruction, indicating that as a person grows older, this internal clock determines the lowering of the optimal functioning of the individual. The genetic make-up of an individual is one of the major factors that determines how an individual is affected by the external environment. While everybody will have problems if subjected to high enough exposures to an environmental hazard, some people are affected at lower exposures due to inherited susceptibility. The following example illustrates the genetic features of an individual.

> He is 23 years old, well educated, looks healthy and is energetic at the time of employment. Within six months of his employment, he starts visiting the clinic with symptoms of fatigue and complaints of not feeling well. A range of blood tests reveals that he is suffering from diabetes. Only at this stage, the health worker asks him about his family history and he reveals that both his parents and two of his siblings suffer from this disease and that he is not surprised that he has also developed the disease.

External environment
The external human environment consists of very basic elements, such as the air we breath, the water we drink, the food we eat, the climate surrounding us and the space we occupy for movement. In addition to this physical component, human beings exist in a social and spiritual (psychological) environment which is of great importance to them. Within this total environment of the human being, two basic factors, namely the predisposing environmental and the genetic factors, lead of an individual developing disease. For example, people who have an inherited predisposition to stress, (A-type personality) may be more susceptible to heart disease if they are exposed to severe stressful situations in the environment.

12.3.3 Ecosystem perspective

The term ecosystem can be described as a system of dynamic interdependence among living organisms and the environment in which they live. It is a bounded entity which has acquired self-stabilizing mechanisms and an internal balance that has been evolving over the course of centuries. Within one stable ecosystem, one species does not eliminate another, otherwise the food supply or the predator species would no longer survive. Ecosystems with well-buffered stability and balance will survive best. An ecosystem cannot sustain massive amounts of materials and energy being consumed by one species without depriving other species and eventually endangering the viability of the entire ecosystem. Similarly, the ecosystem's capacity to absorb wastes and to replenish soil and fresh water is not limitless. At some point an external load can overwhelm the ecosystem's balance, resulting in rapid change or a collapse of the total ecosystem. Just as the concept of homeostasis (the body's capacity to function in a coordinated way to ensure the constancy of its internal functions) is now generally understood and accepted, these complex, compensating mechanisms seem to apply to ecosystems as well.

In every workplace this principle must be taken into consideration and the healthcare professional has a role as educator and conservationist to protect the sources which provide homeostasis to the human population as a whole. Every healthcare professional is concerned with the protection of the natural environment of not only the industry or workplace, but of the total ecology in which people work, play and live.

Ecology is concerned with both the structure and functioning of the organism. It attends to the surroundings as well as that which is surrounded. Ecology, in order to study the interrelationships within an environment, is action-oriented and focuses on what can *be* rather than ending its conceptualization of the human relationship with either what *has been* or what is.

12.3.4 Biosphere

The term *biosphere* refers to the world of living things and is made up of numerous ecosystems. Each ecosystem represents all living and non-living parts that support a chain of life within a selected area and is the sum total of all existing sub-systems.

In each ecosystem, nature provides specific conditions essential for supporting plant and animal life. Each ecosystem is a *circle of life* comprising four principal components:
- Sunlight, water, oxygen, carbon dioxide, organic compounds and other nutrients for plant growth
- Plants, which convert carbon dioxide and water into carbohydrates through photosynthesis
- Consumers of the products of plants: herbivores (cows, sheep), and carnivores (humans and meat-eating animals)
- Decomposed organisms, such as bacteria, fungi and insects.

12.3.5 Environmental health

Environmental health is the control of all those factors in the physical environment of human beings that exercise or may exercise deleterious effects on their physical development, health or survival. Environmental health is a condition of optimal physical and social wholesomeness of the human being's living environment that can have a negative or positive effect on health.

Environmental health is concerned with all forms of life, substances, forces and conditions in the surroundings of people that may exert an influence on their health and well-being. Environmental health embodies the absence or presence of illness, health maintenance, human efficiency and the enjoyment of life.
The WHO (WHO, 1993) defines environmental health as follows:

> Environmental health comprises those aspects of human health, including quality of health, that are determined by physical, biological, social and psychological factors in the environment. It also refers to the theory and practice of assessing, correcting, controlling and preventing those factors in the environment that can potentially affect adversely the health of present and future generations.

There are many parts of the environment in which people work that can produce health hazards, namely biological organisms, toxic chemicals, radioactivity, ineffective waste disposal, noise and other physical and psychological factors. For example, when a person's resistance to disease is not sufficient (through nutritional imbalance, lowered immunity), then the environment (e.g. the bacteria) influences health, and the homeostasis is disrupted.

The objectives of environmental health are the prevention, detection and control of environmental hazards which affect human health. The following aspects include the fundamentals of this process:
- Occupational health and safety programmes
- Epidemiological control
- Air quality management
- Water resource management
- Noise and vibration control
- Heat control
- Chemical hazard control
- Radiation control
- Control of frontiers for the spread of diseases
- Educational activities such as conservation of the natural heritage of human populations
- Promotion and enforcement of environmental health quality standards through legislation
- Collaborative efforts by multi-professionals to study the effects of environmental hazards
- Environmental impact assessment performed in every working environment
- Detection and control of biological agents, such as micro-organisms, arthropods, allergens and toxins from plants and animals.

12.4 Interaction between the human race and its environment

The human race is faced with complex environmental issues which balance health (including physical, social and psychological aspects) against environmental factors such as air pollution, water pollution, noise, surface and ground water disposal, and depletion of natural resources.

Most sources concentrate on the negative effects that air pollution, soil erosion, water pollution, and so on have on the human race. However, the health of individuals, groups and communities are often an indication for conservation. For example, communities who are employed, live healthy lifestyles, work and play in a safe environment, are known also to care for their environment and those of others. In communities where people are subjected to poverty, unemployment, war, violence, crime and a lack of safe facilities such as water, electricity and sewerage disposal, less attention is given to the environment.

Poverty, poor living and working conditions, and lack of education have been repeatedly identified as some of the major impediments to health. Over the years it has become clear that substantial improvements in health could not be achieved without improvements in social and economic conditions.

The environment is especially important in the rural areas (for example where mining activities may occur). The availability of natural resources can play a role, not only in the outcome of every project applied to it, but also in the planning and viability of health and other care projects. For example, many mining companies sponsor and maintain conservation activities (e.g. Sasol bird conservation projects and mining activities, and the implementation of game farming and nature conservation activities). Environmental pollution and degradation have a huge impact on people's lives and many industries are responsible for some pollution. Every year hundreds of millions of people (workers and the broader community) suffer from respiratory diseases associated with indoor and outdoor pollution. Population growth contributes to these factors, especially in the developing countries. Hundreds of millions of people globally are exposed to unnecessary physical and chemical hazards in the workplace and living environment. Half a million die every year globally as a result of accidents. Four million infants and children die every year from diarrhoeal diseases, largely as the result of contaminated food. Hundreds of millions of people suffer from debilitating intestinal parasites. Two million people die of malaria every year, while 267 million are ill with it at any given time. Three million people die each year from tuberculosis and 20 million are actively ill with it. Hundreds of millions suffer from poor nutrition. Potentially, all of these hardships and problems people suffer can be prevented.

12.5 Human needs, health and the environment

Maslow's hierarchy of needs is well known to most people. This need hierarchy is illustrated in Figure 12.1.

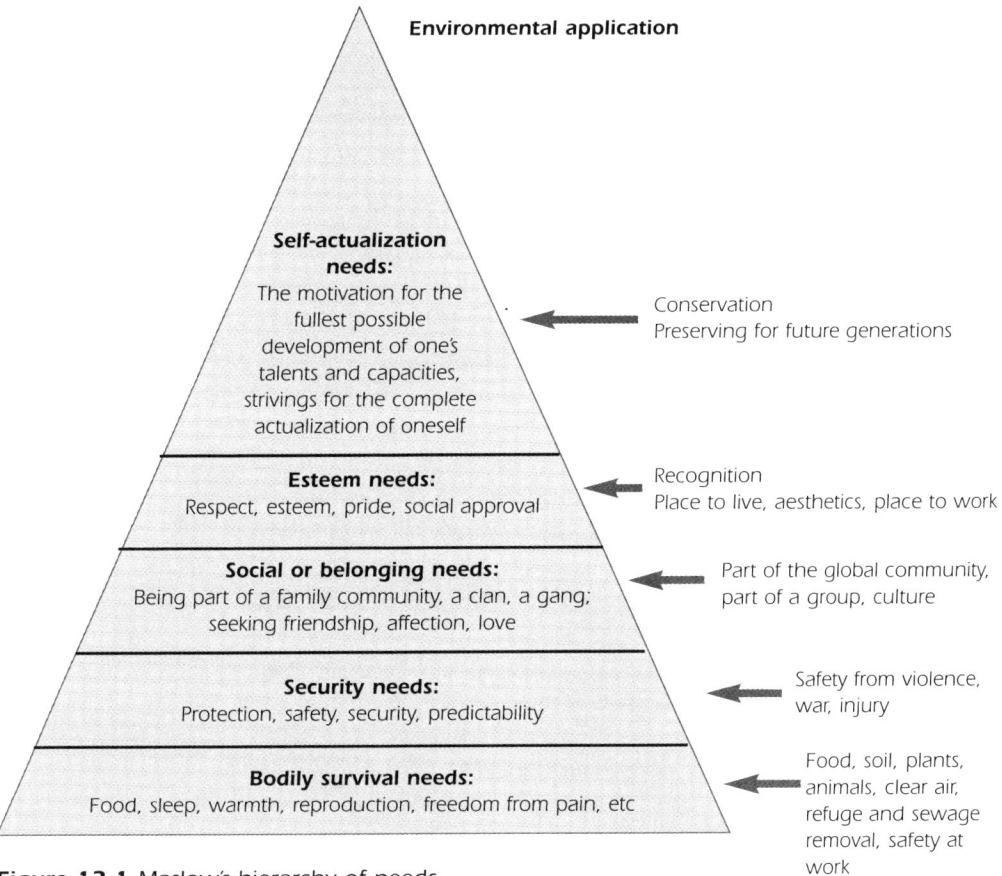

Figure 12.1 Maslow's hierarchy of needs

It is important to remember that merely providing people with basic needs such as clean water, electricity, housing, food, and so on, will not necessarily create awareness of environmental conservation. Education is part of this process – it holds the key to understanding *why* and *what* to protect and preserve. It is for this reason that occupational healthcare professionals combine their efforts to educate and explain. For example, why is it necessary for food handlers to wash their hands after they have been to the toilet? Such seemingly simple information is often taken for granted by healthcare professionals, but is not always understood by the most vital link in the chain of infection, namely the worker him-/herself.

There are also many who do understand the concepts of conservation, they have been taught and educated about the principles of protecting, for example, natural resources but who continue to harm the environment, disregarding all efforts of the conservationists for their own benefit. For these people, harsh rules and legislative aspects are applied and heavy sentences are given. However, only the tip of the iceberg of polluters, destroyers and perpetrators of the environment are caught and charged by the authorities. Others continue on the road of destruction, causing serious health risks for others and depleting our natural resources in the environment. One can regard these people as builders of a road of self-destruction of the human race. An example in industry can be found of those who continue to pollute rivers, streams and the sea by pouring pollutants (e.g. chemicals, raw sewage) into it and causing diseases of humans and aquatic animals.

If the efforts of education and legislation fail, then community efforts must be applied in order to stop this road to self-destruction. It is for this reason that community participation must be enhanced. Every person in the community (and the healthcare professional is no exception) has a role to play in this regard and those who violate the right of people to live a healthy lifestyle must be pointed out by the community.

Every individual in the community and the workplace also has the task of *self-care*. This concept can be applied to environmental health in various ways, for example:

- People with illness and conditions must *care* for others as to not to spread diseases/conditions, for example by educating others who perform dangerous tasks, those who are ill to report their illnesses immediately for timeous treatment.
- People must take *care* not to contract diseases and other health-related problems from their environment, for example by applying hygienic habits, controlling vectors, wearing safety protection clothing and devices.
- People must take *responsibility* for their own immediate environment, for example by not causing pollution.

These self-care and responsibility issues are often disregarded by healthcare and environmental professionals.

12.6 A sustainable environment and development

The concept *sustainable development* addresses the need for a modern economy that does not harm the environment to the extent that it closes off opportunities for future generations. The WHO defines sustainable development as:

> Development that meets the needs of the present without compromising the ability of future generations to meet their own needs. Health, which implies the full development of human potential, requires both an adequate prosperous economy, a viable environment and a convivial community. Economic activity should take these concepts into account. It must not destroy the human and social capacity nor the resources of society. The benefits of the economy must be equitably distributed both within and between nations, societies and communities (Dodds & Middleton, 2002)..

Human health ultimately depends on a society's capacity to manage the interaction between human forces and the physical, chemical and biological environments. It must do this in ways that safeguard and promote human health, while at the same time the integrity of the natural systems on which a healthy environment depends needs to be protected. The physical and biological environments include anything from a home and work environment to regional, national and indeed global environments.

Countries and communities strive for, among others, a supportive environment in which their health targets can be achieved. The focus is on how good environments enhance health rather than on the health impacts of bad environments. This effort involves aspects such as building healthy housing, promoting healthy lifestyles, cleaning up industrial pollution, reducing traffic hazards, reducing tobacco smoking, and changing dietary habits. In poor communities the most important issues may be basic sanitation and water supply, improved maternal and child healthcare, and the control of communicable diseases.

Supportive environments for health imply dealing with determinants of the health of entire populations. It includes:

- Analysis of the role of local environmental factors in the health development of the community
- An enabling and promotion approach as well as health protection
- The creation of equity in health within a community
- Stressing the importance of sustainable development as a health issue
- Encouraging people's understanding of environment in a broad sense
- Giving active and genuine encouragement of people's participation and involvement.

12.7 Environmental concerns

Environmental concerns that affect health include aspects such as air, water, sanitation, pollution, waste disposal, industrial and food safety.

Von Schirnding (in Fuggle & Rabie, 1999:590) identifies two major areas that relate to health.

Developed countries
In industrialized countries, the typical environmental health issues include, for example, radon in homes and schools, lead in drinking water, non-ionizing electromagnetic radiation, asbestos in building materials, pesticide residues in food and indoor air pollution.

Developing countries
In developing countries, the health problems are frequently poverty-related and arise largely as a result of factors such as rapid and uncontrolled urbanization and agricultural and land-use practices.

The following exerpt from 'Epidemiological comments' of September 1999 (Volume 1 Number 3: 13–14) illustrates the relationship and partnership between healthcare and environmental care:

> Trachoma is one of the most common diseases in the world and is still considered the second most common cause of blindness after cataract. It is a contagious disease (caused by Chlamydia trachomatis stereotypes A, B, Ba and C) seen mainly in poor communities, living in overcrowded conditions with poor personal hygiene and insufficient access to water.
>
> In South Africa, trachoma was reported to be a serious health problem in certain areas. It seems that the epidemiological patterns have changed due to a trachoma control programme, better water supplies and changed living standards. It is known that trachoma is found in specific areas or villages. It is necessary that these specific areas should be identified and the necessary trachoma control programme implemented.

The above example illustrates the relationship between health and the sustainability of the environment. This, in turn, indicates what actions should be taken and what planning and policies should be formulated for the protection of the environment to sustain human life. For the successful use of indicators, a reliable and accessible information system is necessary. Sources of information which environmentalists and others may utilize are, among others:
- Vital events such as births, deaths (demographic transitions)
- Population and housing censuses
- Routine health service records
- Disease registers
- Epidemiological surveillance data
- Surveys
- Research data
- Occupational data.

12.8 Demographic transition
Over the last two centuries, a major shift in the health situation of most countries has taken place. In Europe a high-mortality, high-birth rate situation with people suffering from a variety of communicable diseases has given way to a low-mortality, low-birth

rate situation with few cases of communicable diseases and occupational diseases of industrial origin. This change is called the demographic transition of populations. It refers mainly to the crude birth rate and the death rate. When both were high, the population stayed stable. In countries where they are now both low, the population again stays stable. During the transition from high to low there is a period of lowering death rates while the birth rate stays high, and during this period the population will grow. The more death rates decrease in conditions where birth rates remain, the more rapid will be the growth of the population. Examples of this phenomenon can be found in most developing countries. Many developed countries have more or less completed their demographic transition and the death rate cannot be reduced much more.

This pattern may, however, change over the next few years because of the threat of HIV/Aids looming over most developing countries. Demographic transition due to the HIV/Aids pandemic may influence the working population drastically and the consequences may have severe effects of the economies of the world.

Death as an ambiguous event, lends itself well for statistical comparisons of health situations in countries. Nonetheless, mortality rates have their limitations. They tell us little about suffering and loss of productivity related to morbidity. Direct information on the incidence and prevalence of diseases would be a better indicator. But that is only available from surveys of limited temporal and geographical scope. Systems for registering cases of important communicable diseases, such as Aids, yellow fever, leprosy and cholera do exist in most countries. Annual data on cancer incidence are reported to the International Agency for Research on Cancer for participating countries. However, not all cases are reflected in statistics. In war-torn countries, and for example in African countries where the communication networks are not as reliable, statistical data is often questionable.

12.9 Epidemiological transition

The high pre-transition death rate is very much linked to a high level of communicable disease, so the transition in death and birth rates is accompanied by a change in the pattern of the causes of death; less communicable disease and more chronic non-communicable disease. This changed pattern has been called the epidemiological transition.

Transitions are often accompanied by a change in the types of environmental and occupational hazards to which people are exposed. In the pre-transition stage the dominant hazards are what we know to be the traditional hazards of poverty, such as unsafe drinking water, lack of sanitation, poor shelter, indoor pollution from open fires, injury hazards from poor construction, and so on. As the economic development progresses and the transition progresses, the hazards of the modern age begin to dominate, such as air pollution from power stations, industry and cars, water pollution due to mining or industrial wastes, agricultural chemical exposures, and the threat of disasters caused by humans. The term *health hazard transition* has been coined to describe this. All of these concepts can be useful in describing the change that occurs in conjunction with economic and community development.

In Table 12.1 below the causes of death in developed and developing countries are compared.

Table 12.1 Causes of death in developed and developing countries

Causes of death	Developed countries (%)	Developing countries (%)
Infectious and parasitic diseases	1.2	41.5
Chronic lower respiratory diseases	7.8	5.0
Malignant neoplasms (cancer)	21.6	8.9
Maternal causes	0	1.3
Perinatal and neonatal conditions	0.7	7.9
External causes of mortality	7.5	7.9
Other and unknown causes	14.5	16.8

Source: WHO, 1995.

Most of the above factors can also be directly or indirectly linked to industry and the occupational healthcare professional should never regard the above data as 'somewhere out there' that does not concern the industry.

12.10 Mortality rates

Crude mortality rates are declining in many developing countries while remaining steady in developed regions. Life expectancy is a better indicator of trends, as it takes into consideration differences in age structure and shows that improvements have been made throughout the world, although life expectancies are still much lower in developing countries. These trends do concern the occupational healthcare professional, because the working population is getting older and the emphasis is changing from infectious diseases to a population who suffers more from chronic diseases inevitably associated with ageing, for example rheumatism and heart disease. People today are more aware of their own role in staying healthy, for example by changing their eating habits, adopting a healthy lifestyle, and making an effort to stay mentally and physically healthy. However, occupational healthcare practitioners are often not properly informed of the change in focus from the curative aspect of health to the promotive emphasis. This is an aspect that needs to be addressed and added to the healthcare disciplines. In 1994 an effort to reorient healthcare practitioners already in service was made by means of various publications by the South African Government, among others the production of 'An In-Service Training Course for Environmental Health'. This effort was not followed up or supported, however, and the curriculum for environmental health was not revised. Thus, the commendable effort to reorientate personnel was spoiled because practitioners were still trained according to the 'old school of thought' and were not oriented once ready for service.

12.11 Indicators

Indicators are methods used at regional, national and international levels to plan and evaluate healthcare programmes. An indicator could make environmentalists of the state aware of possible sources of contamination or factors that may cause concern for both health and the environment. For example, if the health indicators show an increase in diarrhoeal diseases, such as cholera or gastro-enteritis, then the environmentalists/hygienists/occupational healthcare professionals must, in a combined effort, investigate the possibility of water pollution and look for the sources of the disease. If occupational diseases increase in a certain industry, for example, this may indicate that not only the workers are exposed to the contaminant, but also their families and, in many instances, also the community. Indicators are therefore variables that help to measure change.

An example is the nutritional assessment of workers in an occupational healthcare facility. The nutritional status is a positive indicator because of the availability of measurements to assess the productivity, health status and possibility of disease in the workforce. Weight-for-height is used to measure the current nutritional status and can provide an indication of the extent to which a person is acutely malnourished. Training and education are essential for nutritional improvement, and food supplementation (e.g. adding vitamins to maize or beer), as well as supplementary food programmes (e.g. a discount on food supplied at work) can be implemented as direct measures for providing the workforce with additional food.

The psychosocial development of a person is as important as the physical development. The nutritional status of people is not determined only by the availability of food, but also by cultural values, as well as knowledge and education about food preparation and cultivation.

The role of the environment in the prevention of malnutrition is of vital importance as populations in which malnutrition occurs often have the means to provide adequate food, but the knowledge and insight into the production and preservation of food are lacking. Soil preparation, the utilization of water sources, the production cycles, the type of food to plant and keep, the preservation of the land (e.g. preventing overgrazing, fire control, pollution of water sources, disposal of wastes) often are lacking. Soil is often depleted of essential minerals, and although the food quantity is produced, the quality of the food (nutritional value) is questionable. Food preservation (e.g. storage and the prevention of contamination and exposure to vectors) is often also a problem. Environmental issues such as rain, wind, humidity and climate are aspects that need to be taken into account when it comes to food preservation.

12.12 The burden of disease

Many conditions that are not fatal are responsible for the high prevalence of illness and disability in a population. However, this burden of disease is often a complicated interrelationship of various environmental and genetic factors, as well as a combination of lifestyle and behavioural causes. The burden of disease may be misleading, particularly when comparing disease patterns to various geographical regions. The most vulnerable groups are discussed below.

Children

Children are more vulnerable because they are still developing, they have a smaller posture, their respiratory rate is faster and they are more prone to accidents and injuries. For example, lead causes damage to the growing central nervous system of the child, air pollution causes more damage, and children are more prone to carcinogenetics later in life due to early exposure to agents.

Children are often exploited and as poverty within the house, or the community grows, the more the child loses his/her rights. Child abuse and neglect are often associated with poverty and in many countries child labour is a general phenomenon. It is estimated that there are over 20 million street children in Latin America alone. Children are often forced to prostitution, and the risk of HIV is severe. Children are also prone to be more susceptible to infectious diseases and some diseases, such as asthma, are more prevalent in childhood.

Recognizing the vulnerability of children, the Ministers of Environment of 67 highly developed counties published the '1997 Declaration of the Environment Leaders of the Eight Children's Environmental Health' (Tamburlini, 2002). The declaration highlights the problems of specific hazards such as polluted water, air quality, lead, endocrine-disrupting chemicals, environmental pollution and tobacco smoking as general problems for children. Thus, although children are not part of the workforce, they too concern the occupational health professional because they are susceptible to the emissions coming from industries, may be exposed to chemicals or workplace diseases brought home in, for example clothing, or other means by their parents, family or other working community members and may suffer because of conditions at their caregivers' workplace (e.g. strikes, stress and low pay).

Women

Of the 1.3 billion people living in poverty, 70 per cent are women. The rapid increase in problems arising from the destruction of natural resources, rapid industrialization and urbanization, pollution and population pressures, has a special impact on women. Women have less privileged status in society and less access to resources, although they are often obligated to fulfil multiple roles and function as producers, reproducers and home managers.

Education and training programmes for women have become a high priority in efforts to move towards sustainable development. These programmes must be combined with basic health services, expanded economic opportunities and enforced rights. The following measures are recommended to enhance the health and well-being of women:
- Document and publicize women's vital contribution to development
- Increase women's productivity and remove barriers to productive resources
- Provide family planning and improve the health of women
- Expand education
- Establish equity of opportunity in the workplace for women.

The ageing population
It is a simple fact that the world and thus the workforce is ageing. This has immense implications in, for example, the provision of shelter, healthcare and social support. Elderly people have an increased risk of having diseases. They are more likely to be malnourished than younger people and have a large variety of social, economical, psychological and chronic conditions. Of particular importance is the decrease of the body's ability to cope with hazardous exposures, as well as the fact that they have been exposed to toxic substances over a longer period. An elderly body has less mass, and often metabolizes toxins at a slower rate. Therefore, small doses of substances will have a greater effect on the elderly. The elderly are often exploited by the family and have immense problems in coping with a changing culture within a community.

The disabled
There is an estimated 500 million disabled people in the world today. This number is expected to double in the early part of the twenty-first century. Four out of five live in the developing countries and are subjected to chronic diseases, social problems and a decrease in the body's ability to cope with environmental hazards. Special provision has to be made for the needs of disabled persons in the workplace.

Indigenous people
Often, indigenous people face extreme hardships and they are often not immune to diseases brought in by 'foreigners', such as measles, tuberculosis, poliomyelitis, tetanus and diphtheria. Social problems such as alcoholism and drug abuse also contribute to the problems of indigenous people. Companies that establish industries in foreign countries or geographical areas that are foreign to their own, need to take these aspects into account. Also, the recruitment of foreigners in industries should be carefully considered with regard to the above-mentioned, as they too may expose the normal workforce to diseases that are foreign to them.

12.13 The team approach
For a team addressing health and environmental issues to be successful, the following cardinal aspects must be taken into consideration:
- The sharing of knowledge and information to the benefit of the community
- The sharing of the unique talents of team members to enhance the outlook of the individual members
- The delegation of functions and responsibilities to appropriate members according to their expertise, knowledge and experience
- Meaningful interpretation of the collected data about the community.

12.14 Basic requirements for a healthy environment
There are some basic requirements for a healthy environment. Every industry should strive towards attaining these basic requirements.

The five basic requirements for a healthy environment are:
1. Clean, safe and sufficient water
2. Clean air
3. Safe and nutritious food
4. Safe and peaceful settlements
5. Stable global ecosystem suitable for human habitation.

12.14.1 Clean air

Air is essential for life itself because without it the human race, plant life and animal life would not be able to survive. Air pollution is one of the most serious environmental problems in societies at all levels of economic development. As many as 500 million people are exposed daily to high levels of indoor air pollution in the form of smoke from open fires or poorly designed stoves. More than 1 500 million people live in urban areas with dangerously high levels of air pollution. Industrial development has been associated with large quantities of gaseous and particulate emissions from both industrial production and from burning fossil fuels for energy and transportation. When technology was introduced to control air pollution by reducing emissions of particles, it was found that the gaseous emissions continued and caused problems of their own. Current efforts to control both particulate and gaseous emission have been partly successful in much of the developed world, but recent evidence suggests that air pollution is a health risk even under these relatively favourable conditions.

In societies that are rapidly developing, sufficient resources may not be invested in air pollution control initially because of other economic and social priorities. The rapid expansion of industry in these countries has occurred at the same time as increasing traffic from motor cars and trucks, increasing demands for power for the home, and concentration of the population in large urban areas called mega-cities. The result has been some of the worst air pollution problems in the world.

In many traditional societies, and societies where household energy resources that are considered to be clean are not yet available, air pollution is a serious problem because of inefficient and smoky fuels used to heat buildings and to cook. This causes air pollution both outdoors and indoors. The result can be acute respiratory infections, lung disease, eye problems and increased risk of cancer. Where there is no legislation or standards, particularly in poor and developing countries, workers and the community are particularly exposed.

The quality of air indoors is a problem in many developed countries, because buildings were built to be airtight and energy efficient. Chemicals produced by heating and cooling systems, smoking and evaporation from building materials accumulate indoors and create a pollution problem.

Particles of 10–20 microns or more are trapped in the nasal passages if breathed through the nose and if breathing takes place through the mouth, these particles are retained in the mouth and other passages such as the pharynx and larynx. Particles of 2–10 microns are trapped in nasal passages and bronchial tree, while those less than 2 microns penetrate the bronchiole and alveoli (Fuggle & Rabie, 1999:597). Highly soluble gases such as SO_2 are absorbed largely in the upper respiratory tract, while less soluble gases such as NO_2 and ozone may reach the lower airways.

The general health effects of air pollution are well documented, but the exacerbating pre-existing diseases, as well as the harmful effect of behaviour such as cigarette and dagga smoking, sniffing drugs (cocaine, glue, etc) combined with pollution, are not known.

The general diseases associated with air pollution include:
- Chronic obstructive pulmonary diseases, which include obstructive airway disease, such as emphysema and bronchitis, asthma, acute respiratory infections, cardiovascular diseases and cancers
- Acute respiratory tract infections may occur due to air polluted with NO_2, SO_2
- Throat irritation and headache may occur due to ozone pollution.

12.14.2 Clean, safe and sufficient water

Water, just like air, is essential to the life of all living objects including human beings. We need to drink one to two litres of water per day. After about four days without water, a person will die. In addition, water is essential for plants, animal and agriculture, so throughout human history, people have clustered along the shores and lakes and rivers to get water. Many bloody wars have been fought over water resources. Water also provides natural transportation, is used for disposal of wastes, and plays an essential role in farming, fishing and in the industrial sector.

Although water is regarded as a renewable source, there is a limited supply. Water is also unequally distributed among the counties of the world and the people of the world. In many areas, shortages of water are the main obstacle to food production. The shortages of water lead to poverty and soil degradation, and many cities and agricultural regions are drawing water from underground quantifiers faster than those sources are able to replenish themselves.

Water is also the source of many life-threatening and health-threatening diseases. In fact, more than 80 per cent of all diseases in developing countries is attributed to unsafe water and the inproper disposal of excrement. Nearly half the world's population suffers from diseases associated with contaminated water, affecting mostly the poor in virtually all developing countries. Two thousand million people are at risk from waterborne and foodborne diarrhoeal diseases, which are the main cause of nearly four million deaths each year.

Recently, many parts of the world suffered from floods, and a cholera epidemic was an obvious outcome. Schistosomiasis (200 million people are infected) and dracunculiasis transmit other life-threatening diseases such as malaria (267 million infected), filariasis (90 million infected), onchocerciasis (18 million infected) and dengue fever (30–60 million infected).

Water shortages usually lead to problems such as:
- Water quality polluted with for example sewage
- Industrial wastes
- Agricultural and urban runoff
- Industrial emissions.

These contaminants lead to the breakdown of biodegradable wastes and they dilute non-biodegradable wastes. In many urban and informal settlements there is a lack of control and enforcement of regulations that control industrial emissions and sewers, drains and sewage treatment plants. Another serious contaminant of water resources is the lack of planning of graveyards and the disposal of the dead. These aspects may cause the contamination of underground water sources and thus contaminate the drinking water of those people who depend on boreholes.

12.14.3 Safe and nutritious food

Safe and sufficient food is essential for life. The human being needs between 1 000 and 2 000 calories each day to stay alive, depending on the person's age, height, build and the type of activities he/she performs. Food provides essential nutrients, such as amino-acids, vitamins, inorganic nutrients, essential fatty acids and energy. Most foods contain a variety of nutrients but, as nearly all are deficient in one or more, requirements for essential nutrients are most likely to be met if a wide variety of foods is eaten in moderation. In general, the essential nutrients are found in greater amounts and in more bio-available forms in animal products such as meat, fish, cheese, milk and eggs.

The output of the world's food-producing systems has matched the population growth over the last few decades, and there is no global shortage of food production. However, the distribution of food sources is unequal, for example Africa's food production has not kept pace with the population growth. A large part of the world's population suffers from under-nutrition and infections associated with polluted food and/or a lowered body resistance due to inadequate quality of essential nutrients. The rapid degradation of the soil and water resources also poses an important threat to food production, and many nutrients found in food are absent because the essential elements are depleted from the soil. Poor countries often export their best foods such as vegetables, meat and fruits, leaving those in the country depleted of food sources.

The following are some of the effects of an inadequate diet:
- Starvation or obesity
- Premature and underweight babies
- Weakened immune system resulting in diseases
- Non-infectious chronic diseases such as cardiac, bone and blood diseases
- Unproductive workforce.

With the control of undernutrition, and of infectious diseases in which improved nutrition has played a part in the Western affluent countries, interest in other diseases which may be caused by inappropriate dietary habits has increased. Epidemiological studies show clearly that the cause of some of the most common diseases in Western populations, such as heart disease, stroke and cancer of the breast and bowel, are environmental, since in migrant populations the incidence changes to that of the host country within one or two generations. Diet is one of the environmental factors implicated and a comparison of diets eaten in populations at high risk show that animal protein intake, particularly meat, is strongly associated with risk from colon cancer, fat intake with cancer of the breast, and salt and animal (saturated) fat intake with stroke and heart disease. The association between sugar consumption and tooth decay is well known and a substantial proportion of the population in Western countries is overweight and even obese. All these factors influence the ability of people to perform optimally as a workforce.

Food contamination is also directly or indirectly influenced by:
- Chemical wastes from agricultural chemical residues
- Environmental pollution of the soil by toxic metal and solvents
- Toxins from plants and moulds
- Toxins present in fish and shellfish.

Malnutrition often gets a lot of attention because it is visible, however, foodborne diseases are an equally worrisome public health problem. Not all cases are reported and not all people with such a disease see a doctor. Food is a mixture of chemicals, including nutrients, natural toxins, contaminants and additives. Various toxic substances may affect food intake, and can cause serious diseases and even death in people.

There are several biological contaminants of food, namely:
- Bacteria of which salmonellae, shigellosis, cholera and staphylococci are the most common
- Viruses of which hepatitis A is the most notable
- Parasites may come from the food handler or contaminated water used for food
- Helminths are worms or eggs of worms that contaminate food and water
- Chemical contaminants include lead, cadmium and mercury.

The sources of chemical contaminants are many and include, for example, car emissions which are deposited onto and absorbed by various crops. Mining activities and industrial waste produce poisons that can contaminate water and soil. Contaminants are often found in animals, crops and in the water. Storage or processing foods may also contaminate. Utensils used for cooking have been identified as lead and cadmium sources. Lead-based solder used in food tins is the major source of lead in canned food.

To ensure safe food production it is important to look at the agricultural level and improve the hygienic quality of raw materials. By improving the conditions under which animals are raised, the hygienic quality of raw food products can be significantly improved. Furthermore, the use of pesticides and fertilizers should be taken into account, for example those containing organophosphates. Monitoring is important to identify toxic chemicals which may affect the quality of food and affect health.

Due to increasing trends towards urbanization, greater demands are placed on the foodprocessing process. As consumers move further away from the sources of production, they will require an effective and safe food distribution service.

Food preservation and storage are done to prevent the growth of harmful pathogens during manufacturing so that food will remain safe to eat for longer periods. In order to have bacterial growth a number of conditions have to be met:

- A food item must be present to allow bacterial growth
- A bacteria must be present
- The temperature must allow the bacteria to grow
- The pH water content must be conducive for bacterial growth.

To guard against bacterial growth, at least one of these conditions should be prevented. Food preparation at home is perhaps the most relevant place to combat foodborne diseases. Many bacteria may flourish in food due to the temperature at which it is kept. A refrigerator is one of the most effective tools to stop bacteria from multiplying in food. It does not kill bacteria.

Street vendors often prepare food on the streets or sell prepared food in informally arranged (often cardboard shacks). These foodproducing sectors are often overlooked in food control programmes. Health hazards such as cholera, hepatitis A, typhoid and other diseases of microbiological origin can be transmitted through such foods. Hazardous chemicals such as colourants and preservatives have been found in street-vended foods.

12.14.4 Safe and peaceful settlements

A safe and peaceful place to live and to work in is a necessity for health. Inadequate housing and inappropriately constructed buildings to work in have an adverse effect on the physical, psychological and social health of residents. Other social influences include:
- Low income
- Unemployment or uncertain employment
- Insecurity in residential tenure
- Crime rate
- Lack of facilities for recreation and exercise
- Overcrowding
- Stress
- Lack of space
- Lack of adequate housing
- Sanitation.

Residents are exposed to pathogens (e.g. TB, cholera) and other diseases associated with stress (e.g. ulcers, diabetes), pollutants (e.g. respiratory), violence and trauma hazards (e.g. fires, injuries). Conditions often also lead to psycho-social problems such as drug and alcohol abuse, family violence and breakup, child abuse, rape, suicide, violence to family members, murder and criminal activities.

12.14.5 Stable global environment

Human and ecosystem health are inextricably linked. The following are threats to a stable global environment:
- Long-range transport of air pollutants
- Transboundary movement of hazardous products and wastes
- Stratospheric ozone depletion

- Climate changes
- Loss of biodiversity.

12.15 Ecological issues and their effect on health

Industrial activity is often the result of many ecological changes. When ecological changes occur, it affects the health and well-being of every person on earth.

12.15.1 Deforestation

Deforestation is the large-scale habitat changes that occur during the destruction of natural forests, either through natural causes or through the actions of humans.

Large-scale deforestation is regarded as one of the most serious environmental threats to the ecosystem. More than 10 million square kilometres of wooded and forest areas have already been destroyed, mainly to clear land for agriculture, to obtain fire wood and for financial benefits such as timber for furniture and other uses. Hugo, Viljoen and Meeuwis (1997) write that a recent satellite survey pointed out that the decimation of the Amazon forest exceeds 200 000 square kilometres per year. More conservative estimates put the eradication of the rain-forests on a world-wide scale at a rate of 20 rugby fields per minute, which is equivalent to 12 million hectares or 120 000 square kilometres per year. At this rate, there will be no tropical forests left by the year 2020.

The most serious effect of deforestation is the disturbance of the gas balance of the atmosphere. Once trees and other vegetation have been depleted, the carbon in the plants is released in the atmosphere by oxidation. This increase of carbon dioxide and other gases in the atmosphere will lead to a rise in temperature of at least 2 degrees Celsius as a result of the greenhouse effect. This rise in temperature will have a serious effect on the climate, for example melting of the ice caps and rising of the sea level.

Another serious effect is that the rain forests contain more than two-thirds of the world's 10–15 million species. Eradication of these plants and animals because of the invasion of their habitat by humans is enormous. Certain traditional cultures disappear together with the fauna and flora. Indigenous populations now come into contact with the modern world, which has serious consequences.

The exposure of soil left to erosion reduces the nutritional value they hold. This gives rise to rising river beds and silt deposits, and devastating floods.

Forests are important 'sponge' regions and as a result of water retention, run-off is controlled, uniform and constant. Forests reduce the effect of heavy rain erosion and flooding and planning for agricultural use.

The invasion of non-indigenous species of plants cause serious fire threats and competition with indigenous species, which results in the destruction of indigenous species.

Protected plants indigenous to a specific country, for example South Africa, are often used by indigenous people to make medicine from, with the result that rare and endangered plants are depleted. To conserve both the cultural, medicinal and environmental interests and to preserve the plants, nurseries are planting indigenous plants that can be harvested for traditional medicines. However, perpetrators are still robbing forests of their wealth of plant species, all of which has a negative effect on the sensitive ecosystem.

12.15.2 Desertification

Desertification and drought are caused by human activities in which the carrying capacity of land is exceeded. This is exacerbated by natural or human-induced mechanisms, and results in vegetation and soil deterioration, associated with an irreversible decrease or destruction of biological potential of the land and its ability to support population (Mainguet, 1991:4). Open mining (e.g. diamond mining) often causes large areas of open virgin soil which is washed away and exposed.

Desertification could be a result of natural causes or activated by humans. Briefly, desertification could result from:
- Adverse climatic conditions
- Over-grazing
- Over-cultivation
- Incorrect ploughing
- Poor irrigation
- Salinization
- Ploughing soil not suitable for agriculture
- Periods of drought
- Vegetation clearance
- Deforestation.

Environmental degradation such as desertification brings untold poverty and hardships to many regions of the world which in turn leads to a wide range of diseases. In South Africa, desertification has affected 250 000 hectares and approximately 55 per cent of the country is in danger of desertification. The encroachment of the Karoo as a result of overgrazing in areas of low variable rainfall is also of great concern (Hugo et al., 1997:133). According to these authors, the estimates are that the Karoo veld is shifting eastward at a rate of 1.6 km per year. Large parts (approximately 3 000 000 ha) of the Northern Province bushveld are also in the process of becoming deserts as a result of over-grazing.

If conditions do not improve, South Africa will rapidly feature, like large parts of Africa, on the United Nations Organization's permanent drought list and acquire international beggar status.

Just as serious as nutrient depletion, sanitation and water logging are the effects of toxins (in the form of pesticides and herbicides) and soil erosion. Pollution from pesticides and herbicides is a global problem, it destroys not only the individual organisms in the soil but other wildlife also and is directly harmful to the human population. Denuded soils quickly erode and topsoil loss is a serious problem.

It is a fact that 28.7 billion tons (26 billion metric tons) of topsoil is lost worldwide due to erosion every year. It can take up to 1 000 years to form a layer of soil 0.4 inch (1 cm) thick, yet it can be lost in just a few years as a result of poor management.

12.15.3 Global warming
Global warming or the greenhouse effect refers to the warming up of the lower atmosphere due to the accumulation of greenhouse gases that trap heat near the surface of the earth.

Greenhouse gases are gases such as carbon dioxide, methane and CFCs that are relatively transparent to the higher energy sunlight, but trap low-energy infrared radiation. Greenhouse gases that accumulate in the atmosphere promote global warming.

Ozone is an O_3 molecule. Ozone contributes to air pollution in the troposphere, but is an important natural component of the stratosphere. The stratosphere ozone layer protects the earth's surface from excessive levels of ultraviolet radiation.

The stratosphere is the thermal layer of the atmosphere above the troposphere in which temperature increases with altitude. The ozone layer occurs within the stratosphere.

12.15.4 Climate and weather changes
Scientists from all areas of the world report climate and weather changes that could lead to devastating effects on crops. The consequences of these climate and weather changes include the following:
- Heating of air masses which move over the earth's surface, producing winds, clashing warm and cold fronts, producing more violent conditions
- Tornadoes, hurricanes and dangerous damaging storms
- Changes in overall climatic patterns
- Increased water masses
- Intense droughts and desertification
- Changing rainfall patterns
- Destruction of crops
- The forming of new climate zones
- Modification of paths of ocean currents
- The occurrence of flash floods, with devastating environmental effects.

In the following example the interaction between climate change and tick-born diseases is illustrated.

Ticks belonging to the Ixodidae family have a wide geographic distribution range, which includes parts of the subarctic regions. These ticks are vectors for several disease, such as Lyme disease and tick-born encephalitis. Several animals, like some birds, rodents and deer, act as hosts for these ticks. They may be infected with the pathogen and pass it on to humans through blood-sucking. Ticks, as well as their host animals and habitat, are dependent on changes in local weather conditions. A future climatic change would affect the complicated ecological interactions associated with the transmission of tick-borne diseases. As a result, tick-borne diseases may spread into new areas that are located at higher northern latitudes than present endemic regions.

Some researchers argue that global warming may not be such a bad idea at all, because the increase in the concentration of carbon dioxide in the atmosphere will have benefits that will far outweigh any deleterious greenhouse effects. They say that CO_2 is an essential raw ingredient necessary for photosynthesis in plants. When CO_2 is doubled, the production in plant propagation may increase. This should obviously not be used as a standard argument for ignoring the serious consequences to the human race. What use is it if you have food, but no air to breath? Some also argue that a small amount of global greenhouse warming might not be such a bad idea. This is especially relevant to people who live in regions where harsh winters are experienced. The fact, however, is that global warming will not cause overall weather patterns to become consistently warmer and more equitable – indeed, just the opposite may occur in certain regions.

Intracellular damage occurs as a result of ultra-violet absorption, which may eventually lead to cancers, accelerated ageing and cataracts. Those at greatest risk from the direct effects of UV exposure on skin are people with fair skins who sunburn easily. The human health effects of increased UV irradiation due to ozone depletion include higher risks of non-malignant skin cancer, cataract and retinal degeneration, as well as the possibility of impaired immunological responses.

As the earth heats up, climate patterns will shift and in some places local weather conditions will become much more violent. Cold air currents may be displaced to such an extent that, ironically, regions that are currently relatively warm may experience cold snaps and abnormal winter storms. Due to the shifting air currents caused by increased heating of the earth's surface, cold air masses are displaced from the Arctic regions.

The complex interactive connection of environmental systems leads to the unpredictability of the impacts on human beings. Our individual actions can accumulate and eventually have unseen consequences that are not evident for many years.

A good example is a 1995 landmark study released by the WHO on the effects of global climatic change on human health. The vast majority of research on global climate change has concentrated on the physical impacts, such as the rise in the sea level. But there are growing signs that the potential effects on human health are no less serious. This possibility came to public attention in 1993 when a controversial paper was published where the conclusion was that the 1991 cholera outbreak in South America was related to localized warming of Pacific Ocean waters resulting from global climate changes. The paper argued that the warming had caused the rapid growth of plankton that harbour the cholera bacterium, which led to thousands of deaths.

Though the causes of the cholera incident are still being debated, a number of new studies have identified other potential health impacts of global warming. One predicted impact is that many cities will experience 'killer heat waves' that will increase deaths from bronchitis, asthma, and many other ailments. Many other models show that the incidence of tropical diseases will increase significantly. Global warming is expected to have the most deadly effect on tropical developing nations, which are already suffering from poor sanitation. Epidemiologists (disease experts) predict increased rates of malaria, sleeping sickness, and many other diseases, as shown in

Table 12.2. Each year these diseases afflict more than 500 million people, killing over 2 million.

With global warming, the tropical carriers of these diseases, such as mosquitoes, will spread as tropical conditions, including swamps, expand their ranges. An estimate published in the journal, *Environmental Health Perspectives* in 1995 projected that a global temperature increase of 5.4 °F (3 °C) in the next century could result in 50–80 million new cases of malaria cases per year. A natural 'experiment' provides data that supports such projections: In 1987 the average annual temperature was 1.8 °F (1 °C) above normal; this increase was linked to a 3.3 per cent rise in malaria that year in Rwanda (McKinney & Schoch, 2003:109).

Table 12.2 Major tropical diseases likely to spread with global warming

Disease	Vector	Population at risk (millions)	Prevalence of infection	Present distribution	Likelihood of altered distribution with warming
Malaria	Mosquito	2100	270 million	(sub)tropics	+++
Schistosomiasis	Water snail	600	200 million	(sub)tropics	++
Filariasis	Mosquito	900	90 million	(sub)tropics	+
Onchocerciasis (river blindness)	Black fly	90	18 million	Africa/Latin America	+
African trypanosomiasis (sleeping sickness)	Tsetse fly	50	25 000 new cases per year	Tropical Africa	+
Dengue fever	Mosquito	*	*	Tropics	++
Yellow fever	Mosquito	*	*	Africa/Tropical South America	+

* Estimates not available
As assessed by the WHO Organization: + = likely, ++ = very likely, +++ = highly likely

Even if doubts remain about the probability, magnitude and exact consequences of global warming in the future, it would be foolish to sit back and pursue 'business as usual'.

12.15.5 Planetary toxification

Planetary toxification consists of the deposits of harmful or fatal chemicals in the ecosystem. Acid rain is the precipitation (rain, snow, sleet, etc.) that is more acidic than normal (generally due to human-produced air pollutants).

Acid rains come from air pollution and often these pollutants can be carried thousands of kilometres away from their original sites and fall as acid precipitation in areas where, when it falls on the soil, changes the pH and affects waters in streams and lakes, causing ecological damage. This has caused many deaths throughout the centuries, particularly in rural areas. London is notorious for its smog, and deaths and respiratory ailments are common in all parts of the world. In Tokyo, unpolluted air can be bought in aerosol cans and is used by people indulging in strenuous exercise, joggers in particular. There are even roadside stalls where fresh air can be inhaled. In South Africa, Bloemfontein, Boksburg, Cape Town, Kroonstad and Pretoria pollution exceeds the safety limits set (Hugo, et al., 1997:135).

Air pollution includes gases such as sulphur dioxide, carbon monoxide, ozone and occasionally traces of hydrogen sulphide found in dust from soil and smoke resulting from combustion of coal. When these gases are released into the atmosphere, sulphur dioxide combines with water vapour in the air and causes acid rain.

Acid rain is especially damaging for plant life, weathering of buildings, installations and geographical formations. Lakes and rivers suffer biological damage as their waters become more acidic, and fish species, algae and microbes are sensitive for changes. Most of the great forests in Germany, Canada and Northern Europe are showing severe damage ascribed to acid rain.

Smog is the visible manifestation of air pollution and is known to cause serious respiratory and other illnesses to human, plant and animal life. Air pollution damages the respiratory tract, irritates the eyes and nose, and causes breathing disorders.

It is not only industries and emissions from cars that cause serious problems for the earth's atmosphere, but indoor pollutants are also global toxifiers. Indoor pollution is often greater than outdoor pollution. The cost of health problems from indoor pollution is much greater than those of outdoor pollution. The two indoor polluters mentioned specifically that cause the most harm include radon and cigarette smoke.

Indoor air pollution is a threat to human health for two reasons:

- Indoor environments tend to concentrate pollutants – some toxic and cancer-causing pollutants can reach air concentrations that are 100 times greater than outside air.
- Industrialized nations spend more than 80 per cent of their time indoors, including working hours. Sick-building syndrome refers to chronic ailments such as nasal congestion, headaches, nausea, fatigue, drowsiness, eye irritation, allergic reactions, respiratory difficulties, and other symptoms that are caused by indoor air pollutants. This syndrome is caused by inadequate ventilation, environmental contamination, either from within the building or outside, building materials, humidity, cigarette smoke, noise, static electricity and illumination.

Radon gas, which is the most harmful indoor pollutant, is found in high concentrations in houses built on soil and/or rocks that are rich in naturally occurring uranium minerals and their products. Lung cancer is caused by inhaling these particles, which become lodged in the lungs.

Cigarette smoke is one of the most hazardous indoor air pollutants. Many medical studies have found that smoking causes serious physical diseases such as cardio-vascular diseases, respiratory diseases and cancers.

Rapid urbanization contributes to increases in pollution, and it is essential to deal with the issues that affect health. It is estimated that by the end of this century, half the earth's population will live in cities. The idea behind the Heathy Cities Programme is the improvement of urban health by starting intersectoral action for health at the local level. Therefore the major objective of this programme is to place health promotion high on the political agenda for municipal governments.

The qualities of a healthy city are given as follows:
- A clean, safe physical environment of high quality (including housing quality)
- An ecosystem that is stable now and sustainable in the long term
- A strong, mutually supportive and non-exploitive community
- A high degree of participation and control by the public over decisions affecting their health and well-being
- The meeting of basic needs (food, water, shelter, income, safety and work) for all the city's residents
- Access to a wide variety of experiences and resources, with opportunity for ample interaction
- A diverse, vital and innovative city economy
- The encouragement of connection with the past, with cultural and biological heritage of city dwellers and their other groups and individuals
- A form of city that is compatible with and enhances the preceding characteristics
- An optimum level of appropriate public health and sick care services accessible to all
- High health status (high levels of health and low levels of disease) (WHO, 1995b).

12.15.6 Loss of biodiversity

Biodiversity refers to the multiplicity of species of plants and animals in a biological community and the many ecological niches that they may occupy.

Preserving plants and animals is important for their utilitarian value, however, Hugo et al. (1997:158) state that their ecological value is often lost or not fully appreciated. The health or stability in an ecosystem (habitat) is normally directly related to the number of species and the composition of the associated populations. This is in part because the ecosystem functions more efficiently while different species occupy more niches and extract full benefit from the energy and nutrients available.

If through human or other external influence, the ecological balance is disturbed, it could lead to damage and even the destruction of the ecosystem. Even apparent minor disturbances could result in unforeseen chain reactions. Human-made irreversible change or loss of biodiversity caused by humans may result in as yet unknown risks or damage to the quality of life. The larger the species diversity and therefore the number of links in the food chain, the larger the capacity of the system to adapt to changes in the environment.

Biodiversity also means preserving genetic diversity. Each species and subspecies contains within their genes the result of hundreds of thousands, even millions of years of evolution. The genetic constitution is written onto the DNA, the molecule that conserves the genetic code. It provides the blueprint for the biological adaptation and the characteristics commonly found in these organisms.

People often overlook the multiple interactions required to maintain a stable relationship among living and non-living parts of the environment. A classic example of the lack of an orientation to planning occurred in Borneo with the WHO's mosquito control programme. After a community was heavily sprayed with DDT, the mosquitoes were controlled, but roofs began to be eaten by caterpillars that were unaffected by DDT. The spray killed wasps that previously ate the caterpillars. The problem was further complicated after indoor spraying to control houseflies. However, when the lizards ate the diseased flies, they became debilitated and were easily captured by predators. As the predators disappeared due to the consumption of DDT, which was passed from one animal to another, the rat population boomed, carrying with them fleas, invading houses and buildings and threatening the country with plague. This example shows how easily the balance in nature can be disturbed, with devastating effects for the health and well-being of the human population.

Another example is that dung beetles are becoming extremely endangered as a result of the toxic sprays farmers use. The accumulation of dung causes not only a menace to people, but also holds health risks for animals and humans.

A positive example of biodiversity is among the many forms of species and subspecies in synthesizing unusual chemicals. Snake venoms, pheromones that attract insect mates, squid ink and the light-producing chemicals of fireflies are just a few examples. Plants produce a wide variety of chemicals that could be used to produce medicines. With loss of biodiversity, a huge reservoir of potential useful chemicals may be lost that could be produced in no other way.

Life on earth depends on the unimpeded functioning of natural systems that ensure the supply of energy and nutrients. The ecological limits within which humans should work are not limits to human endeavour, instead they give direction and guidance as to how we can sustain environmental stability (Hugo et al., 1997:158).

The real ecological issue is not whether we should preserve the black rhino as a threatened species, but rather that we should preserve life-giving ecosystems – 'saving' the black rhino is no more important than saving an earthworm. Micro-organisms play an equal part in the preservation and health of the ecosystem and are thus just as important to human welfare as any of the 'Big Five' or any other spectacular species.

> Biodiversity describes the vast wealth of life-forms on Earth: the tens of millions of micro-organisms, animals and plants ... and the intricate ecosystems they function in, which together form the living world (McKinney & Schoch, 2003).

Much of the diversity among species and subspecies, and many of the variations among individual species have direct practical use to human society. They have been the basis of agriculture for many years. Agriculture reduces biodiversity in the long run. Many strains are selected for their greater productivity, resistance to diseases and pests, and their ability to grow in less water. The new strains are planted as a monoculture, a uniform strain or herd of genetically similar or even identical organisms. Once they become infected, the entire strain or herd dies.

12.16 The effects of chemical hazards on health

Industrialization is an essential part of providing in the needs of the global population. It provides the products that we need for living, such as food processing, the production of vehicles for transport, furniture, fuel, mining of minerals, transporting people, and many more. It also provides a place of employment for millions of people throughout the world.

Despite the many forms of research, excellent recording, cleaning-up campaigns and legislative controls on chemical spills and pollution, there is considerable uncertainty about the extent the direct and indirect risks of agents present in the environment, which cannot be seen, or easily detected. The consequences of these toxic substances often go unnoticed, affecting health and the environment, without being given a second thought. Often the safety thresholds are exceeded and the adverse affects are only recognized once they have reached extreme toxic levels or disease outbreaks occur. Most environment-related diseases, however, go unrecognized.

Communities often do not realize that they in fact subsidize the cost of industry to do business, and the costs are not charged back to the industry, for example:
- Human health problems
- Destruction of materials
- Plant and animal damage
- Poor visibility
- Loss of appeal for business and tourists
- Reduced quality of life of residents
- Loss of value of property
- Influence on water quality for human consumption and recreation.

Health hazards associated with chemical exposure may either be acute (with immediate effect) or a long time may elapse before the actual destructive consequences are recognized (for example cancers, asbestosis). Children and small children are especially susceptible and the development of the foetus may be seriously affected by chemicals.

Many diseases caused by hazardous and chemical wastes go unrecognized. The public tends to focus on carcinogens, pesticides and radiation hazards. However, innumerable compounds that do not fall into these categories can pose a treat to the public's safety and health. For example, cancers resulting from asbestos exposure (mesothelioma) affect not only the worker or the person but his/her family too. Other chemicals with adverse effects are arsenic, radon and cigarette smoke in the environment. Often chemicals cause intelligence impairment, for example lead exposure.

An interesting occurrence is the reaction of some people exposed to even small amounts of chemicals. They experience what has been called multiple chemical sensitivity. The symptoms are often vague and non-specific and do not correspond with the known toxic effects of these chemicals. These people often present with allergic reactions that do not clear, so they visit various medical practitioners and often, once a diagnosis has been made, tend to withdraw from society, isolating themselves and exhibiting obsessive-compulsive behaviour. Chemicals found in perfumes, pesticides, solvents, tobacco smoke and food additives are often mentioned.

Pesticides that contain organophosphates are particularly dangerous to animal, plant and human life. When fires break out in pesticide storage places, the consequences are serious because these substances may be converted into even more highly toxic combustion products and substantial amounts of environmental damage (such as water pollution) may be caused.

Strong acids and alkali are commonly found in waste sites and contact with them is dangerous. They cause skin, eyes and mucous burns, as well as lung injury. They may cause a potential explosion and fire hazard. Two of the most dangerous acids are nitric acid (causes pulmonary oedema and bronchial irritation) and hydrofluoric acids (causes deeply penetrating burns of skin and eyes).

At present, very few (about 1 per cent) of the millions of chemicals have been tested as being toxic.

Environmental monitoring and environmental epidemiology research, measure, report and control environmental chemical and other forms of harmful substances. However, exposures of chemical substances are normally mediated by complex environmental pathways and more than one route may contribute to human uptake.

12.16.1 Major chemical contaminants

Some of the major chemical contaminants found in the environment and in the workplace that are seriously detrimental for the environment and for the health and safety of human beings are discussed briefly. This does not imply that others are not of equal importance.

Chemical hazards are usually classified into two major groups, namely inorganic chemicals and organic chemicals, for purposes of indicating their effects on health.

2.16.1.1 Toxic metals

The major toxic metals of concern in industry are lead, mercury, cadmium, arsenic, although chromium, zinc, copper and other metals may be of concern in some areas. These metals are found in the environment as well as in the workplace.

Lead

Lead is the oldest hazard known to society. Residents in urban areas tend to have higher lead levels than those in rural areas. The route of entry is through inhalation of tiny particles or from food or beverages containing it. This is found mainly in old batteries, and soil pollution is often seen with this type of waste. Gasoline, paint, glazes of pottery, food cans, copper drinking-water pipes (due to the solder used on them) also contain lead. Exposure leads to lead poisoning, characterized by kidney damage, acute abdominal pain, nausea and weight loss, and brain damage in children.

Mercury

Mercury is a unique metal, being liquid at room temperature and readily volatizing into gas. The many compounds found in mercury are usually more toxic than the metal element itself. Exposure is through inhalation of vapour or ingestion through contaminated foods, or through absorption through a wound or damaged skin. It is used for goldsmithing, mirror-making, antiseptic and antifungal substances, gold mining and in dental clinics. It accumulates in water and silt, causing polluted water and soil. Health problems include, among others, mouth sores, nervous system damage, visual abnormalities and severe foetal poisoning.

Cadmium
Camium is a metal used for anti-corrosive coating of steel, and in rechargeable electric batteries, and plastics. Water pollution from mines and lead/zinc refineries may cause serious cadmium contamination of water and especially in the irrigation of farm fields. The health risks include kidney damage, osteoporosis and osteomalacia. Cadmium accumulates in the body and the effects only develop after many years of exposure. Fertilizers contain cadmium and may have serious effects on soil and plant production toxicity. This substance is also found in sewage.

Arsenic
Arsenic is a more common element in uncontaminated soil than either lead or mercury. It is also bioconcentrated naturally in shellfish. As a result, many people have small amounts of arsenic in their bodies. Arsenic today does not produce problems as in the past when the compounds were used extensively in antibiotics, especially for the treatment of syphilis, for tanning, green dyes in paper and antiparasitic treatment in sheep dip. Recently it is used in micro-electric applications and may cause a serious health threat to workers. It is a uniquely human carcinogenic, causing skin cancer and lung cancer. It causes various skin rashes. Many famous murders by arsenic poisoning have been recorded, and for this reason it is often regarded by the public as a greater hazard than the other toxic metals.

12.16.1.2 Solvents
Solvents are liquids at room temperature that can dissolve other substances without necessarily reacting with them chemically. Many evaporate easily and are rapidly inhaled, such as chloroform and ether. They cause light-headiness, loss of concentration or errors in judgement, and the person appears as if under the influence of alcohol. It eventually leads to serious brain damage. Cancer could also be a risk and liver damage has been reported.

The term halogen is applied to five elements, namely: fluorine, bromine, chlorine, iodine and estamine. The halogens are a remarkable family of elements, marked by their great chemical activity and unique properties. Stability, non-flammability and a wide range of solvency are but a few of the characteristics imparted by their application. The effects of the halogenated hydrocarbons vary considerably with the number of halogen atoms present in the molecule. Carbon tetrachloride at one end of the scale is highly toxic, acting acutely by injuring the liver, kidneys and the central nervous system.

- Hydrocarbons are basically a string of carbon molecules with hydrogen attached to the carbon molecule. Hydrocarbons include paraffins, methane, ethane, propane, butane pentane, hexane, heptane and octane, among others. Benzene is the most common compound found in the air, water and soil. Because of its potency, benzene is carcinogenic.

- Alcohols are one of the most important classes of industrial solvents and saturated alcohols are widely used as solvents. They are noted for their effect on the central nervous system and the liver but vary widely in their degree of toxicity. Methanol and ethanol are the most widely used alcohols.
- Esters are made up of two hydrocarbon groups held together by an oxygen atom. They are made by combining two molecules of the corresponding alcohol. Esters are characterized by their greater volatility, lower solubility in water and higher solvent power in oils, fats and greases.
- Aldehydes are well known for their skin and mucosa irritations, allergies and their action on the central nervous system.
- Olefin or unsaturated hydrocarbons are molecules that have one or more double bonds between molecules which potentially could be broken down so that hydrogen atoms could be added to the molecule. These hydrocarbons are formed as byproducts of petroleum breakdown. Specific unsaturated aliphatic hydrocarbons include ethylene, propylene, butadiene and isoprene.
- Halogenated hydrocarbons are commonly encountered chemicals found in general use and in industry. Examples are chloromethane, dichloromethane, chloroform and carbon tetrachloride. These chemicals are extensively used in dry cleaning, as industrial solvents and in the production of plastics. In general, the larger and more chlorinated the compounds are, the more the compounds cannot be broken down and therefore remain in the environment. Chlorinated cyclic hydrocarbons are damaging environmentally because they persist for long periods and are consumed and accumulated by wildlife. Besides being persistent in the environment, the bioaccumulation of these compounds and their excretion in human and animal milk pose high risk for infants. Toxic signs of human exposure are central nervous system alterations, developmental delay in children, immune system suppression and a persistent skin rash called chloracne.

Solvents may become hazardous to the public in the form of air pollutants when released outdoors. Solvent hydrocarbons are important compounds in the formulation of photochemical smog. In the presence of sunlight, they react with atomic oxygen and ozone to produce aldehydes, acids, nitrates and a whole series of other irritant and noxious compounds.

The greatest portion of hydrocarbons contributing to air pollution originates from automobiles, but a significant amount also comes from the tons of solvents that are exhausted daily from industrial cleaning and surface-coating processes.

Some solvents are more reactive to sunlight and contribute heavily to the smog problem. The use of such solvents is being curtailed in ore and other areas, especially in the larger cities. Other solvents are less reactive and are exempt from stringent control. The following order of photochemical reactivity is listed as a guide:

- Olefin (unsaturated open chain hydrocarbons containing one or more double bounds) are more reactive
- Aromatics (except benzene)
- Branched ketone
- Chlorinated ethylene (including trichloroethylene, except perchlorethylene)

- Normal ketone (e.g. methyl ethyl ketone)
- Alcohols and aldehydes
- Branched paraffins
- Normal paraffins
- Benzene, acetone, perchlorethylene and saturated halogenated hydrocarbons.

In addition to the smog-related materials, fluorocarbons, such as trichlorotrifluorethane and related materials, catalyze the destruction of ozone by fluorocarbons and other materials, which proves to be significant as the amount of solar ultraviolet radiation reaching the earth's surface may increase. It would impair agricultural production and increase the incidence of skin cancer.

12.16.2 Raw materials
Any type of bulk raw materials that can influence health must be handled carefully. They don't only cause chemical hazards, but also fire and injury are commonly found. An example is chlorine gas, which is stored in large volumes in paper pulp plants.

Cyanides are powerful solvents for gold extraction and metal work. Cyanide is often used in home industries where its use is not controlled. The main problem is leakage in the waterways which will kill fish and other animals.

12.16.3 Threshold limit values
Threshold Limit Values (TLVs) are exposure guidelines that have been established for airborne concentrations of many chemical compounds. TLV refers to the airborne concentration of substances and is believed to represent conditions under which nearly all persons exposed may be repeatedly exposed, day after day, without adverse effect. In other words, it is the tolerable level for exposure.

12.17 The effects of physical hazards on health
The physical environment includes all physical aspects such as heat, light, air, water, radiation, gravity, atmospheric pressure and chemical agents. We have much control over our physical environment through provision of adequate shelter, use of water supplies, treatment or sewage and the use or misuse of fauna and flora. With rapid population growth, our physical environment has become the focus of serious attention, and problems such as the increase in pollution from vehicles, wastes and noise require active intervention.

Problems relating to such things as noise, vibration, temperature extremes, ionizing and non-ionizing radiation, and pressure extremes, as well as all forms of pollution such as air pollution, water pollution, sanitation, hazardous wastes, use of pesticides and contamination of food are among those aspects that cause physical stressors.

Types of physical hazards are described below.

Noise (unwanted sound)
Noise is a form of vibration conducted through solids, liquids or gases. The effects of noise on humans include the following:

- Psychological effects (noise startles, annoys, disrupts concentration, sleep and relaxation)
- Interference with communication by speech and as a consequence, interference with job performance and safety
- Physiological effects include loss of hearing, or aural pain if exposure is severe.

Sound intensity is measured in decibels (dB). Levels are commonly adjusted to reflect how the human ear hears, that is, using the 'A' scale (dB(A)), and measured by a hand-held instrument called a sound level meter. For example, the dB(A) of a shotgun blast, jet aircraft or a firecracker exceeds the human ear pain threshold and is measured as 140 dB(A), whereas whispering is just audible and is measured as 10 dB(A).

Risk of incurring hearing loss according to South African regulations, begins within prolonged exposure to sound of approximately 85 dB, however, other countries have different standards. There are three non-technical rules of thumb to determine if the work area has excessive noise levels:

Firstly, if it is necessary to speak very loudly or shout directly into the ear of a person in order to be understood, it is possible that the exposure limit for the noise is being exceeded.

Secondly, if someone says that he/she has heard noises and ringing in the ears, e.g. after a rock concert or even after work, the person may have been exposed to too much noise.

Thirdly, if someone complains that the sound of speech or music seems muffled after leaving, for example the workplace, he/she may be exposed to levels that cause partial temporary loss of hearing, which can become permanent upon repeated exposure.

Noise control measures include:
- Noise control and monitoring of workers for easy detection of hearing loss
- Acoustical engineering and plant design, engineering control and containment or isolation of noise sources
- Protective clothing and diagnosing and treating of infections as an additional secondary problem
- Responsible behaviour of workers to protect their own hearing and those of others
- Environmental control, including for example building of sound-protective barriers along motorways and highways
- Stringent and set regulations that require enforcement.

Vibration energy

Vibration energy can be transmitted to parts of the body, causing extremely serious physical damage. The use of many tools or hand equipment can result in health effects as a result of arm and hand vibration. The most characteristic effect is vibration vasculitis, also known as 'white finger disease' (Raynaud's phenomenon). This condition is caused by the constriction of blood vessels, which results in reduced sensation to fine touch, vibration or temperature and causes marked pain. It is named for the white appearance of the fingers when the blood vessel constriction occurs.

Vibrations can also be transmitted to the whole body when driving vehicles such as bulldozers, excavators, trucks and cars on rough lands or bumpy roads, damaging the musculoskeletal system (e.g. disc prolapse of the spine).

Temperature

Extremes in temperature could result in exposure to extremes of either heat or cold. These environmental extremes affect the health of millions of people each year. Exposure affects the amount of work people can do and the manner in which they do it. In industry it is more often high temperatures than low temperatures that effect people.

Cold environments

The human body can function best at a temperature of 38–39.°C The body maintains its temperature from food and muscular work or by losing it through radiation and sweating. The reaction if the body to cold is the constriction of the blood vessels. The hypothalamus controls the body heat and conserves and regulates temperature by constricting the blood vessels and sweat glands. Glucose is produced, which makes the heart beat faster, sending oxygen to the tissues. Involuntary shivering begins in an attempt to raise the temperature.

The main focus of cold disorders is exposure to humidity and high winds, contact with wetness or metal, inadequate clothing, age and general health. Physical conditions that worsen the effects of cold include allergies, vascular disease, excessive smoking and drinking, and specific drugs and medicines.

Hypothermia develops in air temperatures between 2–10 °C. However, the wind chill factor must be taken into account, as this may indicate a much lower temperature. It is an acute problem resulting from prolonged exposure and heat loss.

Frostbite can occur without hypothermia when the extremities do not receive sufficient heat from central body stores. It occurs when there is freezing of the fluids around the cells of the body tissues, usually at temperatures at −1 °C or less. This results in damage and loss of tissue, most often resulting in the amputation of extremities, scarring and permanent loss of movement.

The air temperature alone is not sufficient to judge the cold hazard of a particular environment. Heat loss from convection is probably the greatest and most deceptive factor in loss of body heat. When the air in a given environment is −1 °C, the body will feel cool, given the same temperature at a wind of 40 km/h, the air will feel bitterly cold. In essence, the wind blows away the thin layer of air that acts as an insulator between the skin and the outside air temperature.

Heat exposure

The evaluation of heat stress by interpreting information relating to the physiology of a person and to the physical aspects in the environment is not simple or easy. Much more is involved than merely taking the temperature.

Heat stress is the aggregate of environmental and physical activity factors that constitute the total heat load imposed on the body. Environmental factors include temperature, radiant heat exchange, air movement and water vapour pressure. Physical work or activity contributes to the total heat stress by producing metabolic heat in the body in proportion to the intensity of the work. Clothing also affects the heat stress. Heat strain is the series of physical responses to heat stress. The responses reflect the degrees of heat stress. This may lead to heat disorder (e.g. heat stroke) which is a potentially fatal condition because the person is no longer able to adapt to the heat and collapses when failure of the circulation results.

In unprepared or unprotected populations, heat stroke may occur during heat waves, especially when it is humid. The resulting fatalities occur most often in the elderly, the chronically ill and people who are not eating well or drinking enough fluid. Compounding this is the fact that peaks of air pollution due to car exhausts and ozone production at ground level often coincide with heat waves because they often occur during the summer months. The combination of air pollution and extreme temperatures can be serious.

Ionizing radiation

The human body is made up of various chemical compounds which are in turn composed of molecules and atoms. Each atom has a nucleus with its own outer system of electrons. When ionization of the body tissues occurs, some of the electrons surrounding the atoms are forcibly ejected from their orbits. The greater the intensity of the ionizing radiation, the more ions will be produced and the more damage will be done to the cell structures, including DNA. Examples of ionizing radiation are atomic bombings, nuclear testing, nuclear accidents such as Chernobyl, as well as when miners are exposed to radon.

Exposure that exceeds the threshold levels results in skin burns, damage to bone marrow, sterility, radiation sickness and death.

Light consisting of electromagnetic radiation from the sun that strikes the earth is very similar to X-rays and gamma radiation, it differs only in wavelength and energy content. However, the energy level of the sunlight at the earth's surface is too low to disturb orbital electrons and consequently sunlight is not referred to as ionizing, even though it has enough energy to cause severe skin burns over a period of time.

Non-ionizing radiation

Non-ionizing radiation is part of the electromagnetic spectrum that consists of electric and magnetic components. It has varying effects on the body, depending on the particular wavelength of the radiation involved. Examples are microwaves, infrared, lasers and ultraviolet radiation.

The eyes are the organs most vulnerable to injury induced by laser energy. The reason is that the cornea and lens have the ability to focus the parallel laser beam on a small spot on the retina. The fact that infrared radiation may not be visible to the naked eye contributes to its potential hazards.

Pressure

Barometric pressure above and below one atmosphere is part of the conditions of work or play in special environments, such as under water or at a high altitude.

Hyperbaric (greater than normal pressures) environments are encountered by divers under water whether by holding their breath while diving, breathing from self-contained underwater breathing apparatus (SCUBA) or by breathing gas mixtures supplied by compression from the surface.

In tunnelling operations where a compressed gas environment is used to exclude water and mud and to provide support for structures, compression may also be experienced.

Unequal distribution of pressure can result in barotrauma, which is tissue damage resulting from expansion or contraction of gas spaces found within or adjacent to the body, and which can occur either during compression (decent) or during decompression (ascent).

Decompression sickness, commonly known as the 'bends', results from the release of nitrogen bubbles into the circulation and tissues during decompression. If the bubbles lodge at the joints and under muscles, they cause severe cramps. To prevent this, decompression is carried out slowly and by stages so that the nitrogen can be eliminated slowly and without the formation of bubbles. Helium is an inert gas and less soluble in blood and tissue than is nitrogen, so it presents a less formidable decompression problem.

12.18 The effects of mechanical hazards on health

Mechanical hazards include all those immediate or gradually acquired injuries in exposed individuals. It is referred to in many sources as accidents or trauma. The word 'accident' is no longer in use, as this implies that injuries are random, unpredictable, chance type of events. Environmental health specialists believe that most injuries are predictable and preventable and can be studied using epidemiological methods just like any illness or other condition.

Epidemiological data indicates that there are some vulnerable groups in the community who are more exposed to trauma and injury. This depends on the person's age, socio-economic status, kind of work, living conditions, hobbies and interests, culture, etc.

Some cultures believe that injury is the result of fate. In some cultures we view risky behaviour as brave or adventuresome in contrast with too cautious behaviour, which is viewed as dull or cowardly. What type of risk taking behaviour can you identify? Why do you think these individuals or groups display such behaviour?

One way of describing the prematurity of death is the calculation of Potential Years of Life Lost (PYLL). The age at which a death occurs is subtracted from the standard age (usually 65) and the difference is the number of premature or productive years of life that were lost due to the young death. Injuries account for a enormous amount of PYLL even in comparison to other leading causes of death.

12.19 Psychosocial aspects of heath and the environment

Reducing psychosocial problems plays a vital role in health and environmental issues, as the link between psychological and physical health is strong. However, this issue is often disregarded in literature in which environmental management issues, as well as health and environmental aspects, are addressed.

Many of the psychological problems modern people experience are directly or indirectly related to how their environment impacts on them. Not only does poor psychological health make people generally more susceptible to many communicable and chronic diseases, but there are numerous other problems that accompany poor psychological health (for example psychosomatic diseases, suicide, substance abuse, stresses, mental illness and violent behaviours).

Psychological aspects also indirectly influence the environment, for example a depressed person or a highly stressed person often could not care less about preserving and conserving the environment. Children who have not been environmentally oriented and who have not learnt the value of conservation would probably not learn or adapt to conservation ideas when they are adults.

Increasingly, housing in urban settings fails to serve the role of psychosocial havens because overcrowding and the stresses of urban life produce exactly the opposite effect of what one would expect. In fact, urban housing with its model of individual family homes (transplanted from the developed world to communities all over the globe), often tends to break down traditional community structures that existed in rural environments, increasing individual alienation. The urban poor have the additional burden of living in insecure tenant situations and being subject to exploitation in their housing environments. All of these problems are experienced most keenly by those making the transition from rural to urban life. The trend towards urbanization makes this a problem that needs urgent attention.

Occupational stresses, such as noise levels, exposure to traffic, workload, vibrations and unhygienic conditions, to name but a few, contribute to psychological problems which, in turn, create situations which could be hazardous to the person him-/herself and the environment (for example mechanical errors causing potentially dangerous situations, violent behaviour, aggression and the many psychological consequences of stress). All these aspects may in turn lead to physical injury or diseases, or both.

12.19.1 Psychosocial hazards

Uncertainty, anxiety and a lack of feeling in control over one's own life situation or environment lead to what is popularly called stress. The word stress has many meanings.

Stress
Stress is a multidimensional phenomenon. Reducing the detrimental effects of stress is best accomplished by modifying many varied aspects in lifestyle, both occupationally, environmentally and personally. This modification involves reducing the stressfulness of interactions with the environment, other people and self.

Stress is a growing topic of interest because it impacts on both unique high-demand performance environments and everyday settings. There are a large number of applied settings that share the commonality of a potential high-stress, high-demand performance environment. These include, among others, parachuting, military operations, aviation, bomb disposal, diving, firefighting and police work. These stereotypical high-stress environments impose a particularly high demand on those who work or play in them and in which there is a substantial potential for risk, harm or error. It is in the interest of society that individuals who work in these occupations should perform their jobs effectively under the high demands in which they are exposed.

Stress also occurs in more everyday settings, for example working in an office, driving home, going on holiday, attending a funeral, and so on. Stressors that occur in an individual's day-to-day life, include noise, performance pressure, anticipatory threat, time pressure, task load, group pressure, among others. Stress is an unavoidable fact of life. What is more, much of it is *eustress*, or *good stress*, and quite a high degree of it is essential to keep people active and fully functioning.

Burnout
Burnout is the term used for describing the cummulative stress a person experiences. This type of stress could be due to environmental factors such as excessive noise, irritating smells, sights and so on, or could be attributed to interpersonal relations such as work stressors, family stressors and all those 'small' but accumulative aspects that build up in the individual to cause major crises later.

Critical incident stress
This kind of stress is attributed to any overwhelming experience a person has experienced, witnessed or heard of. Examples are stress experienced during war, riots, violence, or acts such as rape, disasters, and so on. Critical incident stress often leads to post-traumatic stress.

Post-traumatic stress
This is a psychiatric condition after experiencing a critical incident. It is a severe and debilitating psychiatric disease and usually long-term psychiatric treatment and care are required.

12.19.2 Maintaining mental health
There is a growing interest in issues of maintaining mental health and reducing the detrimental effects that may lead to stress in the workplace, as well as in the personal life of the community. Attention is now paid to the health (and inevitably the cost) implications of stress of workers within industrial societies, more specifically the susceptibility of individuals involved in the *'dangerous trades'* or *'critical trades'*. Creating optimal conditions at work leads to workers who can face life with competence and hardiness. In turn, *working with joy* is physically healthy, psychologically invigorating and career enhancing, as well as highly beneficial to the employing organization. On the other hand, when optimal conditions do not exist, it is possible to carry on too long and to wear the workforce out to the point of dangerous exhaustion which can destroy their physical, psychological and social health. Thus, the focus is on the creation of optimal conditions by organizations for the promotion of eustress for individuals and groups and the limiting of conditions for distress.

Most descriptions of the term *stress* reveal three statements, namely that stress is:
- A response to a perceived threat, inordinate demands, challenge or change
- A physical and psychological response to any demand
- A state of psychological and physical arousal.

Occupational health

The common element of these definitions is that stress is a response to something in the environment (a stressor). When this environment changes, the individual changes. In addition to the above, stress must be understood in the context of the person–environment relationship, especially the perceptions the individual has of the stressors. The weight of this understanding is placed in the cognitive domain, or how the individual attaches meaning to the environmental stressors that he/she perceives. Stress, in general, is a mind-body arousal that, on the one hand, saves an individual's life, but on the other hand can fatigue the body and the soul to the point of malfunction and disease. Stress is a natural or normal defence mechanism that allows the human species to survive.

Stress is the balance between the external demands (stressors) on an individual and the individual's capacity to cope with those demands at any given time. A person's stress level can be reduced in one of the following ways:
- Decrease the severity of external stressors or
- Increase the ability to cope (compensate).

Although numerous definitions of stress have been advanced, it has been posited that it refers to a disrupted interaction between the environmental demands and the skills needed of the individual (Everstine & Everstine, 1993). Whereas extreme events have not featured extensively in stress research, they do in fact fall within the ambit of the field of stress. According to this view, extreme events constitute a severely disrupted interaction between the environment and the individual. Thus, although the concept of stress has a wider meaning, stress and trauma are not distinct concepts but exist on a continuum with relatively mild events and extreme situations found at either end.

Traumatic events may vary according to their suddenness, controllability, duration of damage and the extent of damage and destruction. The magnitude and type of events are often seen in wars, disasters or overwhelmingly violent or destructive situations.

Trauma reactions differ from stress in that trauma is usually incident-specific or event-specific and depends on the personal significance which the individual attaches to the event. Traumatizing stress is a special kind of stress that places more emphasis on shock and alarm than normal stressful events.

12.19.3 Stressors

A stressor is an event, a situation, a person or an object that is perceived as a stressful element and induces the stress reaction as a result. Stressors can vary widely in nature, ranging from psychosocial and behavioural sources such as frustration, anxiety and overload to bio-ecological and physical sources including noise, pollution, temperature and nutrition. Anticipation and imagination can also act as stressors and trigger the stress reaction. Examples include:
- Exceptionally challenging organizational change, such as renewal processes or radical changes in technology, reorganization, restructuring and re-engineering, produces relentless pressure in volumes of work and lack of job security.
- Large-scale sociopolitical changes (such as in post-1994 South African politics) create inordinate demands through re-alignments of values, social, economical, educational and cultural shifts and transformations.

Many psychosocial factors involved in the environment (e.g. housing) can be encountered, for example:
- Living space provides no privacy, builds no self-esteem
- Unsafe working and living conditions
- Recreational space limited
- Noise and other pollutants
- Violent behaviour
- Economic climate
- 'Life in the fast lane' (vehicles, transportation).

12.20 Biological hazards and their effects on health

Biological hazards include all the forms of life that can cause adverse affects on the health of an individual or a population. These hazards are plants, insects, rodents and other animals, fungi, bacteria, viruses, and a wide variety of toxins and allergens. Often the term 'biohazard' is mentioned – this is a combination of the words 'biological hazard' and refers to plants, animals or their products that may present a potential risk to the health and safety of human beings.

The biological environment encompasses the following:
- Infectious agent of the disease
- Reservoirs of infection, such as human beings, animals, plant matter, soil, water in which infectious agents normally live and multiply – these reservoirs are closely related to the transmission cycle of the agent in nature, in other words, to provide shelter for and to transport the agent to a susceptible host
- Vectors that may transmit diseases, such as fleas, mosquitoes and lice
- Plants and animals which may be sources of food, antigens or medicines.

The identification and classification of biohazards are important tools that health professionals and environmentalists use to decide on the appropriate safeguards and actions in health and environmental issues.

The five classes of biohazard are:

Class 1. These are agents of no or minimal hazard (under ordinary conditions or handling) that can be handled safely without special apparatus or equipment, using techniques generally acceptable for non-pathogenic materials. This class includes all bacterial, fungal, viral, rickettsial, chlamydia and parasitic agents not included in the higher classes.

Class 2. These are agents of ordinary potential hazard and include agents that may produce disease of varying degrees of severity though accidental inoculation, injection or other means of cutaneous penetration, but which can usually be adequately and safely contained by ordinary laboratory techniques.

Class 3. These are agents involving special hazards, or agents derived from outside the country that require special permits for importation. This class requires special handling.

Class 4. These are agents that require the most stringent conditions for containment because they are extremely hazardous to people and may cause a serious epidemic.

Class 5. These agents are foreign animal pathogens that are excluded from the country of origin.

There are some basic agent characteristics that are influential in disease causation, for example:
- Infectivity, which is the ability of the organism to spread rapidly from the host to another organism or host. High infectivity is not necessarily associated with the severity of disease.
- Invasiveness, which refers to the agent's ability to spread within the host.
- Virulence, which is the ability to produce severe disease.
- Dosage, which refers to the fact that multiple organisms invading the host are more apt to overwhelm host defences, whereas smaller numbers of the same organism are frequently suppressed or tolerated without the disease occurring.

12.21 The effects of war

The devastations and destruction of war are known to many in the world. Those who have not been confronted with the terrible consequences of war, cannot begin to realize what it entails. War is one of the most destructive actions of human activity and it is not only people who suffer – the environment becomes a casualty as well. Besides the mortalities due to war injuries, diseases break out and the environment is destroyed.

The following are some of the consequences of war:
- Modern weaponry and warfare strike directly at the economic and logistic ability of a society to make war.
- It is estimated that civilian deaths comprise 90 per cent of total deaths during a war.
- Strategic sources are destroyed during war (e.g. scorched-earth strategies).
- Refugees are used as a strategy of the army to occupy conquered territory (displaced civilians).
- Large movements of distressed people reflect profound human tragedy, create problems of public health and primary healthcare services, lead to overcrowding and overstretched services.
- Education is denied, people grow up in an unstable, often unfamiliar society.
- Scavenging for food and firewood may cause local ecological damage.
- Chemical, biological or nuclear warfare contaminates the environment for generations to come.

Terrorism is a type of warfare that is an increasing concern of the world community. Terrorists injure or kill a relatively small number of people, but they cause a climate of fear that leads to serious psychological problems and social disruption. Terrorists depend on the anxiety of the population to achieve their goals and are becoming more and more sophisticated in their efforts.

The threat of terrorism to health is well illustrated by the incident that occurred in a subway in Tokyo in 1995, where the nerve gas sarin was used and caused the death of more than a dozen people and injured more than a thousand.

Another type of terrorism is emerging, called ecological vandalism. These terrorists take revenge and destroy the ecology, for example the oil fields in Kuwait that were set alight by Iraqi troops after their defeat in the Gulf War. This act of terrorism resulted in massive air pollution.

The degree of imbalance between the needs (psychological, social, security, etc.) of a population and the local services available to meet these needs causes disruption after a war. In fact, for every type of disaster, certain standard problems need to be understood, plans need to be made and standards set to cope with different types of disaster. In the following diagram, the imbalance between a population's needs and the essential services are illustrated.

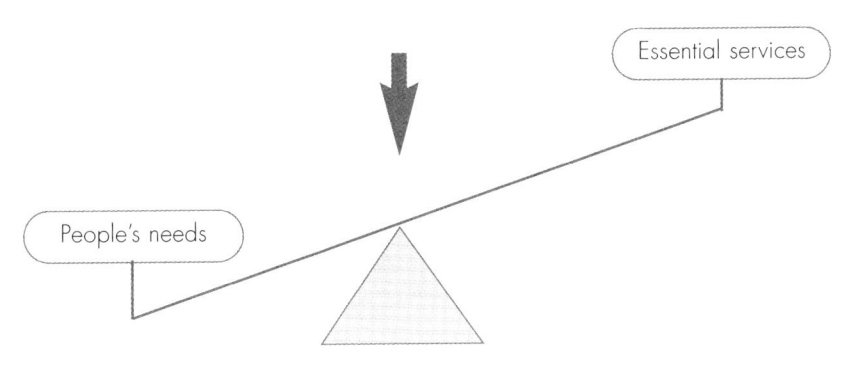

Increase in needs associated with:
- An increase in population
- An increase in morbidity due to insanitary conditions
- Appearance of new needs, for example treatment of war wounds.

Deterioration in effectiveness of services:
- Insufficient means
- Abandonment of facilities by personnel
- Disrupted organization
- Destruction of medical facilities

Figure 12.2 Imbalance between population's needs and the essential services

The untold misery and pain of war, as well as the destruction of plant and animal life, have been highlighted in this section.

12.22 Impact of disasters on health and well-being

A disaster is a catastrophic situation in which the day-to-day patterns of life are disrupted and people are plunged into helplessness and suffering and, as a result, need protection, water food, clothing, shelter, medical and social care, and the other necessities of life.

Natural disasters are extreme or violent acts of nature and can be divided into the following categories, namely:
- Drought
- Famine
- Earthquakes
- Floods
- High winds (cyclone, hurricane, storm, typhoon)
- Landslides
- Volcanoes
- Others (avalanches, cold waves, epidemics, food shortages, heat waves, tsunamis).

Some of the disasters caused by human beings are the following:
- Accidents (transport accidents, structural collapse)
- Technology accidents (chemical, nuclear, mine explosive, chemical atmospheric, oil pollution)
- Fires (forest, bush fires).

Earthquakes result from continuous geological transformations in our planet. According to the latest theories, the tectonic plates of which the world's surface consists are in constant movement. Earthquakes occur near the sites of friction between these plates.

A particularly dangerous phenomenon is the *tsunami* (Marmota), a great wave as much as several metres high that crashes down on the coasts as a result of an earthquake on the ocean bed. Sometimes it engulfs people who have fled toward the beaches. A tsunami may cross the ocean and crash down onto beaches thousands of kilometres away.

The effects of earthquakes are simply and effectively epitomized in scale of intensity.

It is very difficult to foretell the date and intensity of an earthquake but a few recent successes in that regard provide some hope. At present, however, no reliable and generally accepted method of forecasting is available. An earthquake takes place after gradual accumulation of energy connected with subterranean stresses accompanied by important geological changes that may be noted over a period of a few weeks, months or even years before the actual quake. Some phenomena can be observed by the public:
- The water level in wells is subject to sudden fluctuations and there are variations in the temperature, level and turbidity of deep underground water.
- Premonitory shocks (foreshock) may precede the main shock by anything from a few minutes to hundreds of days.

Other premonitory signs can be detected by means of scientific instruments.

Among the types of disaster, floods are by far the most serious in terms of human lives and property. Plains liable to flooding always attract settlement: ease of tillage, water supply, transport and waste disposal. It is because of the concentration of the population on alluvial plains that floods are one of the most deadly natural phenomena. The Yangtze floods of 1931 killed over 3 million people by drowning or famine. The WHO was called upon more recently still – in 1982 – to intervene in the same region. The causes of floods are:

- Rises in stream levels resulting from abundant rainfall or heavy snow melting
- Ice barrages (the piling-up of large masses of ice coming from upstream) that cause stream levels to rise, and the sudden break-up of the masses of ice, which is responsible for flood waves
- Flash floods caused by intense rainfall and sometimes tornadoes
- Tidal waves
- Storm waves, caused by a combination of lunar tides and very high winds.

Hydrologists and meteorologists can forecast floods with a high degree of accuracy. In every zone exposed to flood risks it is possible to know in general terms the time of year, frequency, rate of flow, duration and depth of a rise in the water level. More specifically, a flood can be predicted from a few hours to a few weeks in advance. Various methods of observation make it possible to give warning in various ways: by radio, television, newspapers, telephone message, megaphones, sirens, flags. Continuity of information and keeping the public in areas at risk constantly aware of the danger are very important.

Volcanic activity may range from fumaroles or moderate lava flows up to violent explosions that project various types of material to a great height. The nature of the activity depends on the viscosity of the magma (molten rock) that reaches the surface and on the volume of gases involved:

Streams of lava vary greatly in volume, spread, thickness and speed of progression. Their path depends on the topography; while they are very impressive, they represent very little risk.

Explosions of volcanic domes eject volcanic materials: volcanic bombs, blocks, lapilli, ash and scoria.

Ignimbrite flows, consisting of a mixture of lava, ash and gas, form a cloud that moves at ground level at great speed.

Nuées ardentes or hot avalanches are mixtures of volcanic materials and gases that hurtle down the slopes at over 100 km/h. A *nuée ardente* killed some 30 000 people at Saint-Pierre in Martinique during the eruption of Mont Pelée.

Mud streams, a mixture of debris and water, arising, for example, from the sudden melting of glaciers (23 000 dead in Colombia in 1985) or bursting of the banks of artificial lakes in the crater, flow down the slopes at speeds of up to 100 km/h and may cover stretches of hundreds of kilometres; they are very deadly.

Clouds of volcanic gases (sulfuric, carbonic or fluoric acid) may contaminate water and crops, inflict burns and suffocate human beings and animals.

Volcanic eruptions leave a trail of destruction and death on the path of lava and mud streams and *nuées ardentes* and in areas on which volcanic matter falls. Fires break out, roofs collapse under the weight of the ash, and water and plants are contaminated. Sometimes eruptions are preceded or accompanied by earthquakes.

To envisage the type and intensity of a future eruption, the best approach is to proceed by analogy with previous eruptions of the same volcano. A map of the volcano may make it possible to predict the paths of lava flows. The previous periodicity of the eruptions of a volcano, if any, can serve as a very general guide for predicting a new eruption. Some eruptions are preceded by changes in behaviour of the femoralis or hot springs on the mountain: the appearance of new features, an increase in temperature, changes in the composition of the gases. In other cases there are magnetic changes before an eruption. Some agitation can often be seen among animals. Scientific monitoring of the deformations (upswellings) of the ground and the shocks that accompany volcanic activity is very important. By combining these observations the specialist can predict eruptions, sometime with astonishing accuracy (the eruption of Mauna Loa in Hawaii in 1942).

Tropical cyclones or hurricanes show a regular seasonal tendency. Every year they claim numerous victims and cause great damage. For example, in November 1970 a cyclone laid waste Eastern Pakistan (now Bangladesh), with a death toll of over 300 000. Cyclones originate over the sea in the tropics, particularly towards the end of summer. A cyclone has a central zone, its 'eye', with a diameter varying from 20 to 150 km. Around this calm centre the violent winds move clockwise in the southern hemisphere and anticlockwise in the northern.

The winds generated and accelerated by the difference in pressure between the centre and the periphery may blow at up to 300 km/h. The destructive power of cyclones is due to the force of the winds, to intense and prolonged rainfall, which may also cause watercourses to flood and to tidal waves driven along by the winds to hurl themselves onto the coasts. Cyclones move westwards and die out when they reach land or colder sea surfaces.

Cyclone detection is based on weather radar, satellite data and even messages from airlines. Meteorologists can predict their intensity and path, often with a high degree of accuracy. However, allowance must be made for the possibility of error, since cyclones may follow a very irregular path. In countries liable to cyclones, warning is given by the authorities, generally in radio or television broadcasts. The warnings are followed by bulletins confirming, refining or cancelling them.

Drought and its fearsome consequences, desertification and famine, result from a combination of several factors:
- A reduction in rainfall, causing a shortage of water
- A reduction in vegetation, erosion of the soil, surface evaporation
- An increase in human and animal populations
- Political and technological decisions at national and international levels.

In rural communities, economic factors (type of agriculture) and social elements (nomadism, semi-nomadism, drift of population towards the towns, etc.) affect the health and survival of families and, moreover, have an impact on the desertification process.

It is generally accepted that the struggle against desertification must be waged in two complementary ways: on the one hand, appropriate political and technical measures must be taken at national and international level, and on the other hand there must be a continuous process of information, education and organization in the local communities. As part of this process, the role of the local health personnel is to develop programmes of prevention and to adopt methods of health action based on community participation and self-organization. Voluntary workers and Red Cross workers can make an important contribution here.

Knowledge of the risks to life and health to which the community is exposed can be acquired in various ways and to different degrees of detail. As part of national plans, local plans can be prepared by the community to deal with emergency situations. These plans can make use of special risk maps (e.g. earthquake, hydrogeological or volcanic zoning). In most cases, however, in the absence of plans, the community can ascertain the risks by periodically enlisting the support of various social groups. Even if this does not result in real plans, it is a valid means of preparing for emergency situations, for during these risk-ascertaining activities the problem is also tackled of what would have to be done and what resources would have to be used if the emergency actually arose.

Who carries out the activities?
- Personnel of the public services
- Police and fire brigade
- First-aid associations
- Associations, professional people, organized groups in the community
- The schools.

What risks are envisaged? Each group can consider the risks with which it is most closely concerned, such as:
- The collapse of flimsily built buildings
- The interruption of water in cases of floods, prolonged and heavy rainfall, tidal waves, cyclones, the failure of dams
- Fires (stocks of flammable materials, electrical short-circuits)
- Contamination of the soil, water and air by toxic products, which may spread in the event of an accident or disaster
- Explosions (stocks of gas, petrol or explosives)
- Landslides (in the case of an earthquake or prolonged rainfall)
- Damage from a volcanic eruption (examination of past experience)
- Breakdown of communications (telephone lines, lack of electricity)
- Isolation of the community because of roads becoming impassable.

The local health personnel can cooperate in ascertaining the risks, particularly by helping the groups mentioned above to recognize certain dangers already present in normal times but which a disaster may make more acute:
- Use of contaminated water and food
- Presence of insect disease vectors and rodents
- Poor environmental hygiene (disposal of refuse, sewage, etc.)
- Absence of latrines
- Lack of hygiene (personal, domestic, in markets)
- Harmful eating habits (meals poor in protein)
- Other.

These activities to determine the risks and resources are carried out in the following stages:

- The organizing group meets and discusses the risks it wishes to concern itself with.
- Visits to the sites exposed to risk and information meetings are arranged.
- The risks noted are discussed and possibly indicated on a map of the area visited.
- The resources available to the community in case of disaster are listed.
- Initiatives to reduce the risks envisaged are proposed and efforts are made to put them into effect with the cooperation of other community bodies.

When an area is under an imminent threat of disaster (flood, cyclone, tidal wave, volcanic eruption, mass industrial accident), the competent authorities may order the evacuation of the population. The community's emergency committee will be able to cooperate in the evacuation if it knows the details of how it will be carried out:
- The evacuation routes and the other routes that could be used if one or more of the planned routes became impracticable
- The means of transport by land, water or air
- The sites to which the evacuees can be taken and given shelter
- Arrangements to supply water, food and other necessities.

In the case of evacuation the local health personnel must concern themselves with ensuring, under the best possible conditions and with the collaboration of the families, the marshalling and transport of the sick, the disabled, the handicapped and other vulnerable persons. They will collaborate in providing the population with accurate information regarding the reasons for the evacuation and the ways in which it is to be carried out. They will help to reunite families. They will organize a health post on the site chosen for providing temporary shelter and from the post busy themselves with every aspect of managing the health problems that follow a disaster.

12.23 Multidimensional diagnostic strategies

The ultimate goal of studying the relationship between health and environmental hazards is to do something to reduce or eliminate those hazards. The first step is to assess the effects of exposure of environmental hazards on people, and the potential hazards of the exposure. Many sources refer to this process as risk assessment, which leads to risk management, which in turn is an integrated environmental management approach.

In recent years increased attention has been given to the use of epidemiological principles to eliminate potential health risks. The environmental impact assessment (predictive analysis) and environmental audit (analysis of the existing situation) have become legal requirements in many countries. The health component of these activities is one of the important applications of risk management. Such assessment is also used to predict potential health problems in the use of new chemicals or technologies. The term 'risk management' is applied to the planning and implementation of actions to reduce or eliminate the health risk.

12.23.1 Steps in the assessment of health risk

Identify the hazard

In Figure 12.3 the steps in the assessment of health risks are given. The first step is to identify hazards, as obtained from the epidemiological data and/or the toxicological information relevant to the problem. This is regarded as the quantitative analysis of the problem. During this identification phase, the following information with regard to the hazard is obtained:

- What type of hazard is it? (For example, is it a chemical hazard?)
- If so, which specific chemical (or chemicals) is/are involved?
- Are biological, psychological, accident, physical hazards involved?
- If so, what are they?

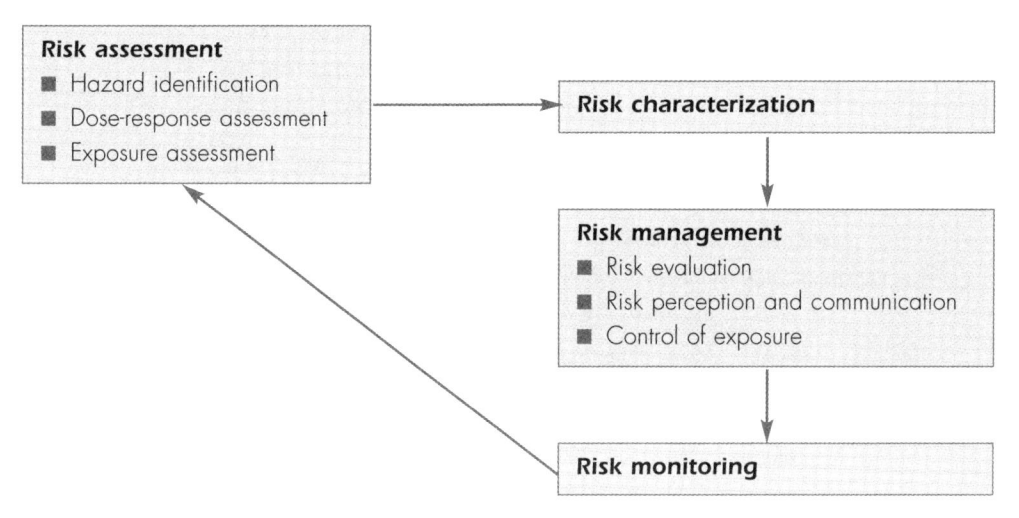

Figure 12.3 *Risk assessment and management framework*

Hazard assessment (also called dose-response assessment)

The second step is the analysis of the type of health effect that each hazard may cause (hazard assessment). The information can be obtained from the following sources:

- Reviewing scientific literature
- Studies completed of people exposed to the hazard
- Epidemiological information
- Animal research studies.

Exposure assessment

The third step is to measure or estimate the actual exposure levels for the people potentially affected (for example in Chapter 4 the TLV of a substance was described), including the general public and the workforce. The human exposure assessment should take into account environmental monitoring, biological monitoring and relevant information about history of exposure and changes over time.

Risk management
From the information received from steps one to four, the action plan is formulated, which is the way forward or the risk management. Risk management involves three main steps. First, estimates of health risk need to be evaluated in relation to a predetermined 'acceptable risk' or in relation to other health risks in the same community. Maximum exposure limits, public health targets, or other policy instruments for health protection are often used in this process. The fundamental question is: Is it necessary to take preventive action because the estimated health risk is too high?

If it is decided that preventive action is needed, the second step in risk management is to reduce exposure. This may involve changing the process to eliminate certain hazards, installing equipment to control pollution, resisting proposed hazardous projects, etc.

Thirdly, risk management also involves the monitoring of exposure and health risks after selected controls have been put into place. It is important to ensure that the intended protection is achieved and that any additional protective measures are taken without delay. In this phase of risk management, human exposure assessments and epidemiological surveys play an important role.

12.23.2 The Health Environment Impact Assessment (EIA)
EIA is a practical process to identify, assess and mitigate the environmental and health effects of major industrial, agricultural and other large developmental projects before they occur. The guidelines have been prepared by various international organizations. Multidisciplinary collaboration is crucial to EIA. It is important to ensure that the health components at each stage of the assessment are addressed.

12.23.3 Evaluating environmental measures
Risk management is a partly scientific quantitative exercise in which the results of a risk assessment are compared with standards, guidelines or comparable risks. From this comparison, and knowing the assumptions, extrapolations and estimates that go into the two numbers in the comparison, an environmental health professional can determine whether a significant risk is present. However, the perception of a risk by the individual or community facing the risk must also be taken into account. The manner in which the risk is communicated will also affect the risk perception as will the effectiveness of communicating the plans for and results of exposure control.

12.23.4 Risk assessment and management framework
After a risk is evaluated, and the exposure is controlled as appropriate, the risk must be monitored. Although sometimes the problem can be solved, usually the process is an iterative one with the risk having to be re-assessed and the community perception re-evaluated on a continual basis. In reality, the risk assessment and management may be carried out simultaneously.

12.23.5 Factors affecting the perception and acceptance of risk
The perception of the public and the health and environmental professionals are often quite different from each other with regard to a health risk. When dealing with

environmental issues, the attitude and feelings of the public must be taken into account at all times.

12.24 Conclusion

Virtually every aspect of the environment may affect the physical and/or mental status of human beings in some way, either positively or negatively. The responsibility of the occupational health provider never ends at the factory wall – indeed as this chapter has shown, it extends far beyond. It is only through knowledge and insight in the global picture of the interaction between human beings and their environment that the total picture of health unfolds.

Health is only possible where resources are available to meet human needs and where the living and working environment are protected from life-threatening and health-threatening pollutants, pathogens and physical hazards. Similarly, if the health team (medical and nursing in particular) focused on secondary healthcare delivery only, the total healthcare provision would be doomed. In the past, preventive medicine and environmental issues received minimal attention compared with the views of today. Attention was mostly directed at the medical model, and very few environmental issues were included in the curricula of medical, nursing and other professional health practitioners.

Lack of response by institutions to organize appropriate retaining courses has disadvantaged practitioners and professionals. A lack of insight to re-curriculate to incorporate the needed courses in order to produce outcome-based products for the tasks on hand is now being corrected, and previously ignored participants in health and well-being, the community, are being brought into the picture. The changed system of education has also led to an awareness among health professionals to work together as a team, whereas previously they worked in their own secluded environments with little effort to collaborate. At last the skills and knowledge of healthcare professionals such as doctors and nurses are being recognized, and healthcare delivery systems, such as the sciences that were not thought to be related are receiving proper attention in the protection of the environment and the prevention of diseases.

12.25 Bibliography

Doods, F. & Middleton, T. (eds.) *Earth Summit 2002: A New Deal*. London: Eartscan.
Epidemiological comments, September 1999 Vol 1 No 3.
Everstine, D. S. & Everstine, L. 1993. *The Trauma Response: Treatment for Emotional Injury*. New York: Norton.
Fuggle, R. F. & Rabie, M. A. (eds.) 1999. Environmental Management in South Africa. Cape Town: Juta.
Hugo, M. L., Viljoen, A. T. & Meeuwis, J. M. 1997. *The Ecology of Natural Resource Management: The Quest for Sustainable Living: A Text for South African Students*. Pretoria: Kagiso.

Last, J. M. 1995. *A Dictionary of Epidemiology.* 3rd edition. Cape Town: Oxford University Press.

Mainguet, M. 1991. *Desertification: Natural Background and Human Mismanagement.* Berlin: Springer.

Maslow, A. H. 1971. *The Farther Reaches of Human Nature.* New York: Viking Press.

McKinney, M. L. & Schoch, R. M. 2003. *Environmental Science: Systems and Solutions.* 3rd edition. Boston: Jones & Bartlett.

Tamburlini, F. 2002. Children's Health and Environment: A Review of Evidence/A Joint Report from the European Environment Agency and the WHO. Copenhagen: Office for official publications of the European Communities.

World Health Organization. 1986. Health Research Strategy for Health by the Year 2000. Geneva: WHO.

World Health Organization. 1995. The National Health Information System of South Africa (NHISSA): from Start to Implementation. Geneva: HO.

World Health Organization. 1993. Community Action for Health. Report and Documentation of the Technical Discussions of the 46th Session of the WHO Regional Committee for South-East Asia. New Dehli: WHO

Addenda and appendices

The following extracts from addenda are included in **Chapter 2** to provide a framework of information for the occupational health worker.

ADDENDUM 1

THE NATIONAL DRUG POLICY

1 INTRODUCTION

A National Drug Policy (NDP) was introduced in January 1996. In this, the Minister of Health states that the goal of the policy is to fully develop the potential that drugs have to improve health status within the available resources in a country. It covers a wide range of activities which contribute to the effective production, supply, storage, distribution and use of medicines.

The NDP was developed to achieve the goal of serving the total community, taking cognizance of the prevailing economic, social and health conditions in this country. The policy has been formulated to ensure an adequate and reliable supply of safe, cost-effective drugs of acceptable quality to all citizens of South Africa and the rational use of drugs by prescribers, dispensers and consumers.

The occupational health professional must have an overall knowledge of the National Drug Policy. He/she must actively participate in the initiation, review and modification of the policy. To be ignorant about the overall policy on drugs and other related health matters has serious ethical and legal consequences for the occupational healthcare worker.

2 OBJECTIVES OF THE NDP

2.1 Health objectives

- To ensure the availability and accessibility of essential drugs to all citizens
- To ensure safety, efficiency and quality of drugs
- To ensure good dispensing and prescribing practices
- To promote the rational use of drugs by prescribers, dispensers and patients through the provision of training, education and information
- To promote the concept of individual responsibility for health, preventive care and informed decision-making

2.2 Economic objectives
- To lower the cost of drugs in both the private and public sectors
- To promote the cost-effective and rational use of drugs
- To establish a complementary partnership between the Government bodies and private providers in the pharmaceutical sector
- To optimize the use of scarce resources through cooperation with international and regional agencies

2.3 National development objectives
- To promote the knowledge, efficiency and management skills of pharmaceutical personnel
- To reorient medical, paramedical and pharmaceutical education towards the principles underlying the National Drug Policy
- To support the development of the local pharmaceutical industry and the local production of essential drugs
- To promote the acquisition, documentation, and sharing of knowledge and experience through the establishment of advisory groups in rational drug use, pharmaco-economics and other areas of the pharmaceutical sector.

3 LEGISLATION AND REGULATIONS
It is envisaged that the Medicines Control Council (MCC) will be strengthened, drug registration will be rationalized, the registration of practitioners will be controlled and the premises where drugs will be kept, will be licensed. Furthermore, the laboratory functions and inspectorate of drugs will be enhanced and other quality assurance measures will be implemented to promote rational drug use, distribution, prescription and control.

3.1 Medicines Control Council
The MCC plays an important and prominent role in facilitating the harmonization of drug regulation and control in southern Africa. This process will include:
- Sharing of review decisions and exchanging of evaluation reports without compromising confidentiality
- Adoption of criteria for drug evaluation and of good manufacturing practice
- Promoting the use of the WHO certification Scheme for the Quality of Pharmaceutical participation and collaboration in international commerce.

3.2 Registration of drugs and supplies
Only drugs which are registered in South Africa may be imported, produced, stored, exported and sold. Licences to dispense drugs will be reviewed annually.

The current drug registration procedure will be adapted to meet the needs within the policy framework. Formal procedures for registration based on quality, efficacy and safety will be upgraded through the introduction or strengthening of:
- A five-year relicensing system for drugs
- Computerization of the evaluation system
- An evaluation report exchange system with reputable regulatory bodies in other countries

- Prioritization of registrations, based on needs – fast-track procedures for essential drugs
- Norms and standards for registration of medical devices.

Special attention will be given to the needs of healthcare providers in primary healthcare environments. This step may include rescheduling of certain drugs to improve patient access to appropriate treatment.

3.3 Registration of practitioners

It is clearly stated in the NDP that only practitioners who are registered with the relevant Council and premises that are registered and/or licensed in terms of the Medicines and Related Substances Control Amendment Act, 1997 (No 90 of 1997) may be used for the manufacture, supply and dispensing of drugs. Medical practitioners and nurses will not be permitted to dispense drugs except where separate pharmaceutical services are not available. In such instances or situations where dispensing by doctors and nurses has to take place, such persons will be in possession of a dispensing licence, issued by the MCC. Criteria for the granting of such licences will include, inter alia, the application of geographic limits.

Special concessions will be granted with regard to certain categories of providers such as occupational health services. Proven competency of such persons to dispense drugs will be by virtue of the successful completion of a suitable training programme. All licences will be reviewed annually. The inspection functions will be delegated to the provinces.

The retail trade in drugs will be confined to a licensed place for the sale of drugs, which by virtue of its staffing can provide a comprehensive pharmaceutical service. Where it is deemed to be in the interests of the public, and provided that comprehensive pharmaceutical care is ensured, ownership of pharmacies by lay persons and other healthcare professionals, will be considered. Where non-pharmacist ownership is permitted, it will still be expected that the pharmacy be under the full-time management and supervision of a registered pharmacist.

Uniform norms and standards pertaining to the dispensing of drugs by different service providers, will be incorporated into one set of regulations.

3.4 Inspection

The MCC will provide an adequate and effective drug inspection service which will be conducted under the drug legislation and regulations. Most inspection functions (e.g. inspection of governmental depots, hospital stores, private dispensaries, dispensing doctors and nurses), will be devolved to provincial authorities, while a few specialized inspectoral functions, such as inspection of manufacturing facilities and wholesale services, will be retained at national level.

3.5 Drug quality control laboratory

A national drug quality control laboratory, linked to the MCC, will be established. The present system of contracting with universities will be retained until such a facility is available. The formal relations with the South African Bureau of Standards will be maintained.

3.6 Quality assurance

The following measures additional to those already described, will apply:

Guidelines for donated drugs to follow WHO guidelines for drug donations. Donated drugs will appear on the Essential Drug List and will be compatible with the overall governmental policy.

The marketing of traditional medicines will be investigated for safety and quality. Norms and standards will be set for medical devices and disposable items which appear on an Essential Equipment List. These items will also be evaluated.

Other information included in this document is drug pricing.

ADDENDUM 2

HIV/AIDS AND EMPLOYMENT: CODE OF GOOD PRACTICE
(Published with permission: AIDS Law Project, Centre for Applied Legal Studies, WITS)

In October 1995, the *HIV/Aids and Employment: Code of Good Practice* was compiled with the objective of including it in the Labour Relations Act, 1995 (No 66 of 1995). It is essential to read widely on HIV/Aids in the workplace (there are many authoritative texts available) and to obtain original publications from which one can determine one's own view. It is the task of the community health professional to keep abreast with developments in this field while taking cognizance of the policy of the industry in which he/she works. A brief discussion of the HIV/Aids Code of Good Practice follows.

1 INTRODUCTION

Aids is becoming a worldwide concern. There is at present no cure for this disease. It is especially important, given the scale of the South African epidemic, to introduce effective strategies to slow and prevent the transmission of HIV. The social impact of the HIV/Aids epidemic has important implications for the workplace as the employment policy should support and reflect the national response to the epidemic. The human immunodeficiency virus (HIV) has no boundaries, does not discriminate against social class, gender, race or creed and is today seen as one of the most serious health problems humanity has to face. It is also one of the most prominent aspects of ethical consideration in society and in the workplace. Yet there are many people in the community who still believe that it cannot happen to them – that they cannot be influenced by HIV/Aids, and there is unusual ambivalence, ignorance, prejudice and stigma surrounding the disease. This attitude not only hurts or influences the person who has Aids, but also his or her family, the community and the employer alike. It is in this light that it is of fundamental importance that HIV/Aids should be treated in all respects like any other comparable life-threatening condition. There is, however, a special obligation of the employer to negotiate and implement appropriate policy with employees and employer organizations.

In the light of the Government's policy on human rights, a committee was formed in 1993 to draft a Code of Practice on HIV/Aids for employers. The final draft of the *HIV/Aids and Employment: Code of Good Practice* is a result of wide-ranging consultation. The Code of Practice has been developed from the point of view of employment law and equity. It is in keeping with international standards, as well as with the prohibition of unfair discrimination on groups of disease or disability.

In this addendum, only a short summary of the *HIV/Aids and Employment: Code of Good Practice* will be given. The policy embodied in the Code can be adapted to meet the specific needs of different companies and industries. By implementing the Code in the workplace, discrimination is eliminated.

2 HIV/AIDS CONTACT

It has been said before that employees or prospective employees with HIV/Aids must not be treated differently from those with comparable life-threatening conditions. They must be treated in a just, humane and life-affirming way. It is therefore essential that these individuals continue their employment and it must be recognized that it may be therapeutic for an employee to be given educational and promotion opportunities.

The committee is of the opinion that in respect of employment capacity, risk of workplace transmission and entitlement to all the employment benefits, there are no relevant differences between HIV and any other life-threatening condition. Therefore, it is envisaged that no special burdens be placed on employees with HIV.

2.1 Recruitment, continued employment and termination of employment

Any medical examination undertaken either before employment (or thereafter) should be solely to determine functional performance, and offer a prognosis on the fitness for work of the prospective employee. In this respect:

2.1.1 An HIV test (or any other test intended to assess the immune/HIV status of the prospective employee) shall not be a precondition of employment and shall not be required under any circumstance or for any occupation, or position.

2.1.2 If a person makes his/her HIV status known voluntarily, it shall not be the basis for refusing to conclude or to continue or to renew an employment contract.

2.1.3 Employees with HIV shall be governed by the same contractual obligations as all other employees.

2.1.4 HIV shall not be used as a justification for the nonperformance of duties agreed to by the parties.

2.1.5 No employee shall be dismissed or have her/his employment terminated merely on the basis of HIV, nor shall HIV status influence retrenchment procedures.

2.2 Promotion, training and development

HIV status shall not be a criterion for refusing to promote, train and develop an employee.

2.3 Ill-health, leave and performance

2.3.1 An HIV test may not form an obligatory part of a medical examination.

2.3.2 Employees with HIV shall be governed without discrimination by agreed existing sick leave procedures. HIV shall not prejudice their entitlement to such leave.

2.3.3 Following an Aids diagnosis the parties concerned may agree jointly on a medical examination to determine the employee's ability to continue to perform her/his duties.

2.3.4 Where it has been decided that an employee with HIV/Aids can no longer perform her/his duties, the following steps may be taken after consultation and agreement:

2.3.4.1 Where possible, an employer should at the earliest opportunity undertake to find a position with duties that the employee can fulfil. The employee's remuneration will be adjusted according to the appropriate rates for the position without discrimination. There should also be a continuing entitlement to company benefits to which an employee was entitled before her/his disability compelled a change in position.

2.3.4.2 Termination of employment due to incapacity may be considered when an employee with Aids is too ill to continue employment, or where a position suitable to the state of health of the employee is unavailable. Should such a situation arise, the employee should continue to be entitled to relevant company benefits.

2.3.4.3 Termination of employment due to incapacity shall be governed without discrimination by the procedures pertaining to agreed conditions of employment.

2.3.4.4 No flags or symbols should be used on an employee's medical, personnel or other records to indicate HIV status.

3 BENEFITS

Employees with HIV are at present affected by unfair, prejudicial and discriminatory benefits policies. Refusing benefits to people with HIV – or other comparable life-threatening conditions – shifts the burden for their care onto the government. This will impact negatively on the economy as taxes will have to be raised to support public systems of care. In view of this, the responsibility falls on employers, employees and the government to create a visible non-discriminatory approach to benefits.

The following steps are critical to protect employees, entitlements and human rights:

3.1 An HIV test should not be a requirement for admission to company-controlled benefit schemes.

3.2 Group life assurance schemes should regard HIV like comparable life-threatening conditions when determining benefits.

3.3 Employees who are known to have HIV/Aids should have non-discriminatory access to employment benefits.

3.4 Employers, the State, private and public institutions are responsible for administering employee benefits such as:
- Medical aid and health-related benefits
- Group life assurance
- Pensions and provident funds – housing benefits
- Unemployment insurance
- Bursaries, training and study subsidies – disability and accident benefits as well as benefits relating to:
- Spouses, children and/or partners and dependants shall be responsible for ensuring that viable non-discriminatory policies are developed.

3.5 Where an employer is unable to ensure that non-discriminatory policies are followed, he/she should seek to ensure that the policies are changed or should find an agency which provides the same benefits on a non-discriminatory basis.

3.6 All relevant authorities shall ensure that delay in obtaining such benefits is reduced to a minimum.

4 GRIEVANCES AND DISCIPLINARY PROCEDURES

4.1 An employee with HIV has the same rights and the same duties as other employees.

4.2 Where discrimination occurs in consequence of an employee's HIV status, that person shall have recourse to agreed mechanisms and remedies for redress.

4.3 The employer of an employee with HIV may as in all other cases, enforce disciplinary procedures against the employee where there is evidence of an infringement of the employment contract.

5 HIV/AIDS AND SEXUALLY TRANSMITTED DISEASES (STDs)

EDUCATION AND PREVENTION: EMPLOYER AND EMPLOYEE RESPONSIBILITIES

5.1 Employers, employees and their respective organizations should agree on HIV/Aids education and prevention programmes and ensure that they are conducted at the workplace. These programmes must be conducted in appropriate languages, and take into account levels of education/literacy of the workforce.

5.2 Educational strategies shall be based on consultation between employers, employees, and their representative organizations and, where appropriate, government and non-government organizations with expertise in HIV/Aids education, counselling and care. Regular evaluation and reviews should be carried out and, where necessary, changes agreed upon by all parties.

5.3 Education is an important way of combating discrimination and irrational responses to HIV/Aids in the workplace. Attendance at such programmes should therefore be compulsory for all employees (including management) and should take place during paid working hours. Educational programmes must utilize strategies that are non-stigmatizing and that promote safe sex practices.

5.4 Education programmes shall inform employers and all employees of the provisions of employment codes on HIV/Aids and the rights and duties of persons with HIV/Aids. The (government-approved) Code of Good Practice should also be available in every workplace.

5.5 Employers and employees have a right to continuing education and information about the models of transmission of HIV, the means of preventing such transmission, the need for counselling and care, and the social impact of infection on those affected by HIV/Aids.

5.6 Special emphasis should be given to the vulnerability of women to HIV, and prevention strategies that can lessen this vulnerability.

5.7 Where possible, and if appropriate, employers should assist in providing education and support systems for the dependants of employees and surrounding communities.

5.8 Employers and employees should ensure that education programmes support the Department of Health's HIV/Aids and STD prevention campaign by making condoms, information brochures and details of local services for persons affected by HIV/Aids, available at the workplace.

6 TESTING

6.1 Pre-employment testing for HIV should not be permitted under any circumstance because it is:
- Discriminatory in that it stigmatizes prospective employees and infringes their human rights by excluding them from productive employment
- Costly and wasteful in that testing is expensive and diverts scarce resources from education and care
- Irrational because many people who are employed may already have contracted the virus or may contract the virus during employment.

6.2 Employers have no right to know the HIV status of an employee and company medical officers shall not be asked to carry out tests to determine this information for the company.

6.3 Testing for HIV shall be done only at request of an employee. Such testing shall be carried out by a suitably qualified person or institution and with observance of the following:
- Express informed consent (as required by the South African Health Professions Council in their Guidelines for the Management of Patients with HIV Infections and Aids) shall be obtained before a test for HIV is undertaken.
- No testing shall be done without pre-test and post-test counselling by a suitably qualified person.

6.4 Any testing for epidemiological purposes must be subject to agreement between employers, employees and their respective organizations and must preserve individual anonymity and not be used to discriminate against any group or category of employee.

7 CONFIDENTIALITY

7.1 Persons with HIV/Aids have the legal right to confidentiality about their HIV status.

Occupational health

7.2 An employee is under no obligation to inform an employer of her/his HWAids status.

7.3 Confidentiality regarding all medical information of an employee or prospective employee must be maintained, unless disclosure is legally required.

7.4 If an employee informs an employer of her/his HIV status this information shall not be disclosed to any other employee (including human resources and medical personnel) without that employee's written and express consent. A breach of confidentiality in this respect should be subject to disciplinary measures, which may include dismissal.

7.5 An employee's HIV status should not be required or reflected on any routine medical or personnel report.

7.6 The law does not require a death certificate to indicate if a person has died of an Aids-related illness. Employers should therefore not attempt to find out whether an employee has died of an Aids-related illness.

7.7 Trustees and administrators of benefit funds may not disclose the identity of a person with HIV to an employer without that person's express and informed consent.

8 COLLEAGUES, MANAGEMENT AND CLIENT FEARS

8.1 There is no medical or scientific justification for refusing to employ or work with someone who has HIV.

8.2 It is the responsibility of an employer in association with employee organizations to ensure that all employees are educated and in possession of facts relating to transmission of HIV/Aids. This will help to minimize discrimination and irrational fears.

8.3 In working areas where there is any possibility of accident, first-aid instructions should be prominently displayed explaining the universal precautions that need to be followed when dealing with blood. There should be proper training of staff to minimize hazards. Safe working conditions should be ensured and latex gloves should be included in all first-aid kits. Employees should be educated to treat every person as possibly HIV positive.

8.4 Refusal to work with an employee with HIV/Aids shall be regarded as a breach of the employment contract. In such a situation an employer shall have the right to institute disciplinary measures, including termination of employment, against such an employee.

9 MANAGEMENT, CARE AND COUNSELLING OF HIV/AIDS AT WORK

9.1 Except on rare occasions of occupational transmission in healthcare and allied professions, where appropriate compensation must be guaranteed, HIV is not a condition that is contracted at the workplace. Transmission is not caused by unsafe working conditions (except in the case of commercial sex work). Employers can generally therefore not be expected to compensate employees or their dependants if an employee contracts HIV.

9.2 However, it should be recognized that HIV/Aids affects, in the main, the economically active and that almost every workplace will be affected by the epidemic. Therefore:
- Employers and employee organizations should, if requested, assist an employee with HIV/Aids and her/his dependants to obtain professional counselling.
- Employers and employee bodies should help to ensure that an employee with HIV has access to appropriate medical care. Medical aid schemes should be pressurized to develop non-discriminatory 'protocols' that will guarantee appropriate and cost-effective care for people living with HIV.
- The cost of such care and counselling should in the first instance be reimbursed or borne by the appropriate medical scheme and/or health authority.
- Employees required to travel should be provided with condoms.
- Employers who depend upon migrant labour or long-distance travel operations should give assistance to HIV prevention work in the communities from where workers originate, or to where they are required to travel.

10 DISPUTE RESOLUTION

10.1 Employers, employees and their organizations are encouraged to develop and refine the principles in this Code of Good Practice into detailed HIV/Aids policies and programmes that are suited to the character of each particular workplace.

10.2 Any dispute between an employer and an employee in relation to or arising from the application of the Code should be subject to the process for conciliation established by the Labour Relations Act, 1995 (No 66 of 1995).

10.3 Where the alleged dispute remains unresolved it should be referred for arbitration to:
- A Bargaining Council if the parties to the dispute fall within the registered scope of that council.
- The Commission for Conciliation, Mediation and Arbitration (CCMA) if no council has jurisdiction.

10.4 Where a dispute concerns an allegation of unfair discrimination, or a question of law, it should be referred to the Labour Court.
- In such a matter the anonymity of the complainant shall, if so desired, be preserved.

ADDENDUM 3

NOTES ON THE PROHIBITION OF PRE-EMPLOYMENT TESTING FOR THE HUMAN IMMUNO-DEFICIENCY VIRUS (HIV) BILL

1 INTRODUCTION

The arguments developed below suggest that legal protection for job applicants with HIV is essential for the following reasons:

- A person with HIV is as fit and healthy as any other job applicant and can live a healthy and productive life for 10, 15 or more years before becoming ill.
- A non-discriminatory approach to HIV/Aids is essential to prevention efforts.
- Transmission in most occupational settings is impossible and where minimal risks exist, these can be eliminated with universal precautions.
- Wide-scale unnecessary testing is a direct infringement on the constitutional rights of prospective employees.
- The scale of the epidemic suggests that it is unjust and unjustifiable to deny up to 25 per cent of our population employment on the basis of their HIV status.

2 WHY IS LEGAL PROTECTION NECESSARY?

Increasingly applicants for jobs in the private sector, and certain parts of the public sector, are being required to furnish the result of an HIV test to their prospective employer, before employment is offered or confirmed. The majority of those who test positive for HIV are disqualified from employment.

Although the decision to have an HIV test should be a voluntary one, and cannot be imposed on any prospective employee, the context in which the test is required amounts to duress. A person who refuses to assent to an HIV test is unlikely to be employed.

As a result, many would-be employees are submitting to an HIV test, with little understanding of the implications of the test. They are being forced to surrender their rights to autonomy, dignity, privacy and confidentiality, and, if they prove to be HIV positive, to gainful employment. This is an affront to the spirit of the Bill of Rights in the Constitution of the RSA 1993 (Act 200 of 1993).

Pre-employment testing constitutes a form of mandatory testing and amounts to direct and unfair discrimination, which, if allowed to continue, will be practised against tens of thousands of people.

3 A NON-DISCRIMINATORY APPROACH

Unlike other life-threatening conditions, HIV/Aids already affects millions of people in our country. The most reliable studies suggest that 1.2 million people in South Africa have HIV. Every day 700 persons contract HIV. In our local townships as many as one in 10 people are estimated to have HIV.

The scale of the epidemic alone suggests that pre-employment testing will deny 10–25 per cent of our economically active population employment. This is not only discriminatory and stigmatizing, but will place an enormous burden on the welfare and social assistance services in the country. Instead, a non-discriminatory environment will assist with reducing risk behaviours and allow persons with HIV/Aids to be treated.

4 IS HIV TESTING EVER JUSTIFIED FOR EMPLOYMENT?

International practice, the policies of enlightened employers and their consultants affirm that pre-employment testing for HIV is unacceptable and irrational. An employer may legitimately exercise the power to request a medical examination to assess:
- The fitness of a job applicant to perform a specified task, or
- Whether an existing employee's incapacity or non-performance is due to ill health.

However, it is medically established that a person with HIV can live a full, productive and healthy life for 15 years or longer after acquiring the virus.

4.1 No risk of occupational transmission
In the vast majority of occupations there is virtually no risk of occupational transmission of HIV (that is, unless persons with HIV, or any untreated sexually transmitted disease, engage in unprotected sexual intercourse with a colleague).

The only situation where a very small chance of occupational transmission exists is in the health and allied professions, i.e. workers who come into contact with the blood of others. However, clear medical and professional guidelines exist for preventing transmission in these.

4.2 Circumstances
In this regard, the Jansen van Vuuren & Kruger (1993 (4) SA 842) decision is instructive. The Appellate Division endorsed expert medical evidence that the risk to healthcare workers (who are almost always exposed to blood) of occupational transmission of HIV was 'small', and that elementary precautions could usually eliminate that risk. Mr Justice Harms stated on behalf of a unanimous five-judge court: Even though the virus is highly infective, it is far less infectious than many other common viruses and can only be transmitted through the exchange of certain body fluids, viz. semen, vaginal fluids and blood. The mode of the spread of the infection generally follows well-defined routes namely unprotected sexual intercourse, the injection of infected blood, and the infection of the unborn foetus whilst in the womb and, in exceptional cases, the infection of a new-born baby through the medium of breast milk.

Not a single case of occupational acquired HIV has been confirmed in South Africa. Although health workers are at risk, the risk is small and arises only if through invasive procedure infected blood enters the worker's bloodstream.

There are many pathogens that are more infectious than HIV, such as Hepatitis B, and a medical practitioner must, in the course of his ordinary practice, take steps to prevent their spread.

4.3 Legal clarity

The legal position is clear. Because the risk of occupational transmission can be eliminated with universal medical precautions, there are no legitimate reasons for exclusionary employment policies on the basis of this, even in the health profession.

4.4 Can HIV affect a worker's performance?

HIV-related stress may affect a worker's performance. However, when a worker does not perform her/his job, the usual procedures for incapacitory misconduct should be followed. Testing for HIV is not necessary, though a worker may of course request such a test for diagnostic purposes. When a worker develops AIDS-related symptoms, the usual procedures for any life-threatening condition should apply.

4.5 If employers invest in training should they not test employees for HIV?

Training of employees represents a significant investment for employers. Because of the scale of the epidemic, HIV will impact significantly on employers, employees and the government. The requirement that job applicants be tested for HIV because of investment in training, is irrational for the following reasons:

- Persons with HIV can live a productive and healthy life for 15 years or more.
- A worker might contract HIV after employment and training.
- A worker who tests negative cannot be bonded to an employer and might leave his employment soon after training.

4.6 Should workers not be tested in their own interest?

Recently, doctors in the service of major employer bodies have suggested that working conditions in certain industries make HIV testing necessary in the worker's own interest. For example, the association of HIV with TB makes it necessary, especially in the mining industry, to test workers for HIV.

All decisions regarding testing for diagnostic purposes should nevertheless be done on the basis of full, free and informed consent. This will respect the constitutional and human rights of employees and safeguard them from employer self-interest masquerading as concern for worker. TB in the mining industry for instance can be eliminated through the creation of a healthy work environment and not through denying employment to, or otherwise discriminating against workers with HIV.

4.7 Informed consent and counselling

In addition to the stigma and injustice of pre-employment testing, the majority of job applicants and workers in employment are tested without informed consent or adequate pre- and post-test counselling. In this regard, attention is drawn to the relevant section of the National AIDS Plan adopted by the Government of National Unity.

- On informed consent the Plan states:

No one should be tested against their will, or without having given their full informed consent. This applies to all sites where blood might be drawn for the purposes of testing hospitals, local clinics or private clinics. Having been informed of what the test involves, any person has the right to refuse to be tested.

- On counselling and confidentiality, the Plan states:

Each person who is about to receive a HIV test, should receive both pre- and post-test counselling from a trained counsellor. Through counselling and the assurance of informed consent, confidentiality must be ensured at all times (National AIDS Plan, Section 2: 23).

4.8 Can pre-employment testing protect benefit schemes?

HIV/Aids will impact seriously on the entire economy but denying employment to persons with HIV will not decrease the costs. In fact, as was learned with apartheid, discrimination carries its own costs. The only justifiable response is to treat HIV/Aids in the same way as all life-threatening conditions and to ensure that benefits are negotiated by employers, the government, the labour movement and the National Convention on Aids in South Africa (NACOSA).

There is no doubt that HIV/Aids will also impact significantly on employee benefit schemes such as medical aid, provident funds and group life assurance. But pre-employment testing will not protect benefit schemes. In fact, the exclusion of as much as 25% of our population from benefits will place an unfair burden on the State and individual taxpayers. This will harm small businesses more than a rational approach in which responsibility is shared by the major stake-holders. As an alternative, the following steps are suggested:

- The Government, the employer bodies, the labour movement and NACOSA should conduct anonymous studies, (unlike sero-revalence studies) for every industry to ascertain the impact HIV/Aids will have on benefits.
- These parties should then develop a national non-disciplinary approach to benefits taking into account the impact of the epidemic.

5 TESTING: MINISTER OF HEALTH'S POLICY STATEMENT

The policy of pre-employment testing for HIV is in breach of international practice and the National Aids Plan as accepted by the Government of National Unity. The previous Minister of Health, Dr Nkosazana Zuma, expressly condemned pre-employment testing in Parliament on 30 August 1994:

> Pre-employment testing for HIV is unacceptable and discriminatory because it stigmatizes prospective employees and infringes upon their human rights by excluding them from prospective employment. It is furthermore costly and wasteful and diverts scarce resources from education and care.
>
> In addition to the above, it is ineffective because of the window period in which the antibodies cannot be traced, and because many people who are employed, may already have contracted the virus or may contract the virus during their employment (Statement to Parliament by Minister Zuma – 30 August 1994).

This statement is based on the best medical, scientific, legal and ethical premises. It is only through a joint non-discriminatory approach to these issues that the social and economic impact of HIV/Aids will be minimized.

6 SHARED RESPONSIBILITY AND NON-DISCRIMINATION

The National Aids Plan recognizes that discrimination against persons with HIV is not only unjust but contributes to transmission of the virus. According to the Plan:

> This is because (discrimination) may encourage denial and risk behaviour, and discourage voluntary testing which would otherwise enable those who either have HIV or are at risk of HIV to be counselled on behaviour change. Combating all forms of discrimination is therefore crucial to preventing or limiting the spread of HIV (NACOSA, Natal Aids Plan, Section 1:45).

HIV/Aids will impact seriously on healthcare provision and costs; employment benefit schemes; insurance and social welfare. In this context, a rational and non-discriminatory approach will assist with reducing HIV/Aids transmission. Such an approach will include sharing responsibility between the Government, employers, trade unions and the National Convention on Aids in South Africa (NACOSA).

Support for the Prohibition of Pre-employment Testing for the Human-Immmunodeficiency Virus (HIV) Bill will ensure that the foundations are prepared for a just, rational and shared approach to the Aids epidemic in the workplace and throughout South Africa.

Appendices

Appendix 6.1

An example of a Company Policy for a specific health issue

XYZ COMPANY LTD

HIV/AIDS POLICY

XYZ Company recognizes that infection with Human Immunodeficiency Virus (HIV) and Acquired Immunodeficiency Syndrome (Aids) represents an urgent problem with broad social, cultural, economic, ethical and legal implications.

The company is committed to address HIV and Aids in a pro-active, supportive and non-discriminatory manner, with the informed support and co-operation of all employees. The same principles that govern other chronic or life-threatening conditions regarding employment apply to HIV/Aids.

The company will communicate with and educate all employees, and where appropiate facilitate the process for their families, local communities on the dangers of, ways to avoid contracting and the treatment of HIV/Aids.

Throughout the organization:

- Applicants for employment need to pass an appropriate pre-placement medical examination, at no time will this include an HIV test.
- No employee will be required to undergo an HIV/Aids test or be asked about results of tests already taken, unless required by law. If any employee wishes to undergo a voluntary HIV/Aids test the company will arrange and pay for such test, should this not be covered by a medical aid.
- Confidentiality and privacy regarding employees suffering from Aids or those with an HIV positive test will be respected.
- Where an employee becomes too ill to perform his/her agreed function, then the standard procedure for termination of service for incapacity will apply.
- Normal sick leave rules will apply.
- The provisions in the Basic Conditions of Employment Act 75 of 97 or the current agreement on Family Responsibility Leave at the workplace will apply.
- Medical assistance will be provided to infected employees, in accordance with the rules of the medical aid scheme. Employees who are not members of a medical aid scheme may receive assistance for healthcare from government, provincial or company clinics, where available.
- If employees are no longer able to continue in employment due to ill health, the appropriate Retirement Fund or Provident Fund rules governing ill health will apply.
- Employees will have access to information and education programmes on HIV/Aids.

All possible assistance will be facilitated for concerned employees to receive expert counselling and advice.

XYZ Company is committed to fair, sound and non-discriminatory employment practices:
- Conditions of service, including membership of pension or provident funds, medical aid, stated benefits, sick leave and training and development will continue, as amended from time to time.
- Employees who develop, disclose or are diagnosed HIV/Aids positive will not be prejudiced, victimized or discriminated against on account of their medical condition.
- Persons in the workplace affected by HIV/Aids must be protected from stigmatization and discrimination by co-workers or clients.
- Employees who are HIV positive should take special precautions and refrain from any activity which might put their fellow employees at risk.

_____   _____
GROUP MANAGING DIRECTOR   DATE

Addenda and appendices

Appendix 6.2
Example of a monthly or annual Occupational Health Service report

XYZ COMPANY OCCUPATIONAL HEALTH SERVICE – ANNUAL REPORT

Total number of employees:_____
Total number of contract workers: _____

Clinic		No.	Remark
1 Clinic attendance	a) Total no of employees who consulted OH Nurse		
	b) No seen by company doctor		
	c) No referred to GP		
	d) No referred to other specialists		
	e) Average attendance per employee per month		
2 Costs in Rands	a) Nursing staff salaries		
	b) Doctor's remuneration p.h. (R.......) x .... of hr		
	c) Medicine/dressings		
	d) Health education, training, seminars, etc		
	e) Total cost of service		
	f) Average cost per employee per year		
	g) Company medical aid contribution		
	h) Compensation for occupational injuries and diseases (monthly assessment cost)		
	i) Other costs		
3 Examinations	a) Pre-placement (baseline) medical examinations		
	b) Number of new appointees (from HR dept. **)		
	c) Periodic medical examinations		
	d) Special/transfer medical examinations		
	e) Exit medical examinations		
	f) Number of resignations/retirees etc.		
	g) Drivers/mobile equipment/locos examinations		
	h) Audiograms		

533

Occupational health

Clinic		No.	Remark
	i) Vision screening		
	j) Chest X-rays and/or lung function tests specify		
	k) Executive medical examinations		
	l) Other (specify) eg. Food handlers		
	m) Biological monitoring		
4 Consultations	**Clinical disease-related consultation (Total)**		
General conditions	Gastro-intestinal and related respiratory tract, specify 'flu, bronchitis. asthma, etc. Tuberculosis, new or chronic		
	Urinary tract and STDs		
	Cardiovascular-hypertension. New cases and chronic cases		
	Endocrine-diabetes – new and chronic		
	Neurological conditions – headaches		
	Musculoskeletal conditions		
	Psychological/psychiatric, e.g. depression Substance abuse		
	HIV positive and Aids sufferers		
5 Occupational related	Injuries-on-duty COIDACT reported		
	First aid cases – not reported		
	Occupational diseases reported specify		
	Other		
6 Social pathology	No of counselling sessions held specify type		
7 Health promotion	Health education sessions – specify topics		
	Special clinics – specify		
8 Workplace inspections	Areas inspected		
	First Aid boxes inspected		
9 Health and safety meetings	Number attended		

Clinic		No.	Remark
10 Absenteeism	Total man-days lost due to ill health		
	Sickness absenteeism rate for the month $$\frac{\text{No of sick absence days} \times 100}{\text{No of employees} \times \text{no of working days}}$$		
11 Comments			

Appendix 6.3 Example of an Occupational Health Service Audit

OCCUPATIONAL HEALTH SERVICE AUDIT	Document	Practice	Value	Remark
1 ELEMENTS				
1.1 Occupational Health Service Philosophy and Policy – available in writing			1	
1.1.1 Reflects commitment and objectives by OHP			1	
1.1.2 Is displayed and utilized			1	
1.1.3 Company Policies displayed			1	
1.2 Organization and staffing				
1.2.1 *Risk managers*, safety officers and line managers address risk, safety and environmental issues			1	
1.2.2 *Occupational Hygienist* – an accredited agent is appointed by risk management for assessments and reports on health risks – forwarded to Occ H Service			1	
1.2.3 *Occ Health Nursing Practioner* appointed registered with SA Nurs C – current receipt on file			2 1	
▪ Professional consultant to company/employees			2	
▪ Neutral in disputes			1	
▪ Occ health nursing qualification			2	
▪ Has specific knowledge of workplace, Occ Hazards, management structure and employee health status. Professional judgement respected			2	
▪ Keeps informed of developments in Occ Health, legislation and the workplace			1	
▪ Formal systems in place – Govt Gazettes, Journals Reference material and Professional membership			1	
1.2.4 *Occ Health Medical Practioner* appointed, registered – SAMDC current receipt on file			2	
▪ Occ Medicine qualification (DOH)			2	

Addenda and appendices

	Document	Practice	Value	Remark
Familiar with workplace and Occ hazards			2	
Keeps up to date with developments in Occ medicine, legislation and workplace			1 1	
Current contract on file				
1.2.5 *First Aiders* appointed ito OHSA/MHSA regulations – available at all times. List available in Medical Centre			2 1	
Trained/registered with accredited First Aid Organization (Dept of Labour) – certificates on file			1 1	
Regular practice/retraining sessions				
1.2.6 *Health and Safety representative* appointed ito OHSA and MHSA – list in Medical Centre OHN serves on H&S committee			1	
Trained to maintain health and safety standards at work, recognize hazards, do inspections and report findings			1	
1.2.7 *Continuing education*				
All members of the Occ Health Team receive on-going education through the attendance of seminars, member of professional bodies, etc.			1	
Records and feedback reports on file			1	
The Occ Health Team have access to current/relevant text books, journals, Internet, etc.			2	
1.3 Health risk identified, assessed and controlled by risk management			2	
1.3.1 A register of all raw materials, products and chemicals in the workplace and their material safety data sheets available in the Medical Centre			2	
1.3.2 The register is kept complete and current through formal risk management procedures			1	
1.3.3 A competent person surveys all areas regularly to identify, assess and document all hazards records available			1	

537

Occupational health

	Document	Practice	Value	Remark
1.3.4 A formal programme for education and training of employees and customers on health hazards is in place and documented			1	
1.3.5 Man-job specifications for each job with health risks and hazard levels are available from Risk & HR depts.			2	
On medical file and used by OHN in medical surveillance			1	
1.3.6 Formal procedures exist and training given and documented in the selection, use, fit, maintenance and testing of PPE			1	
1.4 Medical surveillance programme – guidelines, objectives and annual schedule – available in Policy and Procedure Manual			2	
1.4.1 Schedule for holistic annual examination and test for each employee according to health risks			1	
1.4.2 Results discussed fully with each person, confidentiality ensured – signed by person and OHN			2	
1.4.3 Only statistics are reflected in reports to management – further information only with signed consent of employee concerned			1 1	
1.4.4 Full health assessment ito man-job specification completed *before* employment, transfer, exit or return to work after serious illness or injury			1 1	
1.5 Occupational Health Service Management, Administration and Clinical Practice				
1.5.1 Policy and procedure manual Is available in the Medical Centre Is current and complete, contains			1 2	
■ Title page with introduction to the Company			1	
■ Table of contents with easy referencing			2	

Addenda and appendices

	Document	Practice	Value	Remark
to accommodate amendments and additions			1	
■ OHS philosophy and health policy			1	
■ Company health policy				
■ Company organigram and reporting structure – company doctor for clinical and risk manager for administrative aspects of OHS		*	2	
■ Job descriptions as per PPC Policy for Occ Health nursing/medical practitioners			1	
■ Objectives of the Health Service both long term and short term			2	
■ Current year programme with due dates			2	
■ Guidelines for daily routine – clinic hours etc.			1	
■ List of internal and external contact persons			1	
■ Guidelines for monitoring sick leave			1	
■ Guidelines for monthly reports to risk control manager and management team			1	
■ Guidelines for annual reports to management, Barloworld Occ Health Manager, Director Mineral and Environmental Affairs			2	
1.5.2 Applicable legislation				
■ List of all relevant legislation			1	
■ Summaries of Occ health prescriptions on file:			2	
■ Occ Health and Safety Act 85 of 1993 and regulations			1	
■ Compensations for Occ Injuries & Diseases Act 130 of 1933			1	
			1	
■ Mine Health Safety Act 29 of 1996 and Regulations			1	
■ Medicines and Related Substances Control Act 101 of 1965			1	
■ Employment Equity Act 55 of 1998			1	
■ Labour Relations Act 66 of 1995			1	
■ Occ Diseases in Mines & Works Act 73 of 1978			1	

Occupational health

	Document	Practice	Value	Remark
Mineral Act 50 of 1991			1	
Nursing Act 50 of 1978 as amended			1	
Medical, Dental Supplementary Health Service Professions Act 56 of 1974			1	
The Health Act 63 of 1977			1	
Hazardous Substances Act 15 of 1973			1	
Prevention of Atmospheric Pollution Act 45 of 1965			1	
Basic Conditions of Service Act 3 of 1983			1	
Unemployment Insurance Act 30 of 1966			1	
Other applicable legislation			2	
Formal system for receiving amendments, new legislation, etc. exists				

1.5.3 Responsible appointments – in writing

- Current list of contact persons and tel no's
- Risk manager name and tel no
- Company doctor – name and all tel no's
- Health and safety representatives' names and tel no's
- First-aid team members – Names and tel no's

Values: 1, 1, 1, 1, 1

1.5.4 Health-risk management programme

- Annual programme exists for current year – integrating:
- Environmental monitoring results – used
- Education of the employees re hazards
- Suitable PPE chosen with the employee input
- Medical surveillance results incorporated in future programmes

Values: 1, 1, 1, 1, 1

1.5.5 Planning for emergencies/disasters

- Emergency co-ordinator appointed
- Disaster plan displayed and known to all

Values: 1, 1

540

Addenda and appendices

	Document	Practice	Value	Remark
■ Regular recorded evacuation rehearsals			1	
■ Review of emergency plan – dated and signed			1	
■ Health aspects addressed in emergency plan			1	
■ OHN and First Aiders know emergency procedure			1	
■ Equipment checked regularly – list signed			1	
.5.6 Records and registers				
■ Current, confidential, secure and kept for 30 years			3	
■ *Personnel medical files up to date*			2	
■ Medical surveillance – relevant and up to date			2	
• full medical history and examination			1	
• all previous audiometry, vision, lung function tests, biological monitoring results, etc			1	
■ General health, consultations/reports			1	
• sick certificates and absence record				
■ All injury-on-duty/ Occ Diseases reports			1	
1.5.7 Medicine control				
■ Co Dr responsible for medicines – protocols, checks orders/registers, signs for scheduled Rx			2	
■ *Medicine permit ito Act 101 of 1965 Valid, displayed and on file*			2	
■ Guidelines exist for:				
■ Ordering and disposal of expired stock			1	
■ Secure and correct storage and control			1	
■ Dispensing and labelling			1	
■ Protocols for diagnosing and treatment is drawn up by Co Dr and is available revised and signed regularly for all emergency and general illnesses			1	
1.5.8 Injury-on-duty procedures documented in Policy and Procedure Manual			1	

Occupational health

	Document	Practice	Value	Remark
■ Register and correspondence upo to date			2	
2.5.9 Nursing Procedures and Protocol dated and signed by Occ Health Practioner			2	
■ General clinical procedures (BP, Hb, etc)			1	
■ Occ health clinical procedures (specific tests)			1	
2.5.10 Medical Emergency Procedures – exist			2	
■ Written protocol – dasted and signed by CO.Dr				
■ Liasson with local emergency services ordered			1	
2.5.11 Health protection and promotion Primary Health Care planning				
■ Daily and Specific Clinic schedules on file			1	
■ Referral system on file			1	
■ Diagnosis Guidelines and Treatment Protocol signed and updated by Co physician			1	
2.5.12 Health education/promotion programme				
■ Objectives and Year plan documented			2	
■ Records of sessions and attendees			1	
■ Employee needs identified and addressed			1	
■ Sessions and Programme evaluated			1	
2.5.13 Medical surveillance programme guidelines for:				
■ Audimetry procedures – qualified operator			2	
■ Testing and Reg 171 procedures, referral			2	
■ Calibration of equipment by an accredited technician			1	

Addenda and appendices

	Document	Practice	Value	Remark
Spirometry qualification for Occ. H. P			2	
Procedures for testing, calibration and cleaning of equipment – infection control			2	
Vision screening procedures for			1	
Far, near, colour and peripheral vision			1	
Specific test for drivers, mobile equipment oprerators, etc				
Biological monitoring procedures for			2	
Specific work hazards				
Hexane, lead X-ray, etc				
Ergonomic assessment guidelines on file			2	
Checklists for different work areas			1	
Educatiuon of employees on work design and work area design for maximum effiency			1	

- 2.5.14 O.H.S. Financial Management guidelines in Policy and Procedure Manual — 1
- Current short/lonmg term budget on file — 2
- Current budget balanced — 1
- Average cost per consultation — 1
- Costs per employee per year — 1
- Education, of empl;oyees and O.H.P.'s. — 1
- Including journals, seminar, etc costs — 1
- Medical stock cost per year — 1
- Calibration costs — 1
- Laboratory, X-rays, etc costs — 1
- Injury-on-duty intermediate benefits — 1
- Salaries including benefits per year — 1

2.6 Facilities available
2.6.1 Medical Centre exists, is functional, affords privascy, is clean and in good repair — 3
- It is accessible to employees and emergency vehicles and is sign posted — 1
- Equipment is adequate for possible risks for emergencies, health assesssment, etc — 2

Occupational health

	Document	Practice	Value	Remark
■ Equipment and stocks chaecked daily			1	
■ Regular maintenance			1	
2.6.2 Lecture room, training area is available for health talks, first aid training, etc			1	
■ Adequate size with good light and ventilation chairs and tables			1	
■ Equipment includes board, projector, TV, etc			1	
Total			200	100%
Comments				

Appendix 7.1

MAN-JOB SPECIFICATION

NAME: .... DATE: ....

JOB TITLE: .... DEPT.: ....

BRIEF DESCRIPTION OF JOB: .... FOREMAN: ....

....

....

Mark with an "X"

Male ☐	Physical Work:	Factory Worker ☐		Shifts: Yes ☐
Female ☐	High ☐ Low ☐	Office Worker ☐		No. ☐

Height Requirement: Short ☐ Medium ☐ Tall ☐ N/A ☐ Age Group ☐

WORKING ENVIRONMENT:	YES	NO	PROTECTIVE EQUIPMENT:	YES	NO
Lead Area	☐	☐	Hard Hat	☐	☐
Inside	☐	☐	Earmuffs	☐	☐
Outside	☐	☐	Safety Boots	☐	☐
High Temperatures	☐	☐	Gum Boots	☐	☐
Low Temperatures	☐	☐	Respirator	☐	☐
Noise Zone	☐	☐	Safety Harness	☐	☐
Vibration	☐	☐	Overalls	☐	☐
Elevated Work	☐	☐	Gloves	☐	☐
Confined Space	☐	☐	Eye Protection	☐	☐
Dusty Area	☐	☐	Face Shield	☐	☐
*Toxic Fumes Present	☐	☐			
Wet Area	☐	☐			

PHYSICAL REQUIREMENTS:	YES	NO
Good Hearing	☐	☐
Good Eyesight: Both eyes	☐	☐
Have Colour Distinc.	☐	☐
Good Sense of Smell	☐	☐
Clear Speech	☐	☐
Use of Right Hand	☐	☐
Use of Left Hand	☐	☐
Use of Right Foot	☐	☐
Use of Left Foot	☐	☐
Standing	☐	☐
Sitting	☐	☐
Bending (Frequent Y / N)	☐	☐
Lifting	☐	☐
Walking	☐	☐
Eye/Hand/Foot Co-ordin.	☐	☐
Able to Write / Read	☐	☐

COMMENTS:

*List Chemicals Used / Any Other Specific Hazard

....

....

....

LIMITATIONS FOR EMPLOYMENT:
(To be completed by O.H.N.)

....

....

....

PRESIDENT P.E. 61418

Appendix 7.2

SECTION C				EXIT MEDICAL EXAMINATION		
PHYSICAL		NAD	ABN	COMMENTS:	COMPANY: PPC
Mass (kg)	..........kg				Address:
Height (cm)	..........cm				Tel: Fax:
Pulse rate	........./ min				
Blood pressure	.../..mgHg				Employee name
Urinalysis	Appearance				ID No:
	pH				Date of birth
	Protein				Company No:
	Sugar				Date of appointment:
	Blood				**Job history and hazardous exposure levels**
Haed, face, scalp and neck					
Ears, nose and throat					
Lungs, chest and breast					
Heart (size and sounds)					
Vascular system and lymphatics					
Abdomen					
Neurological (sensory, refelxes)					
Upper and lower limbs					**Compensation record:**
Spine and muscoskeletal					Injury – Date – Claim No – Finalised
Skin and appendages					
SPECIAL MEDICAL INVESTIGATIONS					
Lung function test: (Spirometer)	FVC %				
	FEV %				
	PEFR %				
Hearing test (Screening)	See form 2:46 F02				**Occupational disease record:**
Visual acuity	Far	R	L		LO Class – Date – Claim No – Finalised
	Near				
	Night vision				
Biological monitoring					
Date: ..../......./............ Medical examiner: .... Signature: .... Discussed with, accepted and copy received by employee: .... Signature employee:					**Comments**

Index

Please note: Page numbers in *italics* refer to figures and tables in the text.

a

abdominopelvic injuries 324i325
absenteeism 438
absorption 90, 134
accident/incident 98
   classification of 88
   costs of 98–99
   definition of 87
   factors causing 90–91
   prevention 102–105
   proneness to 439
accident prevention programmes 105
acid rain 488
acne 194–195
activation phase 296–297
acute crisis stage 453
adaptive behaviour 387, 393, 403–404
adjudication 70
adjustment 371
   and defence 404–405
   managing and promotion 441–442
   reactions 403–404
   systemic understanding of 374–375
   techniques 443
adolescence, disorders of 424
adult learners 263
Advisory Council for Occupational Health and Safety 120
ageing population 477
ageing-related disorders 423
agent aspects 348
age psychosis 423
aggression 418
agricultural workers 275–276
Aids, *see under* HIV/Aids
air
   need for clean 478–479
   pollution 488

alarm-and-mobilization phase 388
alcoholism 421, *422*
allergic contact dermatitis 194
American Psychiatric Association 380
analytic studies 359–362
Anglo-Boer War 6
Animal Slaughter, Meat and Animal Products Hygiene Act (1967) 78
annual leave 62
anthrax 207
anthropometrics 112
anxiety 417–418
anxiety-based disorders 415–416
Aphorisms of Hippocrates 341
arbitration 70
arsenic 493
asbestos 178–180, *179*
asphyxiants 330–331
aspirational behaviour, intense 420
assessment
   of mental health 383–385
   of risk *511*, 511–513
   of workplace 293
assistance programmes 271–272
asthma, occupational 180–183
Atmospheric Pollution Prevention Act (1965) 11, 79
atmospheric pressure, abnormal 150–151
A-type personality 392
audiometric testing 250–251
AVPU Scale *302*

b

bargaining council 64
basic conditions of employment 64
Basic Conditions of Employment Act (1997) 9, 59–65
behaviour
   change 442, 444–449
   work and human 377–379
Bill of Rights 26–32

547

biodiversity, loss of 489–490
biological aetiology 423
biological agents 349
biological contaminants 481
biological feedback processes 443
biological hazards 154–155, 195, 503–504
biological monitoring 171–173, 248
biomechanics 112–113
biorhythms, theory of 439
biosphere 467
bleeding 310–312
blind spot syndrome 419
boredom 92
brain
    functioning 423
    injuries 319–320
burnout 411–413, *413*, 501
burns 307–310

c
cadmium 493
Campbell and Cellini's taxonomy *428–430*
cancers, occupational 183–186
cardiac arrest 333
cardiopulmonary resuscitation procedure
    333–334
career development 428
certificates of fitness 59
Certification Committee 11
change
    continuous 441
    in environment 447
    problems of 438
chemical agents 349–350
chemical elements 186–209
chemical hazards 131–136, *133*
    effects of 491–495
  measurement of 135–136
Chernobyl 5
Chief Executive Officer (CEO), duties of 38
child
    labour 64
    welfare 273
childhood, disorders of 424
children and disease 476
chromium 190
chronic crisis stage 453–454
city, healthy 489
claims under COIDA 53–54
climate changes 485–487
clinical nursing guidelines 244
coal workers' pneumoconiosis (CWP) 178
Code of Good Practice, HIV/Aids 519–525

cognitive disorders 423
cohort studies 360–361
cold environments 497
communicable diseases 352
communication and disasters 334–336
community
    health and research 455
    trials 363–364
Community Health Centre model 17
company health policy 21, 531–532
compensation
    to employees 51–52
    injuries and diseases 56–58
    procedure for 53
    for temporary disability 52
compensatable diseases 58–59, *165*
compensation 409
Compensation Board 51
Compensation Commissioner 51
Compensation for Occupational Injuries and
    Diseases Act (1993) (COIDA) 8, 9, 49–55
    Schedule 3 *162–164*
Compensation Fund 50
compulsive organization 436
conciliation 70
confidentiality 48
    HIV/Aids 523–524
conflict 387–390, 430–431
constitutional provisions 32
Constitution of the RSA 26–32
contact dermatitis 54
coping behaviour 387, 388
correlation studies 359
counselling 258, 443
    HIV/Aids 524–525
    approach 449–452
crisis intervention 452–455
critical incident stress 501
cross-sectional studies, *see* prevalence studiesi

d
damage 98
death 339
    causes of *474*
decontamination zone 327–328
defence mechanism 403, 404
deforestation 483–484
delayed hazards 113
demographic transition 472–473
denial 406
dependence 418–419, 421–423
depression 415
depressive organization 437

dermatitis 194–195
  and compensation 196
descriptive studies 358–359
desertification 484
developed countries 472
developing countries 472
deviant acquired behaviour 416
Diagnostic and Statistical Manual of Mental Disorders (DSM) 380, 397–400, 425
diagnostic testing 357
direct defence mechanisms 405
disabled people 477
disaster(s) 279
  of human origin 280, 506
  impact of 505–510
  planning 291–293, 333
  premonitory signs of 506–510
    pre-planning 293–294
  response phases 294–298
disaster management
  provincial and municipal 285–289, 290
Disaster Management Bill (2001) 279, 282
discipline 108–109
disease, occupational 160–161, 424
  burden of 475–476
    diagnosis of 168–169
  distribution of 345
    management of 169–171
  surveillance 354
disease-prone personality 392–393
displacement 408
dispute resolution 70, 525
distressed executives 433
doctor–patient relationship 48
documentation (disasters) 337
Domestic Violence Act (1998) 78
domestic workers 275
dominant influential factors 375
domino sequence 95, 95–96
dose-response
  assessment 511
  relationship *167*
drought 484
drug(s)
  abuse 421, 423
  legislation and regulations 516
  quality assurance 518
  quality control laboratory 517
Drugs and Drug Trafficking Act (1992) 76
dysfunctions, work 380

e
ecological issues 483–490
ecosystem perspective 466–467
education 107–108, 257–258, 267–268
educational approach 266
ego-defence mechanisms 404–405
electrical contact 89
emergency
  care 254–255
  evacuation 333
  management of trauma 304–307
emotional insulation 409
employee(s)
  definition of 86
  duties of 36–37
  participation in workplace 68–70
  relations 395
  and risk management 47
Employee Assistance Programmes 447
employers, duties of 35–36
employment
  practice 108
  procedures 445
  termination of 63–64
Employment Conditions Commission 64
Employment Equity Act (1998) 65–67
engineering revision 107
environment 376
  definition of 465
  extrinsic factors 348
  and health 464–468
  occupational health nurse and 155–156
  requirements for healthy 477–482
environmental concerns 471–472
Environmental Conservation Act (1989) 11, 76
environmental health 467–468
environmental measures 512
environmental monitoring 259
epidemiological dyad *94*, 94–95
epidemiological investigations 358–364
epidemiological study, planning a 367–368
epidemiological transition 473–474
epidemiological triad *93*, 93–95, >*346*
epidemiology 168, 239, 344
  application of 353–364
  sources of data 364
  uses of 364–367
equilibrium 403
Erasmus Commission of Enquiry 8
ergonomic agents 350
ergonomic design 447
ergonomic programmes 114–115, *116*
ergonomics 110–116, 152–153, 202, *202*

essential services 71
ethics 221
   in epidemiological research 368
   and law 26
etiological factors, classification of 386–387
European Economic Community 6
evaluation 266–267, 397–398
   environmental measures 512
   procedures 445
    programme and process 400
executive pathology 431–434
executives and stress 433
exhaustion and disintegration phase 389
exit medical examinations 247–248
experience and inexperience 92
experimental studies 362–364
Explosives Act (1956) 79
exposure assessment 511
external environment 466
external influential factors 396
eye injuries 325–326

f
facial injuries 317
factitious symptoms 425
Factories, Machinery and Building Works Act (1941) 8
faking of symptoms 425
falling objects 88
falls 89
family responsibility leave 62
fantasy 409–410
fatigue 92
fear 417–418
   of failure (FOF) 415
   of success (FOS) 415
Fertilizers, Farm Feeds, Agricultural Remedies and Stock Remedies Act (1947) 11, 166
field trials 363
financial costs management 237
first aid 254–255
First World War 4
fixation 407
follow-up studies, see cohort studies
food
   contamination 481
   need for 480–4482
Foodstuffs, Cosmetics and Disinfectants Act (1972) 78
forced labour 64
frustration 387–390

g
General Federation of Labour (Israel) 6
Glasgow Coma Scale (GCS) *302*
global environment, stable 482–483
global warming 485
grievances (HIV/Aids) 522
group
   dynamics 435
   techniques 451
Group Service Model 17

h
harmful substances 89, 134
hazard(s) 130–155, 166–168
   assessment 511
   classification of 131–156, *132*
   control 46
   effects of *351–352*
   and risks 106
hazardous material accidents 331–333
Hazardous Substances Act (1973) 77
Hazardous Substances Amendment Act (1992) 77
hazardous work 44–45
head injuries 317–321
head-to-toe survey *303*, 303–304
health 7, 464
   assessments 244–248, *247*
   facilities 447
   programme 232–233, 264–266
   promotion 263–264, 270
   safety committees 39
   surveillance 171–173
Health Act (1977) 9, 32–33, 165
healthcare management 447–449
healthcare workers 110, 372–374
Health Environment Impact Assessment (EIA) 512
Health Professions Act (1974) 9
health services
   components of 15, *15*
   development 6–12
   establishment of 230–232, *231*
   scope of 18
hearing
   conservation 139, 142–145
   loss 54, 197–200
heat
   exhaustion 326–327
   exposure 497–498
   illness/stress 148–150
heatstroke 326–327
history, occupational health in 2

Index

histrionic organization 437
HIV/Aids 473
   contact 520–521
   and employment 519–525
   in healthcare workers 54
   prevention of 272–273
   as work problem 427–428
homeostasis 403
hospital and disaster victims 336–337
host (intrinsic) factors 345–346
hostility 418
hours of work 60–70
human(s)
   development and change 391
   and environment 468
   needs 469–470
Human Tissues Act (1983) 79
hygiene
   measurements 46
   occupational 47
hygienist 22
hypertension screening programmes 273–274
hypothermia (cold stress) 149–150, 326–327
hypothesis, formulation of 361

i

'iceberg effect' 100
identification 407
imbalance, needs and services 505
immaturity 418–419
impaled objects 320
impaired executives 433
implementation phase 297
indicators 475
indirect compensation 409
indirect defence mechanisms 405
indigenous people 477
individual(s)
   factors unique to 390–393
   responses 387
   and work 447
industrial accidents 438, 439
industrialization, effects of 3–4
Industrial Revolution 3–4
informal labour sector 274–275
ingestion 90
inhalation 89
injuries on duty 255–256
injury 98
   category of 90
   definition of 88
inquiries 39
inspectors 39–40

insured and uninsured costs 99–102
intellectualization 408–409
interaction process 375
   employee and organization 375
   work and non-work roles 430
Inter-governmental Committee on Disaster Management 283
internal contamination 328
internal environment 465–466
International Health Regulations Act (1974) 75–76, 80
International Labour Organization (ILO) 243
Internet Web sites 22–23
interpersonal skills 443
interruption 98
investigations 39–40, 46–47
ionizing radiation 136, 498
irritent contact dermatitis (ICD) 193–194

j

job
   description 225
   dissatisfaction 410
   factors 96–98
   information 62–63
   satisfaction 410

l

labour relations 447–449
Labour Relations Act (1995) 9, 67–72
latex allergy 196
lead 186–188, 492–493
leadership by employer 105–106
learning, evaluation of 269
leave 62
legal proceedings 65
legionella 208
legislation
   independent nature of 85
   in twentieth century 4
legislative control 84–85
life-change units (LCU) 388
lifestyles, healthy 262–263
lighting 145–147
lung diseases 173–183

m

machinery, users of 37–38
macro-organizational (external) environment 435–441
Major Industry Model 16
maladjustment 419
   to optimality 380

malingering 425
malnutrition 481
management
    by objectives 444
    principles 226–232
    processes 394–396
managers
    functions 45–46
    and stress 431, 432
man–job specification 245
Maslow's hierarchy 469
maternal welfare 273
maternity leave 62
mechanical hazards 153–154, 195, 499
Medical Bureau for Occupational Diseases (MBOD) 11–12
medical emergencies 333–334
medical examinations 49, 246–248
medical practitioners 21–22, 47–48
medical surveillance system 43–44, 47, 244–248
medicine
    control 236–237
    elements of 159
Medicine Control Council 11, 516
Medicines and Related Substances Control Act (1965) 9
Medicines and Related Substances Control Amendment Act (1997) 77, 236
mental facilities 447
mental health 379–380, 382
  assessment of 397–398
  maintaining of 501–502
  problems 385–397, 440
Merchant Shipping Act (1951) 79
mercury 189–190, 492–493
mine, description of 55–56
Mine Health and Safety Act (1996) (MHSA) 11, 41–46
Mineral Act (1991) 79
Miners Phthisis Act (1911) 8
mining industry 42–43
Mining Regulations Commission 6–7
morbidity and mortality 354–358
mortality rates 474–475
motivation, poor 417
motor vehicle accidents 55
multidimensional diagnostic strategies 510–513
multidisciplinary approach 465
multiple trauma 325
musculoskeletal disorders 201–202
musculoskeletal injuries 316–317

n

National Centre for Occupational Health (NCOH) 8, 12
National Committee on Occupational Health 21
National Disaster Management Advisory Forum 283
National Disaster Management Centre 283–284
National Disaster Management Framework 283
National Drug Policy 515–518
National Economic Development and Labour Council (NEDLAC) Act (1994) 72–73
National Health Bill 9, 11
National Health Service model 17
National Occupational Safety Association (NOSA) 117–119
National Research Institute for Occupational Diseases 8
natural disasters 280, 506
neck injuries 321
negative perceptions 410, 417
neurological examination 320–321
neurotic styles 436
Nightingale, Florence 342
night work 61
noise exposure 139–142, 495–496
noise-induced hearing loss 54, 198, *198*, 228
non-ionizing radiation 138–139
non-specific resistance 346
Nuclear Energy Act (1982) 11, 79
nuclear reactor accidents 327–328
nurse, occupational health 220–221
  appointment of 223–224
  nature of functions of 222–223
nursing
  historical background 20
  occupational health 19
  process 259–260
  stressors related to 397
Nursing Act (1995) 9, 242
nursing practitioner 22

o

observational studies 358–364
Occupational Diseases in Mines and Works Act (1973) 8, 11, 55–59, 165
Occupational Exposure Limit (OEL) 135
occupation health
  as discipline 14–15
  organizational models 16
  regulation in SA 13–14
  training 20–21
Occupational Health and Safety Act (1993) (OHSA) 8, 9, 33–41, 84, 119–120
  regulations under 40–41

Occupational Health Service Audit 536–541
Occupational Health Service Report 533–535
occupational hygiene
    definition of 127–128
    legislative control 128–129
    programmes 129–131
off-the-job safety 109–110
organizational environment, internal 435
organizational pathology 436
organizational processes 394–395, 445–449
overtime 61

p

paranoic organization 436
participation in health programme 266
payment 62–63
persistent behaviour 416
personal factors 96
personality 392
    A-type 392
    disorders 416–417
    repertoire 393
personal strategies 442, 443
personnel turnover 438
Pharmacy Council 11
phthisis (pulmonary tuberculosis) 6
physical agents 351
physical ailments, real and 'invented' 424
physical fitness programmes 274
physical handicaps 426
physical hazards 136–153, 195, 495–499
physical health 440
physical illness 370–371
    psychological factors and 414–415
physically disabled 424–425, 426
physiological conditions 93–95
plague 341–342
planetary toxification 487–489
platinosis 183
pneumoconiosis-fibrositis 174
Pneumoconiosis Research Unit 8
policy and procedure manual 233–234
pollutants 488
pollution, indoor and outdoor 488
populations 353
post-disaster management 337–339
post-disaster recovery 289
Post-traumatic Stress Disorder (PTSD) 54, 210–211, 338, 413–414, 501
power factors 451
pre-employment testing, prohibition of 526–530
premonitory signs of disaster 506–510
pressure 498–499

prevalence studies 359–360
prevention of accidents 107–109, 123–125
primary healthcare 252–254, 271
primary survey 300
Private Health Centre Model 17
pro-domal crisis stage 453
productive role fulfilment 452
prohibitions 39–40
projection 406–407
protective clothing and equipment 115
Protestant Work Ethic 377
psychiatric disorders 401–403
psychological conditions 93
psychological disorders 401–403
    DSM axis for 399
psychological factors 209–211
psychological hazards 155
psychological health 370, 371
psychological optimality 381–382
psychological well-being 381
psychological work dysfunctions 401–403, *402*
psychopathology 380–385, 398
psychoses 424
psychosocial agents 351
psychosocial aspects and environment 499–503
psychosocial hazards 500–503
psychosomatic disorders 414–415
Public Finance Management Act (1999) 289
public health 343
public holidays 61
Public Service Coordinating Bargaining Council 87

q

quality assurance 238–239

r

radiation 89, 136
    emergencies 327–328
    exposure 137–138
    pollution 5
radioactive contamination 327
radon gas 488–489
randomized controlled (clinical) trials 362–363, *363*
rationalization 408
raw materials 495
reaction formation 407
'reasonably practicable', meaning of 38
records and reports 48–49, 234–236
recovery phase 297–298
regression 407

Regulations for Hazardous Biological Agents 154–155
rehabilitation 258–259, 289
    workshops 452
repetitive behaviour 416
representation in NEDLAC 73
representatives
    health and safety 38–39
    of workers 22
repression 405–406
research orientation 239
resistance phase 388–390
respiratory emergencies 328–329
respiratory irritants 329
Reviewing Authority 11
Revised Trauma Score (RTS) 302
Rift valley fever 208–209
risk(s) 353–354
    assessment 46, 512
    and hazards 106
    identifying of 280
    legislative control of 282
    management 512
    perception and acceptance 512–513
    predictability of 281

s
safety
    committees 121–123
    definition of 85–86
scalp injuries 317–318
schizoid organization 437
schizophrenic disorders 424
screening tests 248–251
secondary survey 300
Second World War 4–5
sectoral determinations 64
self-assessment by workers 114
self-care 470
self-knowledge 442
self-management strategies 442–443
self-systems 375
self-therapeutic role 444
serious physical harm 88
settlements, safe 482
sexual harassment 66–67
sexually transmitted diseases (STDs) 522–523
shiftwork 211–212
shock 312–316
    classification of 312–316
sickness absence monitoring 237
silicosis 175–178, 177
skills and knowledge 106

Skills Development Act (1998) 74–75
Skills Development Levies Act (1999) 74–75
skin diseases 193–196
skull injuries 318
smog 488
Social adjustment scale 389
social conditions 93
social design 447
socially naïve person 419
social pathology 440
Social Readjustment Rating Scale (SRRS) 388
Social Security Institution model 17
solvents 190–193, 493–494
South African Health Professions Council 11, 22
South African Medicines and Medical Devices Regulatory Authority Act (1998) 76
South African Nursing Council 11
South African Society of Occupational Health Nurses 21
specific resistance 347–348
spill-over effects 430–431
spinal injuries 321–322
spirometric testing 249–250
state of mind 106–107
statutory medical examinations 248
strain and over-exertion 89
stress 209–210, 500–501
    levels in jobs 394
    model 387–390
    reactions 410–415
stressors 502–503
sublimation 408
substance abuse 421–423
Sunday work 61
supervisors and stress 431–434
support
    groups 258
    measures 338–339
suppression 406
sustainable environment 471
symptom-directed mechanisms 405
systems-interactional model 374–375, 376
systems model 375–377

t
'talk and deteriorate syndrome' 321
target groups 257
task demands 394
teaching
    methods 268–269
    plans 269–270
team(s)
    approach 477

Index

disaster management 290
occupational health 21
temperature 147–150, 497
termination of employment 63–64
testing (HIV/Aids) 523
therapeutic approach 449–452
therapeutic techniques 443
thoracic trauma 322–324
Three Mile Island 5
threshold limit values 495
toxic exposure 331–333
toxic materials 134
toxic metals 492–493
toxic substances 328–331
trade unions 5–6, 68–70
training 47, 107–108
and development 446
and experience 243
in health 446
occupational health nurses 20–21
transformation 441
trauma 304–331
treatment service 252
triage 298–304
tropical diseases 487, 487
troubled employee 271–272
tuberculosis 206–207
twentieth century, legislation in 4–5

u

underachievement, criteria for 419
unemployment 438, 439–440
Unemployment Insurance Act (2001) 9, 74
unfair dismissals 71–72
uninsured costs 99–102
unrecognized hazards 252
unsafe acts/conditions 97–98
urgency, tendency towards 420

v

ventilation 151–152
vibration 200–201, 496–497
victims
identification of 299–300
response to 337–338
sorting of 298–299
vision
protection programmes 146–147
screening 251
vulnerable employees 256–257

w

Wallace Rule of Nines 309
war, effects of 504–505
Water Act (1956) 79
water, need for clean 479–480
weather changes 485–487
women and disease 476
workaholism 411–413
work
behaviour, ineffective 444
dysfunctions 382–383, 398, 401, 428–430
habits 106–107
structures 445–449
workers' rights 52
workload 148
Workmen's Compensation Act (1941) 8
work performance
and personality disorders 416
problems 428
workplace, definition of 87
work-related dysfunctions 434441
Work-Related Upper Limb Disorders 203–206
World Health Assembly 14
World Health Organization (WHO) 464
wounds 304, 305–307